The SAGE
Handbook of

Health Care Ethics:
Core and Emerging
Issues

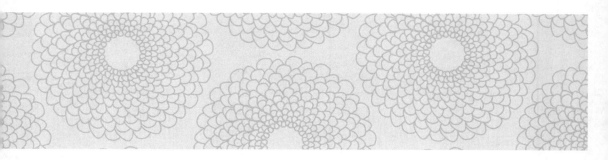

The SAGE
Handbook of
Health Care Ethics:
Core and Emerging
Issues

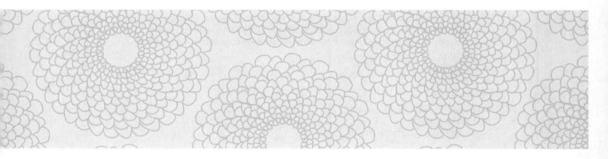

Edited by

Ruth Chadwick, Henk ten Have
and Eric M. Meslin

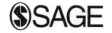

Los Angeles | London | New Delhi
Singapore | Washington DC

1404424

AUG 3 1 2011

First published 2011

SAGE Publications Ltd
1 Oliver's Yard
55 City Road
London EC1Y 1SP

SAGE Publications Inc.
2455 Teller Road
Thousand Oaks, California 91320

SAGE Publications India Pvt Ltd
B 1/I 1 Mohan Cooperative Industrial Area
Mathura Road
New Delhi 110 044

SAGE Publications Asia-Pacific Pvt Ltd
33 Pekin Street #02-01
Far East Square
Singapore 048763

Library of Congress Control Number: 2010941692

British Library Cataloguing in Publication data

A catalogue record for this book is available from the British Library

ISBN: 978-1-4129-4534-9
Typeset by Glyph International, Bangalore, India

Printed by MPG Books Group, Bodmin, Cornwall
Printed on paper from sustainable resources

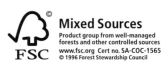

Mixed Sources
Product group from well-managed
forests and other controlled sources
www.fsc.org Cert no. SA-COC-1565
© 1996 Forest Stewardship Council
FSC

Contents

Contributors

Agomoni Ganguli-Mitra is a research fellow at the Institute of Biomedical Ethics, University of Zurich since 2005. She has worked on the ethics of biobanks, as a member of international project in collaboration with the WHO and the University of Geneva. She has also conducted research on the ethics of synthetic biology, as a member of SYNBIOSAFE, one of the earliest EU projects looking into the safety, security and ethical aspects of synthetic biology. She is currently pursuing a PhD in Bioethics at the University of Basel on the Ethics of International Research.

Ahmed Ragab, is a professor of reproductive health at the International Islamic Center for Population Studies and Research, Al-Azhar University. He teaches also at Cairo Demographic Center. He worked as a Professor of Reproductive and Sexual Health at the African Regional Sexuality Resource Center, Lagos, Nigeria. He helped in developing strategies and programmes that aim at reduction of maternal mortality, tackling gender based violence and improving reproductive health in many of the developing countries, mainly in Africa. He is a member of Ethical Committee of the International Islamic Center for Population Studies and Research, Al-Azhar University, a member of the Advisory Committee for African Network for Social Accountability (ANSA) 2006–10 for North Africa, a member of Africa Faith Based Organization, Durban, South Africa and a member of the founding group of the Ethics Society in the Middle East (under construction).

Andrea L. Kalfoglou, PhD, is an Assistant Professor in the Department of Sociology, Anthropology, and Health Administration and Policy at the University of Maryland, Baltimore County (UMBC). She held research positions at the National Human Genome Research Institute, NIH, Johns Hopkins University, and Institute of Medicine prior to joining the faculty at UMBC. She is on the advisory board of the American Journal of Bioethics, is the immediate past Chair of the Ethics Special Interest Group of the American Public Health Association, and has served on a number of committees with the American Society for Bioethics and Humanities. She has published many peer-reviewed articles in bioethics, public health, medical and genetics journals exploring the use of medical and genetic technology on human reproduction. These articles cover topics such as surrogate motherhood, the experiences of oocyte donors, the use of sperm sorting for sex selection and attitudes about the use of genetic carrier testing to make reproductive decisions. She is currently studying women's attitudes about the use of antidepressant medications during pregnancy.

Bartha Maria Knoppers, PhD, O, holds the Canada Research Chair in Law and Medicine (Tier 1: 2001-). Officer of the Order of Canada, she is Director of the Centre of Genomics and Policy at the Department of Human Genetics, Faculty of Medicine, McGill University. Former Chair of the International Ethics Committee of the Human Genome Organization (1996–2004), she is currently Chair of the Ethics Working Party of the International Stem Cell Forum (UK). In 2003, she founded the international Public Population Project in Genomics (P3G) and Quebec's CARTaGENE project. CARTaGENE is a resource of samples and data on the genetic diversity of the population of Quebec.

Bert Gordijn is Chair of Ethics and Director of the Institute of Ethics at Dublin City University. Bert is Editor-in-Chief of a book series, *The International Library of Ethics, Law and Technology* (Springer), as well as two peer reviewed journals, *Medicine, Health Care and Philosophy* (Springer) and *Studies in Ethics, Law and Technology* (Berkeley Electronic Press). He is also Secretary of the European Society for Philosophy of Medicine and Healthcare and founding Secretary of the Irish Chapter of the European Business Ethics Network. He has been appointed to the External Science Advisory Panel of the European Chemical Industry Council and has served on the Scientific Advisory Board of the European Patent Organisation as well as the UNESCO Expert Committee on Ethics and Nanotechnology.

Denise Avard is the Research Director for the Centre of Genomics and Policy and associate professor at the Faculty of Medicine, Department of Human Genetics at McGill University. Her research interests are in the areas of genetic testing and screening relevant to newborn, children, adolescents and persons with disabilities. She has an added interest in knowledge transfer and genetic epidemiology. She obtained her doctorate in social epidemiology from the University of Cambridge, England, and a Master's degree in sociology and a Bachelor's degree in Nursing from the University of Ottawa. Prior to joining the Centre of Genomics and Policy she was researcher in the Centre de la recherche en droit public at the Université de Montreal, Executive Director of the Canadian Institute of Child Health and Assistant Professor in the Faculty of Medicine at the University of Calgary.

Deryck Beyleveld is Professor of Law and Bioethics and currently Head of Durham Law School. He is also Visiting Professor of Moral Philosophy and Applied Ethics at the University of Utrecht. Before joining Durham University in 2006, he was Professor of Jurisprudence at Sheffield University and Director of the Sheffield Institute of Biotechnology Law and Ethics (SIBLE), which he founded in 1993. He co-ordinated the PRIVIREAL project on Privacy in Research Ethics and Law, funded by the European Commission. He has authored or co-authored seven books (including *Human Dignity in Bioethics and Biolaw*, OUP 2001, and *Consent in the Law,* Hart 2007) and co-edited four others, including three volumes on data protection law which were produced in the PRIVIREAL project). His numerous publications cover criminology, multiple areas of law, legal and moral philosophy as well as bioethics. He was Vice-Chair of Trent Research Ethics Committee form 1997–2006. He is a Fellow of the Society of Biology.

Diego Gracia, MD, PhD, is a psychiatrist and Professor of History of Medicine and Bioethics at the School of Medicine, Complutense University of Madrid, Spain. He is honorary professor of the Schools of Medicine of the Universities of Chile, Lima, and Cordoba (Argentina). He is Director of the Master's Degree in Bioethics and an Appointed Member of the Royal National Academy of Medicine, and of the Royal National Academy of Moral and Political Sciences of Spain. He is Fellow of the Hastings Center (New York), Fellow of the National Academy of Medicine of Chile, President of the Board of Trustees of the Foundation for Health Sciences (Madrid), and Director of the Zubiri Foundation (Madrid). His main books are *Voluntad de verdad* (Barcelona, 1986; 2nd edn., Madrid, 2007); *Fundamentos de bioética* (Madrid, 1989; 2nd edn., 2007, Italian translation, 1992; Portuguese translation 2008); *Primum non nocere* (Madrid, 1990); *Introducción a la bioética* (Santafé de Bogotá, 1991; 2nd edn., 2007); *Procedimientos de decisión en ética clínica* (Madrid, 1991; 2nd edn., 2007); *Ética y vida: Estudios de bioética* (4 vols., Santafé de Bogotá, 1998); *Medice cura te ipsum* (Madrid, 2004; Portuguese translation 2010); *Como arqueros al blanco* (Madrid, 2004; Portuguese translation, 2010); *Voluntad de comprensión* (Madrid, 2010); and *La cuestión del valor* (Madrid, 2011).

Dónal P. O'Mathúna, PhD, is Senior Lecturer in Ethics, Decision-Making and Evidence in the School of Nursing at Dublin City University, Ireland. He is an academic member of the Biomedical Diagnostics Institute and the Institute of Ethics at Dublin City University. He is Chair of the Academy of Fellows of the Center for Bioethics & Human Dignity, Illinois and a Visiting Fellow of the UK Cochrane Centre, Oxford. He is the author of *Nanoethics: Big Ethical Issues with Small Technology* (Continuum, 2009) and co-author of *Alternative Medicine* (Zondervan, 2007). He has published several peer-reviewed articles and led funded research projects. He is a member of the herbal sub-committee of the Irish Medicines Board and sits on a number of research and hospital ethics committees.

Donald Chalmers is Distinguished Professor of Law and Director of the Centre for Law and Genetics at the University of Tasmania. He is a Foundation Fellow of the Australian Academy of Law. He is Chair of the Gene Technology Ethics and Community Consultative Committee, Deputy Chair of the National Health and Medical Research Council (NHMRC) Embryo Research Licensing Committee and member of the National Breast and Ovarian Cancer Centre Board of Directors. He was Chair of the NHMRC Australian Health Ethics Committee (AHEC) from 1994 to 2000, member of the NHMRC Human Genetics Advisory Committee from 2005 to 2008 and Law Reform Commissioner for Tasmania from 1991 to 1997. Internationally, he is a member of the Human Genome Organisation Ethics Committee and of the International Cancer Genome Consortium Ethics Committee. His current major research interests are in health law and genetics, research ethics and law reform. His research work involves an examination of the legal and governance arrangements for human tissue biobanks. He has been Chief Investigator on several ARC research grants and an NHMRC program grant.

Eric M. Meslin is Director of the Indiana University Center for Bioethics, Associate Dean for Bioethics and Professor of Medicine, Medical and Molecular Genetics, Public Health and Philosophy. He was previously the Executive Director of the US National Bioethics Advisory Commission (1998–2001) and Program Director in the Ethical, Legal and Social Implications (ELSI) program at the National Human Genome Research Institute (1996–97). He has held academic positions at the University of Toronto (1988–96), at Oxford University (1994–95), and was Visiting Professor-at-Large at the University of Western Australia (2008–2010). He has more than 100 publications on topics ranging from international health research to science policy, and has been a consultant to the World Health Organization, the US Observer Mission to UNESCO, and the Canadian Institutes of Health Research. He sits on several boards and committees including the Institute of Medicine's *Committee on Ethical and Scientific Issues in Studying the Safety of Approved Drugs*; the Stem Cell Oversight Committee of the Juvenile Diabetes Research Foundation; and the Board of Directors of Genome Canada. On May 9, 2007 he was appointed a Chevalier de L'Order Nationale du Mérite (Knight of the National Order of Merit) by the President of France.

Eva Winkler, MD, received her doctoral degree in cancer research from the German Center for Cancer Research in Heidelberg and is a PhD student in Medicine and Healthcare Ethics at the University of Basel. She works as a physician at the Department of Haematology and Oncology at the University Hospital, Munich. She held two Fellowship Positions in Ethics: one at the Division of Medical Ethics, Harvard Medical School and as Faculty Fellow at the Harvard Center for Ethics and the Professions, Harvard University. Her interests in health care ethics focus on organizational ethics, resource allocation and end-of-life decision making. She chairs the medical ethics study group within the Munich Competence Center for Ethics and the Ethics Working group of the German Society for Haematology and Oncology.

Gamal Serour, FRCOG, FRCS, FACOG MD Cairo University 1963; MRCOG 1970; FRCS 1972; FRCOG 1990, FACOG 2009, Professor of Obstetrics and Gynecology, Director, International Islamic Center For Population Studies and Research (IICPSR), former Chairman of Obstetrics and Gynaecology department, and former Dean, Faculty of Medicine, Al Azhar University. He led the work on reproductive heath, population policy, population education, women's and children's rights, empowerment of women and medical ethics in developing countries through projects with UN organizations, NGOS, European governments and USAID. He served as a member of many committees at WHO, UNFPA, UNENSCO, FIGO, IFFS, IPPF and IAB. He has authored and co-authored 368 papers, 28 chapters and 18 books in national and international publications is a reviewer and member of the Editorial Board of several international Ob/Gyn, human reproduction, population science and ethics Journals and has been an invited and keynote speaker in a large number of national, regional and international conferences. Currently he is President of The International Federation of Gynecology and Obstetrics (FIGO) 2009–12.

Georg Bosshard, MD, MAE, is a family physician and geriatrician in Winterthur, Switzerland, and Associate Professor (Privatdozent) of clinical ethics at the University of Zurich. He is a member of the Central Ethics Committee of the Swiss Academy of Medical Sciences (SAMW). Bosshard has published numerous articles and book chapters on ethical and empirical issues in the field of medical end-of-life decisions and assisted dying. His work was awarded the Vontobel-Award for research in Gerontology 2005, and the University of Zurich's Stehr-Boldt-Award for Medical Ethics in 2007.

Henk ten Have is Professor and Director of the Center for Healthcare Ethics at Duquesne University, Pittsburgh, USA. He held positions in the Universities of Maastricht and Nijmegen, the Netherlands. He has been Director of the Division of Ethics of Science and Technology at UNESCO, Paris, France. He is editor-in-chief of *Medicine, Healthcare and Philosophy*. He has published 28 books, including *The ethics of palliative care* (2002), *The UNESCO Universal Declaration on Bioethics and Human Rights: Background, principles and application* (2009) and *Bioethiek zonder grenzen Bioethics without borders*, in Dutch, 2010).

Hongwen Li is PhD (expected in 2012) candidate in Department of Philosophy in Peking University in China. He was awarded BA (2005) and MA (2008) in philosophy and ethics. He was in summer internship program in Yale University's Interdisciplinary Center for Bioethics in 2007, and a research fellow in Institute of Law and Ethics in Medicine in University of Vienna in 2010. His research interests include bioethics and medical ethics.

Jan Helge Solbakk is trained as a physician and a theologian at the University of Oslo. He holds a PhD in ancient philosophy from the same university. Since 1996 Solbakk has been Professor of Medical Ethics at the Section for Medical Ethics, University of Oslo. In the same period he has been Adjunct Professor of Medical Ethics at the Centre for International Health, University of Bergen. From February 2007 to August 2008 Solbakk served as Chief of Bioethics at the UNESCO Headquarters in Paris. At present Solbakk is Chair of ISSCR's Ethics and Public Policy Committee. Since January 2006 Solbakk is member of an Ethics Committee set up by the European and Developing Countries Clinical Trial Partnership and since August 2008 he has also served as member of UNESCO's Task Force of experts set up in connection with the project Assisting Bioethics Committees. Solbakk is also member of the Biomedical Ethics Funding Committee of the Wellcome Trust, UK. Solbakk has published extensively and is involved in several international research projects dealing with ethics teaching and with the ethical implications of biobanking, genetics, nano-technology, synthetic biology and stem cell research.

Jean-Philippe Cobbaut is Director of the Centre of Medical Ethics of the department of ethics, Catholic University of Lille (France). His research concerns clinical ethics, organizational ethics and public health ethics. He is also member of the researcher unit dedicated to disability, aging and participation (HaDePas) at the

Catholic University of Lille and member of the research group HELESI (Health, Ethics, Law, Economics and Social Issues), IRSS, Louvain University (Belgium).

Julie Samuël, LLM, is a lawyer and has a Master's Degree in Law and Biotechnology from the Université de Montréal. Her thesis analyzes the obligation and the liability of doctors in the context of sport doping. She also has a background in Health Law from the Université de Sherbrooke, where she studied the concept of wrongful birth. Ms. Samuël obtained a scholarship from the Canadian Chair of Research in Law and Medicine to do an internship at the International Olympic Committee, in Lausanne. She also obtained an Erasmus Mundus Fellowship to conduct research on paediatric biobanks and genetic testing in sports at the Katholieke Universiteit Leuven, in Belgium. She worked for five years as a Professional Associate for the Université de Montréal (CRDP) and McGill University (CGP). Her research focused on issues related to paediatric research, such as the participation of children in genetic research, biobanks and gene therapy. She is now in-house counsel at the Fonds de la recherche en santé du Québec.

Kadri Simm is a Senior Researcher at the Institute of Philosophy and Semiotics, University of Tartu. Her background lies in philosophy, gender studies and history. She has participated in numerous national and international research projects and her research interests lie in moral and political philosophy, feminist studies, global justice issues, bioethics and science and technology studies.

Kenneth Cornetta, MD, is the Joe C. Christian Professor and Chair of the Department of Medical and Molecular Genetics, Indiana University School of Medicine. Prior to his position as chairman, he directed the Indiana University Bone Marrow Transplantation Program. His research has focused on the production, certification and clinical application of retroviral and lentiviral vectors. He has published over 100 peer-reviewed papers related to gene therapy and hematopoietic stem cell transplantation. He directs the NIH-supported National Gene Vector Biorepository and his laboratory is the site for clinical lentiviral vector production for the NIH's Gene Therapy Resource Program. He previously served as the president of the American Society of Gene Therapy from 2009 to 2010.

Kenneth V. Iserson, MD is Professor Emeritus of Emergency Medicine at the University of Arizona, where he not only practiced and taught medicine, but also directed their very active Bioethics Committee for more than 25 years. With a practice now limited to international and disaster medicine, he was named a Fellow of the International Federation of Emergency Medicine. Domestically, he is Senior Medical Director of the Southern Arizona Rescue Association (search & rescue), a Supervisory Physician with Arizona's Disaster Medical Assistance Team (AZ-1) and a member of the American Red Cross disaster response team. Through numerous NGOs, he has worked clinically, consulted or taught on all seven continents. The author of more than 300 scientific articles on emergency medicine and biomedical ethics, he has also authored numerous books, including *Ethics in Emergency Medicine, Grave Words: Notifying Survivors of Sudden, Unexpected Death,* and the award-winning *Death to Dust: What Happens to Dead Bodies?* His newest book,

Improvised Medicine: Delivering Care with Limited Resources, will be published in 2011.

Kenneth W. Goodman directs the University of Miami Bioethics Program, a World Health Organization Collaborating Center in Ethics and Global Health Policy. He is Professor of Medicine and jointly of Philosophy, Electrical Engineering, Epidemiology and Public Health and Nursing and Health Studies. A Fellow of the American College of Medical Informatics, he has published a number of books and articles on ethics and health information technology. He has also written about ethics and evidence-based medicine and other topics in bioethics, the philosophy of science, and computing. He is co-principal investigator on the Pan American Bioethics Initiative, a US National Institutes of Health Fogarty International Center grant to support research ethics education in Latin America and the Caribbean.

Kris Dierickx is professor of biomedical ethics at the Centre for Biomedical Ethics and Law (Faculty of Medicine, K.U.Leuven). He co-ordinated the GeneBanC project (2006–09) funded by the European Commission. He has published more than 100 internationally reviewed articles and 8 books as author or editor on ethics and genetics, regenerative medicine, biobanks, reproductive medicine and research ethics. He is involved in several European research projects and acts as a reviewer for many international journals. He is member of ethics committees and reviewer for the Seventh Framework of the European Commission.

Lars Johan Materstvedt holds a PhD in political philosophy on the libertarianism of US philosopher Robert Nozick. He is Professor at the Department of Philosophy, Norwegian University of Science and Technology (NTNU), Trondheim, Norway, where he teaches history of philosophy, theory of science, metaethics, normative ethics and medical ethics. As a Postdoctoral Research Fellow with the Norwegian Cancer Society he carried out research on the relationship between euthanasia and palliative medicine, which included conducting interviews with terminally ill cancer patients about their attitudes towards euthanasia and physician-assisted suicide. He chaired the Ethics Task Force on Palliative Care and Euthanasia of the European Association for Palliative Care (EAPC). His most recent publications include Materstvedt LJ, Bosshard G. (2009) 'Deep and continuous palliative sedation (terminal sedation): clinical-ethical and philosophical aspects'. *The Lancet Oncology*, 10; 6: 622–7, and Materstvedt LJ, Bosshard G. (2010) 'Euthanasia and physician-assisted suicide'. Chap. 5.5 in Hanks G, Cherny N, Christakis N, Fallon MT, Kaasa S, Portenoy RK, eds. *Oxford Textbook of Palliative Medicine*, 4th edn. Oxford: Oxford University Press.

Leonardo D. de Castro is Senior Research Fellow at the National University of Singapore's Centre for Biomedical Ethics. He is Editor-in-Chief, *Asian Bioethics Review*. A member of the UNESCO Advisory Expert Committee for the Teaching of Ethics. He is also President of the Asian Bioethics Association, Chair of the Philippine Health Research Ethics Board and Secretary of the International Association of Bioethics. Having previously served as Vice Chair of the UNESCO

International Bioethics Committee, he currently represents the Philippines in the UNESCO Intergovernmental Bioethics Committee.

Margit Sutrop is Professor of Practical Philosophy, Head of the Institute of Philosophy and Semiotics and the founding Director of the interdisciplinary Centre for Ethics at Tartu University. She has studied and worked in the universities of Oxford, Oslo, Konstanz and Tartu. She has published 13 books as author or editor and numerous articles, especially on fiction and imagination, trust in science, ethical frameworks of genetic databases, pharmacogenetics and ethical issues of biometrics. She has held numerous national and international grants from the European Commission (5th, 6th, 7th FP), as well as from UNESCO, *Volkswagen Stiftung*, European Economic Area, NorFa, Nordic Spaces, Estonian Ministry of Education and Research, Estonian Science Foundation, etc. She is a member of the Council of the *Academia Europaea*, independent ethical expert of the European Commission, as well as a member of the Estonian President's Advisory Board, a member of the Estonian Council of Bioethics, and a member of the Clinical Ethics Committee of Tartu University Clinic.

Michael Davis is Senior Fellow at the Center for the Study of Ethics in the Professions and Professor of Philosophy, Illinois Institute of Technology, Chicago, IL 60616. Among his recent publications are: *Thinking Like an Engineer* (Oxford, 1998); *Ethics and the University* (Routledge, 1999); *Conflict of Interest in the Professions* (Oxford, 2001); *Profession, Code, and Ethics* (Ashgate, 2002); *Actual Social Contract and Political Obligation* (Mellen, 2002); *Engineering Ethics* (Ashgate, 2005); *Code Writing: How Software Engineering Became a Profession* (Center for the Study of Ethics in the Professions, 2007); and *Ethics and the Legal Profession, 2nd* (Prometheus, 2009). Since 1990, he has received four grants from the National Science Foundation to help integrate ethics into technical courses.

Michael McDonald is Maurice Young Professor of Applied Ethics at the University of British Columbia and the founding director of the W. Maurice Young Centre for Applied Ethics. McDonald heads the Canadian Network for the Ethical Governance of Research Involving Humans. He was Deputy Chair of the committee that created Canada's policy for research involving humans. He also served as Co-Chair of the Canadian Institute for Health Research's Standing Committee on Ethics and as a member of numerous Canadian committees and research teams on ethics and health research. In 2009, he received a Distinguished Lifetime Achievement Award in recognition of his leadership role in establishing national programs in applied ethics and bioethics. McDonald has published widely in ethical theory, political philosophy, bioethics and business ethics.

Michiel Korthals is Professor of Applied Philosophy at Wageningen University. He studied Philosophy, Sociology, German and Anthropology at the University of Amsterdam and the Karl Ruprecht Universität in Heidelberg. His academic interests include bioethics and ethical problems concerning food production and environmental issues, deliberative theories, and American pragmatism. Main publications: *Philosophy of Development* (Kluwer, 1996 with Wouter van Haaften and Thomas

Wren), *Pragmatist Ethics for a Technological Culture* (with Keulartz et. al.; Kluwer 2002), *Ethics for Life Sciences* (Springer, 2005), *Before Dinner. Philosophy and Ethics of Food* (Springer 2004), in 2006, *Pépé Grégoire, A Philosophical Interpretation of his Sculptures*, Zwolle: Waanders. In 2010 will appear *Genomics, Obesity and the Struggle over Responsibilities* (Springer).

Nina Preto is a doctoral candidate at the W. Maurice Young Centre for Applied Ethics at the University of British Columbia. She practised law prior to pursuing graduate studies in research ethics. She serves on the behavioral research ethics board at the University of British Columbia. Ms. Preto was also a board member of the Provincial Health Ethics Network of Alberta ["PHEN"] for three years, during which time she helped coordinate the development of materials on end-of-life decision making for the Alberta public. Her doctoral work explores how contract research organizations impact the conduct of clinical trials at community-based investigative sites and academic health centers, with a specific focus on the identification and management of ethical issues including conflicts of interest.

Paul McCarthy is a Research Associate and Lecturer at Lancaster University. He is based in Cesagen, Lancaster where he co-leads the research programme on 'Therapies and Enhancement'. This involves a number of researchers at Lancaster and Cardiff University working on projects in Genomics, Food and Agriculture, Translating Research and Genomics and Convergent Technologies. He also manages Cesagen's European projects dealing with issues in Genomics and other novel technological fields and is involved in advising the Commission on ethical issues in the global governance of science. He also leads Cesagen's strategy of developing collaborations in China including work on Traditional Chinese Medicine and other activities, such as public engagement events, with genomic researchers across the country.

Paul Ndebele is Assistant Director for Research Ethics at University of Botswana. He has held Research Ethics related positions at Medical Research Council of Zimbabwe, Michigan State University, University of Malawi and Africa University in Zimbabwe. He is a member of the National Research Ethics Committee for Botswana and he serves as Secretary for the University of Botswana Institutional Review Board, Animal Care and Use Committee and the Hazardous Materials Sub-Committee. Besides his appointment at University of Botswana, he currently serves as an Honorary Lecturer at College of Medicine, University of Malawi; part-time Lecturer at Africa University; and Adjunct Instructor at Michigan State University. Paul has a number of publications in the area of Research Ethics and serves as an Editorial Board member for four journals.

Paul Schotsmans is Ordinarius Professor of Medical Ethics at the Catholic University of Leuven and currently Vice-Dean of the Faculty of Medicine at the same university. He has participated in several European research projects (e.g. on persistent vegetative state patients, on palliative care, on reproductive technologies, and others). He was President of the European Association of Centres of Medical Ethics and Board Member of the International Association of Bioethics. He was also President of the Ethics Committee of Eurotransplant. He is currently President of the Belgian Advisory Committee on Bioethics. He has published mainly in the context of the application of 'personalism' as an ethical model for the ethical integration of reproductive technologies, stem cell research, organ transplantation and end-of-life decision making.

Peter A. Sy is Associate Professor of Philosophy, College of Social Sciences and Philosophy, University of the Philippines, Diliman, Quezon City. He is the Executive Officer of the International Association of Bioethics (IAB) and a research consultant of the Public Assessment of Water Services (PAWS), National Engineering Center, University of the Philippines. He has been a Research Fellow in Ethical Issues in International Research at the School of Public Health, Harvard University.

Pierre Boitte is professor of Medical Ethics at the Medical School and senior researcher at the Centre of Medical Ethics of the Department of Ethics, Catholic University of Lille (France). His research concerns clinical ethics, research ethics, and end-of-life ethics. He is a member of the European Clinical Ethics Network (ECEN) and also a member of the researcher unit dedicated to disability, aging and participation (HaDePas) at the Catholic University of Lille.

Rachel Cooper is Senior Lecturer in Philosophy at the University of Lancaster. Her publications include *Classifying Madness: A Philosophical Examination of the Diagnostic and Statistical Manual of Mental Disorders* (Springer, 2005) and *Psychiatry and the Philosophy of Science* (Acumen, 2007) and she is now working on monographs on the concept of disorder, and on the DSM-V. From 2007 to 2010 she was Honorary Secretary of the British Society for the Philosophy of Science. She is currently co-managing (with Havi Carel, UWE) an AHRC Research Network on Concepts of Health, Illness and Disease.

Rob de Vries studied Biology and Philosophy. He wrote a PhD thesis on the ethics of the genetic engineering of laboratory animals. From 2007 to 2009, he was a postdoctoral researcher at the Department of Ethics, Philosophy and History of Medicine at the Radboud University Nijmegen Medical Centre. There he carried out a research project, funded by the Dutch Program Tissue Engineering, on the ethical aspects of tissue engineering and regenerative medicine. He currently works at the 3R Research Centre of the Radboud University Nijmegen Medical Centre on a project on systematic reviews of animal research.

Roberto Andorno is Senior Research Fellow and Lecturer at the Institute of Biomedical Ethics of the University of Zurich, Switzerland. Originally from Argentina, he holds doctoral degrees in law from the Universities of Buenos Aires and Paris XII, both on topics related to the ethical and legal aspects of assisted reproductive technologies. Between 1999 and 2005, he conducted various research projects relating to bioethics, human dignity and human rights at the Faculty of Philosophy of the University Laval (Canada), as well as at the Universities of Göttingen and Tübingen (Germany). Dr. Andorno served as a member of the International Bioethics Committee of UNESCO (1998–2005) and participated in this capacity in the drafting of international declarations and reports relating to bioethics. He has published extensively on issues at the intersection of bioethics and law, and is a member of the editorial boards of various journals, including Medicine, Health Care & Philosophy, Journal International de Bioéthique, and Bioethica Forum.

Ruth Chadwick is Distinguished Research Professor at Cardiff University and Director of Cesagen. She held positions in Liverpool, Cardiff, Preston and Lancaster before joining the university in 2006. She co-ordinated the Euroscreen projects (1994–96; 1996–99) funded by the European Commission. She co-edits the journal *Bioethics*, and is co-editor of the online journal *Genomics, Society and Policy*. She has published 20 books as author or editor, including the award winning *Encyclopaedia of Applied Ethics* (1998). She is Chair of the Human Genome Organisation (HUGO) Ethics Committee, Fellow of the Hastings Center, New York, and is an Academician of the Academy of Social Sciences. She has served as a member of the Food Ethics Council, the Advisory Committee on Novel Foods and Process (ACNFP), the Standing Committee on Ethics of the Canadian Institute of Health Research, and the Medical Research Council Advisory Committee on DNA Banking.

Ruud ter Meulen is a psychologist and ethicist. He is Chair for Ethics of Medicine and Director of the Centre for Ethics in Medicine at the University of Bristol. Previously he worked as Professor of Philosophy and Director of the Institute for Bioethics at the University of Maastricht. He has published on a wide range of issues in medical ethics, including solidarity and justice in health care, ethical issues of health care reform and health policy, ethics of evidence-based medicine, and ethical issues of long-term care for older people. He was Principal Investigator of a large number of EU projects like the EVIBASE and ENHANCE project, and was member of the Advisory Group of the Science in Society Program of the European Commission. He was member of the Working Party of the Nuffield Council on Dementia: Ethical Issues, and is a member of the Board of Directors of the European Association of Centres for Medical Ethics (EACME).

Teoh Chin Leong is Research Fellow at the National University of Singapore's Centre for Biomedical Ethics, assisting with the development of outreach programs with a special focus on public education and bioethics education in schools. With interests in ethical, political and educational theory and practice, he is currently pursuing his doctoral studies at the Yong Loo Lin School of Medicine at the National University of Singapore.

Thomas Faunce, BA/LLB (Hons), B Med PhD, is an Australian Research Council (ARC) Future Fellow jointly in the College of Law and College of Medicine, Biology and the Environment at the Australian National University. He served as Judges Associate to Justice Lionel Murphy of the Australian High Court and worked as a barrister and solicitor in Australia's two largest legal firms. He then practised intensive care medicine for twelve years in Wagga Wagga, Canberra and Melbourne. His PhD on regulation of the Human Genome Project was awarded the Crawford Prize. He has directed three ARC competitive research grants in the area of health technology regulation. He is an associate editor with Medical Humanities (UK) and edits the medical law reporter for the Journal of Law and Medicine. His latest book with Edward Elgar is on nanotechnology and global public health.

Tsuyoshi Awaya, Bsc, LLM, PhD, is a research professor of bioethics and medical law 'only' in the Department of Bioethics, Graduate School of Medicine, Dentistry and Pharmaceutical Sciences, Okayama University, Japan. He was a member of David Rothman's team, which produced the Bellagio Task Force Report on Transplantation, Bodily Integrity, and the International Traffic in Organs (1997). At present, he is a member of the Board of Directors of the Japan Association for Bioethics and President of the International Society for Clinical Bioethics (ISCB). He has published about 30 books as author, editor or co-author. He has been doing field research on organ trade in the Philippines and in India since 1992 and about the commodification of the human body in the USA since 1996. He consequently wrote *The Human Body Parts Business* (Kodansha, Japan, 1999). The book became a best seller in its field. It was translated into Chinese for sale in Taiwan in 2002. He has been doing field research on transplantation of organs from executed prisoners in China since 1995. In the course of his research, he was expelled from China in 1997. He testified on this topic before the US Congress in 1998.

Vilhjálmur Árnason is Professor of Philosophy and Chair of the Centre for Ethics at the University of Iceland. He co-ordinated the ELSAGEN project (2002–04) funded by the European Commission. He was a board member of the European Society for Philosophy of Medicine and Health Care 2004–10 and of The Nordic Bioethics Committee 2005–10. He is the author of four books on moral philosophy and applied ethics in Icelandic, one of which has been translated into German. He has published numerous articles in the field of bioethics, ethical theory and social philosophy, and edited several books in Icelandic and English. He is a member of the editorial teams of *Medicine, Health Care and Philosophy, Genomics and Society, and Etikk i Praksis – a Nordic Journal.* He is life member of Clare Hall, Cambridge University (2006) and of the Alexander von Humboldt Foundation (1993).

Vittorio Hosle is the Paul Kimball Professor of Arts and Letters in the Departments of German, Philosophy and Political Science at the University of Notre Dame and the Director of the Notre Dame Institute for Advanced Study. He has written or (co-)edited more than 30 books and has published more than 120 articles.

Volnei Garrafa, PhD, Full Professor of the Faculty of Health Sciences of the University of Brasília, Brazil. Chairman of the UNESCO's Cathedra of Bioethics and of the Post-Graduate Programme (Master and Doctorate) in Bioethics of the University of Brasília. President of the Latin-American and Caribbean Network of Bioethics (2003–10); Editor in Chief of the Brazilian Journal of Bioethics; Member of the International Bioethics Committee of the UNESCO (2010–13). Former President of the Brazilian Society of Bioethics (2001–05); President of the Sixth World Congress on Bioethics of the International Association of Bioethics - Brasília, Brazil, 2002.

Yali Cong is Professor and Director of Department of Medical Humanities in Peking University Health Science Center (PUHSC) in China. She got BS (1989) in biology, MA (1992) and PhD (1995) in philosophy of science. She is Vice Director of China-US Center for Medical Professionalism of PUHSC, Secretary of Association of Medical Ethics in Chinese Medical Association, Secretary of Center for Applied Ethics in Peking University and Vice Chair of Education Group of Beijing Medical Ethics Association. She is a member of the Editor Committee of *Chinese Journal of Medicine and Philosophy*. She has written many papers on medical ethics and bio-ethics both in Chinese and English. In recent years, she has made great efforts in developing and construction of Institutional Review Boards at different levels.

Yechiel Michael Barilan is a medical doctor, expert in internal medicine and senior lecturer in the Department of Medical Education, Sackler Faculty of Medicine, Tel Aviv University, Israel. He has published extensively on the social history of bioethical issues, Jewish bioethics, human rights and moral psychology, especially as applied to medical education. He teaches in Israel and Europe and has participated in various national and international bioethical committees.

Health Care Ethics in an Era of Globalisation

Ruth Chadwick, Henk ten Have and Eric M. Meslin

One of the most exciting recent developments in health care ethics is the way that the issues are becoming more international. Discussions about cloning, organ transplantation, reproductive health and health research are now regularly discussed by scholars, governments, advocacy groups, the media and the public in countries around the world. A growing body of research has emerged on comparative international approaches to issues – demonstrating that some of the early foundational work in health care ethics – initially in the U.S.A. and Western Europe, and then expanding to every continent – is now being challenged, amended and applied as countries (and of often different regions within countries) weigh in with different perspectives, strategies, arguments and approaches. IInternational ethics has developed as a field of study in its own right,(Green Donovan and Jauss, 2009; Lavery, Wahl, Grady et al, 2007), suggesting that the implications of the global dimensions of health care ethics, in particular, have been found to merit specific study.

To a significant extent, this phenomenon has informed our choice of topics for inclusion in this *Handbook*. The volume begins with chapters dealing with theoretical perspectives relevant to the field, such as human rights and the ethic of care, and includes a discussion of anti-theory. More traditional areas of bioethics such as reproduction and end of life issues are then discussed. A group of chapters on vulnerable groups considers the principle of vulnerability in addition to specific issues of mental health, children, orphan diseases and poverty. Research ethics is discussed in the international context, and a set of chapters on technologies, including genetics, telemedicine and nanotechnology. The volume concludes with selections that broaden the debate to include environmental health and the pharmaceutical industry's impact on health care. Many anthologies exist covering these topics, of course. No anthology can be fully comprehensive, but we believe that collectively, the selections found in this *Handbook* represent both core and emerging issues in health care ethics in an era of globalization. Therefore, we feel an obligation to explain our rationale.

A WORD ABOUT TERMINOLOGY: MEDICAL ETHICS, BIOETHICS, HEALTH CARE ETHICS

We note that the issues and topics in this volume arose from a much longer tradition in bioethics generally. Indeed, bioethics has been defined in a number of ways. The American cancer specialist Van Rensselaer Potter (1911–2001) is usually credited with coining the term 'bioethics', using it for the first time in *Perspectives in Biology and Medicine* in 1970 (Potter, 1970), and repeating a version of it in the first chapter of his *Bioethics, Bridge to the Future,* published in 1971. Potter identified the need for a new discipline combining science and philosophy arguing that we needed to synthesise our biological knowledge of the science of living systems (hence "bio") and our knowledge of human value systems (hence "ethics"). This synthesis would focus on the basic problems confronting human-kind: population (too many people for a sustainable future on earth), peace (the tragedy of war and violence), pollution, poverty, politics (because of its lack of long-term views) and progress (because of the assumption that science and society will always develop in a positive direction). Potter's called for an interdisciplinary approach was innovative at the time, but it was his global perspective that was especially profound. He argued that we should cross the boundaries between disciplines in order to look for ideas "that are susceptible to objective verification in terms of the future survival of man and improvement in the quality of life for future generations" (Potter 1970, p. 132). In retrospect, as Warren Reich (1994) argued, it is clear that Potter's ideas about bioethics did not occupy much attention in emerging bioethics literature at the time, and yet the residual impact of Potter's thinking could be found in many places. The wealth of activities undertaken by scholars promoting an approach to bioethics both as a new ethics of life sciences and health care and as a new focus of applied ethics could be seen in the growth of research centers around the world and through a growing literature.

Bioethics was new, although it emerged from an established history of professional medical ethics. Its topics were broader than those facing clinicians and patients – often associated with the dramatic developments in medical technology and health care, e.g. reproductive medicine, transplantation technology, resuscitation practices and the emergence of intensive care units in hospitals. In this sense, bioethics included a wider and more challenging set of issues than traditional medical ethics.

The precise range of the term 'bioethics' today remains a subject of scholarly debate – for some, as in its earliest (Potter) usage, it includes environmental issues, but discussion in bioethics still tend to focus primarily on issues in medicine, the life sciences, and new technologies, including those arising out of the Human Genome Project and its aftermath, which have given rise to an extensive discussion in civil society. It remains wider in scope than but still includes *medical ethics* but the term 'Medical Ethics' itself has been challenged in the light of the developing interest in issues related to health care professions other than medicine, in particular nursing.

The development of professional ethics standards in nursing, social work, pharmacy and other allied health sciences and the perception of these professions as accountable in their own right have led to the development of distinct professional ethical standards for each of them. To some extent it is difficult to draw precise boundaries between the different terms, as in common usage they are not infrequently used interchangeably. We have chosen to use the term 'health care ethics' in this volume recognizing that it is not as precise a term as we would like. Below we comment on some of the debates concerning and challenges to bioethics, in so far as they are also relevant to health care ethics.

THE MOVE TO INTERNATIONAL ISSUES

We believe that the increased emphasis on the issues that may affect only one country, to those that affect many countries – and indeed the planet—reflects more than just a change in scope and scale. The move from domestic to international concerns may require a serious reconsideration of the way problems are framed, the way theoretical foundations are defended, and finally the way proposed solutions are assessed (Lansang and Dennis 2004). These effects have an impact on the ways in which particular issues are studied – most obviously for the conduct of health research, and for the distribution of limited health care resources – and also, potentially, on the theoretical foundations for the issues themselves. There are several examples of this phenomenon.

The increasing movement towards data sharing between different national biobanking initiatives, for example, has led to challenges for harmonisation not only in standards for data storage but also in relation to the appropriate ethical guidelines (see Chadwick and Strange, 2009). Similarly, health research is increasingly multi-centre and international, with growing numbers of research subjects recruited in economically developing countries, with more money being spent by more sponsors (government, private sector and philanthropies), more prospects of benefit and more challenges for reviewing and approving studies (Hyder, Dawson, Bachiani et al., 2009).

ENDURING ISSUES AND NEW CHALLENGES

As healthcare issues become more global in their reach, the legal and regulatory schemes to provide adequate governance have not always kept pace. In many cases, guidance differs; in other cases guidelines are absent. As the example of reproductive cloning demonstrated, when a new technology has been developed in one country, it is possible to apply the technology everywhere, even if some countries want to ban its use. This has led to concerns about the phenomena of health care and scientific tourism (Cohen and Cohen, 2010; Delmonico 2009; Turner 2010; Shalev 2010). Accepted rules for transplantation and organ donation, for instance, vary among countries and these different approaches have led to abuses such as organ trafficking and commodification of transplantation practices. Furthermore, the burdens and benefits of scientific and technological advancements are unequally distributed. Poorer countries run the risk of being excluded from the benefits of biomedical progress. What follows from this point of view, health care ethics should not only examine the differences among the moral standards in different countries – the values embedded in their cultures and religions – but also what they share in common.

Despite the fact that core issues continue to be important and that new issues are emerging, there have been a number of criticisms of the field as a whole that need to be addressed.

This anthology will not address them all, but we note a few that are discussed. It is sometimes claimed that bioethics will disappear or indeed that it has already had its day. What does this claim mean? It is difficult to believe that the questions covered by the field will disappear. Although it might be tempting to suppose that we will reach a time when they are 'answered', this is not normally thought to be in the nature of ethical questions – they are re-asked and re-interpreted along with social change.

Where new technologies are concerned, it might be thought, as has been the case with nanotechnology, that ethical issues associated with them simply represent a revisiting of the issues in other debate (see for example Crowe, 2008). Hence discussions tend to focus on whether there is anything different about them. If there is not, then that might lend credence to the suggestion that bioethics might disappear. In every time and place, however, questions will continue to arise about what we should do and how we should live, whether in relation to new technology or in relation to health care and the life sciences more broadly conceived.

Perhaps the claim, however, is not that the *issues* will cease to arise, but that bioethics may not be the appropriate discipline or approach to answering them. Again it is necessary to ask exactly what is meant by this claim. If the questions *constitute* the domain of bioethics then what can it possibly mean to say that it should not be 'Bioethics' that is involved in answering them? One can only give sense to the claim either in terms of bioethics being conceived in terms of one particular disciplinary approach, or in terms of an objection to the notion of some sort of specific expertise that constitutes 'bioethicists' as apart from any other disciplinary approach. There seem to be two distinct possibilities here. First, if bioethics is conceived as a branch of an existing discipline, Philosophy is a strong contender, as Ethics is traditionally a branch of Philosophy. Under this interpretation, criticisms of Bioethics as a field are directed against the monopoly of Philosophy in answering ethical questions and against the *way* in which it asks and answers ethical questions in this field (see below). Second, if Bioethics is not a discipline but a multidisciplinary field of study involving ethical, legal, social and philosophical aspects, things look rather different. The inclusion of both 'ethical' and 'philosophical' aspects here draws attention to the fact that in bioethics some philosophical questions arise that are not ethical e.g. epistemological questions about the limits of knowledge, questions of personal identity and so on.

A potential criticism of this conception is that to constitute such a field *as* a distinct field is a political act. Why should social questions not be addressed by social scientists, legal questions by lawyers, philosophical questions by philosophers? Why is there a need to define bioethics as a distinct field, if not to give a kind of status to those who engage in it? To those who take this view, the attempt to define bioethics by the type of questions covered is insufficient. For some of those who work in the field, however, bioethics is developing as a kind of meta-discipline. It is possible for those who specialise in bioethics to develop different disciplinary approaches to work beyond their home discipline. To engage properly and effectively in bioethics requires the ability to recognise the different and multiple dimensions that ethical questions have, and to be willing to work collaboratively with other disciplinary perspectives and methods.

Misunderstandings are apt to arise concerning the relationship between 'bioethics' and 'bioethicists'. While many people work on ethical aspects of developments in health care and the life sciences (bioethics) then shouldn't those people be called bioethicists?

Agreement on this has been difficult to achieve particularly when 'bioethicist' is taken to mean someone who has privileged expertise on the issues, and excludes others. So let's be clear.

Under an interpretation of bioethics that construes it largely as a branch of [Applied] Philosophy, there are criticisms of bioethics that could come either from within Philosophy or from without. From within Philosophy, it is important to address Alasdair MacIntyre's question as to whether applied ethics rests on a mistake (MacIntyre, 1984). If applied ethics is understood as 'applying' a set of principles, or a theory, to a practical problem or issue, there is a question as to how that question or issue is conceived, and who construes it as a problem. In the health care field, is it for the health care professionals to define the problem or for the philosophers?

While this is an important question, it will only count as a problem for an account of Bioethics that depends on this model of 'application'. Critics of bioethics from outside the field of Philosophy may have similar concerns that 'armchair philosophers' may be trying to apply theories and principles that have very little relevance to real life practice. It is important to disentangle the particular contribution philosophical ethics has to make to bioethics, and the possibility for productive collaboration with other disciplines. On the other hand the external criticism may be based, not on worries about 'application' in general, but on the view that in bioethics particular approaches have been prioritized at the expense of others.

Critics do not always appear to be aware of the diversity of the field. The repertoire of philosophical theoretical approaches is diverse, and yet there is some truth to the idea that there has been a predominantly individualistic focus in bioethics in the first decades of its development. This does not mean, however, that bioethics *itself* is individualistic, and certainly not that it is overwhelmed by an autonomy-based approach. It is possible to find explanations of why bioethics has been primarily (though not exclusively) concerned with the individual to date, and why there is currently a turn to more overtly public health issues. What also has to be borne in mind is that these issues constitute lively debates *within the field*. It would be a mistake to operate with a picture of bioethics as a discrete and unified field being attacked by the critics. As the following quotation shows, there are voices in bioethics who are pointing to two challenges that need to be addressed:

> how to shift to locus of bioethical dialogue to bring to the foreground implicit assumptions that frame central issues and determine whose voices are to be heard and how to sharpen the vision of a global bioethics to include the perspectives of the marginalized as well as the privileged (Donchin and Diniz, 2001,iii–iv)

The point about 'framing' in the above quotation is important, and leads to discussion of the next criticism, which is that any theoretical approach 'frames' the issues in a particular way, drawing attention to what the 'framer' considers to be the salient points of a situation. Such approaches, however, can be blind to the concerns that members of different public and community groups have, whether or not they are key stakeholders in some specific issue e.g. by virtue of being a member of a patient advocacy organisation. This is a crucial question for those who use theoretical approaches in bioethics to address, especially where it is claimed that the roots of a given theoretical approach lie in the 'common morality'. Such concerns have been influential in the 'empirical turn' in bioethics, with social science taking an increasingly important role, leading to discussions about the relationship between the disciplines contributing to the field. This criticism, moreover, is not directed only at academics working in bioethics, but also against members of policy-making committees in the relevant domain, who may, for example, think it adequate to address issues using scientific techniques of risk assessment without having regard to what may be more fundamental social concerns.

Bioethics has increasingly contributed to public policy (Meslin, 2010), yet beyond the discussion of what the role of an ethicist should be in public policy, there has also been criticism of the *performance* of bioethicists in public policy. They are criticised for both trying to 'stop science' and, alternately for not wanting to stop anything. Considerations such as these lead to the need to recognise the desirability and urgency of finding a way for bioethics to facilitate good research rather than perceived as burdensome and bureaucratic. It is also important, if it is to acquire and retain legitimacy that it not be conceived of as a tool to support particular political agendas or economic interests (Meslin and Goodman, 2010).

CAN GLOBAL HEALTH CARE ETHICS RESPOND TO THESE CHALLENGES?

What is distinctive and helpful about taking a global approach to health care ethics? Under one interpretation, it is simply that the issues addressed are global in scope. Health inequalities exist both within societies and between societies: a global ethic will be particularly concerned with the latter. The ways in which, for example, genetic information will be interpreted is closely linked with social conditions: for example, whereas in western countries there has been a considerable discussion about the insurance implications of predictive genetic information; in some countries prospects of stigmatisation may be much more immediate a concern, and may be highly influenced by gender. Discussions of the implementation of 'personalised' genomic medicine look rather different in varying social contexts. Take the issue of food, for example. The problems literally span the spectrum: food security, malnutrition, poverty, food safety are not limited to the impoverished economically developing world of lower and middle income countries. Similarly a poor diet leading to unhealthy lifestyles, obesity and an increase in diabetes are not limited to the economically developed countries of higher income. Worries about food security look different in different countries, although issues of malnourishment can apply in situations of both plenty and scarcity.

However, these examples arguably display a framing that is still *local* in scope – it is just that it shows awareness of differences across the globe which need to be taken into account. To be truly global in scope, the focus should perhaps be on global challenges requiring global *solutions*. Examples of such problems might be global pandemics, such as SARS or H1N1 ("swine") influenza were feared to be. This leads to the suggestion that what distinguishes a global from a non-global ethic is that it applies a global *frame*. Whereas, as Heather Widdows points out, all applied ethics *can* be global (as is shown by the work of prominent philosophers who have contributed to the field, such as Peter Singer and Onora O'Neill), global ethics *must* be global (Widdows, forthcoming, 2012). Global ethics is not concerned with the interests of particular professional groups, it is concerned more with institutional and political factors, which other branches of applied ethics, including bioethics, perhaps take insufficiently into account. Widdows makes the point that global ethicists are more likely to be found in political science departments than are applied ethicists of other varieties, and the priority moral/political concept is likely to be *justice* rather than, for example, autonomy, which has been so predominant in bioethics and health care ethics, at least for a major part of the second half of the twentieth century.

There is a question, then, about the extent to which there are particular theoretical approaches that are relevant in a global context. There have been debates, for example, about whether the 'four principles' of biomedical ethics can be transferred without difficulty from one culture to another (e.g. Holm, 1995). The challenges identified by Donchin and Diniz in the quotation above come from a feminist bioethics perspective, and it might be argued that such a perspective is particularly appropriate for some of the issues of global health ethics. We need, however, to examine the relevance to the present work of the phenomenon of the development of global ethics as a distinct field. Global bioethics poses specific theoretical and practical challenges related to the interaction between globalization and localization. If ethical principles are identified that are valid for all human beings regardless of gender, religion, nationality, race and bodily and mental constitution, how can at the same time the cultural diversity of humankind be taken into account?

The 1990s and 2000s saw considerable discussion about the possibility of a global bioethics, and the extent to which it is possible for principles to have global applicability. Again, however, there are different possibilities to be considered. One is the transferability of a set of ethical principles already alluded to above, and this is what has been at issue in, for example, discussions as to whether the four principles could form the basis of a global bioethic. Another is the question whether a different approach is appropriate. The principle of cosmopolitanism, for example, has been prominent in global ethics *per se*, but has not figured large in bioethics. It may be, however, that global bioethics requires, if not different principles, different priorities.

INTERNATIONAL ORGANIZATIONS

The globalisation of ethical problems and challenges is also reflected in the growing activity of international organizations in the field of bioethics. Nowadays, many of them have programmes and advisory bodies in the area of bioethics. Examples are the European Commission, the Council of Europe and the Arab League. UNESCO started its ethics program in 1993 with the establishment of the International Bioethics Committee (IBC), the first and until now only bioethics committee with a global scope and membership. Its Members States have adopted, unanimously and by acclamation on 19 October 2005, the *Universal Declaration on Bioethics and Human Rights*, affirming the commitment of the international community to respect a set of principles for humanity in the development and application of biomedical science and technology. With this new Declaration, for the first time a political commitment was made towards a set of *universal* principles in bioethics that could and should apply in all countries, regardless of culture, religion and tradition. The Universal Declaration also underscored the requirement to respond to the particular needs of economically developing countries, indigenous communities and vulnerable groups or persons, reminding the international community of its duty of solidarity towards all countries.

What has changed in the last few years is that on the one hand a broader range of relevant ethical principles have been identified and adopted, and on the other hand a wide range of new issues and problems has emerged. The adoption of the UNESCO Declaration marks the evolution of a global perspective in the field of bioethics, since it underlines a broader set of ethical *principles*. The focus is not only on individually orientated principles such as respect for autonomy and human dignity, but also on principles that relate to the social and cultural context, such as the principles of solidarity and social responsibility, and even to the global context, such as the principles of benefit-sharing and protecting future generations. Instead of the critique that ethical principles usually reflect a particular cultural setting (traditionally the western one), there is now emerging agreement on ethical principles that take into account a really global perspective (Ten Have and Jean, 2009).

At the same time, new *problems* are on the agenda of bioethics discourse; – problems that previously were either non-existent or neglected. One example is 'conflict of interest', a concern that existed already but that has been exacerbated enormously due to the neoliberal intertwinement of industry and science. For many developing countries, topics as migration, organ trade, access to health care and medication, clean water and poverty are more pressing, daily problems. Another example is 'dual use', a new issue that has emerged recently as a result of bio-terrorism and security concerns.

Against this background of a broader set of ethical principles and a wider range of issues and topics for analysis and critical consideration, bioethics is in the process of being redefined as global bioethics. Curiously enough, some of the initial ideas of Potter are recurring in this new approach and conception of global bioethics. Potter's emphasis that we need to bridge the present and the future is reiterated in the view of bioethics as a new interdisciplinary approach with a focus on long-term interests and goals that safeguard the survival of humanity. Potter's argument that we also need to bridge nature and culture as well as human beings and nature invites us to regard bioethics as responsibility for the future and as a new ethics that takes into account the science of ecology and regards human beings as interrelated with their environment. Social, cultural and ecological problems are now definitely within the remit of global health care ethics.

ACKNOWLEDGEMENTS

We should like to acknowledge all our contributors, the team at Sage, and the invaluable assistance of Clare Pike and Mel Evans at Cardiff University.

REFERENCES

Chadwick, R. and Strange, H. (2009) 'Harmonisation and standardisation in ethics and governance: conceptual and practical challenges' in H. Widdows and C. Mullen (eds) *the Governance of Genetic Information: Who Decides?* 201–13 Cambridge: University Press.

Cohen, C.B. and Cohen, P.J. (2010) International stem cell tourism and the need for effective regulation. Part I: Stem cell tourism in Russia and India: clinical research, innovative treatment, or unproven hype? *Kennedy Inst Ethics J.* 20(1): 27–49.

Crowe, S. (2008) Understanding the ethical implications of nanotechnology. Highlights of a limited inquiry by the President's Council on Bioethics. Staff paper. http://bioethics.georgetown.edu/pcbe/background/nanotechnology_implications.html (accessed October 26, 2010).

Delmonico, F.L. (2009) The implications of Istanbul Declaration on organ trafficking and transplant tourism. *Curr Opin Organ Transplant.* 14(2): 116–9.

Donchin, A. and Diniz, D. (2001) 'Guest editors' note'. *Bioethics* 15 (3): iii–v.

Gilligan, C. (1982) *In a Different Voice: psychological theory and women's development Cambridge*, Mass.: Harvard University Press.

Green, R.M., Aine D., and Steven A.J. (eds.) (2009) *Global Bioethics: Issues of Conscience for the Twenty-first Century.* Oxford University Press.

Grimshaw, J. (1986) *Feminist Philosophers: women's perspectives on philosophical traditions* Brighton: Wheatsheaf Books.

Holm, S. (1995) 'Not just autonomy – the principles of American biomedical ethics' *J Med Ethics* 21: 332–338.

Hyder, A., Dawson, L., Bachani, A., & Lavery, J. (2009). Moving from research ethics review to research ethics systems in low-income and middle-income countries. *The Lancet* 373(9666): 862–865.

Knoppers, B.M. and Chadwick, R. (2005) 'Human genetic research: emerging trends in ethics' *Nature Reviews Genetics* 6: 75–79.

Lansang, M., & Dennis, R. (2004) Building capacity in health research in the developing world. *Bulletin of the World Health Organization* 82, 764–770.

Lavery, J.V., Wahl, E., Grady, C. and Emanuel, E.J. (eds) (2007) *Ethical Issues in International Biomedical Research: A Case Book.* New York: Oxford University Press.

MacIntyre, A. (1984) Does Applied Ethics Rest on a Mistake? *The Monist* 67(4): 498–513.

Meslin, E.M. (2010) 'Can National Bioethics Commissions Be Progressive? Should They?' In: Moreno, J. and Berger, S. (eds.) *Progress in Bioethics: Science, Policy and Politics* Cambridge MA: MIT Press: 143–160.

Meslin, E.M. and Goodman, K.G. (2010) An Ethics and Policy Agenda for Biobanks and Electronic Health *Science Progress* http://www.scienceprogress.org/2010/02/bank-on-it/

Potter, V.R. (1970) Bioethics, the science of survival. *Perspectives in Biology and Medicine* 14: 127–153.

Potter, V.R. (1971) *Bioethics. Bridge to the future.* Prentice-Hall, Englewood Cliffs, New Jersey.

Reich, W.T. (1994) The word 'bioethics': its birth and the legacies of those who shaped it. *Kennedy Institute of Ethics Journal* 4(4): 319–335.

Shalev, C. (2010) Stem cell tourism – a challenge for trans-national governance. *Am J Bioeth* 10(5): 40–2.

Sherwin, S. (1992) *No Longer Patient: feminist ethics and health care.* Philadelphia: Temple University Press.

Singer, P. and Kuhse, H. (2009) *A Companion to Bioethics.* (2nd ed.), Oxford: Blackwell.

Ten Have, H. and Jean, M. (eds.) (2009) *The UNESCO Universal Declaration on Bioethics and Human Rights. Background, principles and application.* UNESCO Publishing, Paris.

Turner, L. (2010) "Medical tourism" and the global market place in health services. U.S. patients, international hospitals, and the search for affordable healthcare. *Int J Health Serv.* 40(3): 443–67.

Widdows, H. (forthcoming, 2012) 'Global ethics: overview'. In: Chadwick, R. (ed.) *Encyclopedia of Applied Ethics,* 2nd edn. Oxford: Elsevier.

1

Methodology

Vittorio Hösle

INTRODUCTION

Ethics cannot, and does not want to, replace moral life. It is both logically and nomologically possible to be a moral individual without engaging in ethics; and it is also possible to be both a good ethicist and a vicious person at the same time. For ethics is nothing other than the theoretical analysis of the nature of morality: of the values and goods that are to be considered moral; of acts aiming at implementing these values; and of the habits (called virtues) from which such moral acts flow. It is the nature of ethics, as a practical discipline, however, to demand that its insights be acted upon. While engaging in a theoretical discipline like theology or mathematics is an end in itself; the whole end of ethics is to ask for acts in accordance with it. The vicious person who refuses to act according to valid ethical insights is no doubt a possibility and even a reality. But his behavior is condemned by his own insights.

On the other hand, the desire to act morally leads almost inevitably to ethical reflections. In times of rapid social change and institutionalized intercultural encounters, at least, what is morally demanded loses the obviousness that it enjoys in traditional societies. The desire to act morally entails the desire to know what is moral. But, for example in the aforementioned circumstances, such a knowledge cannot be gotten from one's own traditions alone, since their claim to teach what is moral no longer enjoys unquestioned plausibility, challenged as it is by new sets of norms and alternative traditions.

Thus, in both the ancient and modern world, philosophers like Socrates and Kant – who are clearly driven by a desire to act with integrity – engage in ethical research because they regard it as their moral duty to do so. Certainly, ethical and meta-ethical theories can also contradict each other, and this has led anti-theorists to ask for a return to traditional ethics. But this appeal does not solve the original contradiction between the various traditions. The only answer can be to work out an all-encompassing ethical theory that tries to make sense of as many moral traditions as possible. The moral sphere is founded in reason, not in social facts; but social facts have to be interpreted as approximations to the demands of the moral sphere (see Hösle, 2004).

CONSISTENCY IN ETHICS

In some respects, the methods of ethics can be compared to those of jurisprudence. Jurisprudence logically presupposes, and ethics genetically starts from, a set of norms that are accepted by a society (legal norms having the additional property of being enforceable). Since these sets of norms have evolved over time and originate in different sources, they are not always consistent.

One of the first tasks of ethics is thus to eliminate contradictions between concrete applications of what have been called prima facie norms – contradictions at which already the historical Socrates seems to have pointed (at least both Plato and Xenophon ascribe to Socrates' such reflections). Examples of prima facie norms are: 'Do not lie', and 'Do not abet the killing of an innocent'. It is not difficult to find a situation in which both norms contradict each other in application: an innocent person has taken refuge in one's house from murderers who pursue him, and the murderers come to the house asking whether he is hiding in it. Let us assume that one has no chance to ward off the murderers (they may be a group of police agents of a totalitarian state) and that the refusal to answer would be interpreted as a positive answer. What is one supposed to do? Kant's (1797) famous answer is that one is not allowed to lie, since the duty not to lie is a so-called perfect duty, which does not bear exceptions and to which the duty to help other people is subordinated. Whatever one thinks of Kant's answer, the case discussed by him is a typical example of a moral dilemma, where different prima facie norms (or the different goods that are the basis of these norms, namely, human life and truth) seem to lead to contradictory norms for this concrete case: 'You ought to lie' – 'You must not lie'.

The use of terms like 'ought to' and 'must not' is typical of ethics. Even if it is controversial whether norms are originary, as Kant teaches, or themselves founded in values and goods, as the Aristotelean tradition assumed, it cannot be denied that an ethical theory needs deontic operators. Their use characterizes deontic logic, which outlines hypothetical rational commitments with regard to norms – if one accepts the validity of certain norms, then one is obliged to accept the validity of other norms. As Leibniz already understood, the three basic modal operators 'It is necessary', 'It is possible', 'It is impossible' are structurally analogous to the three deontic operators 'It is obligatory', 'It is permissible', 'It is forbidden'.

The system of modal logical that can be given a deontic interpretation is called D (on its logical peculiarities, see Hughes and Cresswell, 1996: 43 ff.). Ethics must not only avoid contradictions (as every rational theory must), for if they are allowed, in classical logic at least, anything can be proven; but, besides logical inconsistencies (A. ~A), ethics must avoid also deontic inconsistencies like O (A). O (~A), i.e. cases in which both A and its negation are obligatory (see Kutschera, 1973: 29 f.). However, the two demands are equivalent, since logical inconsistencies, entailing everything, entail also deontic inconsistencies, and deontic inconsistencies immediately entail logical inconsistencies: If A is obligatory, A is also permissible; and if ~A is obligatory, A is not permissible. Obviously, deontic logic presupposes that statements about norms can have different truth values. This does not preclude ethical statements from also expressing or exciting feelings; but this does not entail, as Ayer (1936) maintains, that ethical propositions have no factual (normative) meaning.

EMPIRICAL KNOWLEDGE IN ETHICS

The elimination of inconsistencies is of course only a necessary, not a sufficient, condition for the rationality of an ethical theory. A popular methodology for science has added empirical knowledge to logic. Would it not be sufficient to do the same for ethics? No doubt the empirical insight that something is a means to an end is of importance for ethics. If certain medical treatments save human lives and have no negative side effects, it is morally justified to engage in them. But of course the latter judgment can be regarded as the conclusion of a syllogism only if a normative or evaluative premise like 'You ought to save human lives' or 'Human life is a value' is added to the descriptive premise 'Certain medical treatments save human lives'. A normative conclusion can never be derived from a set of exclusively descriptive premises; at least one of the premises must be normative or evaluative in order to have a valid normative conclusion.

It is this combination that constitutes a so-called mixed syllogism. It is the merit particularly of George Edward Moore (1903) to have drawn attention to the epistemic difference between statements which claim that something is a means to an end or that something is a consequence of an act (assertions that are open to empirical validation) and statements claiming that something has intrinsic value (which cannot be verified or falsified by experiments). According to Moore, and similarly Max Scheler (1913/16), intrinsic values can only be grasped by a non-discursive value intuition. The main problem of intuitionism is that there is hardly a way in which people with different value intuitions can be brought to an agreement; they will probably end only by reproaching the other with value blindness. Furthermore, the canon of values developed (e.g. by Moore) smacks of the specific limits of his time. Even if, according to Moore, there are no reasons for such intuitions, it is not difficult to find causes why a man linked to the later founders of the Bloomsbury Group defended the values that he set forth in his ethical works.

But could one not try to reduce statements about something being intrinsically valuable to empirical statements, e.g. by claiming that something has an intrinsic value if it enhances the happiness of the person who accepts that value? Before Kant severed the link between ethics and happiness, the millennial eudaimonistic tradition of occidental ethics had usually argued this way and thus avoided some of the typically modern epistemological difficulties. However, that link could be read in two different ways: either as the statement that acting in the morally right way would cause happiness, or as the naturalistic definition of the good as that which is conducive to personal happiness. The ethical tradition before Kant often oscillated between the two positions, and while the first reading made better ethical sense, the second solved the problem of the foundation of ethics by transforming ethics into the empirical discipline of a prudential quest for personal happiness.

But the price is far too high – the latter eudaimonistic conception simply misses the peculiar nature of the ethical demand. There may be an excuse if someone acts against a duty because this would have involved too much of a sacrifice of his/her personal happiness, but this does not entail that the corresponding duty does not exist. One has therefore to pay the price of greater epistemological complexity and recognize that ethics cannot be based solely upon hypothetical imperatives that tell us which means are necessary in order to achieve certain ends, even if the end is as universally shared as personal happiness.

Ethics essentially needs a categorical imperative – so much must be granted to Kant, even if one does not share either the concrete content of his imperative or the formalist nature of his ethics.

LIMITS OF EMPIRICISM IN ETHICS

How does one arrive at basic ethical principles? They cannot be deduced from other principles, since they are the starting points of any ethical deduction; nor can they can be gotten from experience; and the mere appeal to intuition is equally unsatisfying. Let us look at the previous example concerning contradictions between the application of prima facie norms. First, it is obvious that there are various, equally consistent ways of eliminating the contradiction; but hardly all are equally acceptable. Kant's solution to the above-mentioned dilemma is consistent; but it would also be consistent to aver that the protection of an innocent life is of a higher value than sincerity toward criminals to whom we do not owe it. In order to justify one type of solution against another, it is, second, helpful if one can appeal to a principle of higher generality, as e.g. a doctrine about the relation between omissions and actions or a rank order of values. While in our development we start from convictions about the moral nature of certain individual acts and slowly develop more general principles, it would be a misrepresentation of the nature of ethical reasoning if we assumed that such general principles are inductively acquired from a set of original convictions regarding concrete cases. It cannot be discussed here whether the natural sciences are based on induction or not; for the sake of the argument, some form of falsificationism may be granted. But even according to the latter, it remains true that a scientific theory must render justice to each and every relevant fact; a single counterexample destroys the claim that there is a valid law of nature. (I abstract here from the fact that experiments falsify always only a conjunction of hypotheses, never a single hypothesis.)

In ethics, however, an analogous principle does not hold. The normative nature of the discipline entails that ethical claims are not refuted by the fact that the norms they defend are often violated in reality. Even more: not only the wide diffusion of a certain behavior, but also the wide diffusion of the conviction that this behavior is moral is not sufficient to warrant the legitimacy of this belief. This means that, in principle, an ethical theory has the right to be taken seriously even if it violates widespread moral intuitions. (This is one way of interpreting Hume's famous law; see 1739/40: 177 f.) Indeed, as we have seen, moral intuitions have changed – suffice it to mention the attitude regarding slavery or women's political rights.

Thus, an 'inductive' approach to ethical principles from concrete judgments on single cases may render justice to the ontogenetical and phylogenetical moral evolution, but it does not solve the question of the validity of moral principles. Rawls' concept of 'reflective equilibrium' (1971: 46 ff.) rightly insists on the reciprocal adjustment of concrete judgments and general principles, but it does not say enough about the intrinsic criteria that justify general principles. (Rawls himself is seduced by the prospect of inventing a fictitious situation in which rational egoism may be brought to accept principles of justice that he himself regards as valid.) No doubt, an ideal ethical theory will try to satisfy two different criteria: it will not give up widespread moral intuitions without good arguments, but it will be willing to reformulate our moral convictions if this is entailed by principles that are simpler and better connected with general features of our rationality than their alternatives.

THE PRINCIPLE OF UNIVERSALIZABILITY

One such principle is the principle of universalizability: something is obligatory, permissible, or forbidden for a person if and only if, *ceteris paribus*, it is obligatory, permissible, or forbidden for all other persons. The *'ceteris paribus'* is an important limitation, since, of course, every reasonable person recognizes that in a complex society different persons must have different rights. In particular, medical ethics cannot abstract from those asymmetric features of the physician–patient relation that are grounded in the superior knowledge of the physician and constitute a form of vertical responsibility. But in a universalistic ethics the burden of proof is always with those who claim there is a legitimate exception to the principle of equality and symmetry, e.g. because it is in the interest of the patients not to enjoy the same rights that are granted to the physicians.

Limited to all persons within certain groups characterized by the same gender, age, and rank, the principle of equal rights is a basic human principle of justice. But in its universal formulation, this principle is a result of modern Enlightenment. One cannot understand the enormous changes in the legal and political systems brought about in the last three centuries (on these, see Israel, 2001) if one does not interpret them as consequences of this moral principle. Kant has been seduced by the importance of the principle of universalizability to try to reduce ethics to it. But utilitarianism also, the other main modern ethical theory, is committed to it, since in its normative preference relation the utility of each person receives the same weight. The principle is not based on formal logic, since it would not be contradictory to ascribe certain rights only to oneself. But it remains true that a theory is more rational if it is free of indicators like 'me'. It is also true, as discourse ethics has stated, that a universalistic theory can be communicated more widely than a particularistic ethical theory, not to speak of a theory that denies the existence of moral obligations.

Thus it smacks of a performative contradiction to publicly proclaim that nobody has duties toward others, since it cannot be in the interest of the rational egoist to transform people who still accept obligations toward him/her into rational egoists – it is only a sense for universalistic justice that drives him to teach such a doctrine. The idea that any ethical theory that claims to be true must in principle be universally communicable and open to criticism by everyone has been articulated with particular force by Karl-Otto Apel (1973) and Wolfgang Kuhlmann (1985). This, they argue, is the only way to give the principle of universalizability a transcendental foundation. Such a transcendental justification must not be confused with a deduction from axioms.

But even if under conditions of modernity only ethical theories committed to the principle of universalizability can be taken seriously, this does not mean that the principle is a sufficient condition for an ethical theory. It inevitably favors symmetric relations, but does not exclude symmetric brutality. Kant, however, claims in the *Grundlegung zur Metaphysik der Sitten* (1785) that the categorical principle can be formulated in three different, but (as he erroneously thinks) logically equivalent versions. One of these consists in the injunction to treat humanity – whether in one's own person or in the person of any other – never simply as a means, but always at the same time as an end. Now, a symmetrical instrumentalization is not logically incompatible with the first formulation of the categorical principle.

But Kant seems to believe that the categorical nature of the moral imperative, which is not a means to achieve anything else, is communicated to those who are able to act according to the categorical imperative, i.e. persons. They must therefore be regarded as beings with intrinsic value. This conclusion should be also accepted by those who do not share Kant's conviction that persons (whether human or not) are the only beings with intrinsic value. For the latter conviction entails that, e.g. plants, animals, ecosystems, can only have an instrumental value for humans.

MATERIAL GOODS; DECISION THEORY IN ETHICS; INTENTIONALISM

Kant's recognition of the intrinsic value of persons is an important step beyond pure formalism. But it seems necessary to add a list of goods to a concrete ethical theory. However, such an ethics of goods should not be conceived as an alternative to a universalistic ethics: whoever wants to avoid the possible return of a justification of slavery is well advised not to idealize Aristotle, but to integrate the insights of ethical theories based on goods into a universalistic framework. (While Kant rejects the priority of the concept of the good in favor of the concept of duty, he has an elaborate doctrine of virtue. Therefore, an interest in the concept of virtue does not at all recommend a rejection of the Kantian approach.) Some of the basic goods of ethics can be justified with transcendental arguments. Freedom of action and truthfulness, for example, seem indeed to be transcendental presuppositions of any argument (see Gewirth, 1978; Illies, 2003).

One of the major problems of an ethics that recognizes a plurality of goods is how to put them in a plausible hierarchy. The development of comparative concepts is for ethics no less important than the development of classificatory concepts. One basic argument in this context is that a good is more important if it is a necessary presupposition of another good. To give one example: life is more fundamental than property, since property cannot be enjoyed without life. Thus many legal systems do not criminalize the violation of another's property if the violation is necessary to save a human life. It is one of the merits of utilitarianism (compared with Kantianism) that it offers a plausible account of legitimate violations of prima facie norms. But the problem of hedonistic utilitarianism is that it usually assumes that all goods must be reduced to a basic unity, which may be called 'pleasure'. Thus, even if the life of an innocent person is a higher good than, e.g. sexual pleasure, as long as we accept the Archimedean axiom (for all m<n, there is an a such that (a·m)>n), that life will be a lesser good than the appropriate multiplication of that pleasure. In order to avoid this consequence, the introduction of non-Archimedean goods is required.

However, even if one grants that, in principle, a ranking of different goods is possible, every realistic ethicist will grant that tragic conflicts cannot be excluded. There are at least three different reasons for their emergence. First, there may be a conflict between goods of similar rank. Or one can think of situations in which one has, due to a personal commitment, a stricter duty to preserve a lower good than one has the duty to care for a higher good. In fact, universalism need not deny that there are specific duties toward some people (e.g. the members of one's family) that take precedence, as long as one recognizes that every person is in the same predicament with regard to the members of one's family. The third type of a tragic conflict is given when the expected moral value of two possible actions may be very similar, since the action that is intrinsically better may be turned by a probable event into a calamity.

The term 'expected value' stems from decision theory and game theory, which are powerful tools of ethical analysis, even if they are amoral theories. But they are amoral, not immoral; they do not exclude moral preferences and can thus teach a moral agent what action under conditions of risk or uncertainty is the most rational. In the case of decisions under uncertainty, i.e. when no probabilities can be ascribed to the possible events that will determine the different outcomes, there are good moral reasons for exercising the maximin principle, i.e. for choosing the action with the least negative outcome, particularly if the negative consequences threaten people who would not benefit from the advantages in the case of the positive outcome. It is furthermore hard to deny that acts of omission are not on par with other possible actions, insofar as people are less responsible for them than they are for actions. At least this is so in the case where one has not undertaken a concrete responsibility. For example a physician who intentionally omits to save his patient becomes almost as guilty as if he had killed him; but a bystander does not have an analogous responsibility, because he never accepted a concrete obligation as did the physician.

The development of ethical theory in history is not only characterized by an increased awareness of the universalistic nature of any acceptable set of norms. Another dimension of ethical theory that has developed throughout the Middle Ages and modernity is the insistence that the proper subject of moral predicates is the intention of the agent. A physician may cause the death of a person; if his intention was to cure the patient and he could in no way have foreseen that his therapy could possibly cause the death, he is not to be blamed, not even for negligence. But even more: the last source of morality is not to be found in the intention either, but in the motive on the basis of which someone forms his intention. Thus we have to ask: Does someone help another for egoistic reasons, or because he thinks that this is the right thing to do, independently of any advantage for him? As plausible as this point of view is, it seems to have seduced Kant to believe that only acts of the will can be morally evaluated. However, an act of the will is subjectively moral if it aims at something that is objectively right, and if the person competently uses the means that are generally believed to effectively bring about what is objectively right. A comprehensive ethical theory has to recognize a large variety of ethically relevant goods: one of the varieties of goodness, e.g. is medical goodness (see von Wright, 1963: 51 ff.). Furthermore, the general defense of intentionalism should not prevent a person from supporting what is objectively right, even if other people do it for the wrong reasons. In relation to oneself, one has to work on one's motives; but if one can achieve a higher level of public health only by appealing to the egoistic motives of society at large, it would be irresponsible to forego appealing to them.

ABORTION AS AN EXAMPLE

The rejection of the naturalistic fallacy entails only that it is wrong to think that something ought to be only because it exists. It does not at all entail a lack of intrinsic value in something, only because it exists. On the contrary, the evaluative or normative qualities of something supervene on its descriptive qualities (see Hare, 1952: 80 ff.), and one cannot be obliged to aim at the impossible. This has the important consequence that, in order to justify the different moral statuses of two things, morally relevant differences on the descriptive level have to be shown. What 'morally relevant' means is not easy to determine; but this qualification of the differences cannot be renounced, since otherwise the principle of universalizability could easily be circumvented. The racist, for example, would simply say that political rights can only be granted to a person of a certain race. However, it is easy to object that this difference is morally irrelevant.

On the other hand, one may reasonably argue that convicted criminals should be deprived (at least as long as they are in prison) of their political rights, since they have forfeited them through their crimes. The main – purely ethical, not at all religious – issue at stake with regard to the question of the moral legitimacy of abortion is whether one can find a characteristic that applies to human embryos (or even fetuses), but not to human infants. The trait 'not yet being born' seems arbitrary, particularly since it depends on contingent facts of whether someone is born after six or nine months. Moreover, arguments that point to the fact that the embryo could not survive outside of the womb can easily be countered by the claim that infants are equally unable to survive without the help of adults. Even insisting on the fact that consciousness begins only after the first trimester seems unsatisfying, since the conscious life of the fetus, but also the infant, is hardly more complex than that of an adult ape. If one points to the potential development of the infant, this argument applies to the embryo as well. And indeed, the potential development distinguishes the embryo significantly from the patient with irreversible brain death.

The abortion issue, however, is more complex, since the proper ethical issue must be distinguished from the question of what a moral legal system should determine. I do not have in mind the factual legal systems of the various countries, but the philosophical question of how a just legal system should be structured. The tradition has used the term 'natural law' to name such a just legal system, and it is obvious that many questions of medical ethics involve a concept of natural law. For they do not simply ask what the physician – as a benevolent private individual – should do, but also what a reasonable system of public health should enforce by appropriate legal means.

Now, it is clear that not all moral norms can, nor should, be enforced by the state. Thus, the sphere of inner convictions and actions that express it (i.e. religious duties) must not be enforced by the state. Furthermore, since legal enforcement is costly, and the state has a duty to be as parsimonious as possible in using citizens' taxes, the state will have to limit its enforcement actions. Criteria for economic rationality are always appropriate when dealing with scarce resources – and legal enforcement is indeed a scarce resource. Even if someone believes that abortion is morally wrong, and that the state has a duty to protect human life in its early forms, he/she may still hold that, in an age when people can easily go abroad, the possibility of the state to protect the embryo's life against the mother's will is extremely limited and that criminal prosecution is not the most efficient way to achieve this end. (I am speaking of the first trimester when the pregnancy is not yet visible.) In any case, the difference in perspective between ethics and natural law is one of the issues that makes the methods of ethics as complicated as they are. This is unfortunate for the person who desires a quick decision, but fortunate for the professional ethicist trying to draw subtle conceptual distinctions that map the intricacies of the moral world.

SUMMARY

Ethics is a rational discipline. Its first task is to eliminate inconsistencies between the various norms and evaluations one can find in any given culture. This, however, is only a necessary, not a sufficient, condition for the rationality of an ethical theory. How can its norms be positively justified? Within a mixed syllogism, some ethical norms can be deduced from a set of premises including descriptive ones (if the set also includes at least one normative, or evaluative, premise). The most general normative premises are either unjustifiable, or they can be grounded only by transcendental arguments. Such a foundation has been proposed for the principle of universalizability in particular. Clearly, the latter principle is central for any acceptable ethical theory. But theories about material goods, the role of decision and game theory in ethical reasoning, and the difference between the objectively right and the subjectively moral have to be added to a universalistic ethics in order to make it applicable to concrete cases.

REFERENCES

Apel, K.O. (1973) *Transformation der Philosophie*, 2 vols. Frankfurt: Suhrkamp.
Ayer, A.J. (1936) *Language, Truth and Logic*. London: Gollancz.
Gewirth, A. (1978) *Reason and Morality*. Chicago/London: University of Chicago Press.
Hare, R.M. (1952) *The Language of Morals*. Oxford: Clarendon Press.
Hösle, V. (2004) *Morals and Politics*. Notre Dame, IN: University of Notre Dame Press.
Hughes, G.E. and Cresswell, M.J. (1996) *A New Introduction to Modal Logic*. London/New York: Routledge.
Hume, D. (1739/40) *A Treatise of Human Nature*. London: John Noon.
Illies, C. (2003) *The Grounds of Ethical Judgement*. Oxford: Clarendon Press.
Israel, J. (2001) *Radical Enlightenment*. Oxford: Oxford University Press.
Kant, I. (1785) 'Grundlegung zur Metaphysik der Sitten', in Wilhelm Weischedel (ed.), *Werke in zwölf Bänden*, vol. 7. Frankfurt: Suhrkamp.
Kant, I. (1797) 'Über ein vermeintes Recht, aus Menschenliebe zu lügen', in Wilhelm Weischedel (ed.), *Werke in zwölf Bänden*, vol. 8. Frankfurt: Suhrkamp.
Kuhlmann, W. (1985) *Reflexive Letztbegründung*. Freiburg/München: Alber.

Kutschera, Franz von (1973) *Einführung in die Logik der Normen, Werte und Entscheidungen.* Freiburg/München: Alber.

Moore, George E. (1903) *Principia Ethica.* Cambridge: Cambridge University Press.

Rawls, J. (1971) *A Theory of Justice.* Cambridge, MA: Belknap Press of Harvard University Press.

Scheler, M. (1913/16) *Der Formalismus in der Ethik und die materiale Wertethik.* Halle an der Saale: Max Niemeyer.

Von, W. and Georg, H. (1963) *The Varieties of Goodness.* London/New York: Routledge/Humanities Press.

2

Foundationalism and Principles

Henk ten Have

INTRODUCTION

One of the interesting aspects of bioethics today is that it is becoming more and more international. Many clinical trials nowadays are executed in developing countries. When some countries take legal measures against organ trade, the trafficking is displaced to other countries without regulations. Fringe scientists announcing that they have produced the first human clone always do that in areas of the world where it is not explicitly prohibited. Many countries do not have an adequate infrastructure to deal with bioethical issues. They lack expertise, ethics committees, ethics teaching programs, and ethics-related regulations and legislation. Because they are not the drivers of scientific and technological development, they fear to be excluded from the benefits of biomedical progress. At the same time there is the risk of double, or at least different, moral standards being applied in different regions of the world.

It was in this context that in October 2003, based on preliminary feasibility studies of the International Bioethics Committee, UNESCO was mandated by its 191 member states to draw up a declaration setting out fundamental principles in the field of bioethics. Especially the developing countries requested that the organization make normative standards with a truly universal scope. After two years of intense work, the member states adopted, unanimously and by acclamation on 19 October 2005, the Universal Declaration on Bioethics and Human Rights, thus solemnly affirming the commitment of the international community to respect a certain number of universal principles for humanity in the development and application of biomedical science and technology. With this new declaration, UNESCO strives to respond in particular to the needs of developing countries, indigenous communities, and vulnerable groups or persons. The declaration reminds the international community of its duty of solidarity toward all countries.

Unlike the Oviedo Convention adopted by the Council of Europe, the Universal Declaration of UNESCO does not constitute a binding normative instrument in international law. However, the unanimous adoption by the member states is not merely symbolic but gives the declaration moral authority and creates a moral commitment. For the first time in the history of bioethics, all states of the international community are committed to respect and implement the basic principles of bioethics, set forth within a single text. The innovative dimension of the declaration is that it constitutes a commitment of governments to a set of bioethical principles. Previous international declarations, although sometimes very influential (such as the Declaration of Helsinki) have been adopted by professional organizations (such as the World Medical Association). The adoption of the declaration also illustrates that there is now agreement about principles that form the basis of international, multicultural bioethics, itself firmly founded on international human rights (Thomasma, 1997a).

After several decades, bioethics has developed into an established and recognized discipline. During this process of maturation, consensus on fundamental principles has gradually emerged. It is important to note that the rather limited core of four principles that are always recited (the so called 'Georgetown mantra') is now evolving into a coherent set of 15 principles, taking into account not only individual and interpersonal perspectives but also community, social, and even global perspectives. This new constellation of fundamental principles is not only the outcome of a process of internationalization of bioethics, taking into account a wider range of ethical principles that goes beyond the perspective of particular cultures and specific societies. It is also the starting point for a true globalization of bioethics – a global bioethics that cares about issues and problems in all areas of the world and that responds to the needs and concerns of all human beings on this planet. This globalization has reactivated the older debate on the role of principles in bioethics, as well as their foundation.

BIOETHICS AS APPLIED ETHICS

During the last 40 years, a popular and unique view of bioethics as a new discipline has emerged. The growing appeal of this new discipline among public and scientific circles of opinion leaders can be attributed to the empowering combination of two traditional notions from the history of moral philosophy: 'application' and 'principle'.

The dominant conception of bioethics reflected in the mainstream of scholarly literature is that of applied ethics. In Beauchamp and Childress's well known textbook, biomedical ethics is defined as 'the application of general ethical theories, principles and rules to problems of therapeutic practice, health care delivery, and medical and biological research' (Beauchamp and Childress, 1983: ix-x). Instead of the theoretical abstractions of traditional moral philosophy, applied ethics can contribute to analyze dilemmas, resolve complex cases, and clarify practical problems arising in the healthcare setting. The practical usefulness of applied ethics not only manifests itself in biomedicine, but it has a wider scope. In the *Encyclopedia of Applied Ethics*, the following definition is presented:

> Applied ethics is a general field of study that includes all systematic efforts to understand and to resolve moral problems that arise in some domains of practical life, as with medicine, journalism, or business, or in connection with some general issue of social concern, such as employment, equity or capital punishment (Winkler, 1998: 192).

A distinction is made between three major areas of applied ethics: biomedical ethics, business and professional ethics, and environmental ethics. However, the table of contents of the four encyclopedia volumes show a wide range of topics covered, such as archaeo-logical ethics, censorship, divorce, electronic surveillance, gun control, nuclear power, vegetarianism, and wildlife conservation. Applied ethics can extend to almost any area of life where ethical issues arise. 'Application' here has a double connotation: it indicates that ethics is available for what we usually do, it applies to our daily problems; but it is also helpful, practical, in the sense that ethics is something to do; it works to resolve our problems.

The second characteristic of the dominant conception of bioethics is the focus on principles. If ethics is conceived as applied ethics, then subsequent reflection is needed on what is being applied. The emerging consensus that principles should provide the answer to this quest is coherent with the moralities of obligation that have dominated modern ethical discourse, especially since Kant. Behavior in accord with moral obligations is considered morally right. The morality of behavior is a morality of duty. Morality is understood as a system of precepts or rules people are obliged to follow. Particularly in the early days of bioethics, when medical power was strongly criticized, and the rights of patients were vehemently emphasized as requiring respect, the moralities of obligation presented them-selves as a common set of normative principles and rules that we are obliged to follow in practice. As Diego Gracia (1999) pointed out, the Belmont Report in 1978 was influential because it was the first official document to identify three basic ethical principles: autonomy, beneficence, and justice. A basic principle was defined as a general judgment serving as a basic justification for particular prescriptions and evaluations of human actions. From these principles, ethical guidelines can be derived that could be applied to the biomedical area. About the same time, Beauchamp and Childress, in the first edition of their book, introduced the four-principles approach, adding 'nonmaleficence' to the above three principles. In their view, principles are normative generalizations that guide actions. However, as general guides they leave considerable room for judgment in specific cases. Various types of rules are needed to specify the principles into precise action guides.

Although Beauchamp and Childress have considerably elaborated and adapted their theoretical framework in later editions, their work has contributed to the conception of bioethics that has long dominated the practical context in ethics committees, clinical case-discussions, ethics courses, and compendia and syllabi. This conception is sometimes called 'principlism': the focus is on the use of moral principles to address ethical issues and to resolve conflicts at the bedside (DuBose et al., 1994). Belief in the power of principlism is sometimes proselytizing. Raanan Gillon, for example argues that the advantage of the four principles not only is that they are defensible from a variety of theoretical moral perspec-tives, but also that 'they can help us bring more order, consistency, and understanding to our medico-moral judgments' (Gillon, 1986: viii).

Later, Gillon used the principles-approach to develop a major scholarly project, the voluminous textbook *Principles of Health Care Ethics* (Gillon, 1994). Over 100 authors discuss in 90 chapters all possible ethical dilemmas in modern health care, employing the analytical framework of the four principles. In his Preface, Gillon confesses that he is inclined to believe that the four principles approach can encompass all moral issues, not only those arising in health care. Principlism apparently is a universal tool; it provides a method to resolve all moral issues in all areas of daily life, whatever the personal philosophies, politics, religions, cultural traditions, and moral theories of the persons involved.

FOUNDATIONALISM

The emergence of principlism as the dominant approach in bioethics has led to intensive debates on the foundations of moral thought. How can bioethical views be justified, and how can bioethical dilemmas be resolved in a pluralistic and multicultural modern society? Ethical foundationalism is the view that bioethics can identify and produce valid principles because it has a clear theoretical rock bottom. At least some bioethical principles can be based on noninferentially justified beliefs. Such principles can be rationally defended and they apply to all human beings (Thomasma, 1997b). A comprehensive philosophical theory, such as utilitarianism, Kantian deontology, or libertarianism should provide the bedrock for bioethics. Bioethical judgments can only be justified on the basis of an ethical theory that is rational and universal at the same time.

Principlism is criticized because it does not provide such a fundamental theoretical framework. In daily practice, bioethics focuses on mid-level principles – respect for autonomy, beneficence, nonmaleficence, and justice. These principles are applied to dilemmas, cases, and problems encountered in the practice of health care. From a specific principle, guidelines or recommendations can be derived in order to resolve various problematic situations. Yet there is no single rational criterion on the basis of which to decide which principle is overriding; there is no definitive scheme for ordering principles and for choosing between them (Clouser and Gert, 1990). The problem is that as long as the principles of applied ethics are not integrated into some broader theoretical framework they tend to lead to conflicting judgments about which actions and social policies one ought to carry out (Brody, 1988). The lack of agreement on which moral theory to apply on concrete medical cases could make applied ethics counterproductive. Confronting physicians and medical students with a variety of conflicting but plausible theories, applied medical ethics may be seen to give no moral guidance but to reinforce the belief that whatever is done in problematic situations, some moral theory will condone, another will condemn it (Baier, 1985). Because mainstream bioethics focuses on the application of principles and is rather loosely embedded in philosophy providing a clear foundation for moral judgments, it can easily result in a chaos of conflicting moral judgments.

For Beauchamp and Childress this criticism is not relevant. For them, principlism is non-foundationalist. In the earlier editions of their work, theoretical encompassing frameworks are not lacking but they are multiple. The authors can be relatively indifferent to the question of ethical foundations since they argue that the focus should be on mid-level principles. Agreement on such principles can be reached from the point of view of radically different moral theories, like in their own case, utilitarian and deontological theories. Even champions of diverging moral theories can reach convergence on principles. What is sufficient for bioethics is an integrated framework of principles through which to handle diverse moral problems (Beauchamp and Childress, 1983).

In later editions they are more critical about foundational theories because these are one-sided and insufficiently rich to understand the complexities and uncertainties of bioethical dilemmas and cases. The four principles approach is more subtle. It is not a simple deduction of moral judgments from rules and principles but a dialectic process of interpretation, specification, and balancing. The authors reiterate that the justification of moral judgments is provided through an appeal to principles. But there is no single unifying principle or encompassing theory to justify the principles. The framework of principles they present is the theory (Beauchamp and Childress, 1994).

ANTIFOUNDATIONALISM

Antifoundationalism is the view that there are no ethical principles that are certain and universally valid, so that all moral judgment can be firmly grounded on them. In response to the universal claims of principlism, two types of criticism have been advanced.

First, mainstream bioethics has developed within a particular cultural and social context. The fundamental ethos of applied ethics, its analytical framework, methodology, and language, its concerns and emphases, and its very institutionalization have been shaped by beliefs, values, and modes of thinking grounded in specific social and cultural traditions (i.e. primarily Western ones). Nowadays, the bioethics literature serves as one of the most powerful means by which to express and articulate these traditions. However, the literature only rarely attends to or reflects upon the sociocultural value system within and through which it operates. Scholars usually assume that its principles, theories, and moral views are transcultural. Bioethics is a common neutral language, a secular moral grammar, guaranteeing a peaceable society (Engelhardt, 1986). But how neutral is the common neutral language? Is this moral language itself not the expression of a commitment to a certain 'hypergood' (Taylor, 1989), in particular the good of universal and equal respect and self-determining freedom – primal values in the liberal tradition? Such questions assume that the values of mutual respect and individual freedom are not de-contextualized, universal standards but themselves expressions of community-bound agreements.

The second criticism of principlism is focused on its inattention to the particularities of the practical setting. Moral theories and principles are necessarily abstract and therefore not immediately relevant to the particular circumstances of actual cases, the concrete reality of clinical work, and the specific responsibilities of health care professionals. By appealing to basic principles bioethics may fail to realize the importance of concretely lived experiences of health care professionals, as well as patients. The moral agent is taken to have an abstract existence. This point is critically elaborated by contemporary philosophers. Ethics, according to Williams (1988), does not respect the concrete moral subject with his personal integrity. It requires that the subject gives up his personal point of view and exchanges it for a universal and impartial point of view. This is, Williams argues, an absurd requirement, because the moral subject is requested to give up what is constitutive for his or her personal identity and integrity. The idea that knowledge of normative theories and principles can be applied to medical practice simply ignores the fact that moral concerns tend to emerge from experiences in medical settings themselves. A similar issue is raised by Taylor (1989), arguing that morality and identity are two sides of the same coin. To know who we are is to know to which moral sources we should appeal. The community, the particular social group to which we belong, is usually at the center of our moral experience. Even the use of ethical language depends on a shared form of life. The Wittgensteinian notion that our understanding of language is a matter of picking up practices and being inducted into a particular form of life is germane here. Bioethicists should therefore become more appreciative of the actual experiences of practitioners and more attentive to the context in which physicians, nurses, patients, and others experience their moral lives, e.g. the roles they play, the relationships in which they participate, the expectations they have, and the values they cherish (Zaner, 1988). The physician–patient relationship is neither ahistorical, acultural, nor an abstract rational notion; persons are always persons-in-relation, are always members of communities, are immersed in a tradition, and are participants in a particular culture.

In response to these types of criticism new approaches to bioethics have emerged in the 1980s and 1990s: phenomenological ethics (Zaner, 1988); hermeneutic ethics (Carson, 1990; Leder, 1994); narrative ethics (Brody, 1987; Newton, 1995); and care ethics (Tronto, 1993). Furthermore, traditional conceptions have been revitalized, notably the new casuistry (drawing from the classical casuistic mode of moral reasoning) (Jonsen and Toulmin, 1988); and the virtue approach, emphasizing qualities of character in both individuals and communities (Drane, 1988; Pellegrino and Thomasma, 1993).

COMMON MORALITY

Having expressed their skepticism about foundationalism, Beauchamp and Childress have since 1989 been locating the source of bioethical principles in what they call 'common morality'. This is the morality shared in common by all persons in all places. It is the starting point of moral reasoning. Principles have their origin in the common morality. This is not a unified foundation for ethics from which moral judgments can be deducted. Although we are all embedded in common morality, a continuous work of analysis, clarification, interpretation, specification, and balancing is required in order to make a moral judgment on a specific case or problem.

At the same time, Beauchamp and Childress want also to avoid an antifoundationalist point of view. In later editions of their book, they critically discuss all current types of ethical theory, not only utilitarianism and Kantian deontology, but also theories of virtue, rights, community, care, and casuistry. These theories rightly point out that we need to be sensitive to context and community and to individual differences. But they are often too contextual, do not provide certitude, and do not guide conduct. Common morality on the other hand provides a basis for the evaluation and criticism of actions, because it transcends merely local customs and attitudes; in other words 'the principles of the common morality are universal standards' (Beauchamp and Childress, 1994: 101).

Evidently, rejecting foundationalism, Beauchamp and Childress do not want to join antifoundalism either. Otherwise, the universality of bioethical judgments would be lost, principles would no longer work as action-guides, and actions could not be morally justified. Although the principles embedded in common morality are abstract and general, simple deductivism is impossible. A specific moral problem cannot be solved by simple application of the four principles. However, they are universal principles. Common morality in fact is the guiding meta-principle of principlism (Gordon et al., 2009).

Nowadays, common morality has become an important topic of debate (Veatch, 2003). The notion, as explained by Beauchamp and Childress and recently introduced in the bioethics debate, is associated with older ideas from interpretive bioethics. As a particular domain of philosophy, ethics proceeds from empirical knowledge, viz. moral experience. The moral dimension of the world is first and foremost experienced. Moral experience is humanity's way of understanding itself in moral terms (van Tongeren, 1988). Ethics is therefore the interpretation and explanation of this primordial understanding. Before acting morally we must already know, at least to some extent, what is morally desirable or right. Otherwise, we would not recognize what is appealing in a moral sense. On the one hand, moral normativity is pre-given and common to all human beings. The precepts of common morality are universally binding but at the same time historical; they have emerged in the history of humanity because they promote human flourishing. On the other hand, what we recognize in our experience is typically unclear and in need of further elucidation and interpretation. Normativity in bioethics in particular requires continuous specification of principles and balancing against other principles in a specific situation. But in the end, the moral judgment in this situation will be justified by the principles of the common morality. According to some critiques, the four-principle approach of Beauchamp and Childress is therefore foundationalist (Arras, 2009). At least common morality presents a substitute foundation enabling us to make universal and rational moral judgments.

In the debate, many scholars question whether there is a common morality. It is argued that common morality as a universal framework does not exist, that there is no evidence that all cultures and religions have accepted the same common morality. The claim of a universal, cross-cultural common morality is dismissed on empirical grounds (Turner, 2003). Societies differ in the moral norms and values they regard as basic, certainly if we examine them from a historical perspective. Beauchamp (2003) agrees that a distinction should be made between particular moralities and the common morality. The first differ according to history and culture; they express norms unique to particular cultures, groups, and individuals. But there is also a small set of commonly shared principles and norms related to the objectives of morality (i.e. promoting human flourishing). Common morality is not simply a morality among many others; its principles represent at an abstract level the human experience that following them will ameliorate the human condition. Therefore, more important than consensus is justification of principles (relating to the achievement of the objectives of morality). Whether or not there is universal agreement on some principles (which is a matter of empirical study), the question how principles of common morality can be justified, however, is crucial (which is a matter of normative analysis).

CHANGING COMMON MORALITY?

Beauchamp's distinction between common morality and particular moralities locates universality in the first one. Particular moralities present concrete and specific nonuniversal norms that arise from religious traditions, cultural contexts, and professional practices. It is clear that these moralities do develop and change over time. What about the common morality? Beauchamp (2003) argues that in his view common morality is historical and universal. Common morality provides cross-cultural standards. But changes in common morality are not easily imaginable. The normative beliefs embedded in the common morality are there because they contribute to the objectives of the moral system. Changes can only occur if other or new norms better serve those objectives. That makes it rather unlikely that abstract principles are changing. It is more plausible, according to Beauchamp, that common morality is changing because the scope of application of the principles is widening, including more and more categories of moral 'patients' (slaves, women, people of ethnicities, etc.). Although he does not exclude the possibility, Beauchamp therefore is in fact skeptical about historical changes in the common morality itself.

In a foundationalist perspective, the core set of moral beliefs in the common morality is universal and ahistorical. Change, evolution, or progress of such beliefs is a priori out of the question since common morality is the standard against which practices are judged. What is changing is not morality but moral agents and practices. In an antifoundationalist perspective, there are various common moralities, always historical and cultural, thus there is no change but only difference (Wallace, 2009). In a nonfoundationalist perspective common morality is in principle changeable, since the objectives of morality, viz. human flourishing, may evolve over time. Wallace (2009) refers to the notion of universal human rights. This has emerged as a moral notion at a particular point in time and history when human experience has developed in certain ways. The implication, according to Wallace (2009: 63), is that common morality could, in principle, 'be augmented and revised, in light of further experience or changing conditions of human experience'.

This suggestion of changing common morality is interesting now that a broader set of fundamental ethical principles is emerging in the context of global bioethics. Immediately after the adoption of the Universal Declaration on Bioethics and Human Rights, a vigorous debate emerged, especially in regard to the conception of universality underlying the document. Some question the possibility of a transcultural moral approach and universal principles. Others repeat the old argument that so-called universal principles are merely the reiteration of specific, i.e. Western, principles and their imposition onto the rest of the world.

Interestingly, non-Western scholars exposed different views. Jing-Bao (2005) argues that it is necessary to explore non-Western cultures to discover that they advocate universal principles. It is a mistake to assume that such principles (e.g. human dignity) are usually alien to and incompatible with these cultures. It is an example of 'moral protectionism' to assume that ethical principles, even after having emerged and being formulated in Western culture, continue to remain the property of such specific cultures, and therefore not universal but only valid within this specific context. This is exactly the experience within UNESCO. It was explicitly at the request of developing countries that the Organization undertook the drafting of the Universal Declaration, since these countries wanted to have a framework of universal principles in order to put limitations to the tendency of introducing 'double standards' with a reference to cultural diversity. Cultures differ but this does not imply that common standards and universal principles do not exist.

PRINCIPLES AND FALLIBILISM

Wallace (2009) has suggested that there is an association between the possibility of moral reform and human fallibility. Common morality can be improved because as human beings we can never be sure about our moral beliefs. Charles Sanders Peirce's notion of fallibilism implies that none of our moral judgments are absolutely certain; there is always a chance that we might be mistaken. Fallibilism does not exclude universality. As long as universal principles in common morality have not turned out to be wrong we continue to work with them as universal action-guides. This is also the reason why we continuously have to evaluate and possibly revise our moral beliefs. For morality also the famous analogy of Otto Neurath applies: knowledge is like a vessel on the open sea; we cannot bring it ashore in order to caulk and reconstruct it afresh from the bottom; we must repair the ship while sailing and moving on our way. The normative enterprise therefore requires dialectic evolution in order to approach but never to reach an ideal limit. This fallibilistic perspective with the implied need for continuous testing and assessing is also close to the initial ideas of Van Rensselaer Potter when he defined bioethics as 'a new discipline that combines biological knowledge with a knowledge of human value systems in an open-ended biocybernetic system of self-assessment' (Potter, 1975: 2299).

The notion of fallibilism is closely related to the pragmatist perspective that principles are mainly working as action-guides. Rather than looking at the history or origin of principles, we look to the future, i.e. how they actually work to help solving moral problems. The prospective dimension is clear in the work of Beauchamp and Childress. Principles are not recipes or tools providing clear-cut answers to moral dilemmas. They require arduous critical labor; they need interpretation, analysis, specification, and balancing (see, for example Voo, 2009). This labor will be never ending. There is always moral ambiguity and conflict.

The retrospective dimension is apparently less dynamic, since Beauchamp and Childress are reluctant to change in the common morality. But in emphasizing the need for processes of justification, they again require reflective action. Ethical principles do not have a stable and immutable foundation, but they need justification. Moral principles are justified if they contribute to the objectives of morality, such as human flourishing. This process of justification may be undertaken from different theoretical perspectives. In this way, different cultural perspectives can contribute in this validation and revision of the core principles of the common morality (see, for example in resource-poor countries, Azetsop and Rennie, 2010). It certainly leaves room for an expansion or revision of these core principles. Asai and Oe (2005) have reiterated this interrelation between the principles and the objectives of morality in stating that 'the world would be a better place for everyone to live', if human beings would care about the principles expressed in the UNESCO Declaration.

If the quest for foundations is abandoned, we still have to search for common ground, in the application of principles as well as in the justification of principles. These are much more complicated processes than as assumed until now. They require deliberation, negotiation, and compromise. Deliberative democratic processes are replacing the search for universal solutions that can be applied to all human beings. But the significance of deliberation does not restrict the universality of ethical principles. Solutions to moral problems are no longer found and based on fundamental theories but are now negotiated.

REFERENCES

Arras, J.D. (2009) 'The hedgehog and the Borg: Common morality in bioethics', *Theoretical Medicine and Bioethics,* 30: 11–30.

Asai, A. and Oe, S. (2005) 'A valuable up-to-date compendium of bioethical knowledge', *Developing World Bioethics,* Special Issue: Reflections on the UNESCO draft declaration on bioethics and human rights: 5216-19.

Azetsop, J. and Rennie, S. (2010) 'Principlism, medical individualism, and health promotion in resource-poor countries: Can autonomy-based bioethics promote social justice and population health?' *Philosophy, Ethics and Humanities in Medicine,* 5:1 doi: 10.1186/1747-5341-5-1.

Baier, A. (1985) *Postures of the Mind. Essays on Mind and Morals.* London: Methuen.

Beauchamp, T.L. (2003) 'A defense of the common morality', *Kennedy Institute of Ethics Journal,* 13 (23): 259–74.

Beauchamp, T.L. and Childress, J.F. (1983) *Principles of Biomedical Ethics,* 2nd ed. New York: Oxford University Press.

Beauchamp, T.L. and Childress, J.F. (1994) *Principles of Biomedical Ethics,* 4th ed. New York/Oxford: Oxford University Press.

Brody, B. (ed.) (1988) *Moral Theory and Moral Judgments in Medical Ethics.* Dordrecht: Kluwer Academic Publishers.

Brody, H. (1987) *Stories of Sickness.* New Haven, CT/London: Yale University Press.

Carson, R.A. (1990) 'Interpretive bioethics: The way of discernment', *Theoretical Medicine,* 11: 51–9.

Clouser, K.D. and Gert, B. (1990) 'A critique of principlism', *Journal of Medicine and Philosophy,* 15 (2): 219–36.

Drane, J.F. (1988) *Becoming a Good Doctor: The Place of Virtue and Character in Medical Ethics.* Kansas City, MO: Sheed and Ward.

DuBose, E.R., Hamel, R. and O'Connell, L.J. (eds) (1994) *A Matter of Principles? Ferment in US Bioethics.* Valley Forge, PA: Trinity Press International.

Engelhardt, H.T. (1986) *The Foundations of Bioethics.* New York/Oxford: Oxford University Press.

Gillon, R. (1986) *Philosophical Medical Ethics.* Chichester: John Wiley & Sons.

Gillon, R. (ed.) (1994) *Principles of Health Care Ethics.* Chichester: John Wiley & Sons.

Gordon, J.-S., Rauprich, O. and Vollmann, J. (2009) 'Applying the four-principle approach', *Bioethics,* doi: 10.1111/ j.1467-8519.2009.01757.x.

Gracia, D. (1999) 'History of medical ethics', in H.A.M.J. ten Have and B. Gordijn (eds), *Bioethics in a European Perspective.* Dordrecht/Boston, MA/London: Kluwer Academic Publishers, pp. 17–50.

Jing-Bao, N. (2005) 'Cultural values embodying universal norms: A critique of a popular assumption about cultures and human rights', *Developing World Bioethics,* 5 (3): 251–7.

Jonsen, A.R. and Toulmin, S. (1988) *The Abuse of Casuistry.* Berkeley, CA: University of California Press.

Leder, D. (1994) 'Toward a hermeneutical bioethics', in E.R. DuBose, R. Hamel. and L.J. O'Connell (eds), *A Matter of Principles? Ferment in U.S. Bioethics.* Valley Forge, PA: Trinity Press International, pp. 240–59.

Newton, A.Z. (1995) *Narrative Ethics.* Cambridge, MA: Harvard University Press.

Pellegrino, E.D. and Thomasma, D.C. (1993) *The Virtues in Medical Practice.* New York/Oxford: Oxford University Press.

Potter, V.R. (1975) 'Humility with responsibility – A bioethic for oncologists: Presidential Address', *Cancer Research,* 35: 2297–306.

Taylor, C. (1989) *Sources of the Self. The Making of Modern Identity.* Cambridge: Cambridge University Press.

Thomasma, D.C. (1997a) 'Bioethics and international human rights', *Journal of Law, Medicine & Ethics,* 25: 295–306.

Thomasma, D.C. (1997b) 'Antifoundationalism and the possibility of a moral philosophy of medicine', *Theoretical Medicine,* 18: 127–43.

Tronto, J.C. (1993) *Moral Boundaries. A Political Argument for an Ethic of Care.* New York/London: Routledge.

Turner, L. (2003) 'Zones of consensus and zones of conflict: Questioning the "common morality" presumption in bioethics', *Kennedy Institute of Ethics Journal,* 13 (3): 193–218.

Van Tongeren, P. (1988) 'Ethiek en praktijk', *Filosofie & Praktijk,* 9: 113–27.

Veatch, R.M. (2003) 'Is there a common morality?', *Kennedy Institute of Ethics Journal,* 13 (3): 189–92.

Voo, T-C. (2009) 'Editorial comment: The four principles and cultural specification', *European Journal of Pediatrics*, 168: 1389.

Wallace, K.A. (2009) 'Common morality and moral reform', *Theoretical Medicine and Bioethics*, 30: 55–68.

Williams, B. (1988) 'Consequentialism and integrity', in S. Scheffler (ed.), *Consequentialism and its Critics*. Oxford: Clarendon Press, pp. 20–50.

Winkler, E.R. (1998) 'Applied ethics, overview', in R. Chadwick (ed.), *Encyclopedia of Applied Ethics*, Vol. 1. San Diego, CA: Academic Press, pp. 191–6.

Zaner, R.M. (1988) *Ethics and the Clinical Encounter*. Englewood Cliffs, NJ: Prentice-Hall.

3

Anti-Theory

Roberto Andorno

INTRODUCTION

Anti-theory is a broad name for a contemporary movement that is critical of theory as the proper approach to ethics, or at least of certain aspects or forms of ethical theorizing. It is however not a unified camp, as it includes, among others, advocates of neo-Aristotelian virtue ethics, casuistry and pragmatism. Among the claims that have been made by anti-theorists are the following: that our moral lives cannot be reduced to a legalistic application of a set of norms; that the emphasis on theoretical principles to solve concrete practical moral problems is misguided; that some forms of ethical theorizing have a corrupting effect on how to live our moral lives; that ethical theories are inevitably embodied in a particular historical and sociocultural context and therefore it is an illusion to think that there is some neutral standpoint for practical rationality; that some accounts of morality ignore the plurality of goods and the possibility of conflict between them; and that there are no 'moral experts'. These criticisms to ethical theorizing will be briefly discussed, and then some responses to them will be summarized.

THE CRITIQUES OF ETHICAL THEORIES

An excessive emphasis on norms rather than on persons

Among the charges made by anti-theorists is that some moral theories concentrate, in a legalistic fashion, upon obligations to perform or to abstain from certain actions, instead of focusing on moral agents and virtues. The British philosopher Elizabeth Anscombe was a pioneer in pointing out this flaw of what she called a 'law conception of ethics' (1958). Among the theories she criticized for their reliance on obligations were Mill's utilitarianism and Kant's deontology. Taking her inspiration from Aristotle, she called for a return to concepts such as character, virtue and flourishing; that is, for relying on persons rather than on norms.

Accordingly, modern virtue ethicists insist that moral life does not consist in learning some rules and then making sure that each of our actions lives up to those rules. Instead, they stress the paramount importance of developing good habits of character or virtues. The key idea in this view is that ethics cannot be captured in one rule or principle, because ethics is too diverse and imprecise to be codified; moral life is a matter of experience and ability to perceive and to reason practically, not of learning a code of moral norms. The key moral question is not 'what I should do', as Kant puts it, but rather 'how can I make myself a better person?'

In this same line of thinking, MacIntyre (1984) has advocated a radical change in the way we think about morality and for a return to a virtue-centred ethics. He claims that in the world in which we live the language of morality still persists, but it is in a state of 'grave disorder', because we possess just 'the fragments of a conceptual scheme,' parts of which now lack those contexts from which their significance derived; we continue to use many key moral concepts, 'but we have – very largely, if not entirely – lost our comprehension, both theoretical and practical, of morality' (1984: 2). MacIntyre's hypothesis is that the moral schemes that emerged from the Enlightenment philosophers were condemned to fail from the outset because they had rejected Aristotle's idea that human life has a proper end *(telos)*, and ignored the fact that human beings cannot reach this natural end without proper preparation, which consists of an adequate education and of the personal effort in the practice of virtues (MacIntyre, 1984: 51–5).

Similarly, but relying on Plato, Iris Murdoch has challenged moral philosophy to attend more long-term tasks in moral vision and self-cultivation, that is, to focus on lifelong efforts to cultivate patterns of character rather than simply on isolated moments of willing. In her view, moral inquiry in the modern period has been impoverished precisely by its failure to articulate a substantive account of the good as fundamental to human life. Indeed, 'the idea of goodness (and of virtue) has been largely superseded in Western moral philosophy by the idea of rightness' (Murdoch, 2001: 52).

A misguided appeal to theoretical principles

Closely related to the previous criticism is the charge that ethical theories are misguided in their view of morality as a highly abstract set of principles that all agents are expected to use to guide their moral behaviour as well as to evaluate the moral behaviour of others. This is not only because, as stated in the previous paragraph, the central role in morality is played by personal virtues, not by norms; but also because principles are necessarily too vague and general to guide action. Furthermore, it is argued that moral theories do not usually provide any guidance on how to resolve conflicts that may arise between principles.

These criticisms have often been levelled against the so-called 'principlism', as developed in the field of biomedical ethics by Beauchamp and Childress (1989) in the first three editions of their *Principles of Biomedical Ethics*. The proponents of casuistry, for instance claim that absolute moral principles are 'tyrannical', that moral knowledge is fundamentally particular (or case-based) rather than general, and that practical reasoning proceeds by analogy from settled cases to unsettled ones (Jonsen and Toulmin, 1988). Similarly, it has been advanced that the possibility of moral thought and judgement does not in any way depend on the provision of a suitable supply of moral principles (Dancy, 2004: 7). Rather, what is a reason in one case need not be a reason in another case, because whether a feature is relevant or not in a particular case, and if so what exact role it is playing there, will depend on the other features of the case. This means that moral reasons are necessarily holistic, or context-specific: a feature that makes one action better can make another one worse, and make no difference at all to a third (Dancy, 2004: 7).

Also, ethical pragmatism rejects the idea that there are any universal ethical principles. Although it does not preclude ethical theorizing as such, or the appeal to principles in ethics, it insists that moral theories are just social constructs that are to be evaluated in terms of their usefulness. This is why even their most fundamental features must be subject to modification when novel problems encountered in practice demand it. In other words, principles are not seen as absolute fixed moral laws, but rather as provisional tools for guiding action, that is, as mere hypothetical guides. In the specific field of health care ethics, it has been advanced that pragmatism aims 'to reach consensus on good outcomes in cases that pose moral problems by a thorough process of inquiry, discussion, negotiation, and reflective evaluation', in an inductive, rather than a deductive way (Fins et al., 2003: 29, 41).

A dichotomy between moral theory and moral motives

Some accounts of morality are also criticized on the ground that they create a serious dichotomy between their principles and the motives that inspire moral agents. This leads practitioners of such theories to suffer from a 'moral schizophrenia' because they will necessarily have a gap between their values and their motives (Stocker, 1976). Among the ethical systems to which this critique is directed are utilitarianism, hedonism and deontology. In order to illustrate this point, some examples are given: A man committed to utilitarianism believes that an act is moral insofar as it tends to maximize utility. But if he wants to enter into a love relationship, he will find himself in a difficult position, as he will have a tendency not to act for the sake of the beloved, but rather for the sake of the utility or pleasure that such relationship may provide. Therefore, if he would like to enjoy the happiness intrinsic to love, he must willingly submit to the schizophrenic malady and hide from himself the fact that he is a utilitarian.

A similar flaw affects Kantian deontology. A person wanting to act according to the Categorical Imperative who is visiting a sick friend in hospital cannot admit to himself that he is doing so because he enjoys his friend's company, or wants to cheer him up, but is obliged to think that he is acting in this way just because it is his duty (since, for Kant, duty is the only valuable moral motive for action). But the truth is that he is not solely acting for the sake of duty, but mainly for the sake of his friend. Therefore, he will experience an internal conflict between his principles and his motives, and make his moral life schizophrenic. Both examples show, according to Stocker, that what is lacking in these theories is simply love for the other person, which is an essential feature of the most significant human relationships and constitutive of a human life worth living (1976: 456–60). Indeed love, not autonomy, is 'the characteristic and proper mark of the active moral agent' (Murdoch, 2001: 33).

Bernard Williams (1985: 54–70) has made a similar critique by appealing to the notion of 'internal reasons': we cannot have genuine reasons to act that have no connection whatever with anything that we really care about. Thus, mere 'external' arguments that, for example something is unjust would not suffice to that purpose. We will have a reason to act only if there is something contingently about us (our personal education, our psychological states, etc.) such that we are previously motivated to be just. Therefore, there are no independent, universal moral truths which can automatically provide enough reasons for action.

The historical context of practical rationality

An additional criticism to ethical theories is directed to their ambition to develop a moral system which is detached from any particular sociocultural context. According to MacIntyre, every rational justification of moral judgments presupposes some particular conception of rationality. In other words, there is no rationality that is not the rationality of some tradition. Thus, in his view, the Enlightenment's attempt to provide an ahistorical, rationally-grounded justification for universal moral principles was utopian. He illustrates his thesis by examining four philosophers (Aristotle, Augustine, Aquinas and Hume) to show how their different views about practical rationality derive from different sources and the historical contexts in which they lived. He concludes that, since rational justification must be historical, the bearers of justifications are not 'theories' in the abstract, but embodied traditions (1988: 349–54). Nevertheless, his emphasis on culture-specific rationalities does not lead MacIntyre to adhere to moral relativism. On the contrary, he claims that the relativist position is wrong because it fails to admit the timeless character of the truth. In order to solve the problem of how to reach absolute truths from a historically limited position, MacIntyre introduces the concept of 'epistemological crisis', that is, situations in which a tradition finds itself unable to evolve by using its own standards and needs to appeal to the standards provided by another tradition. In doing so, it may find a way to survive such a crisis, but it may also fail. And precisely because the possibility of failure is there, relativism is false (1988: 362–9).

From a different perspective, Williams also has stressed the crucial importance of the historical context for any account of morality. On the grounds that it is impossible to provide 'a general test for the correctness of basic ethical beliefs and principles' (1985: 72), he rejects both Rawls's contractualism and Hare's utilitarianism as they erroneously assume a reflective agent capable of distancing himself from the life and character he is examining (78-92). In contrast to both philosophers, Williams envisions a non-theoretical process beginning and ending with socially and historically conditioned ethical intuitions.

Plurality of goods and moral dilemmas

A common criticism of moral theories is that they present the moral field as unitary, as if all values were commensurable with respect to a single standard. In this respect, Williams (1985: 16–17) asserts that 'the desire to reduce all ethical considerations to one pattern' is characteristic of various moral theories, which 'try to show that one or another type of ethical consideration is basic': the notion of duty in deontological ethics, the best consequences of our acts in utilitarianism, etc. But this is 'a reductive enterprise' which 'has no justification and should disappear', because in real life we weigh different kinds of considerations without reducing them to a single currency of comparison. This is why, he concludes, 'philosophy should not try to produce ethical theory' (Williams, 1985: 17).

A related objection is that moral theorists deny the possibility of irresolvable moral dilemmas. As they claim that all moral values are commensurable with respect to a single standard, they tend to suggest that all moral conflicts are resolvable. But this seems to be false: we constantly experience in our ordinary life various conflicts between different goods that cannot simply, or not always, be resolved by appealing to an overarching value. In this regard, Charles Larmore (1987: 10–11) argues against 'the monistic assumption' of moral theory and claims that sometimes 'we know that ... conflict is irresolvable'. In his view, only when we suspend such assumptions and acknowledge that not everything is good or right to the extent that it is commensurable with respect to any single standard will we be able to recognize how much we need prudential judgment for dealing with particular situations. But in many cases, 'judgment will be powerless to settle the conflict' (Larmore, 1987: 11).

There are no 'moral experts'

Another charge against moral theories is that, since they conceive morality as an axiomatic system of norms that should guide our behavior, it logically follows that there are, or can be, moral experts; that is, people who have an academic training in ethics and know what rules to apply to the case at hand. On the contrary, anti-theorists claim that moral problems are not necessarily best solved by the alleged 'moral experts', because the rule model of decision making they employ does not always, or even usually, illuminate what is at stake in most moral situations (Louden, 1992: 96).

Moreover, moral knowledge (if knowledge is the right word), unlike, for instance, knowledge of physics, is simply not – or not only – theoretical knowledge. As a matter of fact, somebody can be morally wise without having been exposed to any moral theory. There is no reason indeed why a person who has spent time to learn moral philosophy should be more sensitive to moral truths than any other person, and in fact may be worse (McNaughton, 1988: 204). The true training in moral philosophy is not the acquisition of scientific knowledge of what is right and wrong, but the development of the ability to reflect on the nature of our judgements of right and wrong, and to explain how we should account for that wrongness or goodness. In other words, the attainment of moral sensibility does not necessarily result from an academic training. Rather, it can be obscured by such training, especially when it merely consists of the encounter with a multiplicity of opposed and irreconcilable moral theories.

SOME RESPONSES TO ANTI-THEORISTS

In light of the criticisms that have been made against moral theorizing, some authors, while recognizing that some part of truth is contained in such objections, have strongly argued in favour of the possibility and, moreover, of the need for moral theory.

Robert Louden claims that anti-theorists often criticize a caricature of moral theories, which does not correspond to the accounts of morality that some moral philosophers, such as Kant – one of the preferred targets of anti-theorists – have really proposed. Louden agrees with virtue-centred ethicists to say that 'a moral conception that gives priority to being over doing is superior' (Louden, 1992: 28–30). Moreover, he acknowledges that there are indeed bad moral theories, which are too abstract, obfuscatory, contrary to our common moral intuitions, or simply useless. This is why he is sympathetic with the complaint that 'moral theorists tend to be constitutionally disposed towards overly schematic and highly general accounts whose usefulness is a very open question' (Louden, 1992: 126).

But he claims that we do not need to abandon altogether moral theorizing for developing a plausible understanding of morality. We need better theories, not the abolition of theories; we need more, not less, reflection in ethics. He points out that, contrary to what is usually assumed, Aristotle also, no less than Kant, developed a moral theory (Louden, 1992: 99–116). Louden proposes an alternative model of moral theory which is 'empirically informed and less reductionistic than current conceptions' (1992: 139). He notes, however, that such a theory will inevitably need the construction of some principles 'to help people decide what to do and how to live', because morality is not a merely descriptive undertaking, but has a normative dimension (Louden, 1992: 141).

Martha Nussbaum observes that today 'ethical theory is under attack', not from outside as in past centuries, but 'from within' (2000: 227–30). She attempts to respond to such attacks, first of all, by stressing the crucial importance of distinguishing between theories and rules. The criticism of systems of rules does not need to entail a criticism of ethical theory, as anti-theorists assume; rather, on the contrary, it can give us reasons for turning to an ethical theory. It is precisely theory that 'enables us to understand the limitations of general rules in ways we could not do otherwise, therefore to correct the deficiencies inherent in any system or rules' (Nussbaum, 2000: 231). Nussbaum defines moral theory as 'a set of reasons and interconnected arguments, explicitly and systematically articulated, with some degree of abstractness and generality, which gives direction for ethical practice' (2000: 233–4).

On these grounds, she claims that no ethical theory is a system of rules. Theories, unlike systems of rules, offer arguments, reasons, explanations; they address their recipients as reasoning beings (Nussbaum, 2000: 236–40). This distinction does not mean however that ethical theories should dismiss rules as pointless. Most ethical theories, from Socrates onward, draw heavily on the wisdom embodied in rules and conventions. This is understandable, since rules enable us to preserve those general judgments that we regard as especially sound; they summarize the decisions of wise judges, refresh our memory, shape and inform our vision and focus our attention on aspects that we might otherwise have missed (Nussbaum, 2000: 240–1).

But the appeal to some rules is just one element among others of a theoretical account of morality, not the whole morality. At a second stage, Nussbaum responds point by point to the criticisms made by anti-theorists. She argues, for instance that it is simply mistaken to believe that moral theories ignore moral psychology and the importance of emotions. All major theories have a deep interest in the passions, and all have accounts of how institutions and education can contribute to shape the passion so that they are more likely to support good action. This is as true for Kant as it is for Aristotle (Nussbaum, 2000: 243). It is also false to affirm that moral theories ignore moral dilemmas and neglect the plurality of goods. Although Kant and Aristotle do not give prominent recognition to moral dilemmas, their theories are compatible with such recognition as well as with leaving space for local or personal specifications of ends, without renouncing their claim to universality (2000: 244). Anti-theorists are naïve in thinking that the exchange of ethical criticism in everyday life is sufficient to guide our practices. They ignore the brute fact that theory can help our good judgment to prevail by giving us additional opposition to the bad influence of corrupt desires, judgments and passions. This is why we need theory in ethics (Nussbaum, 2000: 252–4).

Similarly, Margaret Little argues that the critiques made by anti-theorists are often 'objections to impoverished moral theory, not to moral theory per se' (2001: 32–3). Moreover, such critiques are in fact not inconsistent with the idea that we can and should build a moral theory. Even Aristotle, who is often claimed as an ally of anti-theorists, 'did not confine himself to commenting on individual cases', but 'insisted that the person of moral wisdom must know the "why", not just the "that"; something that sounds, one might have thought, like a call to theoretical abstraction' (Little, 2001: 32). She makes the case that theory is 'essential to moral life', as we need moral generalizations for guiding and illuminating what our life experience reveals (Little, 2001: 39).

CONCLUSION

The anti-theory movement developed from dissatisfaction with the heavy role that the notions of duty and obligation play in some modern accounts of morality. It also grew out of an objection to the reduction of morality to the mere formal compliance with a set of abstract rules. In this regard, anti-theory represents a refreshing approach to ethics and a call for a more realistic and comprehensive vision of morality. It suggests the need to focus on persons rather on acts, on being good persons rather than on complying with rules.

Nevertheless, some of the criticisms made by anti-theorists go too far when they attack ethical theorizing as such, because philosophy is by its very nature a theoretical enterprise. Ethics, which is a part of philosophy, cannot be explained and justified without the appeal to some concepts and rules, which necessarily involve some degree of abstraction. Practical rationality is after all a form of rationality: the use of reason in the service of action. The challenge consists therefore in developing an account of morality which is not made up of pale abstractions divorced from practice, but rather takes into account how we actually deliberate in our daily lives and tries to identify the rational judgements that are implicit in our search for goodness.

REFERENCES

Anscombe, E. (1958) 'Modern moral philosophy', *Philosophy*, 33: 1–19. [Reprinted in R. Crisp and M. Slote (eds) (1997) *Virtue Ethics*, Oxford: Oxford University Press, pp. 26–44.

Beauchamp, T.L. and Childress, J. (1989) *Principles of Biomedical Ethics*, 3rd ed. New York: Oxford University Press.

Dancy, J. (2004) *Ethics without Principles*. New York: Oxford University Press.

Fins, J., Bacchetta, M. and Miller, F. (2003) 'Clinical pragmatism: A method of moral problem solving', in G. McGee (ed.), *Pragmatic Bioethics*, 2nd ed. Cambridge, MA: MIT Press, pp. 29–44.

Jonsen, A. and Toulmin, S. (1988) *The Abuse of Casuistry. A History of Moral Reasoning*. Berkeley, CA: University of California Press.

Larmore, C. (1987) *Patterns of Moral Complexity*. Cambridge: Cambridge University Press.

Little, M.O. (2001) 'On knowing the "Why": Particularism and moral theory', *The Hastings Center Report*, 31 (4): 32–40.

Louden, R.B. (1992) *Morality and Moral Theory: A Reappraisal and Reaffirmation*. New York: Oxford University Press.

MacIntyre, A. (1984) *After Virtue. A Study in Moral Theory*, 2nd ed. Notre Dame, IN: University of Notre Dame Press.

MacIntyre, A. (1988) *Whose Justice? Which Rationality?* London: Duckworth.

McNaughton, D. (1988) *Moral Vision. An Introduction to Ethics*. Oxford: Blackwell.

Murdoch, I. (2001) *The Sovereignty of Good*. London: Routledge.

Nussbaum, M. (2000) 'Why practice needs ethical theory', in B. Hooker and M. O. Little (eds), *Moral Particularism*. Oxford: Oxford University Press, pp. 227–55.

Stocker, M. (1976) 'The schizophrenia of modern ethical theory', *Journal of Philosophy*, 73 (14): 453–66. [Reprinted in R. Crisp and M. Slote (eds) (1997) *Virtue Ethics*. Oxford: Oxford University Press, pp. 66–78.

Williams, B. (1985) *Ethics and the Limits of Philosophy*. London: Fontana Press.

4

Ethics of Care

Ruud ter Meulen

INTRODUCTION

Since the beginning of the twentieth century average life expectancy has risen significantly in the industrialised world. While average life expectancy in 1900 was approximately 50 years, average life expectancy for the countries of the European Union is presently 78 years, 75 years for men and 81 for women. The rise in average life expectancy is for the greater part the result of improvement in living conditions, food habits and hygiene, as well as the success of modern medicine in fighting diseases, particularly infectious diseases.

However, the increase in life expectancy comes with a price: on the one hand individuals can enjoy a longer life, but on the other hand they have an increased chance of being confronted with a long period of enduring debilitating conditions. While the healthy life expectancy, meaning the period one is free of disease and handicaps, remains the same, and the average total life expectancy increases, a larger part of our life may be affected by disease or handicaps. This is particularly true for women as their healthy life expectancy is around 60 years while their average total life expectancy has risen to above 80 years.

The increased life expectancy can be seen as 'the failure of success': we live a longer life but with an increased period of illness and disability. This development is particularly relevant for the age group 80 years and above, the fastest growing age group in the industrialised countries. This age group will experience a 'compression of dependency', that is, an increased risk to be tormented by physical and mental chronic conditions or diseases like dementia, depression, stroke, osteoporosis, including the risk of fractures, and various kinds of arthritis. Moreover, people of 80 years and above have a high risk of minor, but still debilitating, handicaps like visual and auditory handicaps, urethro-genital problems, poor nutrition and psychiatric problems.

CHRONIC ILLNESS

As a result of increased life expectancy, our societies will have to deal with a higher incidence of chronic illnesses. These illnesses can be characterised as irreversible conditions without the prospects of (full) recovery. They have long duration, can lead to permanent disability and they require special training and rehabilitation of the patient. There is a wide range of chronic illnesses and conditions as a result of chronic illness. Chronic illnesses can be life threatening like cancer; can lead to severe disability like arthritis or stroke; and such people can have permanent symptoms or intermittent periods of symptoms and symptom-free periods. People living with a chronic illness are limited in their functioning, suffer from pain and are dependent on the help of other people. This can be help from professional carers or informal caregivers like family, partner, neighbours or friends. Although people suffering from a chronic illness can participate in our society, many of them feel isolated and in an economically vulnerable position.

While many older people are suffering from chronic conditions, young people can also suffer from a chronic illness like chronic respiratory diseases, leukaemia or rheumatoid arthritis.

Chronic conditions require a different approach from the dominant approach in curative medicine. Curative medicine considers disease as a deviation of a normal condition which needs to be restored as quickly as possible. The practitioner sees his/her task primarily as to combat or remove the cause of a disease. The patient him/herself hardly plays any role in this process: he or she can do no more than to subject him/herself to the medical regime. In caring for chronic conditions we need a different approach: as such conditions are not (fully) curable, patients suffering from chronic illnesses are particularly in need of support and care. Care for people suffering from chronic illness means support of the ill person to manage his/her chronic condition.

An important difference between acute care and care for people with a chronic illness is the type of relationship between the caregiver and the cared-for person. Relationships in curative medicine are generally brief and superficial, usually consisting of brief contact with various professional practitioners. Care is different from cure, as care wants to support people and alleviate their pain and symptoms. Care means a certain attitude, which includes affection, compassion, dedication, patience and involvement.

Although such an attitude is important in curative medicine as well, curative medicine is focused on 'fighting' to heal the patient, not to give up too quickly, to abstain at the moment that further treatment is pointless or futile, etc. In curative medicine, activism is central, trying the best one can to improve the condition of the patient.

As opposed to curative medicine, caring means acceptance by the patient and the caregiver of the limitations of the disease or the handicap of the patient, and trying to make the best of it. Care is much more modest than cure. Cure is continuously trying to fight its own limitations, with the goal to extend life indefinitely. The need for care, on the other hand, is much more limited. Care does not entail a heroic attempt to conquer disease, but it means support and solidarity. Caring is much more fundamental than curing because caring tries to respect the uniqueness and value of a fellow human being.

Care does not just mean an attitude, but refers also to a number of institutions that offer support and treatment where possible and necessary. Such institutions are nursing homes, psychiatric institutions, institutions for home care and other institutions for long-term care. Such institutions have the task to offer safety, comfort and support to the patient to manage his/her illness and disabilities. This can be support and help for activities of daily living like getting into or out of bed, getting dressed or getting shoes on, washing and other bodily care, going to the toilet, cooking and eating, guiding in case of blindness or just having a conversation. The social isolation of people with chronic diseases or needing long-term care is often their biggest and most severe problem. By way of daily help and respectful attitudes one can prevent people with chronic diseases from being alienated from society or losing their self respect.

Due to the increased life-expectancy, the need for physical, social and emotional support for people with long-term illnesses will increase in the near future. This development has important consequences for the allocation of services in our health-care systems, particularly for the so-called 'care–cure' balance. In case of limited resources for health care, we need to make choices between how much we will spend on services to supply long-term care, or services that are focused on treatment of acute conditions. More money for nursing-home care, for care in the community or for care for people with learning disabilities may go at the expense of acute care, or the other way around. Acute care, and that means predominantly care in hospitals, always has a major share in the health-care budget. Even though recently there has been more attention for an increase in long-term care services, curative medicine is still dominant in health care: saving lives by means of impressive medical technology is still seen as the most important task in health care.

The low status of care as opposed to cure is reinforced by the idea that care is seen as ineffective. Curative medicine has a strong bias towards removing the causes of disease. Effective care is care that takes away these causes as quickly as possible. As such, quick and efficient care is not possible in the treatment of chronic diseases; long-term care has a much lower status than curative care in our society. According to Callahan (1990), care is much more modest than 'cure'. Cure is continuously trying to break through its own frontiers, with the goal to extend life into infinitude. As opposed to curative medicine, the need for long-term care is much more limited. Long-term care does not mean a heroic attempt to conquer disease, but to provide support and solidarity.

THE ETHIC OF CARE

To be affected by a chronic condition means, in many cases, a dramatic change in the lives of those who are involved; life plans are aborted, social relationships are disrupted and activities of daily living are seriously hindered. Changes in the body have, above all, serious consequences for one's self-image. The sociologist Katy Charmaz (1987) talks about the 'constant struggle' of people with a serious long-term or permanent condition, needing to fight continuously for their own identity while suffering from pain, handicap and loneliness. In this process, relationships with other persons, and particularly care providers, are of great importance.

Care is in the first place a relationship between individuals. On one side there is an individual who, because of illness or handicap, cannot take care of him or herself and is in need of support by another person. On the other side of this relationship there is somebody who can supply this support: partner, family member, friend, the voluntary or professional caregiver. The reason why these other individuals offer help and support is because they are concerned about the needs of the ill or needy individual; they identify with the needs and predicament of the needy person and they want to do something about that. Usually 'doing' means offering support, coaching, keeping company, caring, bodily caring or having a conversation. The fact that care in many cases is supplied by professional caregivers who get an income out of this activity does not diminish or remove this identification. Good care means a balance between professional treatment and human relatedness.

The relationship between the cared and the carer is a central theme in the so-called ethic of care as formulated by Joan Tronto (1993), among others. She argues that during life we are passing through various periods of dependency and independency, of autonomy and frailty. When we are delivering care, and particularly long-term care, we should recognise the vulnerability and dependency of the person needing care.

According to Tronto, care can be defined as follows:

> [o]n the most general level we suggest that caring be viewed as a specious activity that includes everything that we do to maintain, continue and repair our 'world' so that we can live in it as well as possible. That world includes our bodies, ourselves, and our environment, all of which we seek to interweave in a complex, life-sustaining web (Tronto, 1993: 103).

Tronto (1993) distinguishes four types of relationships as part of the caring process. Each of the four types of relationship presupposes specific ethical qualities. She describes those four types of relationships and qualities as follows:

- caring about. Caring about involves the recognition in the first place that care is necessary. It involves noting the existence of a need and making assessment that caring about is a basic attitude of any caring activity. The ethical quality which is important for this attitude is called attentiveness, meaning being attentive to the needs of others, recognising the needs of those around us. If we are not attentive to the needs of others we cannot possibly address those needs. Attentiveness is opposed to ignorance of others which is so common in our modern society.
- taking care of. Taking care of is the next step of the caring process; it involves assuming responsibility for the needs of the other and determining how to respond to it. It involves the recognition that one can act to address those needs. The central ethical quality in this type of relationship is responsibility. Responsibility has various connotations and various meanings. It depends on a number of factors and is different in every context. As parents we may feel responsible to care for our children or we feel responsible for our elder relatives. We might assume responsibility because we recognise a need for caring and there is no other way that the need will be met except by our meeting it.
- care giving. This is the direct meeting of the need for care. It involves physical work and it requires that caregivers come in contact with the objects of care, as a professional or informally. The ethical quality is competence. Intending to provide care or even accepting responsibility for it means that one is able to provide good care and that the needs for care are met. Including competence as a moral dimension of care is to avoid the bad faith of those who would take care of a problem without being willing to do any form of care giving. Competence means being qualified to provide the care that is needed. But competence does not equate just with professional competence – competence also means to have the moral qualities to provide good care.
- Care receiving. In this phase the person in need of care responds to the care he or she receives. It is important to include care receiving as an element of the caring process because it provides the only way to know that caring needs have actually been met. The perception of the care receiver is decisive for the answer to the question whether care has been provided in a responsible and adequate way. The ethical quality of this phase is called responsiveness. Responsiveness means that the individual who is cared for does not consider her/himself as autonomous and self-supporting. The individual in need of care should

recognise his or her own vulnerability and needs in order to cooperate adequately and responsibly to the caring process. According to Tronto, vulnerability belies that myth that we are always autonomous, and potentially equal, citizens.

The four moral qualities of responsible care are to some extent related to each other; responsiveness presupposes attentiveness, while responsibility takes into account being competent. The four criteria should, in fact, be seen as four elements of one whole. The ethic of care is not a set of strictly described rules or principles. At best it can be described as a practice with specific moral qualities and these qualities do not have the character of specific directives on how to act in certain situations. In fact they should be seen as a 'habit of the mind'.

CARE OR CONTRACT

Marjan Verkerk (1994) places the ethics of care in opposition to the contract perspective that has become dominant in our society. In the contract perspective, society is seen as a treaty between autonomous individuals, each having their own conception of the good life. An individual starts a relationship with another individual when he or she sees an advantage in doing so. The relationship between individuals and between the individual and society as a whole is fully contingent. Such a relationship is always revocable, as soon as the advantages do not outweigh the disadvantages.

The starting point of contract thinking is that society should create equal conditions and opportunities for everybody, no matter whether one is young or old, healthy or ill, poor or rich. The contract perspective is an example of so-called ethics of justice. This is ethics according to which we should treat others as equal by giving them rights and to take care that those rights are fulfilled and not neglected. Ethics of justice should be distinguished from ethics of good. Ethics of good tries to answer the question, what is a good life or what is good care? This branch of ethics is what is known as substantial: it is an ethics that is 'full' of content, as opposed to the ethics of justice which is only dealing with procedures, particularly procedures of fair and equal treatment. Values like responsibility for the other, involvement and solidarity belong to the ethics of the good life. This branch of ethics says something about how we like to shape our lives, how we should relate to our fellow beings and what kind of meaning we can give to our existence as, for example seen from the perspective of religion or world view.

Liberalism tries to separate the ethics of justice and the ethics of good as much as possible. The ethics of justice is the ethics of public life, while the ethics of good belongs to the private sphere. According to liberalism, neither the state nor society should interfere with the choices of people in how they live their lives. Society should limit itself to regulating and protecting communications and relations between people, but in the private sphere people are free to develop their own ethics of good. The state should protect this liberty; nobody should be forced into a certain lifestyle or world view.

In liberalism there seems to exist a balance between the ethics of justice and the ethics of good, in which the first one rules public life and the other has its place in the private sphere. Both kinds of ethics have an equal value but both should limit themselves to their own sphere. In the same way as the ethics of justice belongs to society and should not interfere with relationships between individuals in the private sphere, the ethics of good belongs to the personal life of individuals and has no place in public life. However, one can ask whether public life, and particularly care, is served well with an ethics that is purely based on justice.

As an example we can refer to the contract thinking that has become well established in the care system. By giving patients rights and treating them as equals, as a patient or client they are emancipated and protected against interference in their mental and bodily integrity. The right to equal access, the right to information, the principle of free consent and the safeguarding of privacy can be seen as important rights in our health-care system.

However, relationships between individuals would be impoverished should they be interpreted purely in such terms. According to some, the right to self determination in American psychiatry has resulted in 'a right to rot'. The ideal of freedom and self determination or autonomy is radically explained as the right of individuals 'to be left alone', even if their actual condition makes direct interventions necessary. In the United States, the impact of legal rules on health care has seriously affected the relationship between care providers and patients in a negative way. Doctors and other practitioners are afraid of litigation and take a defensive attitude, limiting themselves only to basic care and only when the patient has explicitly given his or her consent.

The ethics of justice and the contract perspective have resulted in the emancipation of the patient in our health-care system. However, this development has also resulted in a one-sidedness to the advantage of the ethics of justice. Care relationships with care institutions have become less characterised by personal involvement or personal values. These values are seen as irrelevant for the care process. Those relationships that are impartial, distanced, rational and equal fit within the contract perspective. Instead of the ethics of good, we can see how the rules of law and of economy have become dominant within the care system. The ethic of care is one of the ethical theories that try to respond to the one-sidedness of the ethics of justice. As said above, the ethic of care argues that caring relationships are not relationships between equals but in many cases involve a relationship between people who are not equal, between a care giver and a patient suffering from a chronic illness, such as Alzheimer's disease, a stroke or a heart attack. Although the ethics of justice and the contract perspective ought to play an important role in health care, this branch of ethics needs to be balanced by the ethics of good by way of an increased emphasis on responsibility, involvement, solidarity and other values that, for example are promoted by the ethics of care. These are substantial values that do not have a place in the contract perspective but they are values that are fundamental for providing care to persons who are in need.

Virginia Held compares the ethics of justice with the ethics of care:

An ethic of justice focuses on the questions of fairness, equality, individual rights, abstract principles and the consistent application of them. An ethic of care focuses on attentiveness, trust, responsiveness to need, narrative nuance and cultivating caring relations. Whereas an ethic of justice seeks a fair solution between competing individual interests and rights, an ethic of care sees the interests of carers and cared for as importantly intertwined rather than as simply competing. Whereas justice protects equality and freedom, care fosters social bonds and co-operation (Held, 2006:15).

VULNERABILITY AND DEPENDENCY

The ethic of care fights against the exclusion of important moral values like dedication, responsibility and involvement. It argues that these values play an important role in the experience of caregivers, particularly female informal caregivers. Women who are caring for their parents or their partners have the feeling that their moral experiences are excluded from the contract perspective and the ethics of justice. Carol Gilligan (1982) has asked for more attention to be paid to these moral experiences of women and has laid the foundations for a different moral perspective on care. The ethic of care is partly related to a political feminist position which tries to argue not only for the experiences of women to be taken seriously, but also for recognition of their societal position in which caring for others plays such an important role.

However, one should not see the ethic of care as a mere feministic critique on the dominant contractual ethics of justice. The ethic of care is a specific kind of ethics that starts from the fundamental vulnerability and dependency of people. It is an ethics for an era in which we are increasingly confronted with chronic illnesses, and dependency and vulnerability as result of such conditions. It is an ethic that feels responsible for the suffering and needs of the other. The ethic of care does not consider this responsibility as one-way traffic; by dedication to the well-being of the other the care provider enriches her or his own life as well. Caring is not just a matter of giving, but also of receiving. What one especially receives is experience of the insufficiency of our existence. This confrontation should not be seen as threatening, but as a contribution to our self understanding as needy beings continuously searching for autonomy instead of being already autonomous. The ethic of care distances itself from liberal thinking in which individuals are seen as asocial, fully autonomous beings who direct their own lives independently of others. The ethic of care sees man in his/her fundamental relationship and involvement with other individuals.

The ethic of care opposes the concept of autonomy of mainstream health-care ethics which is based on an individualist concept of man. This concept of autonomy does not acknowledge the social relationships and dependencies of every human being. It defines autonomy primarily as rationality, individuality and self determination, ignoring the social structures in which these characteristics play a role. According to Held (2006), the ethics of care works with the concept of persons as relational, rather than as the self sufficient, independent individuals of the dominant moral theories: 'dominant theories can be interpreted as importing into moral theory the concept of the person developed primarily for liberal, political and economy theory, seeing the person as a rational autonomous agent, or a self-interested individual' (Held, 2006: 13). There is an illusion that our society is composed of free, equal and independent individuals who can choose to associate with one another or not.

> It obscures the very real facts of dependency for everyone when they are young, for most people at various periods in their lives when they are ill or old and infirm, for some who are disabled, and for all those engaged in unpaid 'dependency work'. In obscurity innumerable ways persons and groups are interdependent in the modern world … The ethics of care values the ties we have with particular other persons and the actual relationships that partly constitute our identity (Held, 2006: 14).

The liberal concept of autonomy is irrelevant for the care of people with chronic illnesses, where we need a relational concept of autonomy based on a social view of man, a concept that pays attention to the relationships in which the person recognises him or herself.

People with a chronic illness who have become dependent upon the care of others can only realise their autonomy in a relationship that helps them to find their identity and to cope with their condition. This process is not possible in a contractual concept of care that abstracts all personal values and attitudes.

CARE IN THE NURSING HOME

Although many people needing long-term care are cared for at home, there is a large group who will become dependent on permanent care in a care home or nursing home. Examples are people suffering from Alzheimer's disease and who, after being cared for at home for many years, need a level of care that is difficult for family members, friends or neighbours to provide. People who have suffered from a stroke and cannot help themselves any more may become dependent on care in a nursing home. An important risk of permanent stay in a nursing home is so-called hospitalisation. The nursing home is an institution that not only provides care via therapy and basic care; it is also a place where people live for 24 hours of the day. As such, the nursing home can become a place where people become increasingly dependent, not only because of the care that is provided to them in the nursing home, but also because of the regime of daily life. The nursing home can be characterised as a total institution. According to Goffman, a total institution may be defined 'as a place of residence and work where a large number of like situated individuals, cut off from the wider society for an appreciable period of time, together lead an enclosed, formally administered round of life' (Goffman, 1982: 11). An important feature of a total institution is that the life of its inhabitants is programmed by small details. The inhabitant of an institution has no other option than to subject him or herself to the regime of living in, and treatment by, the institution. Abilities that are important for living outside the institution are slowly erased. This is the reason why people who live for a long time in a total institution have great difficulty in leaving such institutions and to build up a life in the outside world.

A nursing home can be considered a total institution as the three areas of living (living, working and sleeping) take place in the nursing home, under one roof and under the same management. All daily activities are executed in a group, where everybody is treated as equal and everybody is expected to do the same thing. The hours of the day are strictly regulated without any room for individual preferences. While the patient is cared for on the one hand, on the other hand he or she experiences a feeling of powerlessness. He/she is helped by, but has not much control over, the caring process or over his/her own life. The feeling of powerlessness may result in severe physical and mental problems on top of the chronic conditions which are already affecting the patient. Long-term stay in a nursing home can lead to mental deprivation, loss of social contacts and lack of any meaningful life.

To counteract such developments, nursing homes put more emphasis on the respect of autonomy and the preservation of dignity of the inhabitants. It is important to know that respect for autonomy should not be limited to dramatic decisions at the end of life, but that it should be considered as a continuous process in daily care. People cared for in the nursing home should have the opportunity to make their own choices about their care and conditions of living. Rosemary Kane and Arthur Kaplan (1990) talk in this context about 'everyday ethics'; particularly in normal daily care there are many opportunities and hindrances for realising one's autonomy. This is particularly true for choices regarding eating, sleeping, going to the toilet, decoration of the room or wearing of specific clothes. Every nursing home needs some kind of a routine, but that should not be at the expense of the social sphere with which individuals can identify and which promotes the development of their autonomy and individuality.

In nursing home care there are many areas where care for the autonomy of the inhabitant falls short because of the need to maintain a regime. Particularly when there is a shortage of personnel, nursing staff try to organise the delivery of care as efficiently as possible. Such a regime may reduce the possibility of individual variation, personal choice and promotion of autonomy. Lack of staff and resources can result in neglect of patients and feelings of powerlessness and superfluity among them.

PROTECTIVE MEASURES

A particular way to limit the autonomy of residents in care homes is by the use of protective measures. Examples are the use of belts and straps to fix patients to their seats or beds; the use of bed frames; the use of psychopharmacological medication; locking the doors to prevent patients from strolling around; removal of objects that may cause harm (razor blades, scissors, matches). Often such measures are taken without the knowledge of the patient or inhabitant. Psychopharmacological medication may be hidden in the food; scissors may be taken away secretly; or electronic tagging devices may be attached to patients' clothes without him or her knowing about it. Particularly in psychogeriatric wards of care homes, such protective measures are frequently taken. The purpose is to protect the person with dementia against him or herself. Examples are prevention of the patient falling, prevention of strolling, the reduction of aggressive behaviour and medical treatment without consent. An important question here is: who is protected by such measures? Is it the demented patient or perhaps his or her family, the caregivers or other patients? In the eyes of the caregiver the protective measures are meant to protect the residents. The resident, however, can experience such measures as a severe limitation of his/her freedom and autonomy.

One can ask whether protective measures result in more safety. It appears that many such measures have a contrary effect as they may result in more accidents and wounds. Protective measures can lead to disorientation, sensory deprivation and increasing hospitalisation. Other harmful effects are: decubitus, incontinence, chronic constipation, cardio stress, lack of appetite and dehydration. While protective measures can have positive results for the resident, these need to be balanced against harm and side effects. In this ethical balance of benefits and harm one should try to respect the autonomy of the inhabitant and obtain his or her informed consent. The inhabitant must be able to indicate which risks he or she wants to take and which of the protective measures against potential harm he or she thinks are acceptable. In case the patient is not able to do so, because of diminished competence, his or her family should be involved in the consent process.

It is important also to respect the dignity of the inhabitant of the nursing home. Care home residents who are fixed by a strap or belt, or have been sedated, lose their decorum as well as their respect and identity. Nursing homes need to respect the dignity of people dependent on long-term care and to prevent people living in such conditions from being harmed by protective or other limiting measures.

CONCLUSION

Due to the increase in life expectancy, we may be confronted with prolonged periods of illness and chronic disease in the final stages of life. Chronic conditions require a different approach and a different ethic than curative medicine; instead of conquering disease, long-term care is focused on support and alleviation of suffering of the dependent person. The ethic of care argues (amongst other things) for an attitude of responsibility and involvement, based on a relational concept of autonomy. Such an attitude should help the dependent person to regain his or her autonomy and to find their identity. However, such a substantial and relational ethics is neglected by the dominant, ethical progression in health care that approaches respect of autonomy from a rational, asocial point of view. Instead of seeing man as an isolated individual, the ethic of care argues that man can only find autonomy in relation with others. This is particularly true in the care for people with chronic illnesses where they are dependent on the support of others and need continuous support to re-establish their autonomy.

REFERENCES

Callahan, D. (1990) *What Kind of Life. The Limits of Medical Progress.* New York: Simon & Schuster.
Charmaz, K. (1987) 'Struggle for a self: Identity levels of the chronically ill', in J. Roth and R. Conrad (eds.), *Research in the Sociology of Health Care,* Vol. 6. Greenwich, CT/London: JAI Press, pp. 283–321.
Gilligan, C. (1982) *In a Different Voice: Psychological Theory and Women's Development.* Cambridge, MA: Harvard University Press.
Goffman, E. (1982) *Asylums. Essays on the Social Situation of Mental Patients and Other Inmates.* Harmondsworth: Penguin.
Held, V. (2006) *The Ethics of Care. Personal, Political, and Global.* Oxford: Oxford University Press.
Kane, R. and Kaplan, A. (1990) *Everyday Ethics. Resolving Dilemmas in Nursing Home Life.* New York: Springer.
Tronto, J.C. (1993) *Moral Boundaries. A Political Argument for an Ethic of Care.* New York: Routledge.
Verkerk, M. (1994) 'Zorg of contract: een andere ethiek', in H. Manschot and M. Verkerk (red.), *Ethiek van de zorg. Een discussie.* Amsterdam/Meppel: Boom, pp. 53–73.

5

Emerging Technologies: Challenges for Health Care and Environmental Ethics and Rights in an Era of Globalisation

Thomas Alured Faunce

INTRODUCTION

The intersections between international human rights, health care and environmental ethics on the one hand, and international trade law on the other, provide one of the great normative challenges for global health policy as we emerge from the era of corporate globalisation. This is particularly so as we attempt to use such norms to achieve not only just and equitable but sustainable habitats. An important case study in this context will be the how we use emerging technologies (for instance, nanotechnology) to rectify global problems such as anthropogenic climate change, the gap between global population and energy and food demand, biodiversity loss and ecosystem pollution.

As we'll see, these intersections provide a challenging background to the aims and content of provisions in instruments such as the United Nations Scientific, Education and Cultural Organisation (UNESCO) *Universal Declaration on Bioethics and Human Rights* (UDBHR), the *Universal Declaration on Human Rights* (UDHR), the *International Covenant on Civil and Political Rights* (ICESCR), the policies and programmes of the World Health Organisation (WHO), United Nations *Millennium Development Goals* *(UNMDGs)*, the recommendations of the *Intergovernmental Panel on Climate Change* *(IPCC)* and *the Copenhagen Accord on Climate Change*, as well as implementation of international treaty and national constitutional provisions on the right to health, sustainable development and environmental protection. They are likely to shape not just issues surrounding the principles and rules governing access to essential medicines, but access to technology-based hospital and health care services as well as emerging technology research, development and transfer. This chapter aims to explore the normative ancestry of these intersections and critique their likely role in some of the key debates and developments in this field.

HISTORICAL BACKGROUND

In the decades following World War II, many hoped that the regime of international human rights (as textually established by the Universal Declaration of Human Rights (UDHR) (UN 1948), the International Covenant on Civil and Political Rights (ICCPR) (UN, 1966a) and the International Covenant on Economic, Social and Cultural Rights (ICESCR) (UN, 1966b)), would become an important means of encouraging states to render respect for the inherent dignity of all human beings, and as a part of that secure the basic preconditions of health (Oppenheimer et al., 2002). Hope grew that such a commitment would mark the start of a process of engagement between the states and international civil society (Sen, 2002). It would lead to government programmes (such as those implementing the UNMDGs) that aimed amongst other things to draw upon new technologies to gradually reduce warfare, poverty, corruption, childhood and maternal mortality and infringements of civil and political liberties (Braveman and Gruskin, 2003). UN human rights institutions and non-governmental organisations (NGOs) were to play crucial roles in this process (Taylor, 2004). So too was the expanding capacity for individual citizens to petition human rights committees and courts concerning violations of patient human rights, but also to achieve negative (removing barriers to access and discrimination) and positive operationalisable standards applicable to multinational corporations involved in health care (Buchanan and Decamp, 2006). Health care ethics was a much less textually crystallised normative discipline than that involved with the human right to health. Three significant and overlapping issues were marginalised from this debate about the normative content and societal impact of global health care ethics and rights. The first involved how ethics and law could best protect the role of the environment in human health as well as its intrinsic value to the health of all life forms. The second concerned the expanding influence of international trade law in shaping influential normative systems largely unresponsive to health care (or environmental) ethics and rights. The third concerned how emerging technologies should be regulated to help resolve some of the great problems facing humanity and its environment.

By way of example, the jurisprudence driving the process of corporate globalisation (and the global distribution of new health-related technologies) was almost entirely constituted by international trade law, a system with few formal connections to international human rights or environmental law and policy. Corporate-driven World Trade Organisation (WTO) agreements, for example, such as those on Trade Related Intellectual Property Rights (TRIPS) and the General Agreement on Trade in Services (GATS) did have provisions that allowed exemption for government policies necessary to protect *public order* and *morality* (articles 27(2) and XIV(a) respectively).

Public order or morals, however, were not defined in such agreements by reference to human rights, such as the right to health or emerging environmental rights like biodiversity and ecosystem sustainability (Chapman, 2002). Trade dispute panels to the extent they were interested in, or were granted the legal capacity to consider implications for public and environmental health, had to rely on reference to the nebulous collection of health care ethical norms and dictionary definitions such as that which defined public morals as 'standards of right and wrong conduct maintained by or on behalf of a community or nation' (WTO Panel Report-*US Gambling*, 2005). Such an approach required that norms of the WTO that were central to the globalisation process have public order and morality exclusions deliberately made vague and unenforceable by the reference to varying cultural, religious and other national contexts, rather than clearly defined rights.

Such a conceptual outcome was in contradistinction to much formative thinking about health care ethics and rights which related to those normative systems to the well established and still valuable intellectual notion of a hypothetical social contract. This concept in broad terms holds that a society's normative foundations are principles and rules emerging (for example, in national legal texts such as the Virginia Declaration of Rights 1776, the American Declaration of Independence 1776, the French Déclaration des Droits de l'Homme et du Citoyen 1789) out of community respect for great social ideals or virtues related to how humans *should* treat each other in ideal conditions (such as justice, fairness, respect for human dignity and self-realisation free from state interference). Many see the culmination of such reasoning on the international stage in the UN's Universal Declaration on Human Rights of 1948 (UN, 1948; Claude and Issel 1998). This is particularly true of Article 1: 'All beings are born free and equal in dignity and rights. They are endowed with reason and conscience and should act towards one another in a spirit of brotherhood.'

The emphasis on evolution towards justiciable and enforceable international human rights as part of any functional global social contract implies a combination of both self-assurance about the universal regulatory and symbolic importance of controlling how humans treat each other, and mistrust of governments to otherwise uphold ethical principles (Hart, 1979; Raz, 1984; Brugger, 1996). At the conceptual heart of any social contract supporting a sustainable global civilisation must be the presumption of contractual type guarantees involving rules about clarifying when any one person's freedom can be interfered with by another's, as well as indicating that consensual statements about the aims of the collective should not unduly infringe those of its members (Rawls, 1976; Dworkin, 1977).

Yet, missing from such jurisprudential discussions has been consideration of how human beings should make basic rules governing their relationship with the environment including how new technologies should be responsive to its sustainability. One exception in practice has been the precautionary principle. This emerged in German regulatory policy during the 1970s and rapidly spread through the international policy arena as a philosophical challenge against free-market policies that demanded an often unrealistic level of scientific certainty about risks before recommending or implementing public health and environment protection measures in relation to the use of new technologies. A well known international enunciation of the precautionary principle is found in Principle 15 of the *Rio Declaration on Environment and Development* (1992): 'Where there are threats of serious or irreversible damage, lack of full scientific certainty shall not be used as a reason for postponing cost effective measures to prevent environmental degradation.'

There is no scientific or economic reason for scholars and policy-makers to make such a comprehensive distinction between the normative foundations health care and environmental ethics and rights. The standard national and corporate policies advocating unlimited economic growth that currently drive the global macroeconomy are increasingly recognised to impinge detrimentally on the finite resources of the global ecosystem and on global public health (Daly, 1990; Ayres, 2008). The argument here is that the hypothetical founders of any social arrangement placed behind a veil of ignorance to shape principles and rules to govern future generations should surely have taken into account species survival and integrity of ecosystems. In terms of the foundational challenges for health care ethics and law, for instance, how technology should be regulated to provide a non-polluting source of fuel and food and create a sustainable biosphere are equally important with equitable access to medicines, medical devices and medical services.

REGULATING HEALTH-RELATED TECHNOLOGIES: FOUNDATIONS IN MEDICAL ETHICS AND INTERNATIONAL HUMANITARIAN LAW

Historically, the development of medical ethics (as a professional subset of general ethics) and human rights are intriguingly parallel systems bearing upon equitable access to new health-related technologies and services. John Locke, a founding father of human rights jurisprudence, was a physician pupil of Sydenham, a great clinical empiricist inheritor of the Hippocratic tradition (Borden, 1967; Dewhurst, 1995; Davey, 2001). Indeed, it is interesting to speculate that a major factor promoting both the corpus of human rights norms, as well as the norms of medical ethics deriving from the Hippocratic Oath, may have been the influence of clinical practice on the humanistic conceptions of Locke, including the inspirational example of Sydenham's loyalty to the coordinating professional virtue of relief of individual human suffering (Faunce, 2007). Influential medical principlists (such as Beauchamp and Childress), however, do not embrace such a virtue-based normative view (Beauchamp, 1995; Pellegrino, 1995; Jonsen, 2000). Medical ethics, until very recently, was silent on the topic of responsibilities to the environment, even indirectly as a means of assuring human health, as well as how existing and new technologies should be equitably distributed to respond to such challenges.

International humanitarian law (IHL) is another source of norms with relevance to global health care ethics that has grown to have complex intersections with environmental and trade law norms. This is particularly true in relation to not only restricting the research, development and transfer of new military technologies, but facilitating reasonable access to new health-related technologies for prisoners and wounded in war. IHL is an aggregation of customary and treaty-based norms concerned with the treatment of the wounded combatants, civilians and prisoners in war. It has many areas of overlap with both medical ethics and human rights law. Its origins may be traced to Henry Durant's attempts to create a regulatory system that would prevent a recurrence of the unrelieved suffering of the wounded soldiers he witnessed on the battlefield after the battle of Solferino in 1859. The Geneva Conventions in 1949, the Hague Convention of 1907 and the Genocide

Convention and Nuremberg Charter, all impose upon states positive duties to permit, and negative duties not hinder, the exercise of medical professionalism amidst armed conflict. These have now achieved status as customary international law (UN, 1949a, 1949b, 1949c; Perrin, 2009).

Medically-related NGOs, such as the International Red Cross, Physicians for Human Rights and Médècins sans Frontières, though often focused on applying medical ethics in the context of armed conflict, are increasingly involved in monitoring, preventing, alleviating and even defining state violations of international humanitarian law including those related to restricting civilian, wounded and prisoner access to necessary health technologies (Rubenstein, 2009). Along with non-physician groups such as Amnesty International and Human Rights Watch, many of their members view themselves as being at the vanguard of a cosmopolitan world order normatively governed by both international humanitarian law and the UDHR. Many weapons of mass destruction and those with indiscriminate lethality, such as nuclear missiles, biological weapons, depleted uranium projectiles and bombs using nanoparticles as projectiles, are new technologies that are prohibited or restricted under IHL as having significant adverse health and environmental impacts.

Proving a breach of the Hippocratic Oath's ethical obligation to 'do no harm' was central to the conviction after the Second World War of the Nazi doctors at the Nuremberg Trials for non-consensual, sterilisation, active non-voluntary euthanasia and experimentation with new military technologies. Those proceedings spurred creation of a tripartite collection of documents that remain central to medical ethics: the Declaration of Geneva (or the modernised Hippocratic Oath); the Nuremberg Declaration on Human Experimentation; and the International Code of Medical Ethics (Nuremberg Code, 1946–9) (Annas, 2005). These international medical ethics documents can be viewed as synergistic with the tripartite international Bill of Human Rights: the contemporaneous UDHR, as well as the later ICCPR and the ICESCR. The former instruments were unambiguously directed at relationships between individuals, the latter chiefly with relations between individuals and states (UN, 1966a, 1966b).

Particularly overlapping with norms of medical ethics in the UDHR were provisions requiring respect for human dignity and equality (articles 1 and 2), as well as the human right to life (article 3). Others resembled components of medical ethics in prohibiting torture, or cruel, inhuman or degrading treatment or punishment (article 5); requiring non-discrimination (article 7); freedom from arbitrary interference with privacy (article 12); and progressive realisation of the human right to a standard of living adequate for health and medical care (article 25). In the same category was the human right to share in scientific advancement and its benefits (article 27) (UN, 1948).

Consent to medical treatment and experimentation is one area of explicit overlap between medical ethics and international human rights related to health technologies (Loff and Black, 2000). Article 7 of the ICCPR provides that 'no one shall be subjected without his free consent to medical or scientific experimentation' (UN, 1966a). Under general comment 20, the UN Human Rights Committee has interpreted this to require 'special protections' – for example, no institutionally nominated surrogate decision making – for persons 'under any form of detention or imprisonment', or those hospitalised on grounds of necessity or involuntarily due to mental illness (UN, 2000). It could extend also to the protection of patients from doctors who were institutionally prevented from providing such 'free consent', even where such physicians were not considered state agents.

HEALTH TECHNOLOGIES: OVERLAP BETWEEN BIOETHICS AND INTERNATIONAL HUMAN RIGHTS

Bioethics, overlapping with medical ethics, might usefully be described as involving the application of moral philosophy to ethical problems in the life sciences. Bioethics as an academic discipline that produces guidelines by groups of eminent persons is an important non-legal regulatory feature in areas of health technology use such as reproductive and end-of-life issues, biodiversity and environmental protection, as well as genetic testing, manipulation and data storage (Faunce, 2005). Its norms also attempt to regulate the conduct of scientific research, access to and quality and safety of medical devices, essential medicines and other preconditions for health (such as access to fresh air, water, fuel and food) that are increasingly dependent on the equitable use of new technologies (Harris, 2001).

Following the work of Rawls (Rawls, 1976) and Dworkin (Dworkin, 1977), many bioethicists endorse the view that principles of what is generally known as 'bioethics' arrived in liberal democracies like legal norms by a process of reflective equilibrium or coherence reasoning from foundational social virtues, such as distributive justice and fairness (Nussbaum, 1999). Influential jurisprudential scholars distrust such ideas as having uncertain and exploitable natural law elements (Kelsen, 1948). It is noticeable that until recently environmental sustainability was not placed in the same jurisprudential category of foundational societal virtues along with justice and equality.

Constitutional human rights and bioethics clearly overlap (UN, 1982; Annas, 2005). International human rights and bioethics do so in the regional European Convention on Human Rights and Biomedicine (CoE, 1997). While in force since 1997, the regulatory impact of this convention on health technology use has been commendable, despite limited ratification, the European Court of Human Rights having referred to, and taken into account, the Convention in dealing with the cases where countries that did not ratify or even sign it were involved (Nys, 2005). It covers matters such as equitable access to health care (article3); consent (chapter II); private life and right to information (chapter III); the human genome (chapter IV); scientific research (chapter V); and organ and tissue removal from living donors for transplantation (chapter VI).

There are now innumerable tribunals, both at national and regional levels, authoritatively interpreting norms of medical and bioethics at least partially in terms of international civil and political human rights. These include the English Court of Appeal and House of Lords, as well as the European Court of Human Rights. In the *Case of D v United Kingdom*, for example, the European Court of Human Rights held that deportation of an HIV/AIDS infected patient to his developing country of origin was state conduct which violated his human right to be protected from inhuman or degrading treatment or punishment. The judges reasoned that such deportation would result in his being denied adequate medical treatment and exposed to poor public health conditions including inadequate access to necessary medicines and medical services (*D v UK*, 1997).

In many other jurisdictions around the world cases concerning access to and cost effectiveness assessment of new reproductive technologies, end-of-life decisions, privacy, and informed consent are now heavily influenced by international civil and political human rights norms, either because of parliamentary or judicial incorporation of human rights into domestic law, or to remedy a common law lacuna, or legislative ambiguity or obscurity.

THE INTERNATIONAL RIGHT TO HEALTH AND EMERGING TECHNOLOGIES

Article 12 of the ICESCR importantly in this context created an international right to health, legally binding upon those parties who have ratified it. An influential analysis has characterised this as involving core obligations to provide the basic preconditions for existence, including food, water, fuel, sanitation, housing, reasonable access to essential health services and products as well as (although not as much discussed) capacity to live in a non-toxic environment (Toebes, 1999; UN General Comment 14, 2000). In 2001, Kinney proposed three approaches to the implementation of the international human right to health: (1) define universal outcome measures that measure compliance with the core state obligations of the human right to health; (2) establish systematic reporting to responsible international bodies to monitor progress on implementation and compliance with international human rights obligations; and (3) highlight civil rights violations, such as discrimination against protected groups that inhibit access to health care services (Kinney, 2001). A UN special rapporteur has reported on these issues (Hunt and Backman, 2009).

The human right to health, particularly in domestic constitutions, has often been interpreted as a largely symbolic, non-enforceable individually, progressively realisable concession to normative decency or attempt to claim political legitimacy. Technical and financial, as well as conceptual limitations, currently prevent it involving a justiciable guarantee for each person of a minimum level of actual health. Progressive realisation of such a right requires effective use of available resources. The minimum content of this core, which cannot be set aside on grounds of progressive realisation, may be conceptualised as a responsibility to reduce serious threats to the health of individuals, or the state's population, according to international standards.

Effective state infectious disease control may be a compelling and justiciable minimum core public health component of the right to health utilising health techonologies. This may allow legally prescribed, non-discriminatory, proportional and least necessary restricions on international civil and political human rights, such as freedom of movement, freedom of thought, conscience or religion, freedom of expression, peaceful assembly and freedom of association. Courts have been prepared to use the right to health in domestic constitutions to make states provide basic treatment to HIV/AIDS patients (CCC, 1992; *Velasquez Rodriguez v Honduras 1988*). In 2002, the South African Constitutional Court (*Minister of Health v Treatment Action Campaign,* 2002) unanimously found the government in breach of ss 27(1) ('right of access to health care services') and 27(2) ('progressive realisation') concerned with the right to health in that Constitution. It held that the government's policy of restricting the anti-HIV drug 'nevirapine' to 18 sites was unreasonably rigid and inflexible, denying babies of HIV-infected mothers outside those sites a potentially life-saving therapy. The court took note of the fact that the drug was apparently affordable, easy to administer and recommended by the WHO (Ngwena, 2003).

In considering the normative intersections between health care ethics, human and environmental rights in an area such as the research, development and use of emerging technologies is important to take into account article 38 of the *Statute of the International Court of Justice* (UN, 1945). This provision identifies international conventions and customary international law, among others, as the sources of international law. Thus, as a declaration, rather than an international convention, the UDHR did not directly create binding human rights norms under international law upon signatory states. Neither did UNESCO's Universal Declaration on the Human Genome and Human Rights and Universal Declaration on Bioethics and Human Rights. The former text pronounces that the human genome represents part of the common heritage of humanity, while forbidding practices contrary to human dignity, such as human reproductive cloning. The latter instrument, though also non-binding under international law, arguably provides, if not certainly a codification, then a promotion of bioethical norms onto the global stage. Particularly important, as we'll see, are norms of technology transfer, benefit sharing and social responsibility in relation to essential medicines that specifically apply to corporations (Kinley and Chambers 2006; Faunce, 2007). Article 14 of the Universal Declaration on Bioethics and Human Rights provides:

2. Taking into account that the enjoyment of the highest attainable standard of health is one of the fundamental rights of every human being without distinction of race, religion, political belief and economic, or social condition, progress in science and technology should advance:

   (a) access to quality health care and essential medicines, especially for the health of women and children, because health is essential to life itself and must be considered to be a social and human good;
   (b) access to adequate nutrition and water;
   (c) improvement of living conditions and the environment;
   (d) elimination of the marginalisation and the exclusion of persons on the basis of any grounds;
   (e) reduction of poverty and illiteracy.

Article 15 – Sharing of benefits provides:

1. Benefits resulting from any scientific research and its applications should be shared with society as a whole and within the international community, in particular with developing countries. In giving effect to this principle, benefits may take any of the following forms:

   (a) special and sustainable assistance to, and acknowledgement of, the persons and groups that have taken part in the research;
   (b) access to quality health care;
   (c) provision of new diagnostic and therapeutic modalities or products stemming from research;
   (d) support for health services;
   (e) access to scientific and technological knowledge;
   (f) capacity-building facilities for research purposes;
   (g) other forms of benefit consistent with the principles set out in this Declaration.

2. Benefits should not constitute improper inducements to participate in research.

EMERGING TECHNOLOGIES: GLOBAL TRADE LAW'S INFLUENCE ON HEALTH ETHICS AND RIGHTS

Since the 1990s in particular, the WTO has been able to create a politically influential, profit-driven global corporate agenda for global governance in health care policy with no explicit requirement to consider norms of international human rights or healthcare ethics concerning trade in health technologies. Multilateral trade agreements, such as GATS and TRIPS, have been influential in this process (Abbott, 2004, 2005).

A state can now elect, as for example have many OECD countries, to place 'hospital services' on its 'schedule of commitments' to be covered by the 'liberalising' rules of GATS. This executive action (often no specific parliamentary scrutiny or democratic mandate was necessary) facilitated a reorganisation of ownership and management of public hospitals on a 'for fee' insurance-oriented model. Under the GATS 'market access' requirement, subsequent (more public goods-minded) governments would be hindered from legislating to regulate the total number or market share of foreign private health care services or suppliers. This has a significant impact on access to the many emerging medical technologies that can only be delivered in hospitals.

The GATS rule of 'national treatment' requires that such a 'liberalising' government could not provide, even unintentionally, more favourable conditions to domestic health care companies than to foreign corporations. The most favoured nation (MFN) rule obligates such administrations to also ensure that the most favourable treatment, in terms of trade, granted to any foreign company was extended to all foreign companies wishing to enter this 'liberalised' sector. The 'domestic regulation' rule likewise makes domestic laws and regulations, including those which protected the public's health and safety (for example, by applying the precautionary principle to restrict marketing of certain new health technologies) subject to challenge and possible elimination if they were determined to be 'unnecessary barriers' to trade, or more 'burdensome than necessary' to assure the quality of a service.

The WTO TRIPS agreement created a revolutionary process of influencing the way states balance public and private intellectual property rights (IPRs) (also now termed intellectual monopoly privileges (IMPs) and societal obligations. This can be seen, for example in its express exceptions to IMP protections over pharmaceuticals, such as compulsory licensing by governments for generic manufacture of medicines (after payment of reasonable compensation to any patent holder) if such medicines were required to be cheaper and more readily available for public health reasons. A public health exception was also allowed in this context for the so-called 'data exclusivity' requirement that otherwise undisclosed pharmaceutical data (revealed to regulators for safety and quality marketing approval) be protected from unfair commercial use or disclosure. Agreed transitional periods postponed full TRIPS obligations for the poorest countries (Sell, 2003).

Yet TRIPS can be viewed as formalising and balancing public knowledge goods generated in the intellectual commons (of, for example publicly funded universities) to deal rationally with the global burden of disease in accord with core components of the international human right to health. This 'ethical' interpretation is supported by the 2001 TRIPS clarification known as the Doha Declaration on TRIPS and Public Health. This declaration affirmed the capacity of WTO members to use the full exceptions in the TRIPS agreement to promote public health by facilitating access to affordable medicines (Gathii, 2002; Abbott, 2005). On 6 December 2006, the WTO also passed a Protocol to amend the TRIPS agreement to enhance the capacity of a state to issue a compulsory licence to provide citizens with cheap access to a medicine essential to public health, even when that country itself lacked manufacturing capacity. Yet the United States Trade Representative (USTR) continues to lobby vigorously against countries such as Thailand and Brazil when they attempt to issue compulsory licenses to facilitate access to essential medicines (Correa, 2002; Abbott, 2004).

Bilateral preferential trade agreements have additionally facilitated the plans of multinational pharmaceutical and managed care corporations to exploit 'liberalised' markets and challenge universalist (taxpayer-funded and egalitarian) domestic health and medicines policies, often on the grounds that they create non-tariff trade barriers, or insufficiently reward health technology 'innovation' defined either in relation to competitive markets (presumably with strong anti-trust laws) or by regulatory systems which scientifically evaluate evidence of objectively demonstrated therapeutic significance (Sell, 2003; Faunce, 2007).

As credible data accumulates, however, it will no longer be acceptable in health policy debates to rationalise widespread deaths among increasing numbers of poor, uninsured patients and those who cannot obtain access to essential medicines or other valuable new health technologies (because of fiercely protected patents or lack of corporate R&D interest in that area) as temporary market failures or 'adjustments' (Holmer et al., 2000; Weissbrodt and Kruger, 2005).

Norms of international human rights, bioethics, medical and environmental ethics are likely to play important roles in developing any new global social contract emerging from such a debate. They might combine, for example, to support the concept of global public goods. These could be defined, not in traditional economic terms, but as providing benefits from which no individual or ecosystem should be excluded (on criteria of global health care ethics or international human rights), spanning national, cultural and generational boundaries. Examples could include emerging technologies facilitating clean air, equitable access to food and energy, peaceful societies, control of communicable disease, transport and law and order infrastructure, as well as sustainable ecosystems. Related global public goods will require international cooperation for their production.

One example could be a treaty (or a WTO-WHO agreement) for rewarding (with sustainable levels of government reimbursement), medicines and medical device 'health innovation' established through internationally harmonised, independent expert assessment of scientific evidence about safety, quality, efficacy and cost-effectiveness, funded by a tax on global financial transactions (Faunce, 2010a). The treaty or administrative scheme creating such a post-market state global regulatory system would list the principles underpinning such assessments. Protecting whistleblowers who provide information about corporate fraud will be an important point of normative intersection between ethics and law in this context. (Laing et al., 2003; Faunce, 2004).

International human rights in general and in relation to new health technologies itself undoubtedly remains highly suspect, particularly in Islamic societies, for its lack of connection with religious law as expressed in the *Quaran* or *Sunna* (Abdullahi Ahmed, 2005). In such societies, norms of international human rights are consistently qualified by *shari'a*-based Islamic criteria and by suspicions that the primary norm-creating bodies in international human rights are dominated by the representatives of developed, northern countries or large corporations with alien social values. Health care ethics may create an important normative bridge in such settings about intense future debates over access to emerging technologies related to access to cheap sources of fuel and food as well as medicines.

Particular challenges for global health care ethics and human rights in the era of globalisation will be the million or so women and girls under 18 trafficked annually for prostitution; the 10 million refugees; or five million internally displaced persons, the victims of any one of the 35 or so wars currently raging across the earth; of state-promoted torture or rape in the guise of 'ethnic cleansing'; or any of the 250 million children exploited for labour, sexual gratification or as soldiers. This in addition to the 1.2 billion people living in severe poverty, without adequate obstetric care, food, safe water or sanitation (Wilson, 2009). Gender discrimination, poverty, famine and displacement by warfare are significant factors in large numbers of children in African countries still failing to receive basic information from health professionals about how to avoid infection with HIV/AIDS, despite often over 20 per cent of the population being seropositive (Fidler, 1998). Yet equally important with considerations about justice and equity in the jurisprudence of health care techonologies should be the development of hard legal norms related to environmental sustainability. It has been argued here that principles and rules governing the research, development and transfer of new technologies will be particularly important in this context.

When sixty three experts, for example, were asked to specify which aspects of nanotechnology could most assist the developing world, the nanotechnologies cited as likely to be important in this context were nanomembranes for water purification, desalination and detoxification, nanosensors for the detection of contaminants and pathogens, nanoporous zeolites, polymers and attapulgite clays for water purification, magnetic nanoparticles for water treatment and remediation and $TiO2$ nanoparticles for the catalytic degradation of water pollutants (Salamanca-Buentello F et al, 2005). Health-related global research efforts such as that involved with artificial photosynthesis will also be important (Faunce, 2010a).

Both international human rights and global health care ethics carry the promise of enlarging the objects of human sympathy and so the applicable range of foundational virtues, principles and rules available to decision makers. But even more than this, foundational environmental virtues, such as 'sustainability' and 'solidarity with endangered species and habitats' respecting the Earth itself as a self-sustaining entity, must now begin in academic and policy discourse to take their place alongside 'justice' and 'equality' in health care debates about the wise use of emerging technologies.

REFERENCES

Abbott, F.M. (2004) *The Doha Declaration on the TRIPS Agreement and Public Health and the Contradictory Trend in Bilateral and Regional Free Trade Agreements*, Working Paper No. 14. New York: Quaker United Nations Office.

Abbott, F.M. (2005) 'The WTO medicines decision: World pharmaceutical trade and the protection of public health', *American Journal of International Law*, 99: 317–56.

Abdullahi Ahmed, A. (2005) 'Human rights in the Muslim world', *Harvard Human Rights Journal*, 3: 13–52.

Annas, G.J. (2005) *American Bioethics. Crossing Human Rights and Health Law Boundaries*. New York: Oxford University Press.

Ayres, R.U. (2008) Sustainability Economics. Where do we stand? Ecological Economics, 67(2): 281–310.

Beauchamp, T.L. (1995) 'Principlism and its alleged competitors', *Kennedy Institute of Ethics*, 5: 181–98.

Borden, E.C. (1967) 'John Locke, physician and author of the first Carolina constitution', *Southern Medical Journal*, 60: 283–8.

Braveman, P. and Gruskin, S. (2003) 'Poverty, equity, human rights and health', *Bulletin of the World Health Organisation*, 81: 539–45.

Brugger, W. (1996) 'The Image of the person in the human rights concept', *Human Rights Quarterly*, 18 (3): 594–600.

Buchanan, A. and Decamp, M. (2006) 'Responsibility for global health', *Theoretical Medicine and Bioethics*, 27: 95–114.

Chapman, A.R. (2002) 'The human rights implications of intellectual property protection', *Journal of International Economic Law*, 5: 861–82.

Claude, R.P. and Issel, B.W. (1998) 'Health, medicine and science in the Universal Declaration of Human Rights', *Health and Human Rights*, 3 (2): 127–31.

Columbian Constitutional Court (CCC) (1992) *Judgment No T–505, 28 August 1992* in 21 *Revista Mensual Jurisprudencia Doctrina* 1101.

Correa, C. (2002) *Implications of the Doha Declaration on the TRIPS Agreement and Public Health*. Geneva: World Health Organisation.

Council of Europe (CoE) (1997) 'Convention for the protection of human rights and the dignity of human beings with regard to the application of biology and medicine', ETS No. 164.

D v United Kingdom, European Court of Human Rights, 2 May 1997.

Daly H. E. (1990) 'Toward Some Operational Principles of Sustainable Development', *Ecological Economics*, 2: 1–6.

Davey L. M. (2001) 'The oath of Hippocrates: an historical review', *Neurosurgery*, 49:554–66.

Dewhurst, K. (1995) 'Sydenham's letters to John Locke', *The Practitioner*, 175: 314–24.

Dworkin, R. (1977) *Taking Rights Seriously*. London: Duckworth, p. 184.

Faunce, T.A. (2004) 'Developing and teaching the virtue-ethics foundations of healthcare whistle blowing', *Monash Bioethics Review*, 23 (4): 41–55.

Faunce, T.A. (2005) 'Will international human rights subsume medical ethics? Intersections in the UNESCO Universal Bioethics Declaration', *Journal of Medical Ethics*, 31: 173–8.

Faunce, T.A. (2007) *Who Owns Our Health? Medical Professionalism, Law and Leadership beyond the Age of the Market State*. Sydney: University of New South Wales Press/Baltimore, MD: Johns Hopkins University Press.

Faunce, T.A. (2010a) 'Innovation and insufficient evidence: The case for a WTO–WHO agreement on health technology safety and cost-effectiveness evaluation', in T. Pogge, M. Rimmer and K. Rubenstein (eds), *Incentives for Global Public Health*. Cambridge: Cambridge University Press, pp. 209–32.

Faunce, T.A. (2010b) 'Regulating plasmonic solar cells and artificial photosynthesis for sustainable energy', Nanotechnology for Sustainable Energy Conference, European Science Foundation, Obergurgl, Austria, 7 July.

Fidler, D.P. (1998) 'Microbialpolitik: Infectious diseases and international relations', *American University International Law Review*, 14: 1–11.

Gathii, J.T. (2002) 'The legal status of the Doha Declaration on TRIPS and public health under the Vienna Convention on the Law of Treaties', *Harvard Journal of Law and Technology*, 15 (2): 291–317.

Harris, J. (2001) *Bioethics*. Oxford: Oxford University Press, pp. 1–4.

Hart, H.L.A. (1979) 'Unitarianism and natural rights', *Tulane Law Review*, 53: 663–80.

Holmer, A.F., Reif, M.C., Schwarting, J.S., Bohrer, R.A., Hayes, T.A., Rightor, N. et al. (2000) 'The pharmaceutical industry – To whom is it accountable?', *New England Journal of Medicine*, 343 : 1415–17.

Hunt, P. and Backman, C. (2009) 'Health systems and the right to the highest attainable standard of health', in A. Clapham, M. Robinson, C. Mahon and S. Jerbi (eds), *Realizing the Right to Health*. Zurich: Ruffer & Rub, pp. 40–59.

Jonsen, A.R. (2000) *A Short History of Medical Ethics*. New York: Oxford University Press.

Kelsen, H. (1948) 'Absolutism and relativism in philosophy and politics', *American Political Science Review*, 42: 906–1002.

Kinley, D. and Chambers, R. (2006) 'The UN human rights norms for corporations: The private implications of public international law', *Human Rights Law Review*, 6: 447–97.

Kinney, E.D. (2001) 'The international human right to health: What does this mean for our nation and world?', *Indiana Law Review*, 34: 1457–68.

Laing, R., Waning, B., Gray, A., Ford, N. and 't Hoen, E. (2003) '25 Years of WHO essential medicines list: Progress and challenges', *The Lancet*, 361: 1723–9.

Loff, B. and Black, J. (2000) 'The Declaration of Helsinki and research in vulnerable populations', *Medical Journal of Australia*, 172: 292–5.

Minister of Health v Treatment Action Campaign, South African Constitutional Court (2002) Case CCT 8/02.

Ngwena, C. (2003) 'Access to health care services as a justiciable socio-economic right under the South African Constitution', *Medical Law International*, 6: 13–23.

Nuremberg Code (1946–9), in *Trials of war criminals before the Nuremberg Military Tribunals under Control Council Law No10*, Nuremberg: Oct 1946–Apr 1949.

Nussbaum, M. (1999) 'Virtue ethics: A misleading category', *Journal of Ethics*, 3: 163–201.

Nys, H. (2005) 'Towards an international treaty on human rights and biomedicine? Some reflections inspired by UNESCO's universal declaration on bioethics and human rights', *European Journal of Health Law*, 13: 5–8.

Oppenheimer, G.M., Bayer, R. and Colgrove, J. (2002) 'Health and human rights: Old wine in new bottle', *Journal of Law, Medicine and Ethics*, 30: 522–32.

Pellegrino, E.D. (1995) 'Toward a virtue based normative ethics for the health professions', *Kennedy Institute of Ethics Journal*, 5: 253–77.

Perrin, P. (2009) 'The right to health in armed conflict', in A. Clapham, M. Robinson, C. Mahon and S. Jerbi (eds), *Realizing the Right to Health*. Zurich: Ruffer & Rub, pp. 157–72.

Rawls, J. (1976) *A Theory of Justice*. Oxford: Oxford University Press.

Raz, J. (1984) 'The nature of rights', *Mind*, 93: 194–201.

Rubenstein, L.S. (2009) 'Physicians and the right to health', in A. Clapham, M. Robinson, C. Mahon and S. Jerbi (eds), *Realizing the Right to Health*. Zurich: Ruffer & Rub, pp. 381–92.

Salamanca-Buentello, F., Persad, D.L., Court, E.B., Martin, D.K., Daar, A.S., et al. (2005) Nanotechnology and the Developing World. PLoS Med., 2:e97.

Sell, S.K. (2003) *Private Power, Public Law. The Globalisation of Intellectual Property Rights*. Cambridge: Cambridge University Press, p. 83.

Sen, A. (2002) 'Why health equity?', *Health Economics*, 11: 659–66.

Taylor, A.L. (2004) 'Governing the globalization of public health', *Journal of Law, Medicine and Ethics*, 32: 500–8.

Toebes, B. (2009) 'Towards an improved understanding of the international human right to health', *Human Rights Quarterly*, 21: 661–79 at 671.

United Nations (UN) (1945) *United Nations statute of the International Court of Justice*. UN Treaty Series, 1: xvi.

United Nations (UN) (1948) *Universal declaration of human rights,* adopted 10 Dec 1948. GA Res 217A (III). UN doc A/810 71.

United Nations (UN) (1949a) *Convention for the amelioration of the condition of the wounded and sick in armed forces in the field*. UN Treaty Series, 75: 31.

United Nations (UN) (1949b) *Convention relative to the protection of civilian persons in time of war*. UN Treaty Series, 75: 287.

United Nations (UN) (1949c) *Convention relative to the treatment of prisoners of war*. UN Treaty Series, 75: 135.

United Nations (UN) (1966a) *International covenant on civil and political rights*, adopted 16 Dec 1966, entry into force 23 March 1976. GA Res 2200A (XXI). UN GAOR supp (no 16) 52. UN doc A/6316 (1966). UN Treaty Series, 999: 17.

United Nations (UN) (1966b) *International covenant on economic, cultural and social rights*, adopted 16 Dec 1966, entry into force 3 Jan 1976. GA Res 2200A(XXI). UN Doc A/6316 (1966). UN Treaty Series, 993: 3.

United Nations (UN) (1982) *Principles of medical ethics relevant to the role of health personnel, particularly physicians, in the protection of prisoners and detainees against torture and other cruel, inhuman or degrading treatment or punishment*. GA Res. 37/194 of 18 Dec 1982.

United Nations (UN) (2000) Committee on Economic, Social and Cultural Rights, *General Comment No 14 on the right to the highest attainable standard of health in Article 12 ICECSR* e/C.12/2000/4 11/08/2000.

Velasquez Rodriguez v Honduras, Inter American Court of Human Rights Judgment, 29 July 1988, (Ser C) (No. 4).

Weissbrodt, D. and Kruger, M. (2005) 'Human rights responsibilities of business as non-state actors', in P. Alston (ed.), *Non-state Actors and Human Rights*. Oxford: Oxford University Press, pp. 315–50.

Wilson, B. (2009) 'Social determinants of health from a rights-based approach', in A. Clapham, M. Robinson, C. Mahon and S. Jerbi (eds), *Realizing the Right to Health*. Zurich: Ruffer & Rub, pp. 60–79.

WTO (2005) Report of the Panel, *United States – Measures Affecting the Cross-border Supply of Gambling and Betting Services*. WT/DS285/R adopted 20 April 2005, para 6.465.

6

Professional Codes

Michael Davis

INTRODUCTION

A professional code is a set of ethical rules or similar standards (usually written) governing members of a profession just because they are members of that profession. Professional codes are distinct from codes of organizational ethics, such as those that apply to employees of a business or members of a scientific or technical society. They are also distinct from codes of ethics that apply to participants in an 'institution', that is, an organized location in which several professions or occupations work together, such as a hospital or research laboratory. Among other names for professional code are: code of professional conduct; rules of professional responsibility; canons of professional ethics; principles of professional practice; and professional guidelines. What matters is not the exact name the rules go by but what their content and relation are to a profession. To explain what a professional code is requires explaining three terms: code, ethics, and profession. Explaining these terms will clarify the importance of professional codes in health-care ethics. (For those concerned with writing a code of ethics for a profession, organization, or institution, see Davis, 2007, especially the extensive references.)

CODE

The word 'code' comes from Latin. Originally, it referred to any wooden board, then to boards covered with wax used to write on, and then to any book ('codex' rather than scroll). That was the sense it had when first applied to the book-length systemization of Roman statutes that the Emperor Justinian enacted in AD 529. Justinian's Code differed from an ordinary digest or other compilation of law in one important way: he had the legal authority to make his compilation law, replacing all that preceded it. Codes always pre-empt (or, at least, are supposed to pre-empt) what they codify.

Justinian's Code was itself part of a larger codification. Along with the Code, Justinian eventually enacted: the Digest, a systematic editing down of Roman jurisprudence (learned opinion); the Institutes, a textbook intended for use in the Empire's law schools; and the Novels, statutes too new to be included in the Code. These documents, known collectively as the Corpus Juris Civilis, replaced the statutes, jurisprudence, and legal textbooks that preceded them. The Corpus Juris Civilis soon became, and remained until a century or two ago, the dominant legal document throughout most of Europe, its terms familiar to most educated people.

For many centuries now, anything sufficiently like the Corpus Juris Civilis, or one of its parts, could (informatively) be called 'a code'. Sometimes the analogy with the Corpus is quite close, as it is, for example in the Code Napoleon or the Illinois Criminal Code. A spy's 'secret code' (cipher) is a code in a more distant sense. While a spy's code is an authoritative system of written rules (and thus resembles law), the rules concern only converting one set of symbols into another (ciphering and deciphering). 'Computer code' is code in an even more distant sense: computer code resembles the seeming nonsense that spies write.

We can see the influence of Justinian on early work in medical ethics. Consider, for example Thomas Percival's (1803) classic *Medical Ethics*. Its subtitle is *A Code of Institutes and Precepts, Adapted to the Professional Conduct of Physicians and Surgeons*. The expression 'Code of Institutes' is not a mere odd choice of words. Percival was working with Justinian clearly in mind. His Preface actually concludes: 'According to the definition of Justinian, however, Jurisprudence may be understood to include moral injunctions as well as positive ordinances' (Percival, 1803: 7). Percival's subtitle was, it seems, intended to tell readers that he was not publishing a code (strictly so called), that is, an authoritative systemization (a systemization with the force of law or something similar). His purpose was to teach rather than legislate; hence, his subtitle's use of 'institutes' and 'precepts' rather than, say, 'laws', 'regulations', or 'duties'. What he published was a 'code' only in an extended sense, a systematic treatment (much like Justinian's Institutes).

There is other evidence for this way of understanding *Medical Ethics*. Percival's Preface tells us that the original title was *Medical Jurisprudence* (suggesting a series of opinions concerning the interpretation of rules governing the practice of medicine). He substituted 'ethics' for 'jurisprudence' because his early readers (many of whom were physicians or surgeons) suggested the substitution. Why they suggested the substitution is not clear. But one scholar has pointed out that, even three centuries before Percival, English physicians often described as 'ethical rules' any regulation specifically concerned with the conduct of their vocation. Whatever the reason for their suggestion, *Medical Ethics*, a text of over 200 pages, is in fact at least as much about law and custom governing medical practice in England as about what we would now call medical ethics. Its nearest relative in today's bookstore is probably the 'how to' book, and not the American Medical Association's (AMA) *Code of Ethics*.

Because Percival lacked the authority to enact rules governing all the physicians and surgeons of England, *Medical Ethics* cannot be a code (strictly speaking). Whether the physicians and surgeons of England could, by adopting the rules of *Medical Ethics*, have legislated the first code of professional ethics is a question we must postpone until we have defined 'ethics' and 'profession'.

Have we been too quick? Could Percival have written a code by putting an unwritten code into writing? That is a question of how far to stretch the analogy with Justinian's Code. There are at least three ways a code might be 'unwritten'. First, the code might have an authoritative but oral form. A code unwritten in this sense is virtually a code, strictly speaking. Anyone who knew it, and how to write, could write it out, and the written form would always be (more or less) the same.

The medical ethics of Percival's time seems not to have been unwritten either in this way, or in a second way rules can be unwritten. This second is the way that the definition of a new word may be 'unwritten' until someone writes it down. The definer has only to write out the (correct) definition for (almost) everyone to recognize it as the one implicitly being followed all along. Though more inventive than the scribe's transcription of the spoken formulation, this sort of writing down of what was before unwritten looks inevitable in retrospect. The disputes of Percival's time suggest that much of medical ethics was not then just waiting to be written down, even in this way. Some of Percival's 'positive ordinances' were controversial.

The last way in which a code might be 'unwritten' is the way in which the English constitution is 'unwritten'. In fact, most of the English constitution, either official (such as Parliamentary statutes) or unofficial (such as learned commentaries), is in writing. The reason the constitution is nevertheless unwritten is that there is no authoritative formulation of it (no codification – as there is of the US or French constitution). There is not even the possibility of an authoritative formulation without considerable negotiation. The English can (and do) disagree about the wording of their constitution (and even which documents are in it). They must offer a construction of its terms whenever they undertake to interpret it.

Before Percival published *Medical Ethics*, medical ethics had no authoritative formulation. After he published, there still was none. Since the point of codification (strictly speaking) is to give law (and, by analogy, any similar system of guidance) an authoritative formulation, a code without an authoritative formulation would seem to be no code at all (or, at best, a possible code). Any code, including any code of professional ethics, must have an authoritative formulation (oral if not written). *Medical Ethics* was not such an authoritative formulation, though it was an important step toward one. Hence, *Medical Ethics* is not a professional code.

ETHICS

Was *Medical Ethics* nonetheless 'ethics'? That depends on what is meant by 'ethics'. Ethics has at least five senses in ordinary English. In one, it is a mere synonym for ordinary morality, those universal standards of conduct that apply to moral agents simply because they are moral agents ('Don't lie', 'Don't cheat', 'Help the needy', and so on). Etymology fully justifies this first sense. The root for 'ethics' (*ēthos*) is the Greek word for habit or character; the root of 'morality' (*mores*) is the Latin word for much the same idea (one's usual way of behaving). Etymologically, ethics and morality are almost twins (as are 'ethic' and 'morale', 'etiquette' and 'petty morals', and even *'ethos'* and *'mores'*).

Ethics in this sense does not apply to members of a profession simply because of that membership.

In four other senses of the word, ethics is contrasted with morality. In one, ethics is said to consist of those standards of conduct that moral agents should follow (what is sometimes also called 'critical morality'). Morality, in contrast, is said to consist of those standards that moral agents generally do follow (what is also sometimes called 'positive morality'). Morality in this sense is very close to its root, *mores*; it can be unethical (in our first sense of 'ethics'). What people believe is morally right (slavery, forced female circumcision, or the like) – morality in this second sense – can be morally wrong in the first sense. Morality (in this second sense) has a plural; each society or group can have its own moral standard; indeed, even each individual can have his or her own. There can be as many moralities as there are moral agents. Even so, ethics remains a standard common to everyone (or, at least, may be such a standard, depending on how we interpret 'critical morality'). Hence, this second sense of 'ethics' is as irrelevant to professional codes as the first.

Ethics is sometimes contrasted with morality in another way. Morality then consists of those standards every moral agent should follow. Morality is a universal minimum, our standard of moral right and wrong. Ethics, in contrast, is concerned with moral good, with whatever is beyond the moral minimum. Ethics (in this sense) is whatever is left over of morality in our first – universal – sense (which includes both the right and the good) once we subtract morality in this third – minimum – sense (which includes only the right). There are two reasons to dismiss this sense of 'ethics' here. First, this ethics of the good is still universal, applying outside the professions as well as within. A profession's ethics, we agreed, applies within the profession, not outside. Second (as we shall see), professional ethics consists at least in part of moral requirements, the right way to conduct one's profession (as in the AMA code) rather than just a good way. Any sense of 'ethics' that does not include the right cannot be the sense relevant to professional ethics.

The second sense of ethics (critical morality) is closely related to the fourth, a field of philosophy. When a course in 'ethics' is offered by philosophers, its subject is various attempts to understand morality (all or part of morality in our first sense) as a rational undertaking (something we should, or at least may reasonably, participate in). Philosophers do not teach morality (in our first, second, or third sense of 'morality') – except perhaps by inadvertence. They also generally do not teach critical morality, though the attempt to understand morality as a rational undertaking should lead students to dismiss some parts of morality (in its second, descriptive, sense) as irrational or to feel more committed to morality (in its first or third sense) because they can now see the point of it. Since a professional code, whatever it is, is not philosophy, we may dismiss this fourth sense of 'ethics' just as we did the preceding three.

'Ethics' can be used in a fifth sense, to refer to those morally permissible standards of conduct governing members of a group simply because of that membership. In this sense (an innovation of the last two centuries), research ethics is for people in research and no one else; nursing ethics, for nurses and for no one else; and so on. Ethics – in this sense – is relative even though morality is not. It resembles law and custom, which can also vary from place to place or group to group. But ethics (in this sense) is not mere law, custom, or mores. Ethics must at least be morally permissible. There can be no thieves' ethics or Nazi ethics, except with quotes around 'ethics' to indicate a mere analogical or perverted use.

Because the term 'govern' may indicate either an achievement (the standards are in fact generally followed) or the mere intent that they be followed (or belief that they should be followed), we may distinguish between actual ethics and ideal ethics (in this fifth sense). Actual ethics are those ethical standards members of the group generally follow, generally use to defend or criticize relevant conduct, and otherwise generally endorse through practice. Ideal ethics are standards that members of the relevant group can recognize as what they would be willing to follow if everyone else in the group (generally) did the same. They are mere ideal standards when they are not part of actual practice. An ideal code of ethics is a possible or model code; an actual code of ethics, a living practice (as well as an ideal one).

This fifth sense of 'ethics' is, I think, the one implicit in the subtitle of Percival's *Medical Ethics* (*Adapted to the Professional Conduct of Physicians and Surgeons*). He has, it implies, done something more than repeat general standards or apply them to medical practice. He has adapted them to the special circumstances of physicians and surgeons. They are, in this respect, special standards ('positive enactments', as he says). The standards are nonetheless (more or less) ideal; Percival was trying to change practice, not just systematize it.

This fifth sense also seems implicit in the claim that a profession has a code of ethics distinct both from ordinary morality and from the code of any other profession. The reason why professions claim this should be clear once 'profession' is explained.

PROFESSION

'Profession' resembles 'ethics' in having several legitimate senses. Profession can, first, be used as a mere synonym for 'vocation' (or 'calling'), that is, any useful activity to which one devotes (and perhaps feels called to devote) much of one's life, even if one derives no income from doing so (or, at least, does not engage in it even in part for the income). If the activity were not useful, it would be a hobby rather than a vocation. In this sense of profession, even a gentleman (in the sense of 'gentleman' still current decades after publication of Percival's *Medical Ethics*) could have a profession, even if only private charity or public service. The opposite of profession in this sense is a trade (or other 'mere money-making calling').

Profession can also be a synonym for occupation, that is, any typically full-time activity defined in part by a 'discipline' (an easily recognizable body of knowledge, skill, and judgment) by which its practitioners generally earn a living. In this sense, we may, without irony, speak of someone being a 'professional thief' or 'professional athlete'. The opposite of 'professional' in this sense is 'amateur' (one who engages in the activity 'for love', not to earn a living).

Profession can, instead, be used for any occupation one may openly admit to or profess, that is, an honest occupation: While athletics can be a profession in this sense, neither thieving nor being a gentleman can be. Thieving cannot because it is dishonest; being a gentleman cannot because, though an honest way of life, it is not a way to earn a living. This has, I think, been the primary sense of 'profession' outside English-speaking countries until quite recently. It certainly is the sense it had, for example, when Durkheim and Weber wrote about professions early in the twentieth century (making their writing on 'professions' more or less irrelevant to understanding professions in the following sense).

Profession can also be used for a special kind of honest occupation. There are at least two approaches to defining this sense of 'profession'. One approach, what we may call 'the sociological', has its origin in the social sciences. Its language tends to be statistical, that is, the definition does not purport to state necessary or sufficient conditions for an occupation being a profession but merely what is true of 'most professions', 'the most important professions', or the like. Generally, sociological definitions understand a profession to be any occupation whose practitioners have high social status, high income, advanced education, important social function, or some combination of these or other features easy for the social sciences to measure.

For social scientists, there is no important distinction between what used to be called 'the liberal professions' (those few honest vocations requiring a university degree in most of early modern Europe) and today's professions (strictly so called). Carpentry cannot be a profession (in the sociological sense) because both the social status and education of carpenters are too low. Medicine certainly is a profession (in this sense) because physicians have relatively high status, high income, advanced education, and important social functions. Business managers also form a profession (in this sense) because they too tend to have high income, high status, advanced education, and an important social function. Nurses may only be 'quasi-professionals' because their income and social status are too low. For most sociologists, it is obvious that Europe and the Americas have had professions for many centuries.

Refuting a sociological definition is not easy. Because its claims are stated in terms of 'most', a few counter-examples do not threaten it. When the counter-examples seem to grow more numerous than the professions fitting the definition, the defenders of a sociological definition can distinguish between 'true professions', 'fully developed professions', or the like and those not fitting the definition ('pseudo-professions', 'quasi-professions', and so on). The only professions that seem to appear on every sociologist's list of 'true' or 'fully developed' professions are law and medicine.

The other approach to defining 'profession' is philosophical. A philosophical definition attempts to state necessary and sufficient conditions for some group to count as a profession. While a philosophical definition may leave the status of a small number of would-be professions unsettled, it should at least be able to explain (in a satisfying way) why those would-be professions are neither clearly professions nor clearly not professions. A definition covering 'most professions' is not good enough.

Philosophical definitions may be developed in one of (at least) two ways: the 'Cartesian' and the 'Socratic' (as we may call them). The Cartesian way tries to make sense of the contents of one person's mind. One develops a definition by asking oneself what one means by a certain term, setting out that meaning in a definition, testing the definition by counter-examples and other considerations, revising whenever a counter-example or other consideration seems to reveal a flaw, and continuing that process until one has put one's beliefs in good order.

The Socratic way seeks common ground between one or more philosophers and the 'practitioners' (those who normally use the term in question and are therefore expert in its use). Thus, Socrates would go to the religious to define 'piety', to soldiers to define 'courage', and so on. A Socratic definition begins with the definition a practitioner offers. A philosopher responds with counter-examples or other criticism, inviting practitioners to revise. Often the philosopher will help by suggesting possible revisions. Once the practitioners seem satisfied with the revised definition, the philosopher again responds with counter-examples or other criticism. And so the process continues until everyone is happy with the result. Instead of the private monologue of the Cartesian, there is a public conversation.

The Socratic method has yielded this definition of 'profession': A profession is a number of individuals in the same occupation voluntarily organized to earn a living by openly serving a certain moral ideal in a morally permissible way beyond what law, market, morality, and public opinion would otherwise require.

According to this definition, a profession is a group undertaking. There can be no profession of one – though there can be just one artist, expert, or inventor of a certain kind. This may seem a small point, but it has the immediate consequence of disqualifying the Hippocratic oath as a code of professional ethics. Since a single person can take an oath whatever anyone else does, the Hippocratic oath cannot, as oath, be a professional code (though its contents may correspond to the contents of a professional code). To be a professional code, the oath would have to bind each and every member of the profession, taking effect only when all have so sworn and remaining in effect only while each new member of the profession also takes the oath and none of the old renounces it. An oath can be an (actual) code of professional ethics only in the context of a complex practice – a practice so complex it probably could not be maintained for long in any large group. Physicians who fall back on the Hippocratic oath for their professional ethics are simply confused (a confusion made worse by the embarrassing content of the oath, for example the requirement to teach children of the physicians without charge).

Members of the group must have an occupation. Mere gentlemen cannot form a profession. Hence, members of any of the traditional 'liberal professions' (clergy, physicians, and lawyers) could not form a profession until quite recently – until, that is, they ceased to be gentlemen, began to work for a living, and recognized the change in circumstance. That seems to be some time after 1850. So, if law and medicine were the first professions, they must (according to this definition) have become professions less than two centuries ago.

The members of the would-be profession must share an occupation. A group consisting of, say, physicians and dentists cannot today be a profession, though physicians can be one profession and dentists another. They cannot because they belong to distinct occupations – occupations so distinct that they have separate schools, degrees, licenses, and organizations. Here, then, is another reason Percival's *Medical Ethics* could not be the first code of professional ethics. In 1803, physicians still constituted an occupation (or, rather, a vocation) different from surgeons. The education, degree, licensing, and organization of surgeons in Great Britain were then still as separate from those of physicians as today the education, degree, licensing, and organization of dentists are from those of physicians.

Each profession is designed to serve a certain moral ideal, that is, to contribute to a state of affairs everyone (every rational person at his or her rational best) can recognize as good to achieve or even merely to approach. So, physicians have organized to cure the sick, comfort the dying, and protect the healthy from disease; lawyers, to help people obtain justice within the law; and so on. But a profession does not just organize to serve a certain moral ideal; it organizes to serve it in a certain way, that is, according to standards beyond what law, market, morality, and public opinion would otherwise require. A would-be profession must, therefore, set special (morally permissible) standards. Otherwise it would remain nothing more than an honest occupation. Among the standards may be a certain minimum of education, character, and skill, but inevitably some of the special standards will concern conduct rather than competence. The special standards of conduct will be ethical (in our fifth sense of 'ethics'). They will govern the conduct of all the group's members simply because they are members of that group – and govern no one else.

These ethical standards will, if effective, be morally binding on every member of the profession simply because of membership in the profession. The best explanation for this power to bind morally follows.

FROM PROFESSION TO CODES OF ETHICS

Members of a profession must pursue their profession openly; that is, physicians must declare themselves to be physicians, nurses must declare themselves to be nurses, and so on. The members of a (would-be) profession must declare themselves to be members of that profession in order to earn their living by that profession. They cannot be hired as such-and-such (say, a physician) unless they let people know that they are such-and-such. If their profession has a good reputation for what it does, their declaration of membership will help them earn a living. People will seek their help. If, however, their profession has a bad reputation, their declaration of membership ('I am a witch doctor') will be a disadvantage. Generally, people will shun their help. The profession's special way of pursuing its moral ideal is what distinguishes its members from others in the same occupation (if there are any).

Because the members of a profession are free to declare their membership, they will (generally) declare it only if the declaration benefits them overall – that is, serves some purpose of their own at what seems a reasonable cost. The purpose need not be selfish or even self-interested. Some members may enter (or remain in) the profession because it seems the best way to help others, even while others enter (or remain) because they like the work, status, or income. Whatever the purposes of a profession's individual members, their membership in a profession identifies them as engaged in pursuing the moral ideal the profession pursues according to the (morally permissible) special standards the profession has adopted.

Where members of a profession declare their membership voluntarily, they are part of a voluntary, morally permissible cooperative practice. They are in a position to have the benefits of the practice, employment as a member of that profession, because the employer (patient, client, or whatever) sought a such-and-such and they (truthfully) declared themselves to be one. They will also be in position to take advantage of the practice by doing less than the standards of the practice require, even though the expectation that they would do what the standards require (because they declared that profession) is part of what won them employment. If cheating consists in violating the standards of a voluntary, morally permissible cooperative practice, then every member of a profession is in a position to cheat (that is, violate the profession's special standards). Since, all else equal cheating is morally wrong, every member of a profession has a moral obligation, all else equal, to do as the profession's special standards require. The profession's special standards are its ethics (in our fifth sense of 'ethics').

A profession's ethics imposes moral obligations (as just explained). These obligations may, and generally do, vary from profession to profession. Indeed, several professions can share a single occupation, one profession being distinguished from another only by its distinctive professional obligations, its special standards. So, for example, physicians (MDs) are one profession of medical healer and osteopaths (ODs) another, even though both claim to serve the same moral ideal (curing the sick, comforting the dying, and protecting the healthy from disease) with much the same knowledge, skill, and judgment. What distinguishes them today are their professional standards (what counts as the appropriate way to serve the shared moral ideal). The special standards of a profession generally appear in a range of documents, including standards of education, admission, practice, and discipline. A code of ethics (whatever it is called) is the most general of these documents, the one concerned with the practice of the profession as such. A 'profession' without such a code (at least a code 'unwritten' in our first or second sense of that term) is at best a nascent profession.

An occupation's status as a profession is then (more or less) independent of license, state-imposed monopoly, or other special legal intervention. Such legal interventions are characteristic of bureaucracy rather than profession. In principle, professions are not the creatures of law; and, even in practice, some professions (such as journalism) do without license, monopoly, and other protection against market pressures.

While professions often commit themselves to obey the law, they need not. Indeed, insofar as the laws of a particular country are unjust (or otherwise fall below the moral minimum), any provision of a professional code purporting to bind members of the profession to obey the law would be void (just as a promise to do what morality forbids is void).

An occupation's status as a profession is also (more or less) independent of its social status, income, and other 'social indexes' of profession. There is, for example no profession of business managers, even though business managers have relatively high social status, income, and education and important social functions. What business managers lack (according to the Socratic definition) is a common moral ideal beyond law, market, ordinary morality, and public opinion – and common standards, including a code of ethics, settling how that ideal should be pursued. There is, on the other hand, certainly a profession of nursing, though nurses typically earn much less than business managers and have much lower social status. The only high status that membership in a profession entitles one to is being regarded as more reliable or trustworthy in what one does for a living than one would (probably) be if that way of earning a living were not organized as a profession. This high status is deserved only insofar as the profession continues to meet the special standards it has set for itself, that is, insofar as it puts its professional code into practice. There seem, then, to be many professions associated with medicine, not only nursing but pharmacy, physical therapy, clinical counseling, and medical administration. These professions may be identified and distinguished by their professional codes.

REFERENCES

Davis, M. (2007) 'Eighteen rules for writing a code of professional ethics', *Science and Engineering Ethics,* 13 (July): 171–89.
Percival, T. (1803) *Medical Ethics; or a Code of Institutes and Precepts Adopted to the Professional Conduct of Physicians and Surgeons.* Manchester: S. Russell.

7

Organizational Ethics

Eva C. Winkler and Russell L. Gruen

INTRODUCTION

Most healthcare systems face challenges relating to changing patient demographics, changes in the public and private sectors, emphasis on effectiveness and efficiency and cost-containment, and changing professional roles. Healthcare organizations (HCOs) often face ethical dilemmas, especially in times of stress and change.

Organizational ethics has the goal of guiding the ethical behavior of organizations. It has done so mainly by focusing on processes that encourage ethical decision making through-out organizations. However, the ethical dilemmas faced by HCOs differ from those faced by clinicians in the care of individual patients. We hold that processes alone are not apt to guide decision making at the board level of organizations involved in health care. We therefore developed a normative framework for healthcare organizational ethics using four guiding principles: (i) provide care with compassion; (ii) treat employees with respect; (iii) act in a public spirit; and (iv) spend resources reasonably.

These principles relate to the different roles that HCOs are expected to play as caregivers, employers, citizens, and managers, respectively, and are based on the specialness of health care as a social good. We anticipate that these principles can clarify tensions between the different spheres of responsibility in HCOs. They add content to the processes that have been proposed in the field of organizational ethics. Content and processes complement each other when tackling ethical problems in HCOs.

ORGANIZATIONAL ETHICS IS CENTRAL TO HEALTHCARE ETHICS

Healthcare organizations, instead of solo and small-group physician practices, have become increasingly important stakeholders in the delivery of health care in many countries. Consolidation and collocation of services have had efficiency benefits as health care has become more specialized and its technology more expensive. The HCO environment is helpful for enabling the coordinated use of expensive and institutionally-based technologies and providing mechanisms for quality control. By necessity, HCOs have multiple levels of management. In previous decades physicians were the principal healthcare decision makers. Now physicians are but one group of professionals – part of the team – who serve the goals of the healthcare organizations.

Clinical ethics has traditionally been oriented towards the individual physician–patient relationship. The focus is on physicians' and patients' rights, their actions, and how treatment decisions are made and justified. Clinical ethics has evolved primarily as ethics for physicians, entertaining only two main participants – the doctor and the patient – who decide jointly and in private on the course of medical treatment.

The emergence of HCOs as important entities in health care has brought with it a need for ethics that deals with more than just the physician–patient relationship. Healthcare organizational ethics requires a perspective that is broader than the clinical and narrower than the societal. For an organization to behave ethically, there must be norms of ethical behaviour relevant to the organization itself to which it can adhere.

ETHICAL PROBLEMS THAT ARISE IN HCOS ARE OF TWO MAIN TYPES

The first type of ethical problem in HCOs arises due to the potential influence of the organizational context on individual ethical behaviour. The focus of clinical ethics on individual agency has not properly recognized the effects that organizational culture – that is, formal and informal rules and expectations – has on an individual's ethical conduct and decision making.

Researchers of organization theory and business ethics have found that ethical conduct by employees can be promoted by leaders who model ethical behavior, reward ethical conduct and punish unethical conduct, and who prioritize fairness in the treatment of employees (Cropanzano, 2003). Ethical conduct is more difficult when there is ambiguity among staff about organizational priorities, lack of role models and insufficient fora for discussing the ethical dimensions of behaviors (Kaptein, 2000; Trevino et al., 1998).

The second type of ethical problem faced by HCOs arises as a result of conflicting obligations of the HCO itself. While clinicians have responsibilities to their patients, organizations have responsibilities to all patients as well as to employees, payers and other stakeholders and must also comply with legal standards and government regulations (Kassirer, 1998). What constitutes ethical behavior for one group of stakeholders can have unintended trade-offs with ethical implications for other stakeholders.

The first type of problem is concerned with the conditions the organization creates for its representatives to act responsibly ('internal' organizational ethics), while the second is concerned with its corporate responsibilities to all of its stakeholders ('external' organizational ethics). While empirical research on behavior in organizations broadens our understanding of organizational ethics, it is necessary to be balanced in apportioning responsibility for decisions to organizational factors and individual's self-determination.

Therefore, a theory of organizational ethics should do justice to both constituents – each individual's decisional discretion and the organizational factors that influence such decisions.

We therefore propose the following definition for Organizational Ethics:

> Healthcare organizational ethics is the study of the moral agency of HCOs:
>
> It delineates processes for decision making about morally contested questions and principles to guide the decision making of HCOs and their employees.
>
> It sets the stage for representatives of the HCO to act in ethically responsible ways.

THE PROCEDURAL APPROACHES OF ORGANIZATIONAL ETHICS

To date, organizational ethics has largely focused on processes for guiding how HCOs promote ethical decision making. Some HCOs have established organizational ethics programs, and others combined them with compliance programs (Blake, 1999; Childs, 2000; Goodstein and Carney, 1999). Most organizational ethics programs have aimed to facilitate ethical behavior by creating a climate that is consistent with the core values and mission of the HCO (Spencer et al., 2000). Such programs have developed processes to clarify and articulate the organization's values, facilitate communication and learning about ethical issues and monitor and offer feedback on ethical performance (Potter, 1996). Administrative case rounds and similar fora have been useful for identifying and discussing conflicts between the interests of the corporation and its multiple stakeholders (Gallagher and Goodstein, 2002; Reiser, 1994).

Approaches to organizational ethics have, therefore, been largely procedural in that they aim to align organizational decisions and behaviors with the core values articulated in the organization's mission statement (Giganti, 2004).

WHY DOES ORGANIZATIONAL ETHICS NEED PRINCIPLES?

Institutionalizing values, however, solves only those problems that result from organizational barriers to enacting values. When values are agreed upon, processes can be developed to successfully institutionalize them. An example is a process that supports advanced directives in order to respect patient wishes.

If problems arise between the HCO's conflicting obligations to different parties, however, processes for resolution are only part of the solution. Debates such as how to balance investments that ensure high quality of care with investor or stockholder payoffs, or how to allocate resources for free care, may be morally distressing and need to be resolved before they can become institutionalized. Thus, to resolve unsettled questions we require substantive principles that will guide deliberation about ethical dilemmas and promote understanding of the broader moral concerns within the HCO setting. In clinical ethics four principles are well known and are labelled beneficence, non-maleficence, autonomy and justice. To date, such principles have not been offered for debate among HCOs.

PRINCIPLES OF ORGANIZATIONAL ETHICS

The principles of clinical ethics are insufficient for the resolution of many of the ethical problems that arise in organizations. In addition to addressing physicians' responsibilities to patients, principles of organizational ethics should address organizations' responsibilities to the entire patient population as well as to insurers, employees, investors and the wider community. We proposed four principles that relate to four major roles that HCOs are expected to fulfill: caregivers, employers, citizens and service managers (Winkler and Gruen, 2005). Using the values and ethical concepts inherent in each role, we propose the existence of four ethical principles (Table 7.1).

Care with compassion

HCOs must protect the patient–physician relationship and ensure that caregivers are able to provide unconflicted patient-oriented care (Crawshaw et al., 1995). At the heart of caregiving is an asymmetric relationship between providers with expert knowledge and skills, and patients who are vulnerable, not only because they are sick, but also because they usually lack expert knowledge and are therefore reliant on caregivers acting in patients' interests.

The nature of the caregiver–patient relationship is based at least on the following fundamental elements: competence, compassion, shared decision making and trust (Emanuel and Dubler, 1995). In an HCO, competence is ensured by setting high standards, promoting continuing professional development, tying incentives to quality of care rather than to costs alone, and ensuring adequate staffing. Compassion and kindness are the appropriate responses to suffering and can be promoted by role models and professional

Table 7.1　Principles of organizational ethics in health care

Normative principles	Care with compassion	Treat employees with respect	Act in public spirit	Spend resources reasonably
Role	Caregiver	Employer	Citizen	Manager
Main stake-holders	HCO[1] as care provider; patients.	HCO as employer; employees.	HCO as citizen; community.	HCO as manager; patients; investors; insurers; the public
Values	Competence; Compassion; Trust; Shared decision making.	Fairness; Empowerment; Participation.	Common good; Community benefit, Accountability.	Quality; Fair allocation of resources; Efficiency; Sustainability.
Field of Ethics	Clinical ethics.	Business ethics; Workplace ethics.	Political ethics.	Business ethics; Political ethics; Distributive justice.

1　Healthcare organization

and informal emotional support (Emanuel and Dubler, 1995). Patient and caregivers should jointly decide treatment by sharing information, understanding each others' values, and following the principles of clinical ethics, especially autonomy and beneficence. It is fundamental that patients are able to trust HCOs and health professionals to provide care that is tailored to patients' needs ahead of the interests of other parties. One way that an HCO can be a trustworthy caregiver is if it enables those actually delivering care to be advocates for their patients and participate, critique and improve organizational guidelines that affect patient welfare (Buchanan, 2000; Shortell et al., 1998).

Within an HCO's caregiving role, therefore, competence, compassion, trust and ethical decision making form the basis of an overarching principle: care with compassion.

Treat employees with respect

While the role of caregiving is primarily informed by clinical ethics, the remaining roles draw on the field of business and political ethics. The duties of employers to their employees are rooted in the trade union movement and workers' rights (Beauchamp and Bowie, 2001). Business ethicists reject the view that employees' labor is simply a commodity subject to the laws of supply and demand, both because this is likely to undermine loyalty to the HCO and, more importantly, because it is fundamentally at odds with the respect owed to any person. Kant's principle of 'respect for persons' is invoked to argue that businesses should treat their employees as ends in themselves, rather than merely as means to increase productivity and profit (Werhane, 1985).

In this sense, the relationship between employer and employee is one of reciprocal accountability, but with a clear power differential in favor of the employers. Their duties include providing fair salaries, ensuring safe working conditions, and rewarding and disciplining fairly. This requires protecting employees from discrimination and persecution in the workplace, and allowing them to voice opinions about policies on ethically contested questions (Gilbert, 1991; Wynia and Latham et al., 1999). Organizations can and should empower their employees to become responsible actors by creating an ethical climate and serving the self-actualization of their members (Hartman, 1996). Such empowerment is a prerequisite for employees taking responsibility for their actions and not hiding behind rules and structures – a challenge that all complex institutions and bureaucracies face (Margolis, 2001).

We incorporate these characteristics within the principle, treat employees with respect.

The first two principles, therefore, focus on the internal organizational setting and may conflict. Consider, for example, a nurse who sustains a needle-stick injury from a high-risk patient, and the patient then refuses to undergo an HIV test. If the patient is HIV-positive, prophylactic treatment may reduce the nurse's risk of HIV infection. If the patient is HIV-negative, prophylactic treatment offers no benefit, is costly, and exposes the nurse to risks of side-effects such as gastrointestinal disturbance, bone marrow suppression, and unnecessary stress. Clinical ethics, with its focus on patients' rights to self-determination, may favor respecting the autonomous decision of the patient to refuse an HIV test. The nurse, however, also deserves respect, and the HCO has a moral duty to its employees to minimize workplace-related health risks. In this case, the duty to an employee may outweigh the patient's right to refuse an HIV test.

Setting limits fairly

Wise stewardship of resources requires using the least costly means for achieving the ends of health care, and allocating the resources fairly. HCO managers are charged with promoting their organization's success within the constraints imposed by the available resources (Repenshek, 2004). Choices must often be made for reasons of both efficiency and equity. 'Stakeholder theory' is often applied in business ethics to discuss the responsibilities of managers and executives when making corporate decisions (Werhane, 2000). HCO stakeholders include patients, insurers, shareholders, business partners, payers, the government and the public. The theory posits that stakeholder claims should be prioritized according to the purpose and mission of the organization. Since an HCO's raison d'etre is to minister to its patients' health, the basic obligation is canvassed in the principle, care with compassion, and is independent of profit-making status.

Economic incentives, however, have led some HCOs to pursue ethically dubious strategies, such as gag clauses for physicians, declining staff-to-patient ratios, and adverse selection of patients by health plans (Kuttner, 1999). Clearly, market forces may be counterproductive to an HCO's core mission, and HCO managers must balance the sustainability and financial success of the organization with its other roles and responsibilities (Pearson et al., 2003). A consensus on guiding ethical principles for HCOs, however, would level the playing field and help to minimize any resulting competitive disadvantage faced by ethical HCOs.

Ultimately these decisions about resource allocation are decisions about limit setting in different domains, and the underlying principle derived from the HCO manager's role is setting limits fairly.

Here, criteria of distributive justice enter the deliberation. The question of how to allocate beneficial resources in a fair way still lacks consensus on what justice requires: equality of opportunities, priority for those in need or those that benefit most (Daniels and Sabin, 2002). In the absence of prior agreement on the criteria or principles for just allocation, additional procedural requirements, such as transparency of the deliberative process, consistency of such decisions over time, and public accountability help to build trust in allocation decisions. Therefore, besides the substance of ethical reasoning the process for ethical limit-setting gains weight and should be deliberative, fair and transparent (Daniels and Sabin, 1997).

Act in public spirit

The HCO is accountable for how it interacts with its multiple stakeholders. Because many people interact in an HCO, and because their interactions are governed by rules and influence one another, an HCO is a 'semi-public' place. This semi-public status bears importantly on the way an HCO should respond to ethical challenges (Winkler, 2005). Unlike an individual doctor's office, where a doctor and patient may reach a private agreement within the limits of the law, any stand an HCO takes on controversial medical practices and ethically contested issues is a public one. An HCO's public engagement with society is analogous to a citizenship role. The citizenship expectations of HCOs originate from three main sources: participation in democratic society, particular responsibilities to society that businesses in general might have and special responsibilities that come with health care.

Analogous to the basic citizenship role, HCOs have duties to obey the law. In return, they benefit from the state's obligations of service, protection, respect for rights and responsiveness to citizens as consumers and taxpayers. Substantively, citizenship is based on interest and participation in the state of affairs and senses of mutuality and reciprocity, whereby citizens offer proportionate returns for goods received (Gutmann and Thompson, 1996).

Corporate citizenship and the social responsibility of businesses have been central to much recent business ethics literature. The perception of business as narrow-minded pursuit of profit to the exclusion of all other considerations has been widely challenged – especially in face of the current financial crisis. Some business ethicists have argued that, in return for granting companies their legal status as separate entities, society is entitled to expect from them a significant net positive contribution to the general good (Kitson and Campbell, 1996).

This is especially true for businesses engaged in providing health care. Health care is a special social good because sick people are vulnerable and because a particular level of health is required for most people to carry out their 'life plans.' Therefore, businesses that provide this kind of good bear special social responsibilities irrespective of their profit-making status (Daniels and Sabin, 1997).

Corporate citizenship in a healthcare system, therefore, refers to the promotion of the optimal health of the community it serves, and its guiding principle is to act in public spirit.

Reasonable ways in which HCOs can be expected to fulfill their citizenship role include advocacy on issues that are in the interests of the public's health, giving a public account of the ethical position the HCO takes on critical issues or provision of outreach and free services for those unable to access care (Repenshek, 2004). Citizen representation on boards of trustees is one way that HCOs can give voice to community concerns (Emanuel and Emanuel, 1996).

ARE THE PRINCIPLES OF HEALTHCARE ORGANIZATIONAL ETHICS GLOBALLY APPLICABLE?

In this discussion we have largely referred to healthcare organizations as stand-alone entities that exist within state or local healthcare systems, and which provide a public good in a market economy. How applicable is this model to the various systems for healthcare provision worldwide, that may be entirely state-run, entirely marketplace based, large or very small in scale? In response to this question, we need to revisit the basic assumptions on which this model is based.

First assumption: Health care is special

Health care, in a dual sense, is a basic social good. First, like food, education and housing, health care is a good that people need in order to thrive and make the most of their opportunities. However, unlike the other social goods any person who is in need of health care must rely entirely on the expertise of others to make their quality and quantity of life better. Second, providing care and compassion have intrinsic value that complements the social dimension of humanity.

Second assumption: The market approach alone cannot do justice to the value of health care

A basic feature of marketplace commodities is, first, that its value is instrumental, not intrinsic. In the market, the transaction of goods itself has no intrinsic value, as the term 'transaction costs' suggest. Therefore the market is ill equipped in figuring the human factor of care into its value-added calculation. Second, market goods are distributed to those who value them the most – indicated by their willingness to pay. If we accept the special importance of health care, it should be made accessible across the board and independent of people's ability to pay.

These assumptions have important implications for the applicability of the four principles as well as for the construction of healthcare systems. Healthcare systems and HCOs need to set the stage for healthcare providers to act as a 'caring profession'. Hereby the principle of 'Care with compassion' leads and it is supported by the other principles. This applies to an entirely state-run system as well as to a market-driven system. Healthcare systems certainly can use the market for optimizing productivity and beneficial competition. However, they need some regulation that ensures universal access for basic health care and which attaches a net value to the 'transaction' of care, for example, by rewarding time for communication, emotional and psychological support that helps the patient coping with his/her illness.

The four principles of organizational ethics provide a framework for discussing the moral obligations of healthcare providers and HCOs. In general, the principles apply to all organizations involved in the delivery of health care. However, the relative weight carried by each principle depends on the type of organization. In provider organizations, care with compassion will figure prominently, whereas in an insurance company, act in public spirit may also be of special importance. The limitations of this framework are those of abstract, universal principles in general. First, agreement on principles alone does not provide a method for resolving conflicts between them. Instead they help to clarify what is morally at stake and identify the irresolvable aspects of a certain situation. Second, the scope of the principles is not defined – for example, how much care for the poor does act in public spirit require? Obviously this depends on many internal and external factors. And third, principles do not obviate the need for good and virtuous character in carrying out in real life what the principles prescribe.

PRINCIPLES AND PROCESS – THE TWO COMPONENTS OF ORGANIZATIONAL ETHICS

Some of the limitations of a principled approach can be counterbalanced by the processes of decision making and communicating values throughout an HCO that have been developed by the field of organizational ethics. Besides the substance of ethical reasoning, the process of how the decision comes about and how it is legitimized is of utmost importance if we take organizations seriously (McMahon, 1994). We have discussed the procedural requirements for decision making of HCOs in morally controversial questions elsewhere in more detail (Winkler, 2005). The most important requirements are that all parties directed by a decision on morally charged practices are represented in the decision making body, that the deliberative process encompasses all of the HCO's obligations reflected by the four principles presented here and that the rationales for the decision are made available, and that there is a mechanism for criticizing and evaluating the decision. Organizational ethics programs previously developed in the field of organizational ethics are likely to ensure the procedural requirements and communicate the values underlying the substantive principles (Blake, 1999; Childs, 2000; Goold et al., 2000; Potter, 1996; Spencer et al., 2000). Thus, content and procedure are equally important in resolving moral disagreement. They mutually enforce the moral soundness of the resolution of the specific ethical challenges.

While the principles apply to all kinds of healthcare systems and HCOs, the processes that ensure conflict resolution on ethical contested questions within an organization depend on the context. They must be very responsive to the setting of the HCOs. For example, in a state-run healthcare system politics might ensure certain ethical standards for HCOs while in a market-driven healthcare system corporate responsibilities of HCOs and benchmarks for ethical conduct might best be defined through a consensus conference or other joint endeavor. This would promote ethical behavior and help to minimize any resulting competitive disadvantage faced by ethical HCOs. HCOs' obligations could then be defined in a form to which managers, administrators, providers and patients could commit. Such consensus also has the potential to promote the public's trust in HCOs.

In sum, basic assumptions about the specialness of health care apply to HCOs across countries and therefore the principles of organizational ethics represent important values independent of the healthcare system. In contrast, processes that ensure the alignment of an HCO with their values vary depending on the healthcare system, HCO, cultural and historical differences. Certainly, the principles represent ideals that HCOs should aspire to while realizing that they do not portray reality. Depending on the healthcare system, funding and political context, it will be more easy or hard work trying to follow these ideals. Still, in living up to those ideals decision making in questions of organizational ethics would be contained within those solutions that do justice to the specialness of health care.

The four ethical principles that should guide ethical decision making in HCOs are derived from the different roles HCOs are expected to play. They reflect different stakeholders' interests, underlying values, and the fields of ethics that inform them.

REFERENCES

Beauchamp, T.L. and Bowie, N.E. (2001) *Rights and Obligations of Employers and Employees. Ethical Theory and Business*, 6th ed. Englewood Cliffs, NJ: Prentice-Hall, pp. 256–65.

Blake, D.C. (1999) 'Organizational ethics: Creating structural and cultural change in healthcare organizations', *Journal of Clinical Ethics*, 3: 187–93.

Buchanan, A. (2000) 'Trust in managed care organizations', *Kennedy Institute of Ethics Journal*, 3: 189–212.

Childs, B.H. (2000) 'From boardroom to bedside: A comprehensive organizational healthcare ethics', *HEC Forum*, 3: 235–49.

Crawshaw, R., Rogers, D.E., Pellegrino, E.D., Bulger, R.J., Lundberg, G.D., Bristow, L.R. et al. (1995) 'Patient–physician covenant', *Journal of the American Medical Association*, 19: 1553.

Cropanzano, R. (2003) 'Deontic justice: The role of moral principles in workplace fairness', *Journal of Organizational Behavior*, 24 (8): 1019–24.

Daniels, N. and Sabin, J. (1997) 'Limits to health care: Fair procedures, democratic deliberation, and the legitimacy problem for insurers', *Philosophy and Public Affairs*, 4: 303–50.

Daniels, N. and Sabin, J. (2002) *Setting Limits Fairly: Can We Learn to Share Medical Resources?* Oxford: Oxford University Press.

Emanuel, E.J. and Dubler, N.N. (1995) 'Preserving the physician–patient relationship in the era of managed care', *Journal of the American Medical Association*, 4: 323–9.

Emanuel, E.J. and Emanuel, L.L. (1996) 'What is accountability in health care?', *Annals of Internal Medicine*, 2: 229–39.

Gallagher, J.A. and Goodstein, J. (2002) 'Fulfilling institutional responsibilities in health care: Organizational ethics and the role of mission discernment', *Business Ethics Quarterly*, 4: 433–50.

Giganti, E. (2004) 'Organizational ethics is "systems thinking"', *Health Progress*, 3: 10–11.

Gilbert, D.R. (1991) 'Respect for persons, management theory, and business ethics', in R.E. Freeman (ed.), *Business Ethics: The State of the Art*. Oxford: Oxford University Press.

Goodstein, J.D. and Carney, B. (1999) 'Actively engaging organizational ethics in healthcare: Four essential elements', *Journal of Clinical Ethics*, 3: 224–9.

Goold, S.D., Kamil, L.H., Cohan, N.S. and Sefansky, S.L. (2000) 'Outline of a process for organizational ethics consultation', *HEC Forum*, 1.

Gutmann, A. and Thompson, D. (1996) *The Sense of Reciprocity. Democracy and Disagreement*. Cambridge, MA: Harvard University Press.

Hartman, E.M. (1996) *Organizational Ethics and the Good Life*. Oxford: Oxford University Press.

Kaptein, M. (2000) 'The empirical assessment of corporate ethics: A case study', *Journal of Business Ethics*, 24: 95–114.

Kassirer, J.P. (1998) 'Managing care – should we adopt a new ethic?', *New England Journal of Medicine*, 6: 397–8.

Kitson, A. and Campbell, A.R. (1996) *Social Responsibilities of Business. The Ethical Organisation – Ethical Theory and Corporate Behavior*. Basingstoke: Macmillan, pp. 138–44.

Kuttner, R. (1999) 'The American health care system: Wall Street and health care', *New England Journal of Medicine*, 8: 664–8.

McMahon, C. (1994) *Authority and Democracy: A General Theory of Government and Management*. Princeton, NJ: Princeton University Press.

Margolis, J.D. (2001) 'Responsibility in organizational context', *Business Ethics Quarterly*, 3: 431–54.

Pearson, S.D., Sabin, J. and Emanuel, E.J. (2003) *No Margin, No Mission. Health-care Organizations and the Quest for Ethical Excellence*. New York: Oxford University Press.

Potter, R.L. (1996) 'From clinical ethics to organizational ethics: The second stage of the evolution of bioethics', *Bioethics Forum*, 2: 3–12.

Reiser, S.J. (1994) 'The ethical life of health care organizations', *Hastings Centre Report*, 6: 28–35.

Repenshek, M. (2004) 'Stewardship and organizational ethics. How can hospitals and physicians balance scarce resources with their duty to serve the poor?', *Health Progress*, 3: 31–5, 56.

Shortell, S.M., Waters, T.M., Clarke, K.W. and Budetti, P.P. (1998) 'Physicians as double agents: Maintaining trust in an era of multiple accountabilities', *Journal of the American Medical Association*, 12: 1102–08.

Spencer, E.M., Mills, A.E., Rorty, M.V. and Werhane, P.H. (2000) *Instituting an Organization Ethics Program. Organization Ethics in Health Care*. New York: Oxford University Press, pp. 151–70.

Trevino, L.K., Butterfield, K.D. and McCabe, D.L. (1998) 'The ethical context in organizations: Influences on employee attitudes and behaviors', *Business Ethics Quarterly*, 3: 447–76.

Werhane, P.H. (1985) *Persons, Rights and Corporations*. Englewood Cliffs, NJ: Prentice-Hall.

Werhane, P.H. (2000) 'Business ethics, stakeholder theory, and the ethics of healthcare organizations', *Cambridge Quarterly of Healthcare Ethics,* 2: 169–81.

Winkler, E.C. (2005) 'The ethics of policy writing: How hospitals should deal with moral disagreement about controversial medical practices', *Journal of Medical Ethics,* 50 (2): 559–66.

Winkler, E.C. and Gruen, R. (2005) 'First principles: Substantive ethics for healthcare organizations', *Journal of Healthcare Management,* 2: 109–20.

Wynia, M.K., Latham, S.R., Kao, A.C., Berg, J.W. and Emanuel, L.L. (1999) 'Medical professionalism in society', *New England Journal of Medicine,* 21: 1612–16.

8

Deliberation and Consensus

Diego Gracia

INTRODUCTION

Decision making is not an optional activity for human beings. We need it in order to remain alive. The role of freedom begins only with the election between different possibilities offered by the diversity of situations. We must choose between them, and therefore we bear responsibility for the choice. But we are compelled by nature to choose. This is the origin of moral life. When we opt between different alternatives, we are first compelled to justify to ourselves the decision made. Conscience is the first tribunal, and we are our primary judges.

THE MORAL POINT OF VIEW

Human acts are always and necessarily moral. They can be either moral or immoral, but not amoral, if they are really human, that is, performed with adequate knowledge and freedom. That is why we all make moral statements, judging things or acts as right or wrong, good or bad, etc. And the first question is: What kind of judgments are moral ones?

How do we make these kinds of judgment called moral? Because they are basic to secure our lives, not only on the spiritual or cultural level, but also on the biological one, it is essential to know how to perform them with the security of doing so correctly.

How do we ensure that our moral judgments are correct? This is a logical question, which can only be answered by taking into account the different ways in which our minds make judgments.

MORAL JUDGMENTS ARE NOT APODICTIC

Some judgments are called apodictic or demonstrative. Traditionally, they were considered typical of mathematical reasoning. When we demonstrate a proposition, we know that it is right, and that all other solutions are necessarily wrong. Demonstration gives us a complete and perfect truth. The Pythagoras theorem is true, and it will remain true forever. Moreover, this theorem was already true before it was discovered by Pythagoras. It is true by itself.

Mathematics is important in human life, but much more important is the right governance of our own lives; therefore, moral judgments are more appreciated by human beings than are mathematical judgments. That is, perhaps, the reason why human beings have always been interested in assuring the rightness of their moral judgments. How? Applying to them apodictic or demonstrative logic, thinking that the logic of the moral reasoning is similar to that of mathematics, and believing that it is possible to demonstrate whether a moral proposition is right or wrong, true or false. This has been the desire – sometimes conscious, other times unconscious – of most Western moral philosophy, from the Stoics, at the end of the classical world, at least until the end of the nineteenth century. The history of philosophy has been essentially 'rationalistic'. Human reason is capable of solving all kind of problems with mathematical exactitude. To make ethics as mathematicians make mathematics was the desire which Baruch Spinoza expressed perfectly when he titled his major work, *Ethica ordine geometrico demonstrata* [Ethics, demonstrated in geometrical order] (Spinoza, 1995).

ARE MORAL JUDGMENTS PROBLEMATIC?

Opposed to the apodictic way of reasoning is the so-called 'problematic' way. Here we face problems with not one solution, but two or more – in some cases, many. Why? Because generally our arguments do not exhaust the reality of the things they are expressing. Things are richer and more complex than our capacity for analyzing and verbalizing them. When we make a judgment, for instance, 'this sheet is white', we are applying a predicate, white, to a subject, the sheet. If the predicate is completely adequate to the subject, the judgment can be true. But a perfect fit is impossible. There are many different types of white which we express with the same word. Empirical judgments are not completely adequate to reality. This is the reason why we must keep reviewing our scientific data and changing our theories. They have been tested experimentally, but empirical trials do not test completely the content of a theory or of a proposition. There is no *experimentum crucis*, no crucial experiment, as Galileo and Newton thought.

In the year 1788 Kant wrote in the conclusion of his *Critique of Practical Reason* about Newton's universal law of gravity:

> The fall of a stone, the motion of a sling, resolved into their elements and the forces that are manifested in them, and treated mathematically, produced at last that clear and henceforward unchangeable insight into the system of the world which, as observation is continued, may hope always to extend itself, but need never fear to be compelled to retreat (Kant, 2002, 204).

Kant thought that empirical experiences, treated mathematically, could produce demonstrative or apodictic judgements, which could be extended in the future, but never retreated. Physical theories could, therefore, be completely true, like the Pythagorean theorem. This was written more than two centuries ago. Today, nobody thinks that empirical judgments can be apodictic. They must be tested continuously. As Karl Popper said, we can say that, in the present state of our knowledge, they are not false, but we cannot say they are true (Popper, 2002).

Moral judgements are empirical. When we say that conduct is bad, or that certain behaviour is immoral, we are making empirical statements. Reasons are not absolute and complete here (Gracia, 2001). There are, for instance, circumstances under which the morality of killing changes, and the same can be said of lying, or of telling the truth, etc. As is well known, Kant wrote an essay criticizing 'a supposed right to lie from altruistic motives' (Kant, 1993). He conceived truth telling as an absolute duty. We already know why he thought this way.

ARISTOTLE ON DEMONSTRATION AND DELIBERATION

The first author who characterized moral judgments as problematic was Aristotle. He called them 'dialectic' (Aristotle, 1831: 100 a–b), because in these fields our mind cannot exhaust reality. We are only capable of giving 'opinions', *doxai*. Opinions are reasons, but not absolute. There are always counter-opinions, 'paradoxes'. In these cases, discussion or dialogue with others is the best way we have to improve our knowledge and to make wise decisions. And this process of exchanging reasons in order to improve our knowledge of things was called by Aristotle 'deliberation' (Aristotle, 1831: 1112 a 18–1113 a 13; 1113 b 5; 1142 a 32–b 34). The goal of this process is always the same: to make wise or prudent decisions. That is why the virtue of deliberating well and reaching right decisions was called by Aristotle *phronesis*, practical wisdom (Aristotle, 1831: 1140 a 23–b 29).

Demonstration is to the apodictic way of reasoning what deliberation is to the dialectic one. In the first, propositions are true or false; in the second, wise or unwise. It is essential to be aware that our moral duty is not to avoid making mistakes, but to avoid being unwise.

Therefore, deliberation is the method of moral reasoning. It is as old as the discipline of ethics itself. But it was immediately forgotten. For centuries, or more correctly, for millennia, it was thought that only some people – popes, priests, philosophers, physicians, and moralists – had the special capacity to know clearly and without any doubt what is right and wrong. They were therefore the moral leaders of societies; this entitled them to lead all the others, who should only respond through obedience. There were two different moral roles, the one of leadership, and the other of obedience. It is no accident that the Greek word for practical wisdom, *phronesis*, would be translated to Latin as *consilium*, counsel. Only a small number of people were entitled to deliberate. All the others should simply obey.

DELIBERATION AND THE MORAL REASONING

Why is deliberation the method for moral reasoning? The first reason is that moral decisions are always, and necessarily, concrete; that is, taken at a specific moment, under certain circumstances, which are different from all other possible situations. Deliberation is the art of including in our judgments all these contingent elements in order to make wise decisions.

But there is also another motive. Moral reasoning is twofold. On the one hand we should have circumstances and consequences of situations, but on the other we must posit moral values, which are abstract and universal – for instance, justice, truthfulness, etc. Traditionally, it was thought that these values or principles were absolute and could be deduced by reason, as in mathematics. This was, for instance, the idea of Kant. His categorical imperative holds, 'Act in accordance with the maxims of a member legislating universal laws for a merely possible kingdom of ends [namely, human beings, beings endowed with dignity and not only with worth]' (Kant, 1968: 439). Thinking on my own, I can imagine the laws which would be necessary in a well-ordered and perfect kingdom of human beings. For instance in this ideal society, values like justice, peace, truth, etc. should be present, because injustice, war, and lying are incompatible with a kingdom of ends in themselves. I can deduce, using my mind, all these values as necessary, without the help of others. Dialogue and deliberation are not needed. Moral principles can be deduced in morals like in mathematics.

When we are thinking of values such as justice, peace, or truthfulness, the previous conclusion is doubtless right. In fact, all cultures agree about regarding these values as positive and about the opposing ones as negative. But there are other cases in which things are not so evident. This is the case, for instance, in religious beliefs. Everyone who has a belief thinks that this belief is the best, and that, in a well-ordered world, everybody should profess his faith. And the same holds with other values: we all think we know the right political ideology which should prevail in a well-ordered human society, or whether women should cover their heads with shawls or not, etc.

NORMATIVE CONSENSUS

The conclusion of this reasoning is that deliberation is not only necessary because we must take into account circumstances and consequences that change quickly in our moral reasoning; it is also necessary, perhaps even more so, because all of us are in need of all the rest of humankind to define the values that should prevail in a well-ordered society. These values are not self-evident, and we must identify them through a complex process of collective deliberation, with all human beings as participants. Rawls stated that what he tried to do with his theory of justice was 'to formulate an ideal constitution of public deliberation in matters of justice, a set of rules well-designed to bring to bear the greater knowledge and reasoning powers of the group' (Rawls, 1971: 359).

Values can only be universalized if all human beings can accept them after a process of deliberation without coercion. Therefore, it is necessary to take all of them into account in the deliberation process. This is what K.O. Apel and J. Habermas call the 'ideal community of communication', which I prefer to call the 'ideal community of deliberation'. Only when all people affected by a specific value are capable of accepting it freely and without coercion, can this value be endowed with normative power; in other words, 'only those norms can claim to be valid that meet (or could meet) with the approval of all affected in their capacity as participants in a practical discourse' (Habermas, 1990: 66), or better, in a practical deliberation. Therefore, only after a general 'consensus' between all the people affected by a rule can this be thought as moral. On this level, deliberation is the way to reach normative consensus and to make rules. When this kind of agreement is impossible, then the values at stake cannot be generalized, and diversity should be respected. The only right way to make rules and norms from values is through deliberation and rational consensus.

WHY IS DELIBERATION SO DIFFICULT?

Deliberation is an intellectual skill. In order to deliberate, it is necessary to offer ourselves reasons when deliberating to ourselves, or to others when the deliberation process is collective. The latter is a very difficult task, because there are different constraints to do it well. At least there is the following:

All members taking part in a deliberative team are compelled by the process itself to provide reasons for their own values. But values are not completely rational: neither religious values, nor political ones, nor aesthetic ones. Values are determined not only by reasons, but also by traditions, history, hopes, fears, desires, feelings, beliefs, etc. Values are not 100 per cent rational or completely justifiable by giving reasons, but they must be reasonable in the sense of reflective, balanced, wise, or prudent. When they go beyond this limit, we enter the field of fanaticism, fundamentalism, sectarianism, etc. Offering reasons for our choice of values is very difficult and always open to discussion.

The second problem is that we do not frequently analyze the rational consistency of our values. We all take for granted that they are absolutely certain and evident. We 'believe' in their consistency so deeply that we try to think they are 'apodictic'. This is the origin of the 'dogmatism' usual not only in religion, but also in politics, and in general in human life. To be aware of the limits of our value election is also difficult.

THE ADVANTAGES OF COLLECTIVE DELIBERATION

Only after we recognize the weakness of our preferences for certain values does collective deliberation begin to be reasonable. It is only at this point that we can begin to think that people with other preferences can be at least as right as we are to defend ours, and that being aware of their motivations can be useful to us in order to be more aware of our options and wiser in our decisions. This is the only way in which we will be open to the reasons of others and capable of listening to them. This is the beginning of a true deliberation process.

Deliberating is a great safeguard against dogmatism. When we are obliged to give reasons about our points of view and our beliefs, we realize that these reasons are less convincing than we thought. We have reasons in favour of them, but they are not absolute or apodictic. Here is another benefit of deliberation: we achieve a better idea of the type of arguments we are using and of their limited value. Others can see the question from different perspectives and give other arguments, which perhaps are contrary to ours. If I know that my arguments are not absolute, I can open myself to the arguments of others and be receptive to them, because they can help me to be wise.

Deliberation is a school of wisdom. But it is a very difficult task. Deliberation is a type of discussion. When we are discussing with others, we always try to gain the upper hand by giving apodictic arguments without possible reply. And due to the fact that generally we do not have this kind of arguments available, we compensate for this weakness with other rhetorical elements: shouting, acting, etc. In this way, discussion changes into arguments. We argue because we like to gain the upper hand. It is a natural behaviour, but not a moral one. Deliberation is a type of discussion, but opposed to arguing. If having arguments is natural, deliberation is moral. We need to learn how to deliberate correctly. This is one of the biggest tragedies of our society that young people are trained to impose their opinion on others, not to deliberate with them.

LEVELS OF DELIBERATION

Deliberation is the method for moral reasoning. In order to do that correctly, it is necessary to go step by step. One step deals with the values to be promoted and implemented in a well-ordered society. This is what can be called the 'value-deliberation' moment. A second role of deliberation is to make adequate duty-judgments by taking into account not only these values, but also the specific circumstances and consequences of every situation. This is the 'duty-deliberation' moment. There are differences between them both, due to the fact that while in the first case we are thinking of an ideal world, the second case takes place in the real, actual world. For instance, I can affirm that in a well-ordered world, truth would be an imperative value, and that there would be no place for lying. This world, which is completely ideal, has nevertheless real consequences in our lives, because it compels us to achieve it. Therefore, we 'should' not lie. But in this real world, there are some occasions in which lying is not only permitted, but necessary. That happens, among other situations, when telling the truth can enter into conflict with other compelling values, as, for example life itself. In this case, we are aware that we 'should' not lie, but at the same time we think we 'ought to' lie. These are the two levels of the moral reasoning, the value-level and the duty-level. They are not identical, among other reasons, because values can enter into conflict between them in specific situations, and in these cases our duty should be to achieve one value, while delaying, or at least postponing, the other. Values and duties are not the same: values are the background of duties, and duties the way of actualizing our values.

Aristotle said that deliberation is the method of practical reason. And this reason deals not only with human 'actions', like the moral ones, but also with the process of 'making' or 'producing' things or 'facts' (Aristotle, 1831: 1139 b 38-1140 a 23). In other words, deliberation is not only related to 'values' and 'duties', but also to 'facts'. If I am thinking how to construct a bridge, I must deliberate to myself, and perhaps with many others, about the way to make it correctly. When I am driving a car, I must be making decisions related to facts, as to when I must turn right or left. And in order to do that in the precise moment and in the right way, I should deliberate, at least, to myself.

Now, we can order the process of moral deliberation. It has no less than three levels. The first is deliberation about facts or factual data, which we can call 'factual deliberation'. Values are always dependent on and supported by facts. The second level is, therefore, 'value deliberation'. And the third and final one is 'duty deliberation'. The end of this process, as we already know, is *phronesis*, practical wisdom, reasonability, prudence.

First level: Deliberation on facts

The distinction between these three levels is very important in clinical ethics. When we are analyzing a clinical case, the first step must be careful deliberation about the 'facts' of the case, in order to make the main medical decisions, diagnosis (what is the disease of this patient?), prognosis (what would be the future of this person with this problem?), and treatment (what can I do for this patient?). In order to make these three decisions, deliberation is needed. This is, for instance, the goal of so-called clinical rounds. Every physician deliberates to himself before making decisions, but when facts are obscure and decisions difficult, physicians open the deliberation process, discussing the case with people with other ideas, experiences, and training, in order to make wiser decisions. Aristotle wrote that 'we call in others to aid us in deliberation on important questions, distrusting ourselves as not being capable of taking decisions' (Aristotle, 1831: 1112 b 10–11). This means that when decisions are difficult, the process of deliberation should be open to other points of view, because in this way we can enrich our own perspectives and make wiser decisions.

This is the logic behind clinical rounds (Gracia, 2003). If medical decisions could be made by an apodictic way of thinking, this method would make no sense. Medical thinking is not apodictic; it is problematic, and that is the reason why the duty of physicians is not to restore the health of the patient, but to take the right measures in order to do that, avoiding all kind of misconduct, negligence, incompetence, or professional imprudence. Imprudence is not a point in space but quite a wide area, within which conduct can differ. During discussions in clinical rounds, diverse medical opinions can be set forth by different professionals, all of them right if they are within the area covered by prudence. The goal of deliberation is not to reach complete agreement between all the participants, but to improve the consistency and wisdom of all the decisions made. A surgeon can diverge from an internist about the treatment of the patient. This is not wrong when both are prudent. The goal of deliberation at this level is to improve the wisdom of our decisions, not to reach a consensus. In clinical rounds, the last word is that of the professional in charge of the patient. He has listened to all the participants in the deliberation process, and perhaps after that he has a better idea of the decisions to be made. But he has the responsibility for his own decision. The sole goal of deliberation is to increase the wisdom of our understanding of reality, not to fit it completely into our opinions, or to reach a full consensus.

This example of the clinical round is important, because it is the most illustrative of a collective and participatory deliberation process about facts, more specifically, about medical facts; and also because this is – or should be – the first step in the deliberation process about ethical problems in a clinical setting. For instance, hospital ethics committees should be deliberative bodies whose first step must always be the analysis of facts, clarifying the diagnosis as much as possible; the prognosis; and the therapeutic measures available in each specific case. The only difference between a clinical round and an ethics committee is that in the latter, factual deliberation is only the first step, followed by other two, one the deliberation about values, and the last the deliberation on duties.

Second level: Deliberation on values

The second step is value deliberation. This is the moment in which the specificity of moral reasoning begins to appear. Facts are data collected mediate or immediately through our senses. What we see, touch, or hear are immediate facts, objective data; and through the mediation of scanners, PETs, or SPECTs, we can perceive hidden elements. We say that facts are objective, because all of us, generally, perceive them in a similar way. There are no major discussions between human beings about facts. Problems begin when we shift from facts to the world of values. Our problems start when shifting from perception to evaluation; from fact perception to value evaluation. Here the diversity of points of view increases dramatically.

The world of values! If they are not facts, what are they? After the positivistic movement of the nineteenth century, it was thought that only facts existed. Values, therefore, were subjective, unreal, erratic, and emotional entities. Nothing rational could be said about them. This was, during the first part of the twentieth century, the point of view of many movements, like Neopositivism, the Vienna circle, Wittgenstein, and his followers, among others.

But values are not as erratic as we are prone to think. A good way of showing this is with the method proposed by G.E. Moore. To the question: 'What things have intrinsic value?' he answered: 'It is necessary to consider what things are such that, if they existed by themselves, in absolute isolation, we should yet judge their existence to be good' (Moore, 1994: 236). Another version of this test is to think what things should be present in a well-ordered human world. We are incapable of thinking this world without justice, peace, truthfulness, happiness, love, friendship, health, life, etc. This means that all these things are valuable 'by themselves', because the lack of them is seen as a great loss.

As we can realize, values are more objective than we think. In fact, we are all continuously valuing things. We cannot see a single thing without valuing it. It can be beautiful or ugly, cheap or expensive, lovely or hateful, but not free of value. There are no value-free things. It was a positivistic misconception to think that scientific facts were value-free. Nobody thinks this way today. Everything is value-laden.

In any case, the objectivity of values is different from the objectivity associated with facts. We all agree about some fundamental values, but not about many others. This means that some values can be assumed reasonably and without coercion by all the people, but others cannot. When a value cannot be assumed freely by all the participants in an equal process of deliberation, it cannot be generalized to the whole of society. It must remain as a private value, not a public one. The first public values generally take legal form, while the last are freely managed by individuals and social groups.

Clinical facts are value-laden, and, to a greater extent, so are ailing human beings. That is the reason why the second step of the procedure must begin with identification of the values involved in the issue. Generally there are many of them; the first, health. Health is a fact, but also a value. Physicians are very aware of the 'factual' dimension of health and disease, but they ignore in general their 'value' dimension. Patients are always concerned about their health problems, because they value health very strongly. But this is not the only value at stake. There are also other values involved: economic values, aesthetic values, religious values, social, legal, political values, etc. The second level of analysis must begin with an accurate identification of the values at stake. After the 'clinical factual history' of the patient, we need to reconstruct his or her 'value history'.

Values are imperatives. This means that all of us have the duty to promote them as much as possible. They are the contents of our moral judgements. The problem is that on many occasions, values conflict. Thus arise 'value conflicts'. When people say 'I have a conflict', or 'I have a moral problem', what they are trying to express is that they have a 'conflict of values'. A moral problem is always a value conflict. In the clinical setting these are very frequent. There are, for instance, conflicts between price, an economic value, and health, a vital one. Others are between justice and autonomy, between autonomy and non-maleficence, etc.

The analysis of the world of values is the goal of the value deliberation step. During this step we must identify the values at stake, and whether they are public and legally compelling, or private and freely self-imposed, and what are the most important value conflicts. In general, they are a few, though at times many. Each one of them is a moral problem. It is impossible to solve all of them at the same time. Each and every conflict needs a specific analysis. Our duty is always to solve every conflict in the best possible way, that is, trying to promote the achievement of both values as much as possible, or doing them the least injury possible. Therefore, this second stage ends by choosing the value conflict we think the most important or, better, that which is more prominent or important for the person who asked for help.

Third level: Deliberation about duties

The problem of the third step is identification of our duties. Our duty is always the same, to do the best. It is a frequent error to think that ethics is the science of the good. It is not true. Ethics is the science of the best. The duty of physicians is to do the best for their patients, not to make decisions which are not the best, but that in any case are not bad. The same can be said of the judge: he must render the best possible judgment. And as in these two examples, so it is in all other human activities. At the beginning of the *Nicomachean Ethics*, Aristotle wrote: 'Like archers, we have a target at which to aim', and the target is always the same, to strike with the arrow at the bull's eye, at the heart of the matter (Aristotle, 1831: 1094 a 23). This is not a pure metaphor. Ethics is always looking for the middle point. This is the idea of *mesotes* that virtue is, in general, in the middle.

In the middle of what? – in the middle of the two opposite and extreme sides. Each conflict can be solved in different ways. These ways are called courses of action. There are two opposite and extreme courses of action, and others between them called intermediate. Our duty must coincide necessarily with one of these courses of action. When conflicts have no ways out, they have no solutions. This is the case of 'tragedies'. Tragedies are as real as human life. Here, deliberation has no possible role.

But many other times, value conflicts do have solutions, and our duty is to find the best way of solving them. This is not an easy task. Our mind is prone to reduce all possible courses of action to two and only two, and to think of them as opposite and extreme. We work like computers, in a binary way, identifying only two values, zero and one, black and white, without any sensitivity for nuances. In this way, we miss the intermediate courses of action, which are, in general, the best from the moral point of view. The 'dilemmatic' mind is the cause of many moral mistakes. There is a dilemma when a conflict has two and only two opposite and disjunctive solutions. True dilemmas are rare; in general, dilemmas are artificial and false, produced by the human tendency to simplify things when thinking. These economies can be very dangerous. In general there are no dilemmas; there are 'problems', conflicts with more than two courses of action. And the goal of this third level of deliberation is to identify all possible courses of action and to choose the best, which is always that which displays the most respect for the values at stake.

Courses of action are concrete, situational, related to specific circumstances and consequences. This means that one course of action can be the best in a specific situation, and not five minutes later. As a general rule, the best courses of action are always to be found in the middle, as Aristotle said (Aristotle, 1831: 1108 b 11–1109 b 26). Only when intermediate courses fail are we entitled to choose as the best, or the least harmful, one of the two extremes.

The end of the process: Wise decisions

The end-point of all this complex process of deliberation is to make a wise decision. This is the answer to the moral question, 'What should I do?' My duty is to do the best. But the best is not a point in the space but an area, as previously said. Different people can identify different courses of action as the best. This is not a problem. The goal of deliberation, as we know, is not to reach complete agreement about the best course of action, but to improve the wisdom or prudence of all the courses chosen as the best, even when there are many.

That is the reason why deliberation cannot be identified or confused on this level with consensus (Rescher, 1993; Bayerz, 1994; Moreno, 1995). Such confusion is a very frequent mistake. Often it is possible to reach consensus through deliberation. But in other cases it is not. Diversity of ideas about the good life and about happiness are usual in a pluralistic society and should command respect. This is also an important value. The goal of morality is not the total convergence of ideas, but to respect all those we can consider wise or prudent. Consensus is needed when we are looking for universal rules or norms, but it is not necessary, and can be impossible, when deciding in view of particular circumstances and specific consequences of an act. Here the goal to be reached is not consensus but practical wisdom, prudence.

LOOKING FOR A DELIBERATIVE SOCIETY

The great tragedy of our society is its lack of deliberation. People are not trained for this goal. Yet it should be the highest objective of any educational programme from the very beginning when people begin their learning, until the end of the process (Gutmann, 1987). A deliberative society is the only truly human society. Humans could be defined as 'deliberative animals'.

Deliberation is also the main concept in medical ethics. It is the essence of the clinical encounter (Emanuel and Emanuel, 1992; Gracia, 2003). And ethics committees should be deliberative bodies (Bulger et al., 1995). Deliberation is also essential in political life (Emanuel, 1994; Gracia, 2005). This is the goal of the so-called 'deliberative democracy'

(Moreno, 1995: 71; Rawls, 1999: 579–81), or 'deliberative politics' (Emanuel, 1994; Habermas, 1996: 315–28; Gutmann and Thompson, 2004).

Deliberation, in short, is the great unknown quantity!

REFERENCES

Aristotle (1831) *Aristotelis Opera*. Berlin: Reimer.
Bayerz, K. (ed.) (1994) *The Concept of Moral Consensus: The Case of Technological Interventions in Human Reproduction*. Dordrecht/Boston, MA/London: Kluwer Academic Publishers.
Bulger, R.E., Bobby, E.M. and Fineberg, H.V. (eds.) (1995) *Society's Choices: Social and Ethical Decision Making in Biomedicine*. Washington, DC: National Academy Press.
Emanuel, E.J. (1994) *The Ends of Human Life: Medical Ethics in a Liberal Polity*. Cambridge, MA: Harvard University Press.
Emanuel, E.J. and Emanuel, L.L. (1992) 'Four models of the physician–patient relationship', *Journal of the American Medical Association*, 267 (16): 2221–6.
Gracia, D. (2001) 'Moral deliberation: The role of methodologies in clinical ethics', *Medicine, Health Care and Philosophy*, 4 (2): 223–32.
Gracia, D. (2003) 'Ethical case deliberation and decision making', *Medicine, Health Care and Philosophy*, 6: 227–33.
Gracia, D. (2005) 'The foundation of medical ethics in the democratic evolution of modern society', in C. Viafora (ed.), *Clinical Bioethics: A Search for the Foundations*. Dordrecht: Springer, pp. 33–40.
Gutmann, A. (1987) *Democratic Education*. Princeton, NJ: Princeton University Press.
Gutmann, A. and Thompson D. (2004) *Why Deliberative Democracy?* Princeton, NJ and Oxford: Princeton University Press.
Habermas, J. (1990) *Moral Consciousness and Communicative Action*. Cambridge, MA: MIT Press.
Habermas, J. (1996) *Between Facts and Norms: Contribution to a Discourse Theory of Law and Democracy*. Cambridge, MA: MIT Press.
Kant, I. (1968) *Grundlegung zur Metaphysik der Sitten, Akademie-Ausgabe Kant Werke IV*. Berlin: Walter de Gruyter.
Kant, I. (1993) *Grounding for the Metaphysics of Morals: With a Supposed Right to Lie Because of Philanthropic Concerns*. Cambridge, MA: Hackett.
Kant, I. (2002) *Critique of Practical Reason*. Cambridge, MA: Hackett.
Moore, G.E. (1994) *Principia Ethica*. Cambridge: Cambridge University Press.
Moreno, J.D. (1995) *Deciding Together: Bioethics and Moral Consensus*. New York/Oxford: Oxford University Press.
Popper, K.R. (2002) *The Logic of Scientific Discovery*. London: Taylor & Francis.
Rawls, J. (1971) *A Theory of Justice*. Cambridge, MA: Harvard University Press.
Rawls, J. (1999) *Collected Papers*. Cambridge, MA: Harvard University Press.
Rescher, N. (1993) *Pluralism: Against the Demand for Consensus*. New York: Oxford University Press.
Spinoza, B. (1995) *Ethics*. New York: Kensington Publishers.

9

Privacy, Confidentiality and Data Protection

Deryck Beyleveld

INTRODUCTION

In many countries, disclosure and use of personal information relating to a person's health is regulated by laws on privacy, confidentiality and data protection. It is neither possible to address here all such regulations in relation to all categories and uses of personal data, nor to comment on all the different conceptions of a right to privacy that have been propounded.[1] I will focus on the provisions of the Data Protection Directive (Directive 95/46/EC) of the European Union (EU), on the right to privacy contained in Article 8 of the European Convention for the Protection of Human Rights and Fundamental Freedoms (ECHR), and on the law on confidentiality in the United Kingdom (UK), with special reference to the use and disclosure of personal data for medical purposes (especially medical research).

Within these confines, I will discuss how confidentiality, privacy, and data protection relate to each other. In all three cases there are duties not to disclose personal information to third parties, in relation to which a central issue concerns the effect of rendering personal information anonymous. Disagreements on this are largely functions of disputes about the scope and nature of the right to privacy. I will argue that in Europe at least, where the ECHR plays a pivotal role both within national laws and European Union (EU) law, the jurisprudence of the European Court of Human Rights (ECtHR) suggests that a broad conception of privacy should be adopted. The importance of consent for the use of personal data is also a matter of some controversy. I will argue that the pivotal role of the ECHR prima facie renders all uses of personal health data without consent of the person to whom the data relate ('the data subject', which is the term used in data protection law) a breach of confidentiality, privacy and data protection law.

This places obstacles in the way of processing health data for medical purposes, which might raise questions about the adoption of a broad conception of the right to privacy.

So, finally, I will comment briefly on the ethical justification of the right so conceived and on conflicts between medical research values and privacy.

PRIVACY, CONFIDENTIALITY AND DATA PROTECTION: PRIVACY IN THE ECHR

According to Article 8.1 ECHR: Everyone has the right to respect for his private and family life, his home and his correspondence.

However, Article 8.2 specifies that there will be no violation of this right if interference with it is in accordance with the law and is necessary in a democratic society in the interests of national security, public safety or the economic well-being of the country, for the prevention of disorder or crime, for the protection of health or morals or for the protection of the rights and freedoms of others.

All EU states, and most others on the European subcontinent, are party to the ECHR. The effect of ratification, however, varies in different states. In 'monist' states (such as France), international treaties are automatically incorporated into domestic law once they are ratified. However, in 'dualist' states (such as the UK) ECHR rights only become part of domestic law if incorporated by a domestic legislative act. In some states, incorporated rights become part of the domestic constitution. In others, they do not, and do not take precedence over domestic constitutional law in cases of conflict. In the UK, where the ECHR is incorporated by the Human Rights Act 1998 (HRA), legislation whenever enacted must (per s.3 HRA) be interpreted so as to be compatible with the incorporated rights[2] (but only if this is not incompatible with conflicting primary legislation)[3] and the courts must not act in ways incompatible with the incorporated rights (again, unless prevented from doing so by primary legislation) (s.6), so must apply the common law so as to be consistent with the incorporated rights. In some states, the jurisprudence of the ECtHR is to be followed, while in others it must at least 'be taken into account'.[4] States also vary in the extent to which they grant the right to individuals against individuals or only regard it as applying in relations between the state and individuals.[5]

Complications are also introduced by the fact that, while the EU is not, itself, party to the ECHR, the values enshrined in ECHR (and other international human rights instruments to which EU member states are party, such as the International Covenant on Civil and Political Rights and the International Covenant on Economic, Social and Cultural Rights of the United Nations) have, through the jurisprudence of the European Court of Justice (ECJ), the supreme court of the EU, achieved the status of fundamental principles of EU law. This is important because the ECJ, at least in principle, considers that a breach of fundamental principles of EU law renders at least secondary legislative instruments of the EU invalid, in consequence of which all EU directives and regulations must be interpreted in ways consistent with the values of the ECHR if at all possible.[6] While the ECtHR is not a court of the EU, its jurisprudence will have strong persuasive force for the ECJ.

The right granted by Article 8.1 ECHR is exceedingly broad in scope. It protects the individual against:

- attacks on his physical or mental integrity or his moral or intellectual freedom;
- attacks on his honour and reputation and similar torts;
- the use of his name, identity or likeness;

- being spied upon, watched or harassed;
- the disclosure of information protected by the duty of professional secrecy.[7]

A narrower view of the right has traditionally held sway in the USA, France, and the UK.[8] Recognising this, the Commission of the Council of Europe stated that [f]or numerous Anglo-Saxon and French authors the right to respect for 'private life' is … the right to live as far as one wishes, protected from publicity.[9]

However, the Commission was adamant that the right to respect for private life does not end there [but includes also the right to: … the development and fulfilment of one's own personality].[10]

For example, the ECtHR has considered Article 8.1 to be engaged in connection with the claimed right of a woman suffering from motor neurone disease to be assisted by her husband in having her life terminated[11] (even though it held that consideration of the protection of the rights of others did not permit the UK to give effect to such a right). In essence, the right to be assisted in taking one's life was declared by the Court to be a right held under Article 8.1, which could be judged to be overridden by considerations specified under Article 8.2.

However, while the right is exceedingly broad it does not amount to a right to human dignity as such. This is because human dignity is, per the Preamble to the Universal Declaration of Human Rights of the United Nations, which the ECHR's Preamble declares the ECHR is designed to implement, the 'foundation of freedom, justice and peace in the world' (hence, of all human rights and fundamental freedoms). Were Article 8.1 to grant such a right it could not be subject to the exceptions specified in Article 8.2 but would be absolute.

Finally, it must be noted that, at least in relation to information about a person's health, there will be a violation of Article 8.1[12] unless a justification can be provided in terms of Article 8.2.

CONFIDENTIALITY

A third party to whom information is given in confidence which has a quality to which confidentiality can attach has a duty to keep it confidential. It is implicit in this statement that not all information is information to which a duty of confidence can attach, that not all such information is given in confidence, and that it is necessary for both conditions to be satisfied for there to be a duty of confidence.

It is difficult to generalise, but at risk of oversimplification, information will possess the necessary quality if the confider has an interest in it that the law recognises as sufficient reason to grant the confider at least a prima facie right to withhold the information from others. So, for example it is generally recognised that sensitive personal information, which includes health data on an individual, can be the subject of a duty of confidence because disclosure of this information to others can in many ways be detrimental to the interests of the individual.

But having this quality is not enough. When qualifying information is disclosed to those who have a duty to keep it confidential, it must have been disclosed to them with the understanding that it is to be kept confidential. What keeping information confidential means is a matter of some controversy: for some, the duty to keep information confidential is simply the duty not to disclose it further without the consent of the confider; for others, it is the wider duty not to use or further disclose the information without the consent of the confider. Furthermore, there is also disagreement about whether the extent to which understanding that it is not to be further disclosed/used needs to be explicit or may be implied by the context (on both of which matters see further below). At any rate, the Hippocratic oath, by which doctors undertake to keep personal information given to them by their patients to themselves, clearly suffices to satisfy the condition that such information is disclosed to doctors in confidence.

The possible bases for granting an action for breach of confidence in relation to data that patients give to their doctors relates to these elements. The duty may be imposed for reasons of fairness or 'equity', because it is manifestly unfair to exploit the position of persons who disclose sensitive information to their physicians because of illness or distress. Alternatively, it might arise out of a contract between the patient and doctor (bearing in mind that such contracts will not always exist). Alternatively, it (as well as the need for doctors to undertake to keep this information confidential) might be dictated by public interest. The reasoning here is that if doctors do not undertake to keep this information confidential and honour this undertaking, patients might become reluctant to seek treatment or to provide complete and accurate information. However, it is in the public interest that those who are ill seek treatment and provide accurate and full information to their doctors: otherwise they will not be properly treated, and so will pass on disease to others, be off work for longer times, or give inaccurate information that contaminates research data.[13]

It should be noted that jurisdictions (and even courts within jurisdictions) vary on the attitude they take as to whether or not a breach of the duty of confidence must be accompanied by some specific harm if redress is to be given. In the UK, for example many judges have held that some significant extrinsic harm must be caused by unsanctioned use or disclosure for the duty to be enforced. Other judges, however, consider the question of harm to be irrelevant, whereas others consider the breach itself to intrinsically constitute harm.[14]

Finally, because 'ought' implies 'can', if information is already in the public domain (which is a matter of degree), no duty of confidence can attach to it, simply because to the extent that the information is public knowledge its use and further disclosure is not within the power of the confidant to control.

CONFIDENTIALITY AND PRIVACY

As normally conceived, for a violation of privacy to occur, it is not necessary for the person who is guilty of the violation to have undertaken (explicitly or implicitly) not to do what constitutes the violation. That is to say, in relation to misuse of private information by a third party it is not necessary for the information to have been imparted to the third party in confidence.

As already stated, the UK HRA requires the UK courts to give effect to the ECHR rights incorporated by the HRA. This has generally been taken to mean that judges are to develop the common law by interpreting existing causes of action (for example, for breach of confidence) in line with privacy. It should be apparent, however, that development of a right to privacy via, for example, an action for breach of confidence is limited if the idea that a breach of confidence requires information to have been imparted in confidence. Nevertheless, there have been some cases where the courts, in order to try to give as much effect to privacy as possible, have come close to suggesting that breach of confidence no longer requires information to have been imparted in confidence.[15]

DATA PROTECTION RIGHTS

The aim of Directive 95/46/EC is to protect the fundamental rights and freedoms of individuals (in particular, privacy) in relation to the processing of personal data (see Article 1).

Central to the Directive are five data protection principles (see Article 6(1)), which require EU Member States to ensure that personal data are:

- processed fairly and lawfully;
- collected for specified, explicit and legitimate processes and not further processed in a way incompatible with those purposes;
- adequate, relevant and not excessive in relation to the purposes for which they are collected or further processed;
- accurate and, where necessary, kept complete and up-to-date;
- not be kept in a person identifying form for longer than necessary for the purposes for which they were collected or (compatibly) further processed.

Member states must grant data subjects a right of access to personal data on themselves (Article 12), a right to object to processing of personal data on themselves for purposes of direct marketing or other legitimate grounds (Article 14) and a right not to be subjected to significant decisions based solely on automated processing (Article 12).

For processing of personal data to be legitimate, at least one of the conditions laid down in Article 7 must be satisfied. These include the unambiguous consent of the data subject, or the protection of the vital interests of the data subject.

In the case of sensitive personal data, which, according to Article 8 includes 'data concerning health', Article 8(1) requires member states to prohibit processing unless certain conditions are satisfied (Articles 8(2)(a)–(e) and 8(3)–8(5)). For the purposes of processing data concerning health, the most relevant conditions are the explicit consent of the data subject (Article 8(2)(a)); the necessity to protect the vital interests of the data subject or another person in cases where the data subject physically or legally cannot give consent (Article 8(2)(c)); necessity for the purposes of 'preventive medicine, medical diagnosis, the provision of care or treatment or the management of health-care services, and where those data are processed by a health professional subject under national law or rules established by national competent bodies to the obligation of professional secrecy or by another person also subject to an equivalent obligation of secrecy' (Article 8(3)); or if specified by national law or the decision of the supervisory authority in the substantial public interest (Article 8(4)), which might cover scientific research (Recital 34).

Consequently, for processing of sensitive personal data to be legitimate it is necessary for at least one condition from Article 7 and one condition from Article 8 to be satisfied;

although satisfying an Article 8 condition such as explicit consent will automatically satisfy the Article 7 condition of unambiguous consent .

Transfer of personal data to countries outside the European Economic Area (EEA) that do not provide a degree of data protection equivalent to that required by the Directive must also be prohibited (Article 25) unless certain conditions are satisfied (see Article 26), such as the unambiguous consent of the data subject.

Last, but by no means least, Article 10 (which applies where data are obtained from the data subject) and Article 11 (which applies where the data were not obtained from the data subject) require member states to impose duties on data controllers (those who determine the purposes of processing) to provide data subjects with information about the identity of the data controller, the purposes of processing intended and any other information needed for processing to be fair. These duties are pivotal, because this information is essential if data subjects are to be able to exercise their rights under the Directive and consent (where applicable) is to be informed (as the Directive requires).[16]

DATA PROTECTION RIGHTS AND PRIVACY

Privacy is only one of the rights that the Directive seeks to protect. Therefore, because the Directive aims to protect fundamental rights and freedoms in general, whether it operates with a narrow or a broad concept of privacy is somewhat moot, for, supposing (contrary to my contention) that it is acceptable to deploy a narrow conception of privacy, although some uses of information held/obtained in personal data might not engage the right to privacy, they might still engage other fundamental rights and freedoms.

However, given that the Directive does seek to protect privacy, the fact that the jurisprudence of the European Court of Human Rights indicates that Article 8.1 ECHR is engaged by any use of health data without the subject's consent, and requires a justification in terms of Article 8.2 ECHR, suggests that the conditions for lifting the prohibition on the processing of data on a person's health specified in Article 8 of the Directive may not be regarded as an open list. If conditions other than explicit consent are to be appealed to then this requires it to be impractical, inappropriate, or disproportionate to seek consent in relation to other competing legitimate objectives of the processing (which must be in line with Article 8.2 of the ECHR).

DATA PROTECTION RIGHTS AND CONFIDENTIALITY

Insofar as data protection rights apply to personal data as such, data protection rights have a broader scope than laws on confidential information. However, laws on confidentiality can be broader in scope than data protection rights because information that is not personal can be imparted in confidence. Furthermore, personal information need not be structured in the way that the Directive specifies for it to qualify as personal data for a duty of confidence to attach to it.

The relationship between data protection and confidentiality is complicated, however, by a requirement that personal data be processed fairly and lawfully. It follows from this that member states must (if they are to implement the Directive properly) render breaches of any of their domestic laws covering the processing of personal data breaches of the first data protection principle.

SECRECY AND THESE RIGHTS

If personal information is already in the public domain then any rights of control over the use of the information that the subject of the information might otherwise have had will be impossible to exercise effectively. Consequently, laws on confidentiality, privacy and data protection all impose a duty on those to whom confidential/personal/private information is disclosed not to further disclose this information without the consent of the data subject (unless special exemptions apply). It follows from this that in all three areas, duties exist for those to whom the applicable information is disclosed to keep the information or data secure or secret (that is, not to disclose them to others beyond that which is necessary for the purposes for which they were disclosed).

In general, however, to keep information securely in this sense cannot be equated with keeping it confidential. This is because information may be disclosed to someone on condition that it be used only for specific purposes even by the person to whom it is disclosed, or at least on the condition that it not be used for specified purposes. Equally, keeping personal data secure in this sense cannot be regarded as sufficient to discharge all duties under the Data Protection Directive for the Directive requires member states to give data subjects control over the purposes of processing and not merely over further disclosures of the data. This, however, raises questions about the effect on the right to privacy, the duty of confidentiality and data protection of rendering personal data anonymous, because, in at least a limited sense, to render personal data anonymous is to keep them secret/secure.

THE ISSUE OF ANONYMISATION RE PRIVACY, CONFIDENTIALITY AND DATA PROTECTION

In 1999, the English High Court ruled that the Department of Health had given correct advice when it issued a letter to health authorities stating that doctors and pharmacists who sold information about the drugs prescribed by doctors to database companies (who intended to sell it on to pharmaceutical companies for purposes of direct marketing of doctors) would be acting in breach of confidentiality unless they had obtained the consent of the patients, despite the fact that the data would be aggregated (and would not disclose the identity of individual patients) before being passed to the database companies.[17] However, the Court of Appeal of England and Wales overturned this decision.[18] The Court of Appeal also declared, in obiter remarks, that the scheme was not in breach of Directive 95/46/EC because Recital 26 of the Directive declares that the principles of data protection do not apply to data rendered anonymous.

THE ISSUE RE CONFIDENTIALITY

The ruling of the High Court was based simply on the idea that patients give their information to doctors for their treatment and that to use it without their consent is to breach confidentiality unless a justification for doing so exists (for example, in the public interest, which the court did not find). In effect, the court held that the duty of confidentiality here is not to use the information outside the scope of what the patient has consented to, and this is very much in line with ECHR jurisprudence if privacy underpins the duty.

On the other hand, according to the Court of Appeal, the duty of confidentiality in relation to personal information obtained by doctors for the treatment of patients arises from a need to treat patients fairly. Consequently, as long as patients are not treated unfairly by so doing, doctors may use or disclose the personal information they obtain for any lawful purpose. In relation to this, the court held that use of this information without consent did not necessarily constitute unfair treatment, because the only interest of the patients engaged by the activities in question was protection of their privacy. This interest, the court held, was fully and completely protected provided only that the patient's identity is fully protected. Given that the database companies were to receive information in a form in which they could not identify patients, privacy was not violated, hence the disclosure was not unfair, and so there was no breach of confidence.

The contention that privacy is protected fully by non-disclosure of the patient's identity reflects a narrow conception of privacy, which does not, as I have pointed out, follow the jurisprudence of the ECtHR, and nor does the claim that to use information on a patient's health without the patient's explicit consent does not constitute unfairness.[19]

RECITAL 26 AND THE DIRECTIVE

In relation to its claim that pharmacists (and GPs) were not acting contrary to the Data Protection Directive, the Court of Appeal focused, quite properly, on Recital 26, according to which the principles of data protection do not apply once data have been rendered anonymous. However, the Court ignored that Recital 26 also says that the principles of protection apply to all personal data. This is important because, under the Directive, processing of personal data is anything that can be done to personal data, and if there might be any doubt that anonymisation of personal data is processing of it, it must be pointed out that the Directive specifies that processing includes alteration and deletion of personal data.

Now, Articles 10 and 11 require data controllers to inform data subjects of the purposes of the intended processing. Anonymisation is a process. Hence, controllers have a duty (subject to exemption) to inform of the purposes of anonymisation and what its effects will be. Also, when data are disclosed to one person in anonymous form they might still be held in personal form by the discloser. In such a case, can the data be said to have been rendered anonymous, or the processing by those who hold them in anonymised form be said not to be processing personal data? Surely not, if Recital 26 is to be followed when it specifies that data are personal if anyone can identify the data subject from them directly or indirectly.

Also, the operative conception of privacy is critical here. If we are to interpret Recital 26 properly then we need to know what is the reasoning behind it. Since the aim of the Directive is to protect fundamental rights and freedoms, in particular privacy, what it says must link to the logic of such protection. But this leaves us with at least two possibilities. First, Recital 26 might merely reflect the idea that once it is impossible to identify the data subject, then the data subject loses the ability to exercise any rights of control over the data that are the concern of the Directive. Alternatively, Recital 26 might reflect the idea that the only interest the data subjects have in their personal data and use of them is in their identities not be disclosed to those who might misuse them. On a broad conception of privacy, which I have argued operates, the latter is simply not a plausible position. In effect, if data are still held in a form in which it would be possible for data subjects to exercise their rights in relation to them, then they cannot be considered to have been rendered anonymous. So, for example when GPs and pharmacists continue to hold data in personal form from which they pass on abstracted information in depersonalised form to a database company, processing by the company is to be considered processing of personal data, because GPs and pharmacists could have informed patients of the scheme when they obtained the data and still could now (for the purposes of consent or at least to give them the opportunity to object).

Indeed, if this is correct then it must be concluded that rendering personal data anonymous without consent might actually constitute a violation of privacy rather than protection of it. Such would surely be the case if rendering the data anonymous prevented their being used for the patient's treatment. And if, as in the present case, no such consequence follows from the disclosure to the database companies, this merely implies that the data have not been rendered anonymous.[20]

PROTECTION OF PRIVACY AND MEDICAL RESEARCH: SOME PHILOSOPHICAL REFLECTIONS

It is apparent that use of a broad conception of privacy creates prima facie obstacles for research and use for other purposes to which the data subject has not consented. There is little doubt that some will find this objectionable on the grounds that medical research and other medical activities aim to protect human life and health, which they will regard as much more important than privacy values, especially if the subject's identity is protected.

In response to this, two points may be helpful.

- The broad conception of privacy does not make consent an absolute right. What it requires is the need to obtain consent for the use of health data unless there are overriding considerations.
- Under a broad conception of privacy, activities that increase life chances and quality of life are activities that enhance privacy. To the extent that medical activities promise/deliver such benefits, they are not in conflict with privacy; and where conflicts do exist they are just as well, perhaps better, viewed as conflicts between privacy values, than between medical values and privacy values. Conversely, it is apparent that the public interest in trust in doctors implies that privacy support is something that supports medical activities, so that privacy should be regarded as at least an instrumental research value.[21]

It should also be apparent that information protection under the broad conception of privacy of the ECHR in effect regards sensitive personal data, such as data about a person's health, sex life, religion, or ethnicity, as constituent elements of the person. Hence to use such data is to use that person. To use such data without consent is to use the person merely as a means and not at the same time as an end in him or herself. Hence the clearest justification for the broad conception of privacy lies in Kantian theory.

However, it should not be thought that only Kantian theory will support such a conception. Utilitarian arguments suggest themselves once the effect of not protecting privacy on public trust in the medical profession and medical science is acknowledged. Utilitarian arguments, I suggest, only appear to argue against placing high value on privacy when privacy is seen as a purely individual interest, when under a broad conception conflicts between privacy and medical values are better viewed as conflicts between different aspects of the public interest.

Finally, it is arguable that the broad conception of privacy, by linking medical research goals to privacy protection, actually makes it easier to argue that persons have qualified duties to participate in well designed and conducted medical research.[22]

NOTES

1 There is a wide selection given at http://www.privacyinternational.org/survey/phr2003/overview.htm (accessed 30 April 2008).

2 The rights of Articles 2-12 and 14 of the ECHR, plus Articles 1-3 of the First Protocol and Articles 1 and 2 of the Sixth Protocol of the ECHR, read with Articles 16–18 of the ECHR (s.1(1)).

3 Higher courts might make a declaration of incompatibility (s.4) but this does not affect the validity of primary legislation or secondary legislation directed by primary legislation (s.3 (3) and s.4), which it is up to the Crown to change through Parliament (see ss.10, 19 and 20).

4 See, e.g. the HRA s.2 (1).

5 For a discussion, see, e.g. Deryck Beyleveld and Shaun Pattinson (2002) 'Horizontal applicability and horizontal effect', *Law Quarterly Review* 118: 623–46.

6 *Second Nold case (Case-4/73)* [1974] E.C.R. 507.

7 Jacques Velu (1973) 'The European Convention on Human Rights and the Right to Respect for Private Life, the Home and Communications', in A. H. Robertson (ed.) (1973) *Privacy and Human Rights*. Manchester: Manchester University Press, pp. 12–128 at 92.

8 Re the UK, see further below.

9 Application No. 6825/74 DR5, 87.

10 Application No. 6825/74 DR5, 87.

11 See *Case of Pretty v. the United Kingdom;* Application no. 2346/02; 29 April.

12 See the case of *M.S. v. Sweden* 28 EHRR 313, paragraphs 34–35.

13 See, e.g. Bingham LJ in *W v Egdell* [1990] Ch. 359 at 419 and 422.

14 See the various judgments in Attorney-General v. Guardian Newspapers (No. 2) [1990] AC 109 at 255, 270, 281.

15 See, e.g. *Campbell v MGN* [2004] UKHL 22.

16 The complexities of, and difficulties with interpreting the requirements of Articles 10 and 11 are discussed in Deryck Beyleveld (2004) 'The duty to provide information to the Data Subject: Articles 10 and 11 of Directive 95/46/EC', in Deryck Beyleveld et al. (eds) *Data Protection and Medical Research Across Europe*. Aldershot: Ashgate.

17 R v. *Department of Health, Ex Parte Source Informatics Ltd.* [1999] 4 All ER 185. For commentary, see Deryck Beyleveld and Elise Histed (1999) 'Anonymisation is not exoneration: R v. Department of Health, ex parte Source Informatics Ltd', *Medical Law International,* 4: 69–80.

18 R v. *Department of Health, Ex Parte Source Informatics Ltd.* [2000] 1 All ER 786. (38) For commentary, see Deryck Beyleveld and Elise Histed (2000) 'Betrayal of confidence in the Court of Appeal', *Medical Law International*, 3/4: 277–311.

19 Had the case been decided after the HRA 1998 came into effect, this ruling would arguably have been in violation of s.6 of the HRA and the duty it imposes on judges to progress the common law in line with ECHR. At any rate it is clear that the judges in the *Campbell* case accepted a broad conception of privacy, Lord Nicholls declaring that the right is wider than the protection of private information ([2004] UKHL 22, para 15) and Lord Hoffmann holding that the right is an aspect of human autonomy and dignity (para 50) in accordance with which Lord Hope declared that breaches are to be measured by what is offensive in the eyes of the individual right-holder, not in the eyes of the reasonable person.

20 The argument for this is more fully spelled out in Deryck Beyleveld and David Townend (2004) 'When is personal data rendered anonymous? Interpreting Recital 26 of Directive 95/46/EC', *Medical Law International,* 6 (2): 73–86.

21 See further, Deryck Beyleveld (2006) 'Conceptualising privacy in relation to research values', in Shelia A.M. McLean (ed.) *First Do Not Harm: Law, Ethics and Healthcare*. Aldershot: Ashgate, pp. 151–64.

22 See Deryck Beyleveld and Shaun Pattinson (2008) 'Moral interests, privacy and medical research', in Michel Boylan (ed.) *International Public Health Policy and Ethics.* New York: Springer, pp. 45–57.

10

Informed Consent

Vilhjálmur Árnason, Hongwen Li and Yali Cong

INTRODUCTION

In this chapter we first briefly discuss historical and moral reasons for obtaining informed consent for therapy and research. Second, we describe and critically evaluate the standard view on what this requirement implies. Third, we discuss some of the practical obstacles in the way of meeting the standard requirements and consider recent attempts to rethink informed consent.

REASONS FOR INFORMED CONSENT

Though it is now widely recognized as one of the cornerstones of the relationship between patient and healthcare professionals as well as between researchers and research participants, the requirement of informed consent for therapy and research is a recent phenomenon. A combination of three main factors contributed to the need to regulate research and to protect human participants. First, the bitter lessons learned from the abuse of people both during the Second World War, and in some outrageous clinical trials and experiments that were brought to public attention (for example Tuskegee and Willowbrook in the US). Second, during the latter half of the twentieth century the general ethos of the patient professional relationship underwent a major change, emphasizing the rights of individuals over their own bodies and to be informed about research and medical procedures. Third, the requirement for informed consent has been engendered by the practice of defensive medicine where the practitioners' purpose is to protect themselves legally.[1]

Regardless of the origin of informed consent, its moral purpose is to protect people against abuse. There are two main strands of moral reasons for seeking informed consent for research participation and medical interventions: autonomy reasons and welfarist reasons.[2]

The former type of reasons prevails in the justification of informed consent. The reasons can be divided into two categories: (1) reasons which emphasize the opportunity for individuals to choose whether or not to undergo treatment or participate in research; (2) reasons which emphasize that people should not be treated as mere means but always as ends in themselves. These different reasons may contribute to different practices but the common goal of autonomy reasons is to ensure that people are not subjected to coercion, deception, or other kinds of manipulation.

Welfarist reasons, on the other hand, refer to the benefits that informed consent may have for the individual subject or for society. Although protection from harm must be an institutionalized task, it is also important to give individuals the opportunity to protect their own well-being and to evaluate what kinds of risks they are willing to take. The social benefits of informed consent can increase trust in science, which may lead to more research participation and possibly valuable research results that can improve the human condition.

ELEMENTS OF INFORMED CONSENT

Standards of disclosure

According to Beauchamp and Childress, medical professionals are obliged to disclose a core set of information, which must include the following five elements: (a) 'those facts or descriptions that patients or subjects usually consider material in deciding whether to refuse or consent to the proposed intervention or research'; (b) 'information the professionals believe to be material'; (c) 'the professionals' recommendation'; (d) 'the purpose of seeking consent'; and (e) 'the nature and limits of consent as an act of authorization'.[3]

Such a list of information only implies what should be disclosed by professionals, but it doesn't answer the question as to whether the information is adequate or not. This question implies that healthcare professionals and biomedical researchers should disclose adequate information to ensure that patients and subjects are informed appropriately. Three different standards have been put forward to guide the disclosure of information.

(1) The professional practice standard or the reasonable doctor standard. Its basic point of view is that a professional community's customary practices determine the disclosure of information. According to this standard, whether a doctor has violated a patient's right to information is judged by the medical professionals' testimony.

There are several problems with this standard. First, it is uncertain whether a professional customary norm exists in many medical situations. A customary standard is a vague notion, and in many clinical practices we cannot find a definite custom to meet this standard. Second, custom cannot always be justified by ethical norms; a custom can give medical professionals a good excuse to avoid their duties. Third, it is also questionable whether doctors have developed skills to judge their patients' best interests. Their professional judgments depend on the personal accumulation of experience in clinical practice. Not every doctor has much experience in medical practice, although many physicians have excellent skills in this respect. Furthermore, experience is not always trustworthy.

Finally, and perhaps most importantly, physicians may ignore the patients' values when they decide how much information should be disclosed.

(2)   The reasonable person standard or the objective patient standard. This is a theoretical hypothesis about what information is pertinent and material as judged by a reasonable person or an objective patient. According to this standard, the judgment power of information disclosure shifts from the medical professional community to a hypothetical reasonable person, that is, from physicians to patients. The notion of 'reasonable person' usually means an average person who has a sound mind, a rational man. The judgments of a rational man meet the expectations of the majority of patients. The 'reasonable person' in this standard is not a specific person, but an abstract notion of the person.

Although this standard has a merit of being patient-oriented, it has some obvious theoretical difficulties. First, the definition of 'reasonable person' is ambiguous. It has never been clearly defined, and different people have different ideas about it. Second, the reasonable person standard is a theoretical hypothesis which has a limited significance for guidance in clinical practice. Physicians can only imagine a reasonable person in theory, but they may not employ this abstract standard effectively in the process of informed consent. In most research situations, however, it is important to ask what most people would find reasonable to know before they participate in research.

(3)   The subjective standard or subjective patient standard.[4] This standard resorts to the individual patient to determine whether the information is adequate. Patients have different needs and values so the information expectation can vary from person to person. This situation requires specific information given according to individual patients' anticipation. The subjective patient standard is an advisable standard, because it admits personal difference of information expectation. This method is context-sensitive, since it considers the specific situation of every individual patient.

It is not enough, however, to depend solely on the subjective patient standard. Sometimes patients do not know what kind of information and how much is relevant and beneficial for decision making, and what information is material for informed consent. Physicians should disclose information according to their professional knowledge and criteria. Then patients can use this information to determine what meets their needs and expectation. This integrates the subjective standard with the professional practice standard, which demands an in-depth communication between medical professionals and patients. Only in this way can professionals know what information patients care to have and what they do not.

In sum, the different standards of disclosure show the standing point shifting from physician to patient, from physician centered to patient centered approach, or from medical paternalism to patient autonomy. Some scholars think the reasonable-patient standard may be ethically sufficient, but the subjective standard is ethically ideal.[5]

GENUINE CONSENT

We have looked at the standards of disclosure of information that is necessary for patients to be informed. We now turn our attention to the consent side of the matter.

Informed consent should at least meet the requirements of competence, understanding, and voluntariness.

(1)   The doctrine of informed consent in medicine requires a voluntary decision from a competent patient. Thus, a crucial question at the outset is how to determine whether a patient is competent or not. Competence means the ability to do what is needed to perform a task. If persons can understand and appreciate the information given by professionals, then they are competent. If they are unable to understand and cannot appreciate the information, then they are incompetent.[6] This definition focuses on intellectual ability. It is instructive to relate this to a situation when a patient refuses treatment. Some patients might understand and appreciate the information given by the medical professionals, but refuse the treatment, even though almost everyone including family members and physicians believe that the patients' refusals are irrational and should be overruled. A typical case illustrates this problem:

Case 1:

A man with an unstable cardiac condition is severely depressed. He is anorexic and has lost a great deal of weight. He will not eat and refuses therapy for his depression. His doctor believes that there is a high likelihood the patient will die from his weakened condition within a few weeks. The patient understands and acknowledges that without treatment he may die and that with treatment he will almost certainly recover. Unlike some depressed patients, he has no 'cognitive distortions'. Nonetheless, because of his depressed mood, he refuses nourishment and potentially lifesaving treatment because, he states, he wants to die.[7]

In this case, although the patient has the understanding ability, he makes an inadvisable decision for his medical treatment. His state of depression undermines his normal capability of clinical decision making. The wrong decision does not come from his cognitive ability, since he has no cognitive distortions. It is the depressive mood that results in negative effects for his self determination. According to the traditional standard, this patient is competent. But we can see that he has made an unwise determination of refusing the treatment. There are good reasons to believe that he has no appropriate competence to make the medical decision for himself in this situation. So, he has no material decision-making capability, and he is incompetent to make the decision.

   This indicates that the traditional definition is inaccurate and that it is necessary to refine the definition: the competence in clinical decision making refers to the ability to make a rational decision.[8] According to this, the patient in our case makes an inadvisable decision, thus he is incompetent according to this new definition. A person who has only cognitive ability and makes an irrational decision is in this sense strictly incompetent. A rational decision is necessary for a competent person. Obviously, there are two essential parts in this new definition: ability and rationality.

   It is important to see the aspect of rationality as an ability of communication which is necessary in the process of informed consent. Medical decisions may need deep consideration over a period of time, especially important critical medical decisions. In the process of deliberation, reasoning capacity is important; this requires patients to imagine the possible consequences of the treatment. In evaluating the risks and benefits, the patients will give these different weight and importance according to their personal values. The notion of rational and advisable choice cannot, therefore, be separated from the patient's own values.

The logic of the term 'competence' is that persons are not globally competent; no one has the ability to do all mental and physical tasks. The conception of competence in civil law is a general conception. It presumes that all sound-minded adults are competent to handle civil affairs and make medical decisions of their own free will. In the legal context, all adults who are in their right mind have the pervasive and global right to medical decision making, except for some incompetent ones, according to the specific rules and laws. However, a person who is incompetent according to civil law may have the capacity to perform some special tasks. For example, some patients cannot understand technically complicated and high-risk surgery, but can understand some that is technically simple and low-risk. That a person is competent in some aspects does not mean that he/she is also competent in other domains. Competence is therefore best understood as task-specific rather than global: it depends not only on a person's abilities but also on how that person's abilities match the particular decision-making task he or she confronts.[9]

The MacArthur Competence Assessment Tool for Treatment is commonly used to evaluate competence which can be crucial, especially when confronting surrogate decision making. In medical decision making and medical research, it is the individual well-being and self-determination that support this general presumption. These two values are important for informed consent. Because when a person is competent to perform normal informed consent, he or she must do that for self-interest in their health care. When he/she is incompetent, it is required by law that a third party as surrogate gives legal and reasonable consent in the best interest of the incompetent person. The consent given by the surrogate should not impair the health and well-being of the patient.

Case 2:

In Beijing, in November 2007, a pregnant woman was sent to an emergency room with high fever, pneumonia. Before she lost consciousness, she looked at her husband, and asked him to decide for her. When the doctor recommended a caesarean operation, the husband didn't agree, for he thought that his wife was there just because of her illness, and that it was not time for delivery of the baby. The hospital asked a psychologist to evaluate whether the husband was competent, and the result was 'yes'. Without the husband's signature, the hospital could not perform the operation, and the pregnant woman and the fetus both died. This case caused hot discussion in China, about revising relevant articles of regulation, about the system, about law and ethics, about the nature and form of informed consent, etc.

In fact, the husband in this case was not competent at that specific time. No tool for evaluation can resolve such problems completely. It is recommended that the ethics committee of a hospital can play some kind of role in such situations, to prevent a tragedy such as happened in the above case. In a medical emergency such a decision by a family member should not be respected.

(2)   Understanding is a vital element of informed consent. With regard to biomedical ethics, the focus has shifted from the physician's or researcher's obligation to disclose information as to the quality of a patient's or subject's understanding and consent. But there are several problems with the definition and nature of understanding. It is commonly accepted that it is difficult to find procedures to make sure that the patients or subjects really understand the information they are given.

A general definition of understanding is that one understands if one has acquired pertinent information and justified, relevant beliefs about the nature and consequences of one's action. Understanding is a subjective process and it is very difficult for us to get an objective approach to measure this inner psychological activity. Understanding is based on background knowledge and beliefs that can be difficult to assess and to correct if necessary.

Disclosure of relevant information is a precondition for informed consent. The professionals' disclosure of information does not mean that the patients or subjects have to be exposed to the total amount of information available regarding the treatment or research. The ethical demand is only that they are adequately informed and have an adequate understanding of the information concerning the treatment or research. In order to achieve this goal, the professionals will have to use their imaginative, empathic, and professional skills. This means that they should be aware of, look for, and try to prevent problems of different kinds that might stand in the way of patients' or subjects' understanding. The duty to disclose material information cannot be overlooked in the process of understanding.

There is no pure and abstract understanding in medical treatments. In order to connect with background knowledge and make understanding possible, the professionals must use comprehensible language, trying to draw analogies between the specialized information and more ordinary events familiar to the patient or subject. Information overload and under-disclosure are two typical barriers to the understanding process. So-called information overload is when the understanding of patients or subjects is prevented by the use of unfamiliar terms, unfamiliar or complicated language. The under-disclosure of information means that the information that is provided is inadequate or not comprehensive enough.

(3)   The voluntary decision of informed consent is first stated in the Nuremberg Code as follows, with regard to permissible medical experiments:

> The voluntary consent of the human subject is absolutely essential. This means that the person involved should have legal capacity to give consent; should be so situated as to be able to exercise free power of choice, without the intervention of any element of force, fraud, deceit, duress, over-reaching, or other ulterior form of constraint or coercion; and should have sufficient knowledge and comprehension of the elements of the subject matter involved as to enable him to make an understanding and enlightened decision.[10]

In order to make a voluntary decision, the individual undergoing medical intervention or participating in research needs to be aware of the possible relevant outcomes of therapy or research. In addition to this requirement of intentionality, the agent must be free of significant controlling influences for a decision to be voluntary.[11] There are three main categories of influence: coercion, persuasion, and manipulation.[12] Some cases of controlling influences are clear, such as deception and coercion. Others are much harder to assess. We can take an example of a poor peasant who 'consents' to an experiment in the hope and expectation of a reward: some money, free drugs, an opportunity to cure his cancer, better health care when involved in the experiment. Are some kinds of rewards proper and permissible in medical researches when professionals get informed consent from a subject? And at what point does reward render informed consent involuntary, making the whole process invalid? The problem of reward is difficult because it involves the question of degree, which is dependent on circumstances.

In some cultures, individual autonomy is not recognized and patients like to make decisions together with their family. In such cases it is important to 'carry out an informed consent discussion in a manner appropriate to the patient's beliefs and understanding'.[13] This does not mean that the principle of autonomy is not valid but that it requires careful application which takes particular cultural aspects into account. This may raise some difficult questions: Can we justly withhold key information from a female research subject in a culture where the husband decides for the woman? Respect for cultural diversity does not outweigh the right of individuals to make their own choices.[14] One way to deal with such an issue is to ask the woman whether she would like to receive the information and make the decision herself or leave it up to her husband. A choice to delegate decision making to someone else can itself be autonomous, but it must be taken by the person herself.

THEORY AND PRACTICE

When the elements of informed consent are properly integrated into medical care and research, they are an essential part of good practice in these areas. Also, most patients want to be given information about medical care and research. However, there are various obstacles in the way of good practice of informed consent. It is quite common to hear criticism of the idea of informed consent from both medical practitioners and researchers, and also sometimes from patients and research participants.

As we have seen, the idea of informed consent implies that patients are informed, that they understand the information, and that they make a voluntary decision. However, often patients are distressed, the information complex, and the hospital environment and the busy routine of health-care professionals not conducive to the kind of deliberation that needs to precede an informed, voluntary decision.[15] As a consequence, the practice of informed consent tends to be reduced to the act of signing an informed consent form. Such a formal act meets some administrative requirements but need not entail any of the elements of genuine informed consent. The experience of this practice has understandably bred cynicism towards informed consent among both patients and practitioners. If the standards of genuine informed consent cannot be met while the practice of medicine and research is largely justified by it, the result will be 'systematic hypocrisy'.[16]

A common response to this dilemma is to emphasize that obtaining informed consent is not an event but rather a communicative process between practitioners and patients.[17] Engaging in communication implies much more than sharing information; it requires listening no less than talking to patients. Communication does not only convey information, it also provides support and thus meets the needs for counseling and comfort that many patients have. Such a communicative approach can thus be sensitive to cultural differences and be understanding of those who do not share common assumptions. To be sure, such conversations take time but they also build mutual trust which can remove many obstacles from the practice of informed consent. If the practical exigencies of medicine make such communicative effort unrealistic, then it amounts to admitting that there cannot be good medical practice.

The situation is rather different in research, especially non-clinical research, which requires a large number of participants. Obviously, it is more difficult in those cases to facilitate dialogical conditions for informing participants than it is in clinical situations. There are several types of research that vary with respect to subject matter, methods, aims and whether they are retrospective or prospective. Also, the nature of participation can range from physical presence in an experiment to analyses of anonymized data. Nevertheless, the tendency has been to take as a standard for all such research on 'human beings' the Declaration of Helsinki, where it is stated that 'each potential subject must be adequately informed of the aims, methods, sources of funding, and any possible conflict of interests, institutional affiliation of the researcher, the anticipated benefits and potential risks of the study and the discomfort it may entail'.[18] There are exceptions from this, for example in retrospective epidemiological studies. Recent developments in genetic research have complicated this situation.

An interesting example that has posed challenging questions about the possibility of obtaining informed consent is population genetic database research.[19] The positions on this matter can be divided into three main categories. First, there are those who argue for the need to inform patients specifically about each particular research project planned in a database. Such specific consent implies that participants will be informed prior to donating their data for research about its objectives, methods, risks, benefits, and other traditional ingredients of informed consent. This means that any research with new questions requires re-contact with the participants. Participants find such continuous re-contact annoying and studies have shown that they are willing to give a wider consent and leave it up to the researchers and regulatory committees to ensure that they are used fairly for the benefit of science and society.[20] Moreover, specific consent requires detailed descriptions in scientific protocols which tend to overwhelm participants' understanding capacity. The paradox is that the more information is provided, the less understanding is obtained, so that the consent procedure tends to become a mere formality.

The second position emphasizes that population databases are resources for genetic research and it is impossible to describe in detail the research that will be performed on the data at the time of collection. If we are to use this resource efficiently, specific consent for database research must be rejected in favor of open consent. By open consent, it is meant here that participants agree that their data will be used for any future scientific research permitted by regulatory institutions. The main emphasis is thus laid upon trust in ethics committees which would evaluate the participants' interests and act on their behalf. However, such open consent does not provide participants with the information necessary for them to make a meaningful choice, i.e. act in a voluntary way on a basic understanding of the matter. It transfers the reflection on population research from the participants to regulatory institutions. Thus motivations for scientific literacy and awareness of the public would be reduced and important benefits related to human agency are ignored.

In order to avoid these pitfalls of specific and open consent, the third position carves out alternatives that are intended to strike a balance between the researchers' need for flexibility and the ethical demand for protection of participants' interests.[21] The main thrust of these proposals, which have different emphases, is that participants should be asked to authorize the use of their data for described healthcare research. They would be informed about the conditions for use of the data, such as how the research will be regulated, how they will be connected to other data, who will have access to the information, how privacy will be secured, and that the data will only be used for the described healthcare purposes. Most importantly, participants would be told that they and/or their proxies will be regularly informed about the research practice and that they can at any time withdraw from particular research projects. In this way, the emphasis on a one-time initial consent is rejected in favor of a dynamic process between researchers and participants.

Such an authorization or permission would both allow participants 'to meaningfully act on their continuing interests in their health information'[22] and provide science ethics committees with a basis for determining further use of the information. Further use can be restricted to comparable research where members of science ethics committees can reasonably argue that the additional research would not have affected the participants' initial decision to participate. Such a policy could maintain the motivation for participants to reflect on their participation in research and to stay informed about how their data are used and for what purposes. An authorization policy might thus contribute to informed research participation that can underpin public trust in research practices. None of these would flow from an open consent policy for database research.

This proposal implies that individuals are offered 'simple and realistic ways of checking that what they consent to is indeed what happens and what they do not consent to does not happen'.[23] If the latter happens, they can opt out. In addition to strengthening the basis for non-deception, this last point aims at securing the purpose of non-coercion, since it implies that participants need not continue with research against their will.[24] In this way interests associated with moral agency and the moral purpose of informed consent can be secured.

This example of consent for participation in genetic population databases is part of recent attempts to rethink the use of informed consent in biomedicine. These attempts are characterized by a search for ways out of the dilemma of either being content with a practice which mainly fulfils formal and administrative requirements or striving to meet the strict standards of genuine informed consent which would require radical changes of the current practices. It has been argued that an account of informed consent which is both practically feasible and morally justifiable requires that the nature of information and communication which forms the basic assumptions of the informed consent discourse have to be reconsidered.[25] Instead of focusing on the disclosure of information as a basis of autonomous decision making, we need to observe whether the epistemic and ethical norms that are constitutive of adequate communication have been observed or not. It follows from this that it is more important to facilitate successful communication than device standardized consent procedures. Good communication is context dependent and although it needs to meet adequate standards it cannot be reduced to standardized and elaborate disclosure, dissemination, and reception of information.

CONCLUSION

In this chapter we have described some of the main elements of informed consent and how they have been translated into practice. We have considered some of the practical obstacles in the way of securing informed consent and shown how the standards of genuine informed consent can place unrealistic and even undesirable demands on the practice of medicine. We have argued that the main objective of informed consent is to ensure that patients and research participants are not deceived, manipulated, or coerced.

Promising reconsiderations of informed consent imply that effective means to reach this moral goal are not rigid compliance with the protocols of informed consent, but relevant and contextually sensitive communicative transactions between the parties. This shift of perspective calls for changes in practices and policies that will hopefully relieve the frustrations of patients and practitioners and improve the quality of both research and clinical work.

NOTES

1 Cf. David J. Rothman (1991) *Strangers at the Bedside. History of how Law and Bioethics Transformed Medical Decision Making* (New York: Basic Books).

2 Sigurður Kristinsson and Vilhjálmur Árnason (2007) 'Informed consent and human genetic database research', in M. Häyry, R. Chadwick, V. Árnason and G. Árnason (eds), *The Ethics and Governance of Human Genetic Databases. European Perspectives* (Cambridge: Cambridge University Press) pp. 199–216.

3 Tom Beauchamp and James Childress (2001) *Principles of Biomedical Ethics*, 5th ed. (Oxford: Oxford University Press) p. 81.

4 Sandy Elkin (2001) 'Informed consent: Requirements for legal and ethical practice', *Physiotherapy Theory and Practice*, 17: 97–105.

5 Albert R. Jonsen, Mark Siegler and William J. Winslade (2006) *Clinical Ethics*, 6th ed. (New York/London: McGraw-Hill) p. 57.

6 Bernard Gert, Charles M. Culver and K. Danner Clouser (1997) *Bioethics: A Return to Fundamentals* (New York: Oxford University Press) p.132.

7 Ibid., p. 134 .

8 Ibid., p. 137.

9 Beauchamp and Childress (2001), p. 70 (see n. 3).

10 Website of the National Institute of Health. Available at http://ohsr.od.nih.gov/guidelines/nuremberg.html, accessed 12 September 2008.

11 Cf. Tom Beauchamp and Ruth Faden (1986) *A History and Theory of Informed Consent* (Oxford: Oxford University Press) pp. 235–69.

12 Ibid., p. 94.

13 Ruth Macklin (1999) *Against Relativism. Cultural Diversity and the Search for Ethical Universals in Medicine* (Oxford: Oxford University Press) p. 122.

14 Cf. The Universal Declaration on Bioethics and Human Rights. UNESCO website. Available at http://portal.unesco.org/en/ev.php-URL_ID=31058&URL_DO=DO_TOPIC&URL_SECTION=201.html, accessed 12 September 2008. See also Beauchamp and Childress (2001) pp. 62–3 (n. 3).

15 Jonathan D. Moreno, Arthur L. Caplan and Paul Root Wolpe (1998) 'Informed consent', in R. Chadwick (ed.), *Encyclopedia of Applied Ethics*, Vol. 2 (London: Academic Press) pp. 687–97, esp. 695.

16 Neil C. Manson and Onora O'Neill (2007) *Rethinking Informed Consent in Bioethics* (Cambridge: Cambridge University Press) p. 25.

17 Stephen Wear (1998) *Informed Consent. Patient Autonomy and Clinician Beneficence within Health Care*, 2nd ed. (Washington, DC: Georgetown University Press) pp. 178–9.

18 Website of the National Institute of Health. Available at http://ohsr.od.nih.gov/guidelines/helsinki.html, accessed 1 September 2008.

19 Cf. Kristinsson and Árnason (2007) (see n. 2).

20 Klaus Hoeyer, Bert-Ove Olofsson, Tom Mjörndal and Niels Lynöe (2004) 'Informed consent and biobanks: A population-based study of attitudes towards tissue donation for genetic research', *Scandinavian Journal of Public Health*, 32: 224–9.

21 Henry Greely (1999) 'Breaking the stalemate: A prospective regulatory framework for unforeseen research uses of human tissue samples and health information', *Wake Forest Law Review*, 34: 737–66;

Tim Caulfield, Ross Upshur and Abdallah Daar (2003) 'DNA databanks and consent: A suggested policy option involving an authorization model', BMC Medical Ethics, 4; Vilhjálmur Árnason (2004) 'Coding and consent: Moral challenges of the database project in Iceland', Bioethics, 18: 27–49; Jane Kaye (2004) 'Broad consent – The only option for population genetic databases', in: G. Árnason, S. Nordal and V. Árnason (eds), Blood and Data: Ethical, Legal and Social Aspects of Human Genetic Databases (Reykjavik: University of Iceland Press) pp. 103–9.

22 Caulfield, Upshur and Daar (2003) (see n. 21).

23 Onora O'Neill (2001) 'Informed consent and genetic information', Studies in History and Philosophy of Biology and Biomedical Sciences, 32: 689–704.

24 Cf. Kristinsson and Árnason (2007) (see n. 2).

25 Manson and O'Neill (2007) (see n. 16).

11

Health Information Technology and Globalization

Kenneth Goodman

INTRODUCTION – TECHNOLOGY AND GLOBAL DEVELOPMENT

The first digital, electronic and programmable computer was developed as an instrument of warcraft. The Colossus was a room-sized collection of racks, pulleys, wires and some 2,400 bottle-sized vacuum tubes built at Britain's Bletchley Park to decipher encrypted German messages (Flowers, 1983; Copeland, 2004). It became operational in 1944 and was used to prepare the D-Day invasion of Normandy. One could argue that it eventually saved more lives than most medical inventions.

Less than a month later, on 1 July 1944 – some coincidences are too pretty to be left out – the Bretton Woods conference convened in New Hampshire. Preparing for a post-war world that would of necessity be interdependent, delegates to what is formally known as the 'United Nations Monetary and Financial Conference'[1] proposed the creation of a number of international organizations, including the World Bank and the International Monetary Fund. Here is what they said:

> This Conference at Bretton Woods, representing nearly all the peoples of the world, has considered matters of international money and finance which are important for peace and prosperity. The Conference has agreed on the problems needing attention, the measures which should be taken, and the forms of international cooperation or organization which are required. The agreements reached on these large and complex matters are without precedent in the history of international economic relations. (UN, 1944)

While it would be some time before information technology, health and economic development would be interwoven in any substantial way (Cortada, 2004), it is reasonable to acknowledge that the threads were spooled out during a ghastly war and represented both technological creativity and benign, if not progressive, attempts to address the economic disparities that so often lead to human conflict.

What we now call 'globalization' – too often the mostly unregulated quest for free trade opportunities – is apparently unguided by the values expressed at Bretton Woods. At its best, health information technology under globalization could reduce economic disparity and improve public health around the world. At worst, computational resources could be used to perpetuate disparity and provide new tools for the exploitation of the developing world. In either case, the use of information technology raises an array of important, interesting and difficult ethical issues.

In what follows, we will (1) identify core duties in health or medical informatics; (2) plot these against the needs of global health; and (3) suggest an ethically optimized approach to guide the use of global health information technology.

ETHICS AND HEALTH INFORMATION TECHNOLOGY

Nearly three decades of literature on ethics and health informatics have tended to emphasize privacy and confidentiality; appropriate uses and users of decision support systems, or computer programs that help render diagnoses or prognoses, or help guide treatment; the role of the internet and World Wide Web; bioinformatics, or the use of information technology to collect, store, analyze and transmit genetic information; and so on. Put differently, ethics-and-informatics scholarship has emphasized issues of great importance in mostly Northern, mostly Western and mostly developed regions of the world.

This is to be expected: the modern medical center has become an information-intensive place, with great ferment surrounding the development of electronic patient records, of very large databases for treatment, analysis and research and of tools for digitizing an otherwise overwhelming amount of patient information. The most recent issue of note concerns personal health records, or applications that patients themselves can use to store health information and to communicate with health professionals, among other functions. Even garden-variety clinics and community physicians' practices are becoming electronic – if for no reason other than to improve the efficiency with which patients and other payers are billed for services.

Much of this is of little or no value to most people on Earth.

The world's healthcare landscape is, as ever, shaped more by poverty than privacy, more by inadequate public health infrastructure than digitized genetic data, more by woefully lacking resources for basic primary care than the latest device in radiology, cardiology or orthopedic surgery. In the nearly three-quarters of a century since Bretton Woods, in other words, health and development in what are sometimes called 'low resource countries' are still distant goals. But that uncontroversial observation serves as a powerful lens by which to examine the ways in which information technology might *contribute* to health and development; and if that is the case, then we will be pointed in a direction that will help us uncover duties commensurate with that ability. That is, rather than savor only the challenges posed for 'high resource countries' by the tools of health informatics, it is also necessary to analyze the moral obligations elicited by the availability of these tools, or versions of them, in the developing world.

We can approach this from another direction. In common experience, ethics is misused as a means by which to pass judgment or unfurl a warning: Stop, slow down, don't do that. It is too often the case that the term 'concern' follows 'ethics'. Make no mistake – there is no shortage of bad behavior and bad actors, and any credible system of morality will be able to identify them as such and without much ado. But ethics, *qua* branch of philosophy, is at ground about the analysis of moral claims, about critical thinking applied to human action. Among the consequences of this standard view of what constitutes ethics is that a proper analysis will disclose duties as well as prohibitions.

When it comes to health information technology, the idea that it might be blameworthy to *fail* to use an intelligent machine was articulated in the first sustained treatment of ethical issues in health computing (Miller et al., 1985). The authors, a physician, a philosopher and a lawyer, were not concerned with the use of computers in the developing world, or the effect of Western information technology on low-resource countries. But their point is a crucial one for our purposes. It is this: if there are reasons to believe information technology (or any technology or tool, for that matter) will improve human health and well-being, then there can be identified a commensurate duty to test and, as appropriate, use the technology. Health science would stagnate if this or something like it were not true.

IDENTIFYING GLOBAL VALUES IN INTERNATIONAL HEALTH COMPUTING

Those who use computers for education, research, commerce, and so on have found they are indispensable; and the utility of information technology for health care in the developed world is, generally, a settled matter. In resource-poor countries, there is growing evidence that health informatics is or will be a necessary component of public health, clinical care and health research. There is in fact a growing research program to develop and/or assess various kinds of computational tools in the developing world for primary care (Hannan et al., 2001; Tierney et al., 2002; Kamadjeu et al., 2005; Siika et al., 2005); research (Royall et al., 2005); health information seeking (Renahy and Chauvin, 2006); and other purposes.

The Open Medical Record System (OpenMRS), for instance was established in 2004 as an exemplar of:

> ... the best way to help patients within developing countries through a robust and extensible medical record system foundation. The unrelenting pandemic of HIV/AIDS along with the burden of malaria and drug-resistant tuberculosis demand coordinated and rapid responses. Working together, we hope to reduce the amount of redundant efforts in collecting and managing medical information in these settings. We've found several tools available within the open source community that can enhance communication and collaboration.[2]

This and other initiatives are undergirded by the premise that the disease burden in the developing world is so great, and the means of relieving it so information-intensive, that it would be morally and socially irresponsible *not* to develop and provide adequate health information resources (Goodman, 2008). While the phrase 'digital divide' was originally applied to disparities in access to personal computers in the United States, it is at least as apt in describing the health information technology chasm that separates the developed and developing worlds (cf. Baur, 2008).[3]

Disparities in access to health care, including services customarily provided by public health organizations, represent civilization's greatest ethical challenge. One might be forgiven for overlooking this point, given the attention focused in the developed world on end-of-life care and the appropriate use of sophisticated medical technology, genetics and pharmacogenomics, cloning and embryonic stem cell research, neuroethics, nanotechnology and the rest. These issues and technologies are of great ethical interest and importance, even as they are unlikely to be of interest to or importance for most people in the world. Compared to vector-borne diseases, the health consequences of malnutrition and lack of sanitation, and, say, transmission of the HIV virus, the applications and implications of genetic data bases and stem-cell-driven 'regenerative medicine' support what has been called 'boutique ethics', or the emphasis on issues and devices of comparatively little use or interest to most of the world's people (Goodman and Prineas, 2009 [1996]).

Assuming only a rudimentary appreciation of the role and significance of health justice and resource-allocation challenges, it follows that anything that can reduce health disparities should be given at least as much attention as other issues. Given, then, the evidence suggesting that more fully fledged health information systems can improve primary care and public health in the developing world, we can identify in medical informatics a strikingly under-represented, or overlooked, source of opportunity – to reduce disparities on the one hand and as a locus of novel ethical issues in itself on the other.

In this way, ethical issues raised by the tools of health information technology recapitulate those raised by traditional technologies:

- If a device or intervention can improve or, as appropriate, lengthen life, why do we do such a poor job sharing it?
- Even if we share it (more or less) fairly, do pre-existing economic or social conditions seed the ground for use of the technology to exploit vulnerable populations?
- Is the technology being studied first among those likely to benefit from it last?

Consider for instance the adoption of telemedicine and other 'e-health' utilities. Promoted for more than a decade as a way to reduce disparities between urban and rural populations in North America and in Europe, there has long been concern that applications of 'remote presence healthcare' have been advocated before they have been demonstrated to be effective, and that what rural citizens might actually need is a good doctor or nurse and not a computer-mediated video hookup to the nearest academic medical center (Goodman, 1998; Bauer, 2003). In the developing world, the same concerns have been raised in light of challenges related to health system accountability and poorly supported public health infrastructures (Litewka, 2005).

We can recast this challenge in the following way: The demands of globalization are shaped at least in part by the need for sustained growth. This leads to efforts to expand global markets for products and services of the dominant cultures' industries. This in turn fosters the temptation, if not the imperative, to sell products of questionable or provisional utility to resource-poor countries. Putting matters this way helps also to make clear the close relationship between science and ethics in health care. Many uncertainties about the appropriate use of health information technology and, indeed, any technology, are in part empirical uncertainties. These uncertainties are reduced by more and better science. The demands of evidence-based health science therefore run parallel to the challenges of global ethics: The question whether any device, intervention or policy is morally defensible is in part a function on whether it works as intended and whether the guiding intentions themselves enjoy ethical warrant (Goodman, 2003a).

As above, then, if the intention is, for instance to reduce health disparities and if there is adequate scientific justification to suggest that a proffered device, approach or policy will help realize that potential, then one can make the case that failure to use the device (or adopt the policy, etc.) is or might be blameworthy; or, in the opposite direction, its use might be obligatory.

As we've seen, there is at least some evidence that a variety of health information tools could in fact improve the health of people in resource-poor countries. It remains for us to lay out some of the ethical challenges posed by the use of these tools, and suggest putative guidelines for their ethically optimized use.

TOWARD AN ETHICAL 'STANDARD OF CARE' IN INTERNATIONAL HEALTH INFORMATION TECHNOLOGY

Appropriate use of a medical tool is plotted by a number of factors, including training, sustainability and the needs of the population it purports to serve. It should cause no controversy to point out, apropos these three factors, that those who use health information tools should be adequately instructed in their use, that it is usually a mistake to begin an intervention that cannot be completed and that the tool(s) should be tailored to the population one intends to help. Regarding this last, consider that the people of Haiti, say, will benefit much more from computer systems to track and study vaccinations than computer systems to track and study allocation of solid organs for transplantation. In other words, we must ensure that a health information system of any type serves the community in which it is deployed – and not, for instance the professional or academic aspirations of the system designers or of investors. This corresponds nicely to a recommendation regarding human subjects research in developing countries offered in the United States by its National Bioethics Advisory Commission (NBAC):

> NBAC understands the principle of justice to require that a population, especially a vulnerable one, should not be the focus of research unless some of the potential benefits of the research will accrue to that group … U.S. and international research ethics require not merely that research risks are reasonable in relation to potential benefits, but also that they respond to the health needs of the population being studied (NBAC, 2001).

In some respects, the NBAC was responding to the growing pressure of a global pharmaceutical industry in search of lower research costs, diminished or absent regulation and drug-naïve populations. The challenge is not that the science is not in itself worthwhile, but that it is often more worthwhile to investigators and investors than to the populations selected for study.

Fortunately, we face a somewhat different situation with health information technology. Global economic forces, anticipated only dimly at Bretton Woods, have internationalized electrical engineering and information technology enterprises while doing comparatively little to reduce disparities in access to health computing and other resources in the world's poorest regions. Unlike pharmaceutical research in the developing world, the deployment of health information technology offers no corresponding market offset. There is, to put it differently, little or no money to be made in helping resource-poor countries do a better job of managing health data. This means the motivations for doing so will engender fewer conflicts of interest. This is not to diminish the importance of responding to local needs – only to suggest that the obligations of research and development might suffer somewhat fewer temptations for such distractions.

In what follows, we identify five provisional values intended to foster a set of international standards and best practices and to guide the study and application of health information technology resources in an era of globalization.

Reduce disparity

The overarching moral challenge in the health professions – including health informatics – is the reduction of disparities. If that can be achieved by broader access to information technology, then reducing disparities in access to effective computational resources is a correlate duty. Such a duty, however simply stated, is in fact a nuanced and complex undertaking requiring an assessment of the needs of the target population including the motivations of those who seek to meet those needs, as well as of the adequacy of resources for realizing the goals of the project.

This might be read as a warning against overreaching and against acting merely on a naïve or untutored desire to help others in need. More computers will no more improve the health of populations than will more drugs. What is needed in addition to a putatively helpful technology is the development of appropriately trained professionals and adequate social infrastructure to use and assess that technology. Some countries or regions, for instance will require a reliable supply of electricity before they can take full advantage of computational resources.

The process of globalization has many moving parts. The globalization of information technology offers up a number of opportunities, although these are conditioned on the availability of related resources. A system to support primary care[4] requires primary care providers, and they need a supply of standard tools to do their job; a vaccine tracking system is useless without both the availability of vaccine and a community's willingness to be vaccinated; a computer system to store something as basic as vital statistics is no more useful than a box of wires if it is populated with inaccurate data, or the host community either fails to appreciate or is unable to act on the significance of information related to birth, nutrition, death and so on.

Improve public health

Public health begins with education and basic measures for sanitation – matters about which a fair amount of knowledge is already available. Public health authorities in even the most resource-poor settings are essential allies in any attempt to improve the health of populations. The point of suggesting that to 'improve public health' should be counted among our 'provisional standards for the study and application of health information technology' is only to emphasize that while individual patients can be the source of a great deal of data that requires analysis, the greatest economies of scale in health and wellness are to be realized when data are collected from several sources and analyzed *ensemble*.

The tools of public health informatics are fundamental to any effort to improve the health of populations. That is, data volume and complexity require the tools of information technology for the creation and use of registries for screening, tracking and other purposes.

The evolution of computational epidemiology itself raises a number of ethical issues, and these might vary in content or focus depending on location. These issues include privacy and confidentiality, error management, risk communication and decision support (Goodman, 2003b).

Manage intellectual property

The computer industry poses interesting and important challenges to traditional views of intellectual property in health care and other domains. At least as much as with any other international industry, one could make the case that copyright, patent and other restraints on free use of potentially life-saving technology require redoubled efforts to ensure that developing populations enjoy the benefits of the technology while developers enjoy the benefits of having created it.

To this end, there is growing interest in 'open source' medical utilities, that is, software applications freely available without patent or copyright restrictions (e.g. Fegan and Lang, 2008). The open source movement began among software writers and engineers and is based on the value that (at least some) information is necessary for human well-being and progress, and should therefore be easily available even to those who cannot afford to pay for it.

In a globalized health information technology environment, the opportunities promised by open source tools need additional exploration, along with research on the consequences of enforcing putative intellectual property rights for potentially life-saving technology.

Protect privacy

One might be forgiven for detecting in some quarters the stance that privacy is a Western value or one worth protecting only for those in societies with highly evolved legislative and legal mechanisms affording such protections. In addition to its circularity, such a position fails to recognize the universal appreciation for and insistence on rules or other mechanisms to restrict the disclosure of personal information.

Attention to the rights of individuals and groups to control access to their health information will help build trust, which is essential for the kinds of data sharing on which health information systems rely. That is, people who are sources of health information will not trust the health professionals and researchers who need the information if those professionals and investigators cannot safeguard the information from inappropriate disclosure. Disclosures are, generally, inappropriate if they are not approved with knowledge of the consequences of disclosure. That people fear bias, stigma or the loss of health benefits as a result of certain disclosures underscores the interrelatedness of healthcare systems and privacy protections – when health benefits are withheld from sick people because they are sick, or have 'pre-existing conditions,' it dissuades them from making the information available in the first place.

When information is aggregated in databases, there is the further risk that entire groups will lose benefits or be stigmatized. This has led to elaboration of the concept of 'group privacy', especially in the context of stored genetic information (Alpert, 2000). This points to the need for a global privacy ethic that parallels globalization's economic imperative.

Foster appropriate uses and users

We saw earlier that one of the first insights to emerge from ethical analyses of health information technology was that it might be blameworthy to fail to use an intelligent machine if doing so will improve the health of individuals or populations. It follows that any ethical standard of care for globalized health information technology should guide professionals in demarcating appropriate uses and users from inappropriate ones. For instance establishing a database to help a government do a better job of discriminating against people with HIV ought to be found to be inappropriate; a tracking system to help identify those who have been overlooked by a vaccination program requires endorsement; a decision-support system that guides professionals in crafting clinical or public health interventions will be appropriate or not according as users are adequately trained, understand the probabilistic nature of health computing, etc.

This means that the identification of appropriate uses and users governs or supervenes on the previously postulated ethical standards. Surely, 'reduce disparity' or 'protect privacy' are appropriate – though they are so obvious they deserve separate itemization. We still require this 'foster appropriate uses and users' standard for less obvious or more nuanced cases. It should perhaps go without saying that none of these standards, especially this one, can be adopted or succeed without a concomitant program of ethics education and the development of adequate curricular tools.

The very process of globalization, including its effects on international computing in general and health information technology in particular, affects so many aspects of life for so many people – and is so controversial in so many ways – that any particular industry or profession or development goal will surrender only reluctantly to a comprehensive non-partisan ethical analysis. The attempt here has been to cast a little light on a particularly important suite of globalization-related health tools and to try to make the case that, in the decades since the optimism of Bretton Woods, there is still a great deal of work to be done.

NOTES

1 While the United Nations' Charter was approved in San Francisco in 1945, the precursor entity of that name was in operation during the war. According to the UN, 'The name "United Nations", coined by United States President Franklin D. Roosevelt, was first used in the "Declaration by United Nations" of 1 January 1942, during the Second World War, when representatives of 26 nations pledged their Governments to continue fighting together against the Axis Powers'. Available at http://www.un.org/aboutun/history.htm, accessed July 2010.

2 http://openmrs.org/wiki/Community. OpenMRS is a multi-institution, nonprofit group led by the Regenstrief Institute at Indiana University (http://regenstrief.org). According to the OpenMRS website, 'Our world continues to be ravaged by a pandemic of epic proportions, as over 40 million people are infected with or dying from HIV/AIDS – most (up to 95%) in developing countries. Prevention and treatment of HIV/AIDS on this scale requires efficient information management, which is critical as HIV/AIDS care must increasingly be entrusted to less skilled providers. Whether for lack of time, developers, or money, most HIV/AIDS programs in developing countries manage their information with simple spreadsheets or small, poorly designed databases ... if anything at all. To help them, we need to find a way not only to improve management tools, but also to reduce unnecessary, duplicative efforts'. Available at http://openmrs.org/wiki/OpenMRS_Overview, accessed July 2010.

3 In the United States, a report by the National Telecommunications and Information Administration in 2000 ('Falling Through the Net: Toward Digital Inclusion') said, '… schools, libraries, and other public access points continue to serve those groups that do not have access at home. For example, certain groups are far more likely to use public libraries to access the Internet, such as the unemployed, Blacks, and Asian Americans and Pacific Islanders. … Internet access is no longer a luxury item, but a resource used by many' (p. xviii). Available at http://search.ntia.doc.gov/pdf/fttn00.pdf, accessed July 2010; an earlier version of the report was titled 'Falling through the Net: Defining the Digital Divide'.

4 Research on health equity has demonstrated the importance of primary care and associated policy development (see Starfield, 2006, and the references cited therein), making in part the obvious point that attempts to reduce health disparities must generally occur in a socially and scientifically diverse and complex environment.

ACKNOWLEDGEMENT

Work on this chapter was supported in part by a grant from the Fogarty International Center of the U.S. National Institutes of Health (Pan American Bioethics Initiative, R25TW008186).

REFERENCES

Alpert, Sherri A. (2000) 'Privacy and the analysis of stored tissues', in *Research Involving Human Biological Materials: Ethical Issues and Policy Guidance, Vol. II: Commissioned Papers*. Rockville, MD: National Bioethics Advisory Commission.

Bauer, K. (2003) 'Distributive justice and rural healthcare: A case for e-health', *International Journal of Applied Philosophy*, 17 (2): 241–52.

Baur, C. (2008) 'An analysis of factors underlying e-health disparities', *Cambridge Quarterly of Healthcare Ethics*, 17 (4): 417–28.

Copeland, B.J. (2004) 'Colossus – its origins and originators', *Annals of the History of Computing*, 26 (4): 38–45.

Cortada, J.W. (2004) 'How did computing go global? The need for an answer and a research agenda', *Annals of the History of Computing*, 26 (1): 53–8.

Fegan, G.W. and Lang, T.A. (2008) 'Could an open-source clinical trial data-management system be what we have all been looking for?', *PLoS Medicine*, 5 (3): e6 doi:10.1371/journal.pmed.0050006.

Flowers, T.H. (1983) 'The design of colossus', *Annals of the History of Computing*, 5 (3): 239–52.

Goodman, K.W. (1998) 'Bioethics and health informatics: An introduction', in Kenneth W. Goodman (ed.), *Ethics, Computing and Medicine: Informatics and the Transformation of Health Care*. Cambridge and New York: Cambridge University Press, pp. 1–31.

Goodman, K.W. (2003a) *Ethics and Evidence-based Medicine: Fallibility and Responsibility in Clinical Science*. Cambridge and New York: Cambridge University Press.

Goodman, K.W. (2003b) 'Ethics, information technology and public health: Duties and challenges in computational epidemiology', in P.W. O'Carroll, W.A. Yasnoff, M.E. Ward, L.H. Ripp and E.L. Martin (eds), *Public Health Informatics and Information Systems*. New York: Springer-Verlag, pp. 251–66.

Goodman, K.W. (2008) 'Ethics and health informatics: Focus on Latin America and the Caribbean', *Acta Bioethica*, 11 (2): 121–26.

Goodman, K.W. and Prineas, R.J. (2009 [1996]) 'Ethics curricula in epidemiology', in Steven S. Coughlin, Tom L. Beauchamp and Douglas L. Weed (eds), *Ethics and Epidemiology* (2nd ed.). Oxford: Oxford University Press, pp. 283–303.

Hannan, T.J., Tierney, W.M., Rotich, J.K., Odero, W.W., Smith, F., Mamlin, J.J. and Einterz, R.M. (2001) 'The MOSORIOT medical record system (MMRS) phase I to phase II implementation: An outpatient computer-based medical record system in rural Kenya', *Studies in Health Technology and Informatics*, 84 (Pt. 1): 619–22.

Kamadjeu, R.M., Tapang, E.M. and Moluh, R.N. (2005) 'Designing and implementing an electronic health record system in primary care practice in sub-Saharan Africa: A case study from Cameroon', *Informatics in Primary Care*, 13 (3): 179–86.

Litewka, S. (2005) 'Telemedicine: un desafío para América Latina' [Telemedicine: A challenge for Latin America], *Acta Bioethica*, 11 (2): 127–32.

Miller, R.A., Schaffner, K.F. and Meisel, A. (1985) 'Ethical and legal issues related to the use of computer programs in clinical medicine', *Annals of Internal Medicine*, 102: 529–36.

National Bioethics Advisory Commission (NBAC) (2001) *Ethical and Policy Issues in International Research: Clinical Trials in Developing Countries*, Vol. 1. Bethesda, MD: National Bioethics Advisory Commission.

Renahy, E. and Chauvin, P. (2006) 'Internet uses for health information seeking: A literature review', *Revue d'épidémiologie et de santé publique*, 54 (3): 263–75.

Royall, J., van Schayk, I., Bennett, M., Kamau, N. and Alilio, M. (2005) 'Crossing the digital divide: The contribution of information technology to the professional performance of malaria researchers in Africa', *African Health Sciences*, 5 (3): 246–54.

Siika, A.M., Rotich, J.K., Simiyu, C.J., Kigotho, E.M., Smith, F.E., Sidle, J.E. et al. (2005) 'An electronic medical record system for ambulatory care of HIV-infected patients in Kenya', *International Journal of Medical Informatics*, 74 (5): 345–55.

Starfield, B. (2006) 'State of the art in research on equity in health', *Journal of Health Politics, Policy and Law*, 31 (1): 12–32.

Tierney, W.M., Rotich, J.K., Smith, F.E., Bii, J., Einterz, R.M. and Hannan, T.J. (2002) 'Crossing the "digital divide": Implementing an electronic medical record system in a rural Kenyan health center to support clinical care and research', Proceedings of the Symposium of the American Medical Informatics Association, 792–5.

United Nations (UN) (1944) 'Conference at Bretton Woods: United Nations Monetary and Financial Conference at Bretton Woods. Summary of Agreements, July 22, 1944'. Published as Pamphlet No. 4, 'Pillars of Peace: Documents Pertaining to American Interest in Establishing a Lasting World Peace: January 1941–February 1946', Book Department, Army Information School, Carlisle Barracks, PA, May 1946. Available at http://www.ibiblio.org/pha/policy/1944/440722a.html, accessed July 2010.

12

Abortion

Y. Michael Barilan

INTRODUCTION AND HISTORICAL BACKGROUND

Abortion has always been morally problematic and has always been linked to the liberties and empowerment of women in general. The most ancient canon of Western medical literature, the Hippocratic writings, contains a prohibition on abortifacient drugs in its oath and a story about a doctor who induced abortion in a prostitute-slave upon the behest of her owner.

Opposition to abortion has often protected the life of women. Saint Basil condemned abortion as murder because of the destruction of the fetus and because 'most women who make such attempts die'. The second century gynecologist Soranus wrote that the Hippocratic Oath forbade abortion because it endangers the life of women. The very same reading was shared by a late-nineteenth-century Iraqi rabbi (Barilan, 2009-10:154). The British medical establishment of the nineteenth century was unanimous in judging abortion 'suicidal' and of lower efficacy, should the mother survive (Keown, 1988: 35).

The fact that numerous women all over the world have struggled to procure abortion tells us that the medical risk of their pregnancy was even higher, or that the choice to abort was not theirs, or that cultural circumstances pushed them to risk their lives rather than have the child.

The contemporary moral debate on abortion is not symmetric. The 'pro-life' camp maintains that abortion is murder or similar to murder and must always or nearly always be prohibited. Moderate 'pro-life' would endorse abortion only due to *serious* and *objective* causes such as protection of the mother's health or rehabilitating her from the trauma of rape. Notwithstanding the severity or leniency of the objective criteria meriting abortion, this approach relies on legal and medical regulations, leaving no room for personal valuation, feelings and choice (Women can only choose to keep the child supererogatorily). There is no respect for the cultural and religious background of the woman (i.e. antiabortionist legislations do not allow women from minority cultures to follow their own traditions).

On the other hand, 'pro-choice' is not synonymous with 'pro-abortion'. Rather, abortion is never taken as an achievement, but as the lesser evil. 'Pro-choice' people believe that the decision should be the woman's, and that only women broadly empowered can deliberate each situation of abortion with the appropriate earnestness.

The debate on abortion has been conducted along two intersecting lines of reasoning. The first deals with the moral status of the unborn; the second with conflicts of rights and the ethics of self-defense. This chapter will not trace the first line of argumentation, because resolution of the debate on the moral status of embryos and fetuses is far from being exhaustive of the moral question of abortion. Not being a person does not entail permission to abort, as owners of rare animals and works of art do not have permission to neglect and destroy them at will; being a full person morally, even within the special relationship between child and mother, does not confer unconditional protection, since with the exception of the official doctrine of the Catholic Church, at any stage of pregnancy, all known moral and legal systems permit abortion that is necessary to save the life of the mother.[1]

In this chapter I skip the imperative discussion on the private deliberation of abortion – how to talk with women who seek counseling prior to making a choice. I set aside as well abortions requiring technologies unavailable to much of humanity – genetics, prenatal diagnosis and infertility care. Instead, I will present the moral problem of abortion from a global perspective, focusing in particular on the restriction and accessibility of safe abortions.

First, I will present the problem of abortion for the sake of saving the mother's life. This tragic dilemma occurs most commonly during childbirth in times and places where modern obstetric surgery is not available. This would be the background for surveying the history of abortion and its regulation. Then I will discuss philosophical arguments on life-saving abortions, abortion following rape and lessons from these and related issues (e.g. slavery, prostitution) that might be relevant to the abortion debate in general.

A SOCIAL HISTORY OF THE ETHICS OF CHILDBIRTH AND ABORTION

In pre-modern times, over 5 per cent of women died due to maternal causes. This tragic figure still reflects current maternal mortality in countries such as Chad, Cameroon, Malawi, Nigeria, Laos, Nepal and Afghanistan, where 1–2 per cent of childbirths are fatal to the mother.

Global maternal mortality in 2005 is estimated at four deaths in 1000 births (0.4 per cent). It is only 4/100,000 in the affluent countries. Over half a million women die each year from childbirth.

These women die mainly from infection, bleeding and obstructed labor (fetus stuck in the birth canal). These pathologies are interrelated. Every problem invites intervention which is potentially infectious, and every delay of intervention might produce uncontrollable bleeding.

Poor adolescent mothers and women with disabilities and health problems are especially at risk. The pelvis of a 16-year-old girl who suffers from nutritional deficiencies is unlikely to support normal delivery. Multiparous women are also at risk, as repeated pregnancies tend to weaken their muscles beyond the capacity to sustain healthy delivery. In the

absence of safe abortion or cesarean surgery, pregnancy becomes a gamble on life, typically of vulnerable women – the very young and those already blessed and burdened with
many children. This is true also regarding women affected by rheumatic heart disease and
many other medical conditions as well as those women carrying malpresenting fetuses or
malformations, such as hydrocephalus.

At least one fourth of humanity still cannot afford safe obstetric surgery and other
technologies essential for dealing with such crises of pregnancy and labor (Schofeld, 1986;
De Browere, 2007; Hill et al., 2007).

Until the nineteenth century, cesarean surgery was almost universally fatal. Mortality
rates reported from different European hospitals during the nineteenth century ranged
above 50 per cent (Newell, 1924: 5).

In the beginning of the twentieth century, a prominent American obstetrician reported 3–5
per cent overall maternal death in the United States. We may safely assume that poor societies then and now do not fare better relative to his candid words (Bledsoe, 2002: 300):

> The highest mortality that befalls the human race in one day occurs on the day of birth … 5% of children
> are still-born, dying during labor, and 1.5% die shortly after birth, the result of the trauma of labor … in Paris
> 9% die …
>
> [Birth] kills thousands of women every year … leaves at least a quarter of the women more or less invalided,
> and a majority with permanent anatomic changes of structure.

In emergencies of labor, Jewish law *requires* the active destruction of the fetus (embryotomy/
craniotomy) whenever the mother's life is in danger. Moreover, since the Middle Ages,
Jews have abstained from so-called post-mortem cesarean surgery for the sake of saving
the life of the baby. Sensitivity to maternal life was so high as to risk the loss of potentially
healthy babies in fear of cutting dying mothers a little too early (Barilan, 2009-10).

The official doctrine of the Catholic Church takes the other extreme, teaching that
from conception the embryo should be counted as a human person which must never be
deliberately killed even for the sake of saving life (with two debated exceptions of ectopic
pregnancy and cancerous uterus).[2]

Consequently, since the eighteenth century, many theologians have appealed to the
'principle of double effect' in order to encourage cesarean section on parturient mothers in
spite of the risk. Foreseeable but indirect death of mothers was less deplorable than the
deliberate butchering of babies (Berroit-Salvadore, 2000; Ryan, 2002). Symphysiotomy
was another mutilatory and dangerous operation which was introduced in the late-
eighteenth century as a substitution for life-saving abortion during childbirth (Wright-
St Clair, 1963).

Common Law, Islam, cultures of the far East and virtually all indigenous societies of
Africa, America and Oceania practiced a middle way between the Jewish prohibition on
sacrifice and self-sacrifice of pregnant women, and the Catholic prohibition on killing
fetuses, even those who are not likely to survive and even when this was the only way to
save the life of a healthy mother.

Whatever reasons societies have harbored for the regulation of abortion, be it concern
over the strength of society (e.g. communist Romania), population control (Maoist China),
discouragement of licentious behavior (e.g. post-bellum United States) or public health
and respect for developing human life (e.g. most Western nations nowadays), most people
and peoples have endorsed, practiced and openly condoned abortion under a wide variety

of conditions. Saving the mother was chief among them. Once birth became difficult, people all over the world tended to see the 'promised fruit' as a 'source of evil' – a threat to be removed by the care-givers by all means (Sargent, 1982; Gelis, 1991: 142). Most such decisions regarding 'secrets of women' – from menstrual pain to childbirth – were made within intimate circles of feminine self-care, which were quite removed from written records and the direct scrutiny of law and government.

The waning of feminine management of labor occurred early in the West. Already in the Middle Ages learned physicians imputed the death of many infants to female midwives (Park, 2006: 96). From the early modern period, when possible, folk-midwives would call the barber surgeon when surgical removal of the presumably dead or doomed child was necessary. In many places it became illegal for female midwives to possess and to use surgical instruments (King, 2007: ch.2).

When in the nineteenth and twentieth centuries obstetrics was incorporated in mainstream academic medicine, doctors debated the indications for cesarean section and embryotomy (Keown, 1988: ch. 3). Maternal death was not the only concern. A choice between killing a child and the irreversible loss of fecal continence is another typical dilemma which haunted all of humanity until less than a century ago and still afflicts women in such places as Sierra Leone (Pigott, 2004).

Although moral condemnation of abortion is traceable to the very early phases of Western civilization, in the Roman Empire, abortion and infanticide were common and legal. Concern over decline in the demographic power of the Roman nobility was behind the first anti-abortion edicts in Rome. However, it was the nascent Christian religion which launched an uncompromising attack against abortion, infanticide, blood sports, sexual use of slaves and other lethal and abusive practices central to pagan life in the classical world. Like most pre-modern societies, the classical world did not distinguish among abortion, neonaticide and abandonment of babies. The commonplace notion that each and every human child is a full human being worthy of care, respect and spiritual fulfillment is the product of the centuries-long Christian campaign which was conducted on behalf of young children, many of whom had very little chance of survival (Bakke, 2005).

In pre-modern Europe, the legal regulation of abortion hinged on the concept of quickening, which is the first maternal sensation of fetal movements (around the twentieth week). In the absence of modern medicine, until that point, pregnancy was never a definite reality. Hence, on technical grounds it was practically impossible to take action against early abortion, which could as well be cast as a therapeutic removal of a tumor, an already dead fetus or other pathology. Although no official body in Europe accepted Aristotle's view that the embryo was not animated (ensouled) before quickening, many women and 'irregulars' (folk healers) availed themselves of this teaching upon trying to deal with an unwelcome situation. In the eyes of society early abortion was stigmatized by a strong association with prostitution, fornication and infanticide; sources on early abortion among 'reputable' women are skimpy and controversial.

The surviving evidence from Europe indicates a principled taboo on abortion combined with practical tolerance and vagueness of language. Therapies that 'restore menstruation' were rife (Riddle, 1995: 122–6). Surgeons taught and practiced abortion, induction of early labor and embryotomy 'of dead fetuses' – a very elusive diagnosis for anybody lacking stethoscopes and modern monitors, let alone electricity.

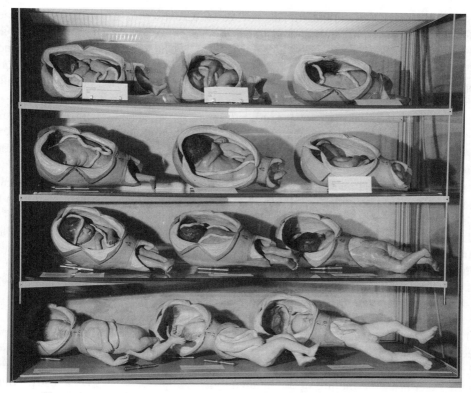

Plaster casts of 'children who stayed with their mothers' (i.e. both died in childbirth). The Anatomy Museum, Bologna

These are silent monuments to the myriads of women who died because of the taboo on embryotomy, more strictly observed in Papal academic centers. We can see that some of these babies got stuck due to lethal malformations.

All of this changed along with the rise of science, technology, the modern state system and the Enlightenment's ethos of universal values and personal responsibility. At the same time a few European nations were assuming domination over the globe and were casting a tight net of rational governance over family life, from child labor to battery of women and abortion (Miller, 1998).

During the seventeenth century European governments began to crack down on infanticide (Wiesner, 1993: 48–53; Ruff, 2001: 147–99). This probably revived interest in the dangerous practice of abortion. English law criminalized early abortion in 1803. The Napoleonic Code did so in 1810. In 1837, English law abolished the distinction between early and late abortion and aggravated the punishment for the former. In 1861, the law changed once again, turning early abortion from a misdemeanor to a felony punishable by imprisonment for life. In 1869, Pope Pius IX declared abortion of nonquickening fetuses an excommunicable crime. During the nineteenth century abortion entered the criminal codes of other European countries as well as in the United States. More significantly, colonialism spread European laws and regulations all over the world.

Parallel to global de-colonialization and the rise of the Civil Rights movements, and the 'sexual revolution' in the 1960s and 1970s, most democratic countries relaxed their abortion laws (as well as divorce and illegitimacy laws) considerably. Today, in virtually all affluent nations, any woman with a few hundred dollars may procure early abortion easily, safely and privately. Many countries, including France, Israel, Japan, China and India subsidize abortion.

The United States is the only country in the world recognizing a constitutional right to abortion as such, but in the first two trimesters only. Among the rich nations, the United States offers the least legal and material support to mothers, either married or single. In dozens of cases American courts have ordered forced surgeries and treatments of pregnant women in the third trimester, some of whom went into hiding. In one case a court ordered a *lethal* cesarean surgery on a terminal patient in order to save her barely viable fetus (Daniels, 1993). Where living wills have legal power, pregnant women have no right to restrict life-saving treatments (Sperling, 2005). The polarization of the abortion debate has rendered it the only bioethical controversy generating murderous terrorism, mainly in the United States, where legal abortion clinics have been bombed.

The communist revolutions in Russia, China and other countries legalized abortion as a right of the working person. Some communist regimes restricted abortion in order to boost their working and fighting power.

Colonialism has gone, but its grip still clutches the fate of millions. The 'abortion revolution' skipped the former colonies in which the restrictive legislations of their former rulers are still in power. Ironically, countries such as Egypt still follow the 1938 British law and not the lenient teachings of Islam (permitting abortion in the first four months under specific circumstances). Senegal and Niger also adhere to the older French law, allowing abortion only for the sake of saving the mother. In Nicaragua abortion is prohibited even for the sake of saving the life of the mother, whereas for a few decades already, both in France and Spain, early abortion has been available to all.

The only sources of modern health care in many postcolonial nations are Western charities. These enterprises often shun sexual education, contraception, abortion (even when legal) and life-saving embryotomy. Lack of each of these services cost the lives of many women (Epstein, 2007:172 ff; Sedghe, 2007.).

ABORTION AND THE RIGHT TO LIFE

Permissive abortion policies are ethically supported by three separate modes of reasoning.

Utilitarians present the staggering rates of women's morbidity and mortality as being due to 'black' abortions (Grimes, 2006). Besides, mainly due to difficult births and to a chronic shortage of wet-nurses in the pre-modern West, orphan mortality rose from an annual baseline of between 15 and 30 per cent to over 80 per cent (Lomax, 1993; Heywood, 2001: 147–57). The situation has not changed much in the poor countries of the world. Too often, abstaining from abortion does not save the life of the future child.

Liberal feminists promote the woman's self-determination over her own body, particularly in matters of sexuality and regarding the often harmful, painful and always invasive and holistic events which are pregnancy and birth. They also underline the value of equality of feminine life and liberty relative to men's. In the absence of contraceptive and abortion care, millions of women are entrapped in poverty, dependence, lack of education and vulnerable health.

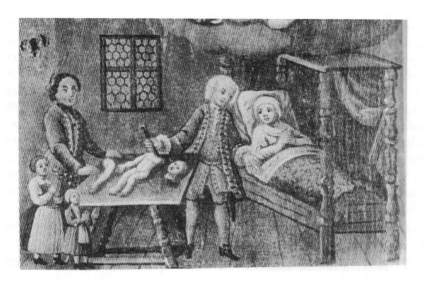

An ex voto following embryotomy that saved the life of the mother
On the left we see the midwife and the children whose mother was almost dying.
In the middle stands the surgeon
Swabia, 1759 (National Museum of Bavaria, Munich)

Many societies practice embryotomy as a 'last measure' to save the life of the mother. European authors usually explained that their instructions for embryotomy were for use only for already dead fetuses. Pre-modern medicine could not diagnose fetal death reliably. But such a diagnosis was psychologically, legally and morally helpful to everybody involved. As late as the nineteenth century, there was no practical distinction between stillbirth and neonaticide and death from pre-maturity. Rose, L. *Massacre of the innocent: infanticide in Great Britain 1800–1939* London, Routledge & Kegan Paul, 1986; ch. 14.

Last, considerations regarding the moral status of the embryo imply the permissibility of abortion of embryos that have not yet reached the person-defining stage as well as for weighty reasons.

Although each of these lines of argumentation has produced a rich body of literature, the difficulties are still glaring.

The utilitarian balance may shift depending on sociopolitical circumstances. Utilitarianism may also fail to provide protection for some of the most vulnerable – retarded women who cannot procure even illegal abortion, for instance.

The vigorous discourse on women's right to self-determination is somewhat offset by alternative feminist narratives that find in the recognition of pregnancy a call for maternal responsible care for her defenseless and voiceless child. It may also be argued that promotion of gender equality does not justify killing.

Most significantly, any theory about the formation of the human person is not likely to coincide with two very widely and firmly held convictions – that as late as at childbirth itself, maternal life takes precedence over the fetus', and that from the moment birth is complete, the baby has a right to life like any other human person. If an embryo becomes a moral person sometime during pregnancy, how is it possible in crises of labor to give preference to the life of the mother over his/hers?

The debate as to whether the fetus is a person is also shrouded in ambiguity. One formulation of the problem inquires whether the fetus could be a victim of personal harm who is capable of suffering the loss of his or her life. Being the recipient of such harm arguably entails a minimum level of neuropsychological maturity that does not exist in early stages of pregnancy (DeGrazia, 2007). This line of inquiry suits the liberal mind-set, which discerns right from wrong *only* through the perspective of harm and justice towards morally considerable entities (Haidt, 2007).

However, many people and moral systems regard the fetus as a person *because* it is intrinsically valuable, and regardless of (or in addition to) its capacity to suffer harm personally. It does not seem reasonable that human life in any of its manifestations and stages of development deserves less public concern than wildlife and archeological sites, whose protection is associated with significant discomfort and financial losses to numerous people.

Against these complex sets of ideas stands the tenet that from conception (or within days from conception) until birth the embryo is a human being with a right to life equal to that of born people. Health care professionals have always felt that their special mission is the protection of life from its beginning to the inevitable moment of death.

Alas, conflicts of life and death are unavoidable as well.

The defense from necessity and duress has long been established as a justification for killing under extremely unusual and tragic circumstances. Many legal systems, ethicists and theologians resort to it when abortion is the only way to save the mother's life, either during pregnancy or in childbirth. However, this framework best suits conflicts among *equal* claimants to life, such as seamen trapped in a lifeboat or conjoined twins (Barilan, 2003).

Hence, in the context of childbirth, the defense from necessity is expected, depending on the particularities of the event, to allow the sacrifice of *either* mother or child. Besides, the defense from necessity does not create obligations, merely excuses or agent-relative permissions only. Those who seek active preferential protection of pregnant mothers from conception until birth are in need of a different paradigm.

Moral or natural human rights are special moral (normative) properties of individual people, protecting and promoting their very basic interests, such as life, bodily integrity and freedom of consciences (Barilan and Brusa, 2008). Nobody has a right to life, which by *its own nature* is incompatible with respect for the life and bodily integrity of another person. Proclamation of such a right will render one's right principally stronger than another's – a conclusion that is incompatible with the value of equality that is fundamental to human rights (Barilan, 2005).

The very nature of fetal life is an invasive and precarious existence of one human being within another, always on the verge of disrupting the harmony between them. If we place fetal life and well-being in the center of our moral deliberation, by necessity we prime ourselves to pushing aside the life and health of the woman. This, mothers willingly do. They usually welcome their pregnancies and sustain them with much devotion and self-sacrifice. But sometimes women decide that their own life and health should be preserved at the expense of fetal life (they often do so out of responsible care for other family dependants).

Since only the woman had benefited from the right to life prior to getting pregnant, and since human rights are stable, inviolable and hard to lose, and since conferring a right to life to the unborn often infringes on the right of the woman, endowment of a right to life to the unborn goes against this very logic of human rights. It will suspend the absoluteness of a woman's right to life each time she conceives a child; even worse still, as it would be especially unfair to suspend the absoluteness of her right to life for the sake of somebody who threatens her life. Only full consent of the person who is requested to submit her life and body allows the needy person to use them for the sustenance of his/her own life.

In the same vein, a patient's right to life does not grant him/her the right to a compulsory kidney donation from a matching donor. As a matter of fact, even aspiration of bone marrow, which is relatively pain-free and non-mutilatory, is not carried out by force even when the proposed donor is the only person whose marrow can save the life at stake. Organs from the *dead* are not harvested non-consensually (presumed consent is sometimes sufficient) for life-saving transplantations anywhere in the world. As a matter of consistency, women should not be coerced and their rights trampled to save the lives of their embryos.

Although self-sacrifice is sometimes praiseworthy, and although many ethicists believe that certain patients have a right to pledge an organ donation and even to choose euthanasia, a binding and irrevocable contract to future-self sacrifice and to alienation of the right to life and bodily integrity are not considered valid by any known ethical system. Consequently, the initial responsibility of a woman for her pregnancy cannot oblige her to carry it in the future when things develop quite substantially for the worse.

The argument from human rights may be reformulated in the language of the ethics of doctor–patient relationship. It is universally accepted that the physician is committed to the well-being of his or her patient only and that there is no permission whatsoever to direct the care of one patient with the intention of benefiting another. Since there is no way to care for the fetus without dealing with the mother, any action done for its benefit, from administration of vitamins to intra-uterine surgery, must have her full consent and possibly must comply with her well-being as well. It is absurd to claim that although the mother had been a patient until conception, this event (or any other morally relevant milestone during pregnancy) dissolves her absolute status as a patient. The fetus has never been a patient (it did not exist at all) prior to conception, so making it wait until birth for becoming one is not inconsistent with the very basics of the doctor–patient relationship. Only when the fetus exists in a manner that allows full and undivided commitment of a doctor will it become a patient of medicine.

Synthesizing the arguments we may say that the life of the unborn is too much implicated with the life of their mothers, not allowing the degree of individuation necessary for benefiting from human rights. This is the problem of compactedness, which bears also on the ethics of multiple-pregnancy (fetal-fetal conflicts) (Barilan, 2004, see Kamm, 2007:20). Additionally, the very nature of prenatal life is invasive, exploitative and potentially life-threatening. Such mode of existence cannot benefit from a right to life in a morally consistent way. In this particular respect the unborn have a weaker moral standing relative to survivors in a life boat that cannot sustain all of them. All of the survivors had been independent humans with the right to life prior to the accidental shipwreck; they all compete equally for a place on the boat. The position of the fetus is doubly weaker. First it had never had a right to life, but the mother do have it; second, the fetus is not competing with the mother over a neutral resource such as the boat, but it needs her body and life. In this light we may conclude that when one life is by necessity exploitative of another person's life, and full and undivided care cannot be provided to both, the right to life of the supportive person takes priority over the value of life of the dependent one, especially when the dependent one has never benefited independently from a right to life.

Another way to look at this line of reasoning is through reflection on Marquis's argument against abortion (1989). Marquis invokes the Golden Rule, underlining abortion as an act that deprives somebody of a 'future like ours'. It is immoral to take one's future for reasons we believe do not justify the taking of our own future. (This argument does not address abortion for the sake of saving maternal life, but it may *require* abortion of fetuses who expect a life of extreme suffering.)

The precept in the Golden Rule contains two elements: 'Do not do unto (1) your fellow (2) that which you do not wish be done unto yourself'.

Evidently, deprivation of a 'future like ours' meets the second element. The question asked is whether an embryo could be considered 'your fellow'. As we have seen, DeGrazia maintains that embryos who cannot be victims to deprivation are not 'fellows' in a manner relevant to abortion. This brings us back to the debate on the moral status of the unborn, now in the disguise of the philosophy of victimhood. But Marquis has a subtler argument, saying that whoever has a human future waiting for him, is a 'fellow' to the Golden Rule argument on abortion as deprivation of human future. In other words, anybody with a continuity of identity overarching the time of harm and realization of "future like us" is a relevant fellow, at least in terms of expectance of the same kind of future (Marquis, 2007, 2008).

The line of reasoning proposed in this chapter first attacks the first element in the Golden Rule, the identification of "having a future like ours" with being "your fellow" regarding prenatal life. Indeed, there is one segment in the future of embryos which is morally very much different from our kind of future life. It is the remaining intra-uterine existence within another person as an invasive potential threat to that person. Such existence is incompatible with enjoyment of a right to life. If being a potential threat to life and health is not a relevant consideration, why should there be potential benefit from the good of post-natal life?

All this said and done, we must keep in mind that the denial of rights to the unborn as well as denial of the status of a person does not entail an automatic permission to abortion (see Fletcher, 1980: 136–7).

Contenders may argue that the fate of any human being must not be dependent on the perceptions and goodwill of another human being. Hence, in situations of conflict, proportionate and fair decisions must follow clear objective criteria, such as a medical diagnosis of a serious illness (the no-choice in the moderate 'pro-life' tenet). They might also argue that the lives of both mother and child embody the same fundamentally inviolable value and that in life-and-death conflicts we never kill intentionally with our own hands. This is the Catholic 'pro-life' version, whose origins, indeed, are in the ethics of personal salvation, and virtue, and not within the paradigm of human rights.[3]

As a matter of fact, some deontological and virtue-based ethics regard passive inaction that lets innocent people die as the better alternative to action that directly kills the innocent as a means to save the life of others. Alas, typically, when pregnancy becomes life-threatening to the woman, she depends on active intervention to save her live (abortions, embryotomy). If human physiology and anatomy were different, inaction on behalf of third parties (doctors) would be enough to let the fetus die and thus save its mother.

Suppose, for example that humans laid eggs as do birds, in life-and-death conflicts between mother and egg, the same natural law and virtue ethicists would allow passive abortion (avoid sitting on the egg) for the sake of saving the life of the mother. It is very difficult to see why the lives of women and children should depend on the purely technical or biological relationship of action/inaction among rescuers, threats and victims.

One answer might be that people should never engage themselves in killing other innocent people, that letting die is less disruptive of self and identity than active killing; that humans must never decide that a person should die, even for the sake of saving another (Rhonheimer, 2009: 42). But it is also difficult to see why the personal integrity of the agent is a weightier consideration than the life of the victim, and why people's lives should be at the mercy of the brute forces of nature, rather than be decided by the best medical and ethical standards.

Contemporary virtue ethics tends to underline ideals of conduct which have developed within historical traditions. As abortion is never part of an ideal vision of anybody, the regulation of abortion is better informed by official and practical attitudes of tolerance and intolerance that have been part of the same historical traditions. As we will see in the next section, moral traditions that cannot tolerate abortion have been quite tolerant with slavery, marital rape and prostitution of destitute women and of victims of rape (many of whom were adolescents). Other traditions have not. Interestingly, these other traditions accepted abortion as a possible course of action in circumstances of rape.

ABORTION FOR NON-MEDICAL REASONS

The UN 'Program of action on Population and Development' regarding women's reproductive health, ratified in 1994, prohibits abortion as a method of family planning, and requires the dealing with the health impact of unsafe abortions.[4]

In 2003, the African Union published the first document ever to mention a right to abortion in the context of international law. This landmark charter proclaims a right to abortion in cases of health risk to the mother and following rape or incest.[5]

How is it possible to justify abortion of a healthy pregnancy merely because of the circumstances, however vile, surrounding the conception of the fetus? If abortion is justifiable by non-medical reasons, could it be upheld and actively provided on grounds other than rape and incest?

As rape is a kind of assault, one may begin exploration of the issue through reflection on self-defense. Debates abound regarding the kinds of relationships required between the two sides to a permissible act of self-defense ('shifting harm' in the philosophical jargon). On one extreme in philosophic hypotheticals stands a villainous murderer; on the other, an innocent threat (e.g. a fat man who has been pushed from a cliff and is about to smash somebody). Particularly controversial is the question whether it is possible to conceptualize maternal–fetal relationships within the framework of self-defense (Davis, 1984; Huffman, 1993).

Suppose one concedes that when two people find themselves in a relationship which is morally equivalent to that which exists between fetus and mother, it might be immoral for the strong party to 'abort' the dependent one. More problematic still would be the position of a third party, say a doctor, who is solicited to perform the 'abortion' by the strong party and is simultaneously pleaded with to desist by the dependent person (see Thomson, 1971; Himma, 1999; Barilan, 2003). Especially tasking is the search for convincing analogies – is unwanted pregnancy similar to an imposition of minutes, months or years of imprisonment (Rajczi, 2009)?

In the previous section it has been argued that, notwithstanding the immense value of pre-natal life, the unborn cannot benefit from the special protection of the right to life. So we do not need at all to resort to self-defense in cases of abortion following maternal–fetal conflicts. But the doctrine of self-defense is helpful in obtaining a perception of the kind of infringements that are incompatible with *acquisition* (not the ongoing exercise) of rights.

I maintain that a substantial difference exists between entrance into a life-and-death conflict from a position of a right to life, and entrance into such a conflict from a position of non-existence (hence – no right to life). Born people do have the right to life even when it accidentally coincides with the right to life of others, so conflicts of self-defense are indeed conflicts of rights that are ordinarily compatible with each other, but in very unusual and unexpected circumstances they collide. However, since the unborn do not have a right to life, the moral status of the embryo is weaker than the position of all other people who are potential targets of killing in the name of self-defense (or 'shifting harm'). In other words, the right to life [of the mother] trumps over the value of fetal life, as the very power of human rights lies in their power to trump non-rights' interests and values.

To the argument against the logical impossibility of granting rights to the unborn, we may or may not add the propositions that the embryo is not a moral person (practically, most abortions following rape and abortions for non-medical motivations are carried out as early as possible during pregnancy), and that self-defense justifies violation of the right to life of anybody who becomes a physical threat.

Consequently, it may be concluded that, although maternal–fetal conflicts might differ significantly from situations of self-defense, interests justifying homicide in self-defense of people with a right to life certainly justify, and possibly even create, a moral duty to perform abortion of fetuses that cannot benefit from the protection of the right to life. It might make sense to argue that pre-natal life deserves every measure of protection up to the limit of violating human rights of the kind that merit killing in self-defense.

The ethics and laws of self-defense hold that rape and other 'extreme intrusions on the freedom of the person' are proportionate interests to life itself (Uniacke, 1994:40; Kopel et al., 2008). In 97 per cent of cases, rape does not involve physical harm other than the sexual act (Cleck and Sayles, 1990). The gravity of rape is not related to the risk of impregnation either, as rape of a prepubescent girl and an old woman is as offensive as any other kind of rape. Rape is a special case indeed, as it creates no objective harm such as disability or loss in life expectancy. Rape is equally reprehensible when it generates no pain or discomfort, as may happen when the victims are feeble-minded or stupefied by drugs.

The crucial factor constituting the difference between a most loathsome offense worthy of lethal self-defense and a most wonderful life-bringing joy is the absence or presence of the *subjective* state of mind of consent. This is so because sexuality is a domain of human action in which personal voluntariness is as fundamental as the valuation of life itself. For a sexual relationship to be non-rapacious, active ongoing and full consent is always mandatory. Precisely here the sexual integrity of the person and his or her life bear similar and unique normative implications. Submission to sex and self-sacrifice of life and limb are never acceptable without full consent in real time. Promises to 'give sex' and to donate organs become void once the promise-giver changes her or his mind (Barilan, 2011).

Abortion following rape is a recently recognized problem in European law and morals. Until the era of modern medicine, impregnation was taken as 'medical' evidence to female enjoyment of and cooperation in sex (Crawford, 2007:154). Any event of miscarriage or neonatal death of *illegitimate* children or by 'disreputable' women was considered criminal, unless they were able to produce convincing evidence to the contrary. Pregnant victims of rape have been treated as offenders rather than sufferers who deserve help and compassion (Ruff, 2001: 140 ff.).

The most common causes leading to prostitution and abortion were the interconnecting factors of dire poverty and social marginalization, often by means of rape (Rossiaud, 1984: 28–9). It has been calculated that about one half (!) of urban males in certain early modern European communities committed rape at least once in their lifetime (Rossiaud, 1984: 21). Augustine, Thomas Aquinas and numerous theologians and jurists called for public tolerance of prostitution as the lesser evil for the sake of fending off 'sodomy' and 'corruption of decent women'.[6] Never did they express toleration of abortion.

It is not a historical coincidence that the relaxation of the abortion laws in the West went in parallel to the recasting of rape as non-consensual sex rather than sex under irresistible violence, to the criminalization of marital rape and to the acceptance of no-fault divorce as a civil right. The notion that consent to marriage on behalf of the woman constitutes an irreversible submission of her body (so-called 'The Hale doctrine', based on 1 Cor., 7:4) is now condemnable worldwide (Glendon, 1987; Martin et al., 2007). Marital rape was a criminal offense in both Jewish Law and Roman Law. It was a novelty of Canon Law (and later Common Law) not to regard marital rape and rape of "dishonest" women as a crime (Brundage, 1982: 144). So, in law and history, enforcement of sex on women was tolerated and institutionalized, whereas women's reaction against the outcome of this reality was persecuted as if it was murder. Women could principally recourse to lethal self-defense only as a means to thwart off the rape, not to rid themselves of its outcome. Obviously, they had much better chances of procuring abortion than overcoming their male aggressors. Not only was this situation unfair and abusive, it was internally inconsistent as well.

In this section, I contend that pregnancy and labor are inseparable elements in the phenomenology and ethics of sexuality, being holistic and extremely powerful experiences of the body and person. Consent to pregnancy must be at least as powerful and endurable as consent to sex.

Undeniably, one may desire sex on Sunday, abstain on Monday and consent to it again on Tuesday; a woman cannot abort on Sunday and keep the child on Monday. Refusing sex is harmless, while abortion costs the life of a developing human. Some victims of rape choose to have the child; some who conceived willingly develop a powerful alienation from their pregnancy later on. Therefore, the mind-set constituting a genuine wish for abortion must be endurable, thoroughly premeditated and possibly as intense as the intent to repel sexual assault. This is certainly one of the most vexing moral decisions humans can make. Like sex, marriage and uses of the body such as in labor and medicine, decisions on abortion should never be made by third parties, no matter how authoritative, wise, well intentioned and powerful they might be. For sex and pregnancy to be considered moral, a genuine and ongoing consent of the person is mandatory.

This centrality of subjectivity in the condemnation of rape brings forth the analogy of slavery or serfdom. We can imagine two men working in the field. One does so willingly. The other performs the very same tasks, but he is a slave. His master supplies him with ample food, shelter and even recreation. He suffers no abuse, as his slavery is a kind of noble servitude endorsed by Aquinas (Sigismund, 2003: 222; Finnis, 1998: 184–5) and many other theologians from the monotheistic religions. The only thing lacking is the slave's freedom to go away and an immunity from the arbitrary will of his master. This is enough to qualify his condition as an evil worthy of self-defense.

Although the fetus never strikes a relationship of enslavement with the mother, society does so (albeit only up to 9 months and for a very noble cause) when it refuses to grant her an opportunity to terminate pregnancy, thus subjecting her responsible personal judgment and her mental and physical well-being to the interests of her developing child.

Imagine a retarded man attempting rape. Being mentally deficient, he is innocent. If you believe that it is permissible to kill him in self-defense of rape, then abortion of innocent babies could be moral as well. If you condemn therapeutic abortions and abortions following rape, you should also expect people to submit to rape by innocent retarded attackers rather than kill them.

Now imagine a slave in charge of his master's baby. He notices a unique opportunity to escape, yet at the price of the baby's life. If you think he has the right to freedom even in this situation, then abortion may also be moral. Since the unborn does not have a right to life, and their person status is questionable, you may even object to abandoning the baby and still justify abortion.

Still today we find Natural Law ethicists who hold that 'at times a slave might be required by other responsibilities to endure with patience even the injustice of the condition of slavery' (Grisez and Shaw, 1988: 164). This is reminiscent of their teachings on abortion. The circumstances of pregnancy may be predatory and profoundly traumatizing; even so, the woman is expected to submit to her role as an expectant mother and not to destroy innocent human life.

The abolition of slavery in the West was initiated by some protestant radical sects and Enlightenment activists in the late-eighteenth century. The Vatican joined them only a hundred years later and only when the last country in the Western hemisphere, Brazil, liberated its last remaining slaves. Pius IX, the Pope who declared early abortion excommunicable, supported the Confederacy and was the only state leader to exchange ambassadors with the South (Capizzi, 2004). A contemporary Catholic historian explains, 'The Catholic Church found the tendencies of the North [secularism] more dangerous than slavery' (Johnson, 2005).[7]

The Southern Baptist Church was a staunch supporter of slavery in the nineteenth century and the only contemporary major Protestant church in America to prohibit abortion (with the exception of 'saving the physical life of the mother').[8] Among world moral traditions, there is a consistent correlation between tolerance of slavery and objection to abortion following rape. The Vatican and other religious denominations create far more headlines reporting their fight against abortion and stem-cell research than against the abuse of women. One third of women world-wide are bitten at home; women between the ages of fifteen and forty four are more likely to be maimed and die from male violence (which is obviously linked to men's interest in sex) than from cancer, malaria, traffic accidents and war combined (Halpern, 2009:36). The Church's struggle against abortion care stifles desperately needed gynecological care in poor countries (Kristof and WuDunn, 2009:132).

Slavery and sexual slavery are not fossils from past history; nor are they abstract legal concepts. The international trade in women, mainly refugees and poor, is an epidemic of globalization. Rape in war zones is rampant worldwide. One third (!) of women report their first sexual intercourse as being forced (Jewkes et al., 2002). Most of them were teenagers at the time and living on less than $1 a day, having no access to contraception and safe obstetric care. This level of poverty is the lot of one quarter (!) of the world's teenage population.[9] When these girls are raped (or 'tempted'), they usually have no other choice in society but to accept the rapists as husbands and be further subjected to their sexual advances and other needs and desires. Women who are 'given in marriage' by their fathers (or clansmen) do not fare much better. In the absence of economical independence and option for divorce, their situation is nothing but enslavement for life. Not only do these social maladies produce numerous situations of abortion, but they also offer a broad framework of reference for the morality of abortion in general.

SUMMARY

A consensus exists in the discourse on self-defense that protection of the sexual integrity of the person is a value proportionate to life itself. This extension inevitably leads from a near universally accepted duty to perform abortion for the sake of saving life, to permissions for abortion for some other reasons. Most intuitively, the extension covers pregnancy conceived through rape.

Working within the paradigm of rights, the aim of this chapter was to offer a philosophical argument, compatible with different theories on the wrongness of killing and on the moral status of the embryo, and which is acceptable even by those who disapprove of killing innocent persons in self-defense.

Though most often maternal and fetal interests do not collide, granting the unborn with rights is incompatible with unconditional respect for the rights of their mothers. From a non-violable value, maternal life will thus become contingent on the natural course of pregnancy and its unpredictable vicissitudes.

Respect for the right to life of accidental violators (scenarios of self-defense) is controversial; conferring a status of inviolability (human rights) to obligatory violators (the unborn) is a moral contradiction. Allowing rightholders (women) to die or to suffer equivalently (violation of sexual integrity) in the name of the value of life of threats (the unborn), who never existed without being exploitative of the life of others, is incompatible with the notion of human rights.

Even when innocent human life is at stake, self-sacrifice and self-submission to invasive and sexual uses of the body are universally stipulated on consent in real time. It is unclear why abortion should be the only exception.

Respect for the diversity of human moralities claims the empowerment of women, particularly those whose life, health and integrity are threatened by realities beyond their control, by men they could not resist and by unborn babies whom they might wish to beget lovingly, but now threaten their health and life. Ethicists and theologians are welcome to address women thus empowered and to convince them to subscribe to their respective teachings.

All of us must be committed to fight the most common conditions behind women's wishes for abortion – poverty and exploitation.

NOTES

1 A significant, if not the main, line in Shiah Islam prohibits life-saving abortions (after 4 months) save in circumstances whereby (1) both mother and fetus will die if the mother is not saved immediately; and (2) the double-effect rule is applicable (Sekaleshfar, 2008).

2 The encyclicals *Human Vitae*, 1968, and *Evangelium Vitae*, 1995. See also Noonan (1970) and Ellingsen (1990). Rhonheimer surveys the Catholic debate on the management of obstructed labor and ectopic pregnancy, concluding that only if the child is doomed to die anyhow (or live a 'negligible period of time' in a life-threatening situation that he 'provoked'), is it permitted to kill it for the sake of saving the mother's life (Rhonheimer, 2009: 29).

3 Some Catholic authors hold that Aquinas justified the killing of the innocent in self-defense (Noonan, 1970: 24–6). Other theologians taught that it was moral to kill in defense of 'property of great importance' (1970: 40). Consequently, it has been suggested that the Natural Law taboo on abortion is derived from theological rather than moral considerations. See Ellingsen (1990) and Noonan's (1970) contention that the Vatican's objection to abortion for the sake of saving the mother's life is derived from the 'pastoral role' of the Holy See, not from rational argumentation. Indeed, some Catholic theologians oppose the official position of their church by endorsing life-saving abortions (e.g. Farley, 1974; Farley et al., 1984; McCormick, 1989). The *Magisterium*, however, endorses life-saving abortions *only* within the confines of the 'principle of double effect'.

Besides, until the twentieth century, Church doctrine held that abortuses and unbaptized children go to Hell. They were not allowed burial in consecrated ground. This terrified people to the point of preferential attempts to save the children, at least until baptized, even at the expense of their mothers, who were not at the risk of eternal damnation (Orme, 2001: 125–6). On the theological debate on the Limbo of infants, see the Catholic Encyclopedia. Available at http://www.newadvent.org/cathen/09256a.htm.

4 Available at http://www.unfpa.org/icpd/icpd_poa.htm#20 clause, 8.25.

5 The African Charter on Human Rights and People Rights on the Rights of Women in Africa. Available at http://portal.unesco.org/shs/en/ev.php-URL_ID=3963&URL_DO=DO_TOPIC&URL_SECTION=201.html.

6 Thomas Aquinas, *Summa Theologica*, 2.2. 69.2. This exposed them even further to rape, since rape of a prostitute was not punishable by Canon law. In many places license for practicing prostitution was given from the age of 12 and on condition of already lost virginity (Pike, 1972: 205). Most prostitutes were recruited between 15 and 17 years of age. In Paris and other cities, prostitutes constituted about 1 percent [sic] of the population. This title covered low-class single women who fended for themselves, usually resorting to occasional or full-time trade in sex (Richards, 1991: ch. 6).

7 Pius IX condemned the slave trade in the beatification of Peter Claver, 40 years after it had been criminalized by European nations. Available at http://www.angelusonline.org/modules.php?op=modload&name=News &file=article&sid=80&mode=thread&order=0&thold=0.

8 Resolution on Abortion and Infanticide, adopted at the SBC convention, May 1982. Available at http://www.johnstonsarchive.net/baptist/sbcabres.html.

9 UNFPA. *Fast facts*. New York. Available at http://www.unfpa.org/adolescents/facts.htm.

REFERENCES

Bakke, O.M. (2005) *When Children became People: The Birth of Childhood in Early Christianity*. Minneapolis, MN: Fortress Press.

Barilan, Y.M. (2003) 'One or two? Re-examination of the recent case of the conjoined twins from Malta', *Journal of Medicine and Philosophy*, 28: 27–44.

Barilan, Y.M. (2004) 'Ethical issues in multiple-pregnancy: A non essentialist point of view', in I. Blickstein and L.G. Keith (eds), *Multiple Pregnancy: Epidemiology, Gestation and Perinatal Outcome*, 2nd ed. London: Parthenon, ch. 51.

Barilan, Y.M. (2005) 'Speciesism as precondition to justice', *Politics and the Life Sciences*, 23: 22–33.

Barilan, Y. M. (2009–10) 'Her pain prevails and her judgment respected: abortion in Judaism' *Journal of Law and Religion* 25:97–186.

Barilan, Y. M. (2011) 'The biomedical uses of the body: lessons from the history of human dignity and rights' in C. Lenk, K, Beier and C. Wiessemann, eds. *Human Tissue Research: a Discussion of The Ethical and Legal Challanges from a European Perspective*. Oxford: Oxford University Press, ch. 1

Barilan, Y.M. and Brusa, M. (2008) 'Human rights and bioethics', *Journal of Medical Ethics*, 34: 379–83.

Berroit-Salvadore, E. (2000) 'The discourse of medicine and science', in G. Duby, M. Perrot, N. Zemon-Davis and P. Schmitt-Panel (eds), *A History of Women in the West: Renaissance and Enlightenment Paradoxes*. Cambridge: Cambridge University Press, pp. 381–3.

Bledsoe, C.H. (2002) *Contingent Lives: Fertility, Time and Aging in West Africa*. Chicago, IL: University of Chicago Press.

Brundage, J. A. (1982) 'Rape and seduction in medieval Canon Law" in V. L. Bullough and J. A. Brundage, eds. *Sexual Practices and The Medieval Church*. Buffalo: Promotheus.

Capizzi, J.E. (2004) 'For what shall we repent: Reflections on the American Bishops, their teachings, and slavery in the United States, 1839–61, *Theological Studies*, 65: 767–91.

Cleck, G. and Sayles, S. (1990) 'Rape and resistance', *Social Problems*, 37: 149–62.

Crawford, K. (2007) *European Sexualities 1400–1800*. Cambridge: Cambridge University Press.

Daniels, C.R. (1993) *At Women's Expense: State Power and the Politics of Fetal Rights*. Cambridge, MA: Harvard University Press.

Davis, N. (1984) 'Abortion and self-defense', *Philosophy and Public Affairs*, 3: 175–207.

De Browere, V. (2007) 'The comparative study of maternal mortality over time: The role of the professionalisation of childbirth', *Social History of Medicine*, 20: 541–62.

DeGrazia, D. (2007) 'The harm of death, time-relative interests and abortion', *Philosophical Forum*, 38: 57–80.

Ellingsen, M. (1990) 'The Church and abortion: Signs of consensus', *Christian Century*, Jan: 12–15.

Epstein, H. (2007) *The Invisible Cure: Africa, the West and the Fight against AIDS*. New York: Farrar, Straus and Giroux.

Farley, M.A. (1974) 'Liberation, abortion, and responsibility', *Reflection*, 71 (May): 9–13.

Farley, M.A., Chervenak, F.A., Walters, L., Hobbins, J. and Mahoney, M. (1984) 'When are third trimester pregnancy terminations morally justifiable?', *New England Journal of Medicine*, 310: 501–4.

Finnis, J. (1998) *Aquinas: Moral, Political and Legal Theory*. Oxford: Oxford University Press.

Fletcher, G. (1980) 'The right to life', *The Monist*, 63: 135–55.

Gelis, J. (1991) *History of Childbirth*. Boston, MA: Northwestern University Press.

Glendon, M.A. (1987) *Abortion and Divorce in Western Law*. Cambridge, MA: Harvard University Press.

Grimes, D.A., Benson, J., Singh, S., Romero, M., Ganatra, B., Okonofua, F.E. et al. (2006) 'Unsafe abortion: The preventable pandemic', *The Lancet*, 368: 1908–19.

Grisez, G.G. and Shaw, R. (1988) *Beyond the New Morality*, 3rd ed. Indianapolis, IN: Notre Dame University Press.

Haidt, J. (2007) 'The new synthesis in moral psychology', *Science, 316*: 998–1002.

Halpern, S. (2009) 'Breaking conspiracy of silence' *New York Review of Books* 56(18)33–40.

Heywood, C. (2001) *A History of Childhood*. Oxford: Polity.

Hill, K., Thomas, K., AbouZahr, C., Walker, N., Say, L., Inoue, M. et al. (2007) 'Estimates of maternal mortality worldwide between 1990 and 2005: An assessment of available data', *The Lancet*, 370: 1311–19.

Himma, K. (1999) 'Thomson's violinist and conjoined twins', *Cambridge Quarterly of Healthcare Ethics*, 8: 428–39.

Huffman, T.L. (1993) 'Abortion, moral responsibility and self-defense', *Public Affairs Quarterly*, 7: 287–301.

Jewkes, R., Garcia-Moreno, C. and Sen, P. (2002) 'Sexual violence', in E.G. Krug, L.L. Dahlberg, J.A. Mercy, A. Zwi and R. Lozano (eds), *World Report on Violence and Health*. Geneva, WHO, ch. 6. Available at http://www.who.int/violence_injury_prevention/violence/world_report/en/full_en.pdf.

Johnson, P.G. (2005) 'The Catholic Church and the confederate states of America', *The Angelus*, 28 (6).

Kamm, F.M. (2007) *Intricate Ethics: Rights, Responsibilities and Permissible Harms*. Oxford: Oxford University Press.

Keown, J. (1988) *Abortion, Doctors and the Law: Some Aspects of the Legal Regulation of Abortion in England from 1803 to 1982*. Cambridge: Cambridge University Press.

King, H. (2007) *Midwifery, Obstetrics and the Rise of Gynaecology*. Aldershot: Ashgate.

Kopel, D. B., Gallant, P. and Eisen, J. D. (2008) 'The human right of self-defense', *BYU Journal of Public Law*, 22: 48–176.

Kristof, N. D. and WuDunn, S. (2009) Half The Sky: *Turning Oppression into Opportunity*. New York: Knopf.

Lomax, E. (1993) 'Diseases of infancy and early childhood', in K.H. Kiple (ed.), *Cambridge World History of Human Disease*. Cambridge: Cambridge University Press, pp. 147–57.

McCormick, R.A. (1989) 'Abortion: The unexplored middle ground', *Second Opinion*, 10: 41–51.

Marquis, D. (1989) 'Why abortion is immoral?', *Journal of Philosophy*, 86: 183–202.

Marquis, D. (2007) 'Abortion', in B. Steinbock (ed.), *Oxford Handbook of Bioethics*. Oxford: Oxford University Press.

Marquis, D. (2008) 'Abortion and human nature', *Journal of Medical Ethics*, 34: 422–6.

Martin, E.K., Taft, C.T and Resick, P.A. (2007) 'A review of marital rape', *Aggression*, 12: 329–47

Miller, P. (1998) *The Transformation of Patriarchy in the West, 1500–1900*. Bloomington, IN: Indiana University Press.

Newell, F.S. (1924) *Cesarean Section*. New York: Appleton & Co.

Noonan J.T. (1970) 'An almost absolute value in history', in J.T. Noonan (ed.), *The Morality of Abortion*. Cambridge, MA: Harvard University Press, pp. 1–59.

Orme, N. (2001) *Medieval Children*. New Haven, CT: Yale University Press.

Park, K. (2006) *Secrets of Women: Gender, Generation and the Origin of Human Dissection*. New York: Zone.

Pigott, R. (2004) 'Sierra Leone silent sufferers', BBC, 18 June. Available at http://news.bbc.co.uk/2/hi/africa/3817009.stm.

Pike, R. (1972) *Aristocrats and Traders: Sevillian Society in the Sixteenth Century*. Ithaca, NY: Cornell University Press.

Rhonheimer, M. (2009) *Vital Conflicts in Medical Ethics: A Virtue Approach to Craniotomy and Tubal Pregnancies*. Washington, DC: Catholic University of America Press.

Richards, J. (1991) *Sex, Dissidence and Damnation: Minority Groups in the Middle Ages*. London: Routledge.

Riddle, J.M. (1995) *Contraception and Abortion from the Ancient World to the Renaissance*. Cambridge, MA: Harvard University Press.

Rossiaud, J. (1984) *Medieval Prostitution*. New York: Barnes and Noble.

Ruff, J.R. (2001) *Violence in Early Modern Europe*. Cambridge: Cambridge University Press.

Ryan, C.G. (2002) 'The chapel and the operating room: The struggle of Roman Catholic clergy, physicians, and believers with the dilemmas of obstetric surgery, 1800–1900', *Bulletin of the History of Medicine*, 76: 461–94.

Sargent, C. (1982) 'Solitary confinement: Birth practices among the Barber of the Peoples of the Republic of Benin', in K.M. Artschwager (ed.), *Anthropology of Human Birth*. Philadelphia, PA: F.A. Davis, pp. 193–210.

Schofeld, R. (1986) 'Did the mothers really die? Three centuries of maternal mortality in "the world we have lost"', in L. Bonfield, M. Smith and K. Wrightson (eds), *The World We Have Gained: Histories of Populations and Social Structure*. Oxford: Oxford University Press

Sedghe, G., Henshaw, S., Singh, S., Åhman, H. and Shah, I.H. (2007) 'Induced abortion: Estimated rates and trends worldwide', *The Lancet*, 370: 1338–45.

Sekaleshfar, F.B. (2008) 'Abortion perspective in Shi'a Islam', *Studies in Ethics, Law and Technology*, 2 (3): art. 3. Available athttp://www.bepress.com/selt/vol2/iss3/art4, (accessed 12 July 2010).

Sigismund, P.E. (2003) 'Law and politics', in N. Kretzman and E. Stump (eds), *The Cambridge Companion to Aquinas*. Cambridge: Cambridge University Press.

Sperling, D. (2005) 'Do pregnant women have (living) will?', *Journal of Healthcare Law and Policy*, 8: 331–42.

Thomson, J.J. (1971) 'In defense of abortion', *Philosophy and Public Affairs*, 1: 47–66.

Uniacke, S. (1994) *Permissible Killing: The Self-defence Justification of Homicide*. Cambridge: Cambridge University Press.

Wiesner, M.E. (1993) *Women and Gender in Early Modern Europe*. Cambridge: Cambridge University Press.

Wright-St Clair, R.E. (1963) 'History of mutilating obstetric operations', *New Zealand Medical Journal*, 62: 468–70.

13

Ethics of Genetic Counseling

Gamal I. Serour and Ahmed R. A. Ragab

INTRODUCTION

Genetic counseling has become an important part of medical genetics. The demand for genetic counseling will likely increase as knowledge accumulates about the genetic component of commonly occurring disorders. With the tremendous advances in the field of genetic techniques and genetic diagnoses, ethical aspects involved in genetic counseling are now emerging as major issues. Exploring some ethical aspects of genetic counseling will assist health providers, policymakers and program managers in ensuring that genetic information and services will be provided in an ethically acceptable way.

Research into the structure and function of genes is increasing our understanding of their role in maintaining health and causing disease. Over the last half century, our understanding of genetic disorders has increased spectacularly. The knowledge generated has already created, and will create further, opportunities and sound reasons for genetic testing. The knowledge gained from discoveries in human genetics since the advent of recombinant DNA technology has the potential for making significant improvements in health when applied probably at the individual, family and community levels (El-Hazmi, 2004). Genetic counseling programs and services are critical for adequate genetic testing.

Genetic counseling is defined as the process by which patients or relatives, at risk of an inherited disorder, are advised of the consequences and nature of the disorder, the probability of developing or transmitting it and the options open to them in management and family planning in order to prevent, avoid or ameliorate it (Evans et al., 2004; Lea et al., 2005). It is viewed as a therapeutic interrelationship between genetic counselors and their clients.

EVOLUTION OF GENETIC COUNSELING

Over the last few decades, a major change in the field of medicine has been observed, due to the development of the science of human genetics. The traditional focus on diseases themselves has now turned towards the risk of illness. This evolution made possible the understanding, treatment or even prevention of some diseases.

Although genetics as a formal discipline emerged after the rediscovery in 1900 of Mendel's nineteenth-century experiments, genetic diseases had been described in the scientific literature long before then (UNPC, 1983).

In this regard, clinical genetic and thus genetic counseling evolved into a profession in parallel to the advancement in diagnostic tests. As the profession grows, the definition of genetic counseling and genetic counseling procedures also continue and will continue to evolve.

The first American genetic counseling center was probably the Eugenic Records Office in Cold Spring Harbor, New York, founded by Dr Charles B. Davenport in 1915. The heredity clinic was established in 1940 at the University of Michigan, USA (WHO, 1985). Since then many such centers have been opened around the world. In 1947, Sheldon Reed, a geneticist at the University of Minnesota, introduced the expression 'genetic counseling'. The role of the genetic counselor was 'to explain thoroughly what the genetic situation is but the decision must be a personal one between the husband and wife, and theirs alone'. The year 1959 was identified as the birth year of clinical genetics, with convergent achievements in molecular, biomedical and cytogenetic research.

By the 1960s, great strides had been made in understanding human genetics. The new information gave counselors a broader and more scientific basis for informing families about the recurrence risks and inheritance patterns of an increasing number of diseases. The development of genetic tests based on blood and cell samples introduced in the field of prospective counseling helped shift counseling from a primarily nonmedical setting to screening programs involving public health officials, physicians, nurses and other health providers, often working in specialized genetics centers in hospitals and universities (USPC, 1983).

Currently, clinical genetics has expanded from the diagnosis and prediction of rare, often untreatable conditions, to the prediction of common, often treatable conditions. With increasing genomic and post-genomic knowledge, there are hopes of being able to screen individuals for a wide variety of susceptibility genes and gene variants causing late-onset diseases, and to adopt preventive strategies based on dietary measures and a control of environmental factors.

Terminology

It is important that, to avoid misunderstandings and false impressions about the implication of genetic counseling, both the counselor and the subject are very clear about terminology in this rapidly expanding field. The international Declaration on Human Genetic Data (UNESCO, 2004) agreed on the following terminology:

- Human genetic data: Information about heritable characteristics of individuals obtained by analysis of nucleic acids or by other scientific analysis.
- Human proteomic data: Information pertaining to an individual's proteins including their expression, modification and interaction.
- Consent: Any freely given specific, informed and express agreement of an individual to his or her genetic data being collected, processed, used and stored.

- Biological samples: Any sample of biological material (for example blood, skin and bone cells or blood plasma) in which nucleic acids are present and which contains the characteristic genetic make-up of an individual.
- Population-based genetic study: A study which aims at understanding the nature and extent of genetic variation among a population or individuals within a group or between individuals across different groups.
- Behavioral genetic study: A study that aims at establishing possible connections between genetic characteristics and behavior.
- Invasive procedure: Biological sampling using a method involving intrusion into the human body, such as obtaining a blood sample by using a needle and syringe.
- Non-invasive procedure: Biological sampling using a method which does not involve intrusion into the human body, such as oral smears.
- Data linked to an identifiable person: Data that contain information, such as name, birth date and address, by which the person from whom the data were derived can be identified.
- Data unlinked to an identifiable person: Data that are not linked to an identifiable person, through the replacement of, or separation from, all identifying information about that person by use of a code.
- Data irretrievably unlinked to an identifiable person: Data that cannot be linked to an identifiable person, through destruction of the link to any identifying information about the person who provided the sample.
- Genetic testing: A procedure to detect the presence or absence of, or change in, a particular gene or chromosome, including an indirect test for a gene product or other specific metabolite that is primarily indicative of a specific genetic change.
- Genetic screening: Large-scale systematic genetic testing offered in a program to a population or subsection thereof intended to detect genetic characteristics in asymptomatic people.

Genetic counseling

This is a procedure to explain the possible implications of the findings of genetic testing or screening, its advantages and risks and where applicable to assist the individual in the long-term handling of the consequences. It takes place before and after genetic testing and screening. When conducting genetic counseling, both the counselor and the individual should be very clear about the terminology used during counseling. Genetic data should be protected and the purpose of its collection identified with the prior, free informed consent of the subject.

Each individual has a characteristic genetic make-up. Nevertheless, a person's identity should not be reduced to genetic characteristics, since it involves complex educational, environmental and personal factors and emotional, social, spiritual and cultural bonds with others and implies a dimension of freedom.

Provision of information about 'genetic' test and 'genetic counseling' is not synonymous. Genetic counseling encompasses both information giving and discussion of the implications for the individual in a contextual framework that is unique in each person. In addition, genetic counseling is a communication and, in some cases, a psychotherapeutic process, while the others are diagnostic or prognostic services (Biesecker and Marteau, 1999).

PROTECTION OF GENETIC DATA

Human genetic data are very special because they can be predictive of genetic predispositions concerning individuals. They may have a significant impact on the family, including offspring, extending over generations, and in some instances on the whole group to which the person concerned belongs.

They may contain information the significance of which is not necessarily known at the time of collection of the biological samples; they may have cultural significance for persons or groups.

Due consideration should be given to the sensitivity of human genetic data and an appropriate level of protection for these data and biological samples should be established.

PURPOSE OF COLLECTING HUMAN GENETIC DATA

According to the UNESCO declaration (UNESCO, 2004), human genetic data and human proteomic data may be collected, processed, used and stored only for the purposes of: diagnosis and health care, including screening and predictive testing; and medical and other scientific research, including epidemiological, especially population-based genetic studies, as well as anthropological or archaeological studies, collectively referred to as 'medical and scientific research'.

THE AIMS OF GENETIC COUNSELING AND ITS PROCESS

Requests for genetic testing are increasing each year. The challenge is to ensure that genetic testing is delivered as efficiently and appropriately as possible, and to the highest scientific and ethical standards. Currently, genetic counseling goes beyond mere presentations of risk facts and figures to the prevention and cure of disease, the relief of pain and the maintenance of health (WHO, 1985; Evans et al., 2004; Lea et al., 2005).

The process of genetic counseling has changed dramatically over the past three decades, and instead of being based on purely clinical findings, the identity of many disorders can be proven because their genetic or chromosomal basis is known.

The process of genetic counseling involves an attempt by one or more appropriately trained persons to help the individual or family to: comprehend medical facts, including the diagnosis, probable course of the disorder and the available management; appreciate the way heredity contributes to the disorder, and the risk of recurrence in specified relatives; understand the alternatives for dealing with the risk of occurrence; choose the course of action which seems to them appropriate in view of their risk, their family goals and their ethical and religious standards, to act in accordance with that decision; and to make the best possible adjustment to the disorder in an affected family member and/or the risk of recurrence of that disorder (Robinson and Linden, 1993). The availability of an ever-increasing number of laboratory tests allows more accurate diagnosis, and often gives the opportunity for pre-symptomatic or prenatal diagnosis to family members who prefer to use it. However, it must not be overlooked that the availability of such tests also poses psychological and ethical questions which are difficult to resolve (DeLozier-Blanchet, 2007).

The first step in the genetic counseling process is to establish an accurate diagnosis, which involves the collection and review of medical records and family history information. Receiving a diagnosis of a genetic disorder can have a profound impact for both patients and their family members, thus a supportive type of counseling is required.

Clinical evaluation is performed by a clinical geneticist and involves a detailed physical examination and the documenting of any unusual physical features. After a diagnosis is made, the natural history of the disorder, the prognosis, and the available management or treatment options are discussed with the client or his/her guardian (WHO, 1985; Evans et al., 2004; Lea et al., 2005). In cases where a diagnosis cannot be established, the client may be asked to return to clinic after a period of time.

The preferred language of the person or couple should be determined and an interpreter provided if required; the interpreter should ideally be a trained health interpreter rather than a family member. Support is also a very important component of this process, which focuses on promoting informed decision making for patients who are often in very difficult situations (Schneider, 2005). The active listening, and counseling skills practiced by the genetic counselor are as important as the process itself. It is essential that the counseling process allows time for discussion and reflection. Multiple counseling sessions may be needed and an appropriate amount of time should be allowed between the provision of counseling and performance of the test/s.

Genetic counseling is an expanding and evolving field. Based upon recent findings about the counseling process, changes can be expected to continue as the role of genetic counselor assumes an increasing role in health care. Genetic counseling is generally required before and after pre-symptomatic or predictive tests, following a positive genetic carrier test and following abnormal results on prenatal diagnostic or screening tests.

The genetic counseling process involves multiple steps that may include, but are not limited to, gathering and assessment of information, establishment of a diagnosis or risk of disease, and discussion of the implications as well as available options to address risk for family members. Evaluating family history in the process is important; it is generally useful to record the cultural background of the family, including race, religion, occupation and age and state of health of first, second and third relatives (WHO, 1985; Evans et al., 2004; Lea et al., 2005).

It is mandatory that the process of genetic counseling needs to observe the ethical codes and the prevailing traditions and beliefs of the community in all steps of its process.

APPROACHES FOR GENETIC COUNSELING: DIRECTIVE OR NONDIRECTIVE

Genetic counseling should be nondirective. Nondirective genetic counseling is understood to imply the client is given all relevant information and then left to make his or her decision. Nondirectiveness is based on the desire to uphold the personal nature of reproductive decision making and the reluctance to pass judgment on the worthiness of the life of a person affected with a genetic condition.

The nondirective approach involves the presentation of facts in an unbiased manner, leaving the entire responsibility of decision with the client, while directive genetic counseling has a positive impact on the client's decision. The major difference between directive and nondirective counseling is whether or not the counselor actively participates or helps the client to make a decision (Kaushal et al., 2006). It is argued that the cornerstone of the practice of genetic counseling is that it is nondirective. The autonomy of the client and the right of the individual to make decisions based on his/her own values and beliefs is important. Aston (1998) affirmed that genetic counseling 'must' be nondirective. He argued that many parents do not want to undergo tests that might lead on to the abortion of their child, or even that many parents, having had positive test results, will feel able to value their child's life, whether or not there may be a handicap.

However, Thorpe et al. (1995) argued that nondirective counseling can have biases. The belief of the counselor would be reflected in his/her expressions, including the tone of voice and facial expression, which might end in prompting a directive approach. Rentmeester (2001) argued that the underlying assumption of value-free genetic counseling is theoretically unfounded. Traditionally, the professional duty of doctors is not confined merely to disclosing medical information for the patient but also to giving advice about what to do (Bernhardt, 1997). A directive approach may be more appropriate in cases where the life, health or well-being of the client needs to be preserved (BMA, 1998).

The popular view of nondirective genetic counseling limits the counselor's role to providing information to clients and assisting families in making decisions. It is argued that nondirective genetic counseling is shown to be incomplete, as with fuller understanding of what it means to respect autonomy, merely respecting clients' choices does not exhaust this duty. Moreover, the genetic counselor–client relationship should also be governed by the counselor's commitment to the principles of beneficence and autonomy. When nondirective counseling is reexamined in light of both these principles, it becomes clear that there are cases in which counselors should attempt to persuade clients to reconsider their decisions.

In between the directive and nondirective approaches, an emerging approach is the shared decision-making approach. This approach allows genetic counselors to contribute their professional knowledge while acknowledging the importance of the client's wider value system. In this regard, the genetic counselors and clients should share information about decisions to be made and come to an agreement for which they share responsibility (Elwyn et al., 2000).

FACTORS INFLUENCING GENETIC COUNSELING

The genetic counselors' and clients' social and cultural backgrounds strongly influence decision-making processes and outcomes in genetic counseling. Awwad et al. (2007) investigated influences of culture and acculturation on the prenatal decision-making process of native Palestinians and Palestinian Americans. Five major issues were investigated: influence of family history of an inherited condition on premarital decisions; perceptions of nondirective genetic counselor statements regarding options; role of gender in prenatal decisions; gender differences in emotional expression; and role of family and society in prenatal decisions. The study found several similarities and differences between native Palestinian and Palestinian American responses. Genetic testing for an inherited condition is commonly requested by both groups. However, in the perception of nondirective coun-seling, the role of gender in prenatal decision and emotional expression are different in the two groups. Similarities appear to be due to common cultural roots, while differences may be due to acculturation.

OBSTACLES TO EFFECTIVE GENETIC COUNSELING

Genetic counselors are faced by tests of varying predictive values and reliability, unfair testing distribution mechanisms and tests for conditions where no treatment exists. The main obstacles to effective genetic counseling are lack of knowledge of genetics and biol-ogy, emotional conflicts (Clarke, 1991), and presenting the counselor knowledge in an unbiased manner (Kaushal et al., 2006). Studies have demonstrated that genetic counseling primarily involves the provision of genetic information and its implications but pays rela-tively little attention to the social, emotional and familial aspects of the information (Michie et al., 1997).

It is difficult for a counselor to impart unbiased information because of the clients' ethnic background, reproductive history (e.g. abortions, stillborn or dead siblings and the age, sex and health of living children). This may lead the counselor to adopt a directive rather than nondirective approach to genetic counseling (Clarke, 1991; Kaushal et al., 2006).

Is there is a need for a universal model for genetic counseling?

In all cultures, from the inception of humanity, medical practice was regulated by codes of ethics. According to each society's condition, the ethical attitude of the individual may be influenced by the attitude of society, which reflects the interests of theologians, legislators, sociologists, economists, physicians, ethicists, demographers and policymakers in the country (Serour, 1995, 2000a). It is therefore not surprising to find what is ethical in one society might not be ethical in another. It is mandatory for the counselors to be aware of such background before they make their judgment on different ethical problems (Serour, 2006).

Genetic counseling is an understanding of a set of facts according to the counselors' frame of reference, background in the science of genetics and previous training and expe-rience in effectively communicating with clients (Kaushal et al., 2006). It depends heavily on community sociocultural background (including religion and education level, for example); the legal system of the country (abortion laws, for instance) and the advancement in genetic testing and its availability and affordability (Serour, 2000b).

Consequently, it is difficult to have a universal model for genetic counseling in the world of today with its increasing diversity in culture, religion and social background. As indi-cated in the Universal Declaration of Bioethics and Human Rights (UNESCO, 2006) and adopted by the international community, cultural diversity and pluralism, solidarity and cooperation, social responsibility and health, sharing benefits, protecting future genera-tions and protection of the environments, biosphere and biodiversity should be respected and applied.

IMPACT OF GENETIC COUNSELING

The focus of clinical genetics, and thus genetic counseling, is forecast to expand from the diagnosis and prediction of rare, often untreatable conditions, to the prediction of common, often treatable or preventable conditions (Holtzman and Marteau, 2000). Molecular medicine has introduced into clinical practice an unprecedented form of prognosis, based on the ability to identify susceptibility genes. This improves the potential of informing a patient that, at some point in the future, with some probability or with near certainty, he or she will suffer from a disease of greater or lesser severity (Kaplan, 2002; Valet et al., 2006).

The ability to test for susceptibility genes will precipitate into the world of medicine millions of individuals who have no personal experience of any disease. While a proportion of these will benefit from the information, many will not. Those are individuals who are neither patients under treatment nor non-patients free of any medically relevant condition (Valet et al., 2006).

This new class of individuals, watching and waiting for a sign of disease, will be advised to subject themselves to systematic clinical and instrumental monitoring, and some of them may develop psychosomatic symptoms (Valet et al., 2006).

ETHICAL ASPECTS OF GENETIC COUNSELING

Ethical discourse is necessary for any society to form its responses to any scientific or medical innovation (Serour, 1995, 2000b). It is ethically imperative that when genetic testing and counseling are being considered, the importance of cultural diversity and pluralism should be given due regard. However, such considerations are not to be invoked to infringe upon human dignity, human rights and fundamental freedom. Genetic counseling should be nondirective, culturally adapted and consistent with the best interest of the person concerned.

When human genetic data or human proteomic data are collected for the purposes of forensic medicine or in civil, criminal and other legal proceedings, including parentage testing, the collection of biological samples, in vivo or post-mortem should be made only in accordance with domestic law consistent with the international law of human rights. Genetic counseling and testing is governed by the universally accepted set of ethics that are applied to medicine (UNESCO, 2006).

The four principles of bioethics – autonomy, beneficence, non-maleficence and justice – first proposed by Tom Beauchamp and Childress (Beauchamp and Childress, 1989) have their rational basis and truth only within the wider set of moral principles (Finnis and Fisher, 1994). However, with expanding medical knowledge, technology and the wider application of multi-centric medical research, globalization, medical tourism, transfer of technology and advancement in communication systems, the four principles alone, though highly valuable, became inadequate to cover all aspects of ethical issues arising in the application of new technologies on human, particularly genetic and proteomic, data.

In October 2005, the general conference of UNESCO adopted by acclamation the Universal Declaration on Bioethics and Human Rights (UNESCO, 2006). In dealing with ethical issues raised by medicine, life science and associated technologies as applied to human beings, the declaration covered a much larger scope of principles including the principles of: human dignity and human rights; benefit and harm; autonomy and individual responsibility; consent, and persons without the capacity to consent; respect for human vulnerability and personal integrity; privacy and confidentiality; equality, justice and equity; nondiscrimination and non-stigmatization; respect for cultural diversity and pluralism; solidarity and cooperation; social responsibility and health; sharing benefits; protecting future generations and protection of the environment's biosphere and biodiversity.

The ethics of genetic data were covered in several international treaties and conventions and in other international human rights instruments adopted by the United Nations and their specialized agencies (UNESCO, 2004). Several international and regional instruments, national laws, regulations and ethical texts relating to the protection of human rights and fundamental freedoms and to respect for human dignity as regards the collection, processing, use and storage of scientific data, as well as of medical data and personal data, were implemented.

The International Declaration on Human Genetic Data (UNESCO, 2004) recognizes that genetic information is part of the overall spectrum of medical data and that the information content of any medical data, including genetic data and proteomic data, is highly contextual and dependent on the particular circumstances. Furthermore, human genetic data have a special status on account of their sensitive nature, since they can be predictive of genetic predispositions concerning individuals, and given that the power of predictability can be stronger than assessed at the time of deriving the data, they may have a significant impact on the family, including offspring, extending over generations, and in some instances on the whole group; they may contain information the significance of which is not necessarily known at the time of the collection of biological samples; and they may have cultural significance for persons or groups.

Genetic data and proteomic data, regardless of their apparent information content, should be treated with a high standard of confidentiality. With the expanding and rapid development in the field of genetic and proteomic data there has been increasing importance on human genetic data for economic and commercial purposes. In this regard, one cannot ignore the special needs and vulnerabilities of developing countries and the need to reinforce international cooperation in the field of human genetics.

The collection, processing, use and storage of human genetic data are of paramount importance for the progress of life sciences and medicine, for their applications and for the use of such data for non-medical purposes. The growing amount of personal data collected makes genuine irretrievability increasingly difficult.

UNESCO's (2004) declaration on human genetic data placed the interests and welfare of the individual above the rights and interests of society and research. It reaffirmed that the principles established in the universal declaration on Bioethics and Human Rights (UNESCO, 2006), as well as the principles of equality, justice, solidarity and responsibility as well as respect for human dignity, human rights and fundamental freedoms, particularly freedom of thought and expression, including freedom of research, and privacy and security of the person, must underlie the collection, processing, use and storage of human genetic data.

Prior free informed consent

Prior, free, informed and express consent, without inducement by financial or other personal gain, should be obtained for the collection of human genetic data, human proteomic data or biological samples, whether through invasive or non-invasive procedures, and for their subsequent processing, use and storage, whether carried out by public or private institutions. Limitations on this principle of consent should only be prescribed for compelling reasons by domestic law consistent with international human rights law.

When, in accordance with domestic law, a person is incapable of giving informed consent, authorization should be obtained from the legal representative, in accordance with domestic law. The legal representative should have regard to the best interests of the person concerned.

An adult who is unable to consent should as far as possible take part in the authorization procedure. The opinion of a minor in proportion to age and degree of maturity should be taken into consideration as an increasingly determining factor.

In diagnosis and health care, genetic screening and testing of minors and adults not able to consent will normally only be ethically acceptable when it has important implications for the health of the person and has regard to his or her best interests.

When human genetic data, human proteomic data or biological samples are collected for medical and scientific research purposes, consent may be withdrawn by the person concerned unless such data are irretrievably unlinked to an identifiable person. Withdrawal of consent should entail neither a disadvantage nor a penalty for the person concerned.

When a person withdraws consent, the person's genetic data, proteomic data and biological samples should no longer be used unless they are irretrievably unlinked to the person concerned.

If not irretrievably unlinked, the data and biological samples should be dealt with in accordance with the wishes of the person. If the person's wishes cannot be determined or are not feasible or are unsafe, the data and biological samples should either be irretrievably unlinked or destroyed.

The right to know

When human genetic data, human proteomic data or biological samples are collected for medical and scientific research purposes, the information provided at the time of consent should indicate that the person concerned has the right to decide whether or not to be informed of the results. This does not apply to research on data irretrievably unlinked to identifiable persons or to data that do not lead to individual findings concerning the persons who have participated in such a research. Where appropriate, the right not to be informed should be extended to identified relatives who may be affected by the results.

USE OF GENETIC INFORMATION

Every effort should be made to ensure that human genetic data and human proteomic data are not used for purposes that discriminate in a way that is intended to infringe, or has the effect of infringing human rights, fundamental freedoms or human dignity of an individual, or for purposes that lead to the stigmatization of an individual, family, group or community.

In this regard, appropriate attention should be paid to the findings of population-based genetic studies and behavioral genetic studies and their interpretations.

Any debate on the social, legal and ethical issues surrounding genetic counseling must consider the new genetic tests and their implications within the general context of health care. In providing this new technology one must respect the dignity of human beings, security of human genetic material, inviolability of the person and necessary quality of services (Serour and Dickens, 2001). This technology, while increasing the amount of information and the number of options an individual has, can lead to some complex ethical situations. It is the role of genetic counseling to assist clients as they grapple with these complex situations (Evans et al., 2004).

Numerous ethical theories exist, but no ethical theories, principles or decision-making models provide an absolute guide to good action (Lea et al., 2005). They do, however, provide a framework for working through decisions by seeking to define the limits of morally acceptable behavior and by elucidating guidelines for making decisions within those limits. In other words, they assist with *how* to make a decision, but not always with *what* decision to make (Lea et al., 2005).

It is ethically imperative that human genetic data and human proteomic data be collected, processed, used and stored on the basis of transparent and ethically acceptable procedures. States should endeavor to involve society at large in the decision-making process concerning broad policies for the collection, procession, use and storage of human genetic data and human proteomic data and the evaluation of their management, in particular in the case of population-based genetic studies. This decision-making process, which may benefit from international experience, should ensure the free expression of various viewpoints.

Independent, multidisciplinary and pluralist ethics committees should be promoted and established at national, regional, local or institutional levels. Where appropriate, ethics committees at national level should be consulted with regard to the establishment of standards, regulations and guidelines for the collection, processing, use and storage of human genetic data, human proteomic data and biological samples. They should also be consulted concerning matters where there is no domestic law. Ethics committees at institutional or local levels should be consulted with regard to their application to specific research projects.

When the collection, processing, use and storage of human genetic data, human proteomic data or biological samples are carried out in two or more states, the ethics committees in the states concerned, where appropriate, should be consulted and the review of these questions at the appropriate level should be based on the principles on the ethical and legal standards adopted by the states concerned.

It is ethically imperative that clear, balanced, adequate and appropriate information shall be provided to the person whose prior, free, informed and express consent is sought. Such information shall, alongside providing other necessary details, specify the purpose for which human genetic data and human proteomic data are being derived from biological samples, and are used and stored. This information should indicate, if necessary, risks and consequences. The information should also indicate that the person concerned can withdraw his or her consent, without coercion, and this should entail neither a disadvantage to nor a penalty for the person concerned.

ETHICAL PROBLEMS IN GENETIC COUNSELING

Ethical problems arise not only from the current state of knowledge about genetic risk factors and utility of genetic tests but also result from conflicts that can arise when the needs of the client are not in unison of others within the family or society (Lea et al., 2005). A major ethical problem is the tendency to ignore the underlying socioeconomic or environmental causes of disease in favor of a genetic approach to disease prevention. This can result in using more and more advanced technology, and consequently diverts limited resources to the study of more and more trivial issues, while the major population causes of diseases are ignored. Poverty is responsible for most deaths worldwide. Poor inhabitants of the population are more likely than those with higher incomes to live near polluting areas. In addition, poorer groups/countries are explicitly targeted by those marketing unhealthy products, which in turn leads to more health problems, including genetic diseases.

In contrast to other medical screening tests, genetic testing in prenatal clinics is focused on individual reproductive decision making rather than the management of clinical disease (Lea et al., 2005). Genetic counseling might result in difficult choices, among them abortion choices, fetal sex selection and sterilization (Serour and Dickens, 2001).

Families affected by genetic disorders have educational, social, medical and psychological needs that require attention. Within this context, many of the ethical dilemmas that would result, for example the probability of carrying an affected child till term, abortions and rights for childbearing regardless of the impact on offspring and the possibility of predicting future diseases/health risks, need answers (WHO, 1985; Evans et al., 2004; Lea et al., 2005).

Some genetic tests do not identify all the possible genetic mutations that can cause a particular condition, or they have limited predictive value, which can lead to uncertainties for patients and clinicians. For instance, the cause of birth defects can only be determined in approximately 40 percent of affected children (Evans et al., 2004). In addition, because some genetic tests are screening tests, some will generate false-positive and false-negative results. This means that a woman who is screened as negative may have a false-negative result and have a baby born affected by a genetic disease (Lea et al., 2005). In addition, a genetic test can only indicate a susceptibility to the disease, with no certainty of the illness developing. Despite much research, genetic susceptibility to complex disease such as heart disease, cancer and obesity has proved difficult to identify, with many poorly reproducible results. Except in a small percentage of cases, genes are poor predictors of future health (Holtzman and Marteau, 2000). These issues raise real ethical concerns for a counselor. Many clients need help in understanding the meaning of a statistical probability.

Genetic testing can lead to identifying specific conditions but not others; and at present, not all the conditions can be treated. Therefore, one ethical dilemma that occurs is whether a newborn should be tested for disorders that cannot be treated (Lea et al., 2005).

One important ethical concern is the fact that it is becoming possible through extensive genome analysis to gather information on individual sequence variation, and ultimately unveil one's genetic fate. This represents a risk of intrusion into individual privacy if the genetic information is not kept scrupulously confidential (Kaplan, 2002). For instance, there is a risk of discrimination when a third party (insurance companies, employers) claims to require access to this information.

Medical information always changes over time, leading to revisions in diagnosis, refinements in treatment or improved carrier testing or prenatal diagnosis (Evans et al., 2004).

Over-concentration on research on genes and their heath implications could lead to neglect of the effects on human health of other factors, such as the physical, social and economic environments in which people live.

During the process of genetic counseling, there could be other findings, such as fetal sex, which might put the counselor in an ethical dilemma if the process was not related to X-linked disorders (Dickens et al., 2005). If genetics is used for purposes of identifying paternity and the findings disclose false paternity, what can the counselor do in this regard?

SUMMARY

Genetic counseling is defined as the process by which patients or relatives, at risk of an inherited disorder, are advised of the consequences and nature of the disorder, the probability of developing or transmitting it and the options open to them in management and family planning in order to prevent, avoid or ameliorate it.

It is important that both the counselor and the subject are very clear about terminology in this rapidly expanding field, to avoid misunderstandings and false impressions about the implication of genetic counseling. Genetic data should be protected and the purpose of its collection identified with the prior free informed consent of the subject.

Human genetic data are very special because they can be predictive of genetic predispositions concerning individuals. They may have a significant impact on the family, including offspring, extending over generations, and in some instances on the whole group to which the person concerned belongs. They may contain information the significance of which is not necessarily known at the time of the collection of the biological samples, and which may have cultural significance for persons or groups.

When human genetic data or human proteomic data are collected for the purposes of forensic medicine or in civil, criminal and other legal proceedings, including parentage testing, the collection of biological samples, in vivo or post-mortem should be made only in accordance with domestic law consistent with the international law of human rights.

Prior, free, informed and express consent, without inducement by financial or other personal gain, should be obtained for the collection of human genetic data, human proteomic data or biological samples, whether through invasive or non-invasive procedures, and for their subsequent processing, use and storage, whether carried out by public or private institutions. Consent may be withdrawn by the person concerned unless such data are irretrievably unlinked to an identifiable person. Withdrawal of consent should entail neither a disadvantage nor a penalty for the person concerned.

Every effort should be made to ensure that human genetic data and human proteomic data are not used for purposes that discriminate in a way that is intended to infringe, or has the effect of infringing, human rights, fundamental freedoms or the human dignity of an individual, or for purposes that lead to the stigmatization of an individual, family, group or community.

REFERENCES

Aston, R. (1998) 'Genetic counseling must be non-directive', *British Medical Journal*, 317 (July): 82.

Awwad, R., Veach, P.M., Bartles, D.M. and Levroy, B.S. (2007) 'Culture and accumulation influences on Palestinian perceptions of prenatal genetic counseling', *Journal of Genetic Counseling*, 17 (Feb): 101–16.

Beauchamp, T.L. and Childress, J.F. (1989) *Principles of Biomedical Ethics*, 3rd ed. New York: Oxford University Press.

Bernhardt, B. (1997) 'Empirical evidence that genetic counseling is directive: Where do we go from here?', *American Journal of Human Genetics*, 60: 17–20.

Biesecker, B. and Marteau, T. (1999) 'The future of genetic counseling: An international perspective', *Nature Genetics*, 22: 133–7.

British Medical Association (BMA) (1998) *Human Genetics: Choice and Responsibility*. Oxford: Oxford University Press.

Clarke, A. (1991) 'Is Non-directive genetic counseling possible?', *The Lancet*, 338: 998–1001.

DeLozier-Blanchet, C.D. (2007) Genetic Counseling in <a href= 'http://family.jrank.org/pages/697/Genetic-Counseling.html'>Genetic Counseling</a>.

Dickens, B.M., Serour, G.I., Cook, R.J. and Qiu, R.Z. (2005) 'Sex selection: Treating different cases differently', *International Journal of Gynecology & Obstetrics*, 90 (2, Aug): 171–7.

El-Hazmi, M. (2004) 'Ethics of genetic counseling – basic concepts and relevance to Islamic communities', *Annals of Saudi Medicine Journal*, 24 (2, March–April): 84–92.

Elwyn, G., Gray, J. and Clarke, A. (2000) 'Shared decision making and non-directiveness in genetic counseling', *Journal of Medical Genetics*, 37 (2): 135–8.

Evans, M., Bergum, V., Bamforth, S., and MacPhail, S. (2004) 'Relational ethics and genetic counseling', *Nursing Ethics Journal*, 11 (5, Sep): 459–71.

Finnis, J. and Fisher, A. (1994) 'Theology and the four principles: A Roman Catholic view', in R. Gillon (ed.), *Principles of Health Care Ethics*. Chichester: John Wiley and Sons, pp. 31–44.

Holtzman, N.A. and Marteau, T.M. (2000) 'Will genetics revolutionize medicine?', *New England Journal of Medicine*, 343: 141–4.

Kaplan, J. (2002) 'Genomics and medicine: Hopes and challenges', *Nature*, 9 (11, June): 658–61.

Kaushal, P., Malaviya, D. and Roy, A. (2006) Ethical aspects in genetic counseling. Available at: http://www.ias.ac.in/currsci/nov25articles9.htm

Lea, D., Williams, J. and Donahue, M. (2005) 'Ethical issues in genetic testing', *Journal of Midwifery Women's Health*, 50 (3): 234–40.

Michie, S., Bron, F., Bobrow, M. and Marteau, T. (1997) 'Nondirectiveness in genetic counseling: An empirical study', *American Journal of Human Genetics*, 60: 40–7.

Muller, R.F. and Young, I.D. (eds.) (2001) 'Mathematical and population genetics', in *Erney's Elements of Medical Genetics*, 11th ed. Edinburgh: Churchill Livingstone, pp. 113–26.

Rentmeester, C. (2001) 'Value neutrality in genetic counseling: An unattained ideal', *Medicine, Health Care and Philosophy*, 41: 47–51.

Robinson, A. and Linden, M.G. (1993) *Clinical Genetics Handbook*, 2nd ed. Cambridge: Blackwell, p. 5.

Schneider, G.H. (2005) *Genetic Counseling Process: Encyclopedia of Genetics, Genomics, Proteomics and Bioinformatics*, Part 1 Genetics 1.6 Genetic Medicine and Clinical Genetics. Chichester: John Wiley and Sons.

Serour, G.I. (2000a) *Ethical Implications of Human Embryo Research*. Rabat, Morocco: ISESCO.

Serour, G.I. (2000b) 'Reproductive choice: A Muslim perspective', in J. Harris and S. Holm (eds.), *The Future of Human Reproduction*. Oxford: Clarendon Press, pp. 191–202.

Serour, G.I. (2006) 'Religious perspectives of ethical issues in art: Contemporary ethical dilemmas' in F. Shinfield and C. Sureau (eds.), *Assisted Reproduction*. Colchester: Informa Healthcare.

Serour, G.I. and Dickens, B.M. (2001) 'Assisted reproduction developments in the Islamic world', *International Journal of Gynecology & Obstetrics*, 74 (Aug): 187–93.

Serour, G.I., Aboulghar, M. and Mansour, R. (1995) 'Reproductive health care policies around the world: Bioethics in medically assisted conception in the Muslim world', *Journal of Assisted Reproduction and Genetics*, 12 (9): 559–65.

Thorpe, J.M., Weiss, S.R., Bowes, W.A., and Cfalo, R.C. (1995) 'Integrity, abortion and the pro-life perinatologist', *Hasting Center Report*, 25 (1): 27–8.

UNESCO (2004) International Declaration on Human Genetic Data. www.unesco.org/shs/ethics.SHS/BIO/04/

UNESCO (2006) Universal Declaration on Bioethics and Human Rights. www.unesco.org/shs/ethics/shs/EST/BIO/06/1

United States President's Commission (UNPC) (1983) President's Commission for the Study of Ethical Problems in Medicine and Biomedical and Behavioral Research. *Screening and Counseling of Genetic Conditions: A Report on the Ethical, Social, and Legal Implications of Genetic Screening, Counseling and Education Programs*. Washington, DC: US Government Printing Office, p. 122.

Valet, G., Murphy, R., Robinson, J., Tarnok, A. and Kriete, A. (2006) 'Cytomics – from cell states to predictive medicine', in A. Kriete and R. Eils (eds.), *Computational Systems Biology*. Amsterdam: Elsevier, pp. 363–81.

World Health Organization Advisory Group (WHO) (1985) *Community Approaches to the Control of Hereditary Diseases*. Geneva: WHO.

14

Regulating Reproductive Technologies

Don Chalmers

THE DEBATES ON REPRODUCTIVE TECHNOLOGY: THE PROTAGONISTS

Assisted reproductive technologies (ART) have enabled many people unable to conceive to have children. Following the publicity of the first IVF births at the end of the 1970s, official enquiries were conducted in many countries throughout the 1980s. ART is now an established procedure. A member of the International Committee for Monitoring Assisted Reproductive Technologies (ICMART) presented data from 56 countries to the European Society of Human Reproduction and Embryology (ESHRE) conference in 2006 that estimated that there are now some three million ART children world wide accounting for an estimated 2–3 percent of annual births (http://www.eurekalert.org/pub_releases/2006–06/esfh-tmb062106.php#). These procedures have also raised fundamental, social, ethical and legal questions about the essence of personhood and humanness (Cusine, 1988; McLean, 1989; Mason, 1990; Lee and Morgan, 2001).

The inevitable change in social and moral attitudes about aspects of ART starkly reflects Professor Somerville's tripartite timescales; fast-moving science time precedes the slower, deliberative public discussion in ethics time, which is followed by the gradual move to regulation in law time (Somerville, 2000). After the first successful IVF birth in 1978, ART science time moved noticeably and quickly into cryopreservation, donor gametes surrogacy, embryo experimentation, cloning, gamete intra-fallopian transfer (GIFT), intra-cytoplasmic sperm injection (ICSI), stem-cell technology and pre-implantation genetic diagnosis, all of which were the subject of scientific advances and heated debate. As science developed further, the debate shifted to ethical issues surrounding ART, particularly embryo research activities and stem cells and somatic cell nuclear transfer. These ethics time debates have been global, highly contentious and polarised with many of the organised churches involved. Feminist critiques and accounts of ART have been sustained and significant (Firestone, 1970; Arditti et al., 1984; Corea et al., 1985; Corea, 1986; Wikler,

1986; Stanworth, 1987). However, feminisms' (Davies, 1994; Morgan, 2001) responses to reproductive autonomy, exploitation and surrogacy and genetic privacy were diverse (Shultz, 1990; Rothenberg, 1996). A prolific literature has developed around the ethical, legal and social implications of each development in ART and medical ethics generally (Toulmin, 1982), which has enlivened debates in philosophy and ethics in particular.

The rise in ART programs was linked to the rapid decline in the number of children available for adoption in western countries. For example, there has been a drop of some 70 percent over 10 years from 9,798 in 1971–72 to 3,072 in 1982–83 in Australia (Szoke, 1999: 240). This decline in adoption in developed countries is attributable to social acceptance of single parenting supported by welfare payments and, second, an increase in terminations of pregnancy.

REGULATION OF ASSISTED REPRODUCTIVE TECHNOLOGY GENERALLY

The divisions in views about ART have resulted in a diversity of policies (Bleiklie et al., 2003) reflected in a diversity of regulatory schemes (Vayena et al., 2002; Gunning and Szoke, 2003). These diverse regulatory systems reflect fundamental cultural and social differences in approaches to the family and family law in different countries. Some of these differences are also 'constituted by our choosing or deciding to think a certain way' (Mackie, 1977: 30). These distinctions are pronounced in the regulatory framework for research involving human embryos. ART regulation can be broadly classified into licensing, statutory and guideline schemes.

Licensing schemes

The United Kingdom established the first carefully regulated licensing authority, the Human Fertilisation and Embryology Authority (HFEA) in 1990. The HFEA licenses IVF clinics and sets standards for reproductive procedures, gametes storage, success rate reporting and monitoring. New Zealand follows a similarly strict approach, with the Human Assisted Reproductive Technology Act 2004. In 2004, Canada introduced the Assisted Human Reproduction Act, which establishes a federal agency to regulate ART (s. 21). This Act prohibits a number of practices including payment for gamete donors (s. 7), surrogacy (s. 6), sex selection (s. 5(1) (e)) and the introduction of any inheritable change to the genome (s. 5(1) (f)). Three states (Victoria, South Australia and Western Australia) have statutory oversight bodies that govern the licensing of IVF facilities (Chalmers, 2002). Arguably, these countries have developed their regulatory schemes as part of their comprehensive legislative public health systems (Nelson, 2006).

In 1994, France introduced bioethics laws that also regulated ART through the National Council on Reproductive Medicine and Biology, which advises the Minister on the approval, renewal and withdrawal of licenses. Licensing may be a means of revenue raising or a means of limiting the numbers of ART practitioners, but ART licensing aims for quality assurance standards and monitoring.

Statutory schemes

In Germany, there is a form of regulation by reason of the prohibition on all embryo research. The German Embryo Protection [Embryonenschutzgesetz] Act 1990 introduced severe penalties for the transfer of more than three embryos to a woman (s. 1(3); egg donation or the creation of embryos for research purposes (s. 2); sex selection for non-medical reasons (s. 3); and posthumous IVF (s. 4(3)). These penalties limit the type of activities that can be undertaken in ART facilities and reflect German attitudes to research and a highly protective view of human embryos (Gottweis, 2002: 441). Specific offences include It is also an offence to allow eggs to develop past syngamy where those embryos will not be transferred to the woman (s. 2(2)).

Sweden was one of the first countries to introduce legislation, with the Act on fertilisation outside the body (SFS 1988:711). This 1988 Act introduced access rights to donor identifying information (s. 7). Spain also regulates ART and research by statute (*Law 14/*2006). Italy has moved from an unregulated to a regulated system. Originally, Italy had little regulation and offered ART to women beyond the biological age of procreation. In 2003, *Law 40* (Fenton, 2006) was introduced, limiting ART to heterosexual couples of childbearing age, excluding single parents and same sex couples (article 5). This Act also regulates research (article 13); restricts to three embryos the number of eggs transferred in one procedure (*Law 40*); regulates posthumous artificial insemination by donor (AID), pre-natal genetic diagnosis (article 13) and storage of embryos (article 14). The Minister of Health and the Higher Institute of Health authorise clinics under *Law 40*, article 11.

Guidelines

Clinical practice guidelines are an effective approach to regulation in many countries.

Guidelines have been able to set standards for the quality and development of procedures (Haagen et al., 2006). Both Japan and India regulate ART by non-statutory bodies and guidelines. The Japanese government has ART guidelines, developed by the National Society of Obstetricians and Gynecologists (Takeshita et al., 2003). India's ART services are regulated by the *National Guidelines for Accreditation, Supervision and Regulation of ART Clinics in India* (Allahbadia and Kaur, 2003). Many other Asian countries also regulate ART by 'ministerial regulation or guidelines issued by their medical councils or associations (Kumar in Gunning and Szoke, 2003: 40). Singapore, for example conducts ART within guidelines issued by its Ministry of Health that provide for licensing of ART centres, counselling of parties involved and donation of gametes.

The United States has relatively little regulation, generally organised at state level. It has been argued, however, that there is significant regulation of ART through the Federal Fertility Clinics Success Rates and Certification Act 1992, the enforcement of laboratory standards, the various NIH and FDA regulations, the Medicare and Medicaid Services and the Department of Health and Human Services policies (Adamson, 2005: 727). However, only five states, New Hampshire, Pennsylvania, Louisiana, New Mexico and South Dakota, have regulatory schemes dealing with embryos in the context of ART. Generally, US law does not require licensing or accreditation of ART clinics and there are few regulations on embryo research (Ouellette et al., 2005). The President's Council on Bioethics has described the regulatory landscape as 'patchwork, with authority divided among numerous sources of oversight' (2004: 75), and has proposed an increased level of regulation, including further studies on the long-term effects of ART on offspring.

Some Australian States and Territories (NSW, Queensland, Tasmania and the ACT) apply the guidelines developed by the National Health and Medical Research Council which have been adopted by the Reproductive Technology Accreditation Committee (RTAC) – the industry body that formally accredited ART clinics (Chalmers, 2002).

Effect of different regulatory regimes

The differences in regulatory regimes reveal concomitant differences in clinical practice. For example, in a comparative study between Germany and the United States, differences in drugs used and eggs retrieved were noted, with German practice favouring the use of small amounts of hypo-stimulating drugs with fewer eggs retrieved. German practice utilises ICSI far more and there is evidence of higher pregnancy success rates in the United States (in the year 2000, IVF pregnancy rates were 28.4 percent in Europe compared with 30.2 percent in the USA (see Society of ART and the American Society for Reproductive Medicine [Robertson, 2004]).

There are still differences in practice between countries in the number of embryos transferred. Some countries limit embryo transfer to two or three to reduce the possibility of multiple births, an ongoing problem. Some clinics now prefer the transfer of one embryo only. But restrictions on multiple egg transfer do not necessarily reflect the liberality of the regulatory regime. Belgium, which has a liberal regulatory regime, restricts transfer to one embryo (Jain et al., 2004).

COMMON THEMES IN THE REGULATION OF ART

The Australian state of Victoria produced the first ART legislation (Infertility (Medical Procedures) Act 1984) and, in the same year the widely cited *Report of the Committee of Enquiry into Human Fertilisation and Embryology*, 1984 (Cmnd 9314, the Warnock Report) was published (Lee and Morgan, 2001: ch. 1; 2). In the 1990s, the Royal Commission of Canada into Reproductive Technologies was one of the longest running enquiries. These are some of the many reports that resulted in ART regulation. Many of these reports made essentially consistent recommendations. Some general themes can be identified.

Consent

There is an accepted requirement for consent of the parties involved in ART procedures consistent with principles of medical consent generally (Spar, 2007). Where the donation of gametes is undertaken, the express consents of the recipient and donor parties are required and the availability of counselling is generally considered best practice. Counselling often aims to provide accurate factual information about the procedures and outcomes. Consent is the central principle in ART and the ESHRE Task Force Consent has highlighted it (Shenfield et al., 2002).

Use of donor gametes

Generally, donor gametes are permitted in western ART programs (Annas, 1980; Stepan, 1990; Bennett, 1993). However, many South American, Muslim and African countries have restrictions on donor gametes (Wardle, 2007). The ethical approach to ART in India presents a mixture of 'customary social practices within the community, conventional human rights, and sometimes religious law' (Chakravarty, 2001: 10). Clinical practice is varied. The use of donor sperm is not restricted in law, provided that there is full consent from the participating couple and the use of donor eggs is restricted to circumstances where there is little chance that the female can conceive without ART (Chakravarty, 2001).

AID is regulated by religious values and some Islamic decrees prohibit the procedure (Chakravarty, 2001). While there were fewer concerns about ART for married couples, the extension of ART to donor gametes generally involves some restrictions. For example the ART guidelines and professional standards in Japan allow access for married couples, but ban the use of donor gametes (Gunning, 2003; Takeshita et al., 2003). There are general restrictions on the sale of gametes as part of the general 'no commerce' rule in human tissue. Under s. 7 Assisted Human Reproduction Act 2004 in Canada, gametes may not be purchased, offered for purchase or advertised for purchase either by a donor or a person acting on behalf of the donor. Purchase or sale includes exchange for property or services. In New Zealand, the Human Assisted Reproductive Technology Act 2004 also prohibits the commercial supply of human embryos and human gametes (s. 13). However, there is evidence that many eggs are sourced from poorer, less-developed countries and the sums, described as reimbursement of out-of-pocket expenses may be small in developed countries but considerable and attractive sums in the sourced poorer countries (SEED, 2005).

Status of children

Generally, where donor gametes are involved, legislation clarifies the legal doubts about the status of children born as a result of ART procedures (Stepan, 1990; Lee and Morgan, 2001: ch. 9). Legislation generally establishes consent requirements and that the recipient couple, rather than the biological parent/s, are the legal parents of the child. In Australia, under the Family Law Act 1975 (Cth) (s 60H), a child born to a married woman as a result of an artificial conception procedure during the marriage is the child of the woman and her husband, provided the procedure was carried out with the consent of the couple and any person, including the spouse, who donated gametes (Chalmers, 2002). The effect is to establish an irrebuttable presumption of legitimacy. Legislation avoids technical legal concerns that the use of donor gametes could amount to adultery (*MacLennan v MacLennan,* 1958 SC 103; *People v Sorensen* 437 P 2d 495). The status of the child under Article 8 of the Italian law, *Law 40,* is that of a legitimate child or a child born of a cohabiting couple (as the ART is restricted to married or cohabiting couples). Where there is an illegal fertilisation, the spouse of the mother has paternal rights and obligations rather than the natural father (Boggio, 2005: 1155).

Access to programs

Many countries restrict access to ART to married or cohabiting established de facto heterosexual couples, including India, Italy, Japan and Singapore. The restrictions to married or de facto heterosexual couples supports the view of the traditional nuclear family This position reflects the view of the UK Warnock Report that 'as a general rule it is better for children to be born into a two-parent family... although we recognize that it is impossible to predict with any certainty how lasting such a relationship will be' (1984: para 2.11). In Italy, *Law 40,* Article 5 restricts access to heterosexual married or cohabiting couples, of a potentially fertile age, with both partners currently living. Also, the Patient Selection chapter of the *National Guidelines for Accreditation, Supervision and Regulation of ART Clinics in India* (ICMR, 2005) excludes single parents or homosexual couples from access to ART. In Japan, guidelines restrict the availability of ART to married couples (Takeshita et al., 2003: 261). There are similar restrictions in Austria, the Czech Republic, Denmark, France, Germany, Hungary, Iceland, Norway, Poland, the Slovak Republic, Switzerland, Portugal and for the most part, the Commonwealth of Australia (Schenker, 1997). This restrictive access regime extends in general to South American nations, Muslim nations and much of Africa (Wardle, 2007).

Access is also limited generally by reference to the definition of medical infertility: a 'couple' not being able to conceive after 1 year of unprotected intercourse or the inability to carry pregnancies to a live birth. This excludes infertility by reason of the person's social or sexual status. Similarly, in some jurisdictions, infertility has been legislatively provided as not being based on a specific age. A widely publicised case of a 66-year-old Romanian woman giving birth prompted the Romanian Parliament to prohibit infertility treatments on post-menopausal women, on the basis that the best interests of the child would not be served by elderly parental conceptions (Storrow, 2005).

The issue of restricted access to infertility services has been challenged in the courts, often on the basis of discrimination against single sex couples (*JM v QFG, GK and State of Queensland* [1997] QSC 206) or single parents (*Pearce v SA Health Commission* (1996) 66 SASR). The Canadian *Royal Commission on New Reproductive Technologies* (1994) also supported a more liberal approach and stated: 'excluding single women or lesbians from DI programs not only contravenes their equality rights it also puts their health at risk, by forcing them to resort to unsafe practices ... if a service is to be available, women should be treated equally, unless there is good evidence that the best interests of the child will suffer' (RCNRT, 1994: 457).

Donor anonymity

There are differences between regulatory schemes in respect of donor anonymity. Generally, a child reaching his/her majority is entitled to *non-identifying* information on any gamete donor. This is the case in India where the child has a right to access certain information about genetic parents, if the child is the result of donor gametes, and if such information relates to the child's health. The New Zealand *Human Assisted Reproductive Technology Act* 2004, s. 50 allows the offspring of donor conception access to both non-identifying and identifying information that is relevant for medical purposes. So too in India, it is the legal right of a child born through the use of donor gametes to see any available medical or genetic information about the donors that may be relevant to their health (ICMR, 2005: 70). Similarly, the Victorian *Infertility Treatment Act* 1995 (ss. 79–80; 72–75) provides a comprehensive scheme for access to information for the child. In Victoria, an adult person born as a result of 'donor treatment' may apply to the infertility treatment authority for identifying information subject to counselling requirements (ss. 79, 80(2)(a)).

The Victorian Act also establishes the principle that access to *identifying* information is subject to the consent of the donor and the child's parents (s. 72(3)). Similarly, in Canada, disclosure of information that could reasonably be expected to be used in the identification of the donor cannot be disclosed without the donor's written consent (s. 15(4)).

A common theme in ART reports was the standard of 'the best interests of the child'. This internationally accepted, but Delphic, principle requires that the best interests of the child, rather than the interests of the parents, guide decision makers. This principle has expression in the requirement to maintain records. Comparisons were often drawn with adoption where there has been a move towards greater access to information about the relinquishing parent or parents for the adopted child. Many adopted children were unable to trace their biological parents, which led to psychological distress, labelled 'genealogical bewilderment' (Triseliotis, 1973). By analogy, it was argued that similar precautions should be in place in ART to avoid any 'genealogical bewilderment' and protect children born of donated gametes.

There was evidence from Sweden that the introduction of the requirement to retain and provide information on the donor to the child led to a reduction in the number of willing sperm donors as well as a shift from young student donors to older married sperm donors (Burrell, 2005: 10–11). The supply of gametes must be balanced with the interests of the parents, donor and child rather than practical concerns.

The trend is towards the greater legislative recognition of an ART child's right to access to information, with the consent of the donors. Growing public discussion of human genetics, children's rights and the parallels between adoption and ART have been influential components in this trend. However, many countries, particularly the under-regulated US states allow donor anonymity. This can be a factor in reproductive tourism choices.

Keeping of information and records

Access by the parties, particularly the offspring, to records is important. Apart from access to records, the maintenance of quality health records on donors and parents is an important aspect of regulation for long-term follow-up studies. Many countries require that information and records of individuals involved in ART programs using donor gametes should be maintained on a central register. In India, clinics are required to 'maintain records in an appropriate pro forma to enable collation by a national body' (ICMR, 2005: 60). In the United Kingdom, HFEA lays down stringent requirements for registering data about IVF success rates, multiple births and birth defects. This provides a critical epidemiological research tool. In addition, ART children can use this registered data to access information about the donors. The provision of statistical information to the HFEA is a requirement for licensed ART clinics in the United Kingdom.

In Australia, data on reproductive technology pregnancies and births is provided to the National Perinatal Statistics Unit in Sydney. Similarly, Canadian information regulations (s. 14 Assisted Human Reproduction Act) require the donor to provide health reporting information. Donors are informed of the retention, use, provision to other persons and the destruction of the donated human reproductive material or *in vitro* embryo. Under s. 11 of *Law 40*, the Italian Higher Institute of Health is required to collect information on donors and recipients as well as other aspects of ART.

Codes of practice

Generally all ART clinics, even if they are required to be licensed, will be regulated by professional codes of practice. Generally, the law can only establish a regulatory frame-work and cannot define appropriate or effective details for regulating medical or laboratory practice. In ART, codes of practice and professional guidelines have provided the necessary practice guidelines. Broadly, these cover the following areas:

- A national body usually publishes the code of practice, for example, the *National Guidelines for Accreditation, Supervision and Regulation of ART Clinics in India* (Allahbadia and Kaur, 2003). In Australia, the National Health and Medical Research Council (NHMRC) published the *Ethical Guidelines on the use of Assisted Reproductive Technology in Clinical Practice and Research* in 2004.
- The clinic must follow prescribed clinical and professional standards that will cover all the aspects of treatment, counselling, patient care and record keeping. In Australia, for example the Fertility Society of Australia (FSA) has a code of practice for ART clinics (http://www.fsa.au.com/rtac/index.htm) and has a Reproductive Technology Accreditation Committee (RTAC) to assess and accredit clinics in conformity with its code on a 3-year accreditation cycle. RTAC also adopted the NHMRC guidelines in their accreditation requirements.
- Written consents should be obtained from the parties involved. If donated gametes are involved, consent must also be obtained from the donors and spouses.
- The clinic should maintain records including the signed consent forms, and the outcome of the procedures (pregnancies, births, miscarriages).
- Counselling should be provided.
- Certain procedures may be excluded, such as cloning, mixing of gametes, and research on embryos; or sex selection except for medical reasons to avoid a genetic disease.

The development of codes of clinical practice and standards is a significant aspect of the regulation of ART clinics. In more regulated areas, standards of clinical practice may be imposed by the regulatory authority (Storrow, 2007). Guidelines are not a uniform approach. The regulatory range spans the spectrum from an essentially free market approach (Robertson, 2004) to systems employing rigid licensing legislation. In both cases, professional self-regulation and codes of practice play an important role. There are ongoing discussions in academic literature and between policymakers about the cost and propriety of the rigid legislative model of legislation, particularly in the international free market (Johnson and Petersen, 2008).

Sex selection: Pre-implantation genetic diagnosis

Some ART programs also experience criticisms over pre-implantation genetic diagnosis (PGD) (Wertz and Fletcher, 1989; Scott, 2005) and the potential of this procedure for sex selection or eugenics. The term 'eugenics' is often referred to in debates on PGD (Galton, 1908: 312) and is generally restricted to use for medical diagnoses. Canada prohibits sex selection except where prevention, diagnosis or treatment of sex-linked diseases or disorders is concerned. This is also the position in India under their *National Guidelines*, Germany under the Embryo Protection Act, Italy under *Law 40* and New Zealand under the Human Assisted Reproductive Technology Act. Deliberate selection of desired genetic characteristics, physical attributes or the like are not possible at this stage of development, much less the use of techniques to genetically enhance human characteristics (Marteau et al., 1995). However, PGD raises serious ethical issues, where sex selection is offered in some ART programs in some Asian countries (Chappell, 1997).

Litigation in ART

Litigation in ART has increased and many of the cases have attracted media attention. Problems involving the disposition of embryos have resulted in litigation where parents separate, change their minds about transfer or one or both die. Two American cases illustrate the problems arising from situations. In *York v Jones* 717 F Supp 42 (ed) Va 1989 and *Davis v Davis* 842 SW 2d 588 (Tenn) 1992 disputes were heard, respectively, about refusals to transfer a frozen embryo to another institution or to transfer embryos to a divorced spouse. The state Supreme Courts considered arguments on contract, constitutional rights, and authority over pre-embryos and procreational autonomy. Some legislation, for example the Infertility Treatment Act 1995 (Vic s. 53) and the Human Reproductive Technology Act 1991 (WA s. 26) deal with such disposition problems. The potential inheritance rights of embryos (Atherton, 1986) were considered in the *Estate of the Late K* J (Chalmers, 1996). In that case a right of inheritance for the embryo was recognised.

Human rights have often been argued in litigation in the ART. In *R v HFEA ex parte Blood* (1997) 2 *Fam* 401, the UK Court of Appeal upheld the refusal by the HFEA to refuse Blood's request to be inseminated with her dead husband's sperm. Eventually the European Court of Justice allowed Blood not only to export the sperm but also to have a posthumous insemination in a less restrictive country in Europe. The prohibition on posthumous transfer of embryos has been upheld by the French Court of Cassation in the *Pires Case* (McGregor and Dreifuss-Metter, 2007: 122). In *Evans v UK* (2008) 46 EHRR 34, the woman claimed the reproductive autonomy to have an embryo transferred to her despite the refusal of the partner (Thornton, 2008: 330). The European Court of Human Rights Grand Chamber upheld a refusal to the appellant's application for implantation of the embryo. This refusal was held not to constitute a violation of any of the rights under the

European Convention of Human Rights. The Evans case raised genuine legal and ethical disputes about the extent of the reproductive autonomy (Priaulx, 2008).

SURROGACY

Surrogacy generated something of a 'moral panic' (Freeman, 1989) after the publicity on the American 'Baby M' case (1987, 13 *Fam L. Rep* (US) 22, 2001) and the English 'Baby Cotton' case (1985, FLR 846; Cotton and Winn, 1985). The early consensus viewed surrogate motherhood as unacceptable. Some countries moved to ban surrogacy. In Germany, for example the practice is effectively prohibited under their legislation (s. 1 *Embryo Protection Act*). Surrogacy is not permitted in Italy (article 12(6) of *Law 40* punishable with imprisonment and a fine of up to one million euros).

Gradually, a distinction has been drawn between altruistic surrogacy and commercial-for-fee surrogacy. Most countries declare that commercial surrogacy is not acceptable. This is the position in the United Kingdom under their Surrogacy Act, 1985. Commercial surrogacy is also banned in some US states.

Similar legislation has been introduced in Australia, despite the fact that few couples are involved in surrogate births. Canada has followed the no-commercialisation view and in s. 6 of the Assisted Human Reproduction Act 2004 the payment or acceptance of consideration to or by a female for surrogacy is prohibited, as is advertising or arranging surrogacy. All states and territories in Australia prohibit commercial surrogacy (Queensland, Surrogacy Parenthood Act 1988 and Tasmania, the Surrogacy Contracts Act 1993). In New Zealand, a surrogacy arrangement is not enforceable by or against any person (Human Assisted Reproductive Technology Act 2004, s. 14). Other countries have a disapproving but tolerant attitude. Israel allows state-controlled surrogacy. The Approving Committee is empowered to authorise surrogacy, according to the legitimacy of the need and religious dictates (Schenker, 2003).

In some US states, surrogacy services are not only available but the contracts involved are enforceable. In California and in some other states, surrogacy contracts are enforceable (Spar, 2005: 531–4). The Australian Capital Territory Substitute Parent Agreements Act 1994 allows limited altruistic surrogacy but only about 10-12 procedures per year are carried out in the Australian Capital Territory (ACT). Surrogacy disputes have occasionally been litigated in the courts, which have invariably referred to the best interests of the child test and have generally awarded custody to the biological mother (*Re Evelyn* 23 Fam LR 53; *Re W (Minors) (Surrogacy)* [1991] 1 FLR 385; *Re Q (Parental Order)* [1996] 1 FLR 369).

ART AS A GLOBAL BUSINESS ENTERPRISE

ART is an international mega-business involving not only the provision of ART services but also the development of drugs and devices used in the programs and the sale of gametes and surrogacy services. There is a global industry supplying fertility services (Carbone and Gottheim, 2005). ART remains a service that is generally delivered in the private medical 'business' sector (Brazier, 1999) and many companies have entered the ART market. Regulation of the ART industry includes the practical hurdle of internationalisation of trade and services. Denmark's largest sperm bank exports internationally and the United States is one of the world's leading suppliers of both cryo-preserved eggs and sperm (Heng, 2007), with Cryo-Eggs International Inc. and Donor Egg Bank both providing services. This egg market has been partly caused by policy in such countries as the United Kingdom, which allows for reimbursement of expenses only to donors rather than a negotiated sale price. The tendency for women to delay reproductive decisions until later in life also contributes to the shortage in egg donors. Egg shortage is one of many reasons for cross-border reproductive tourism.

Reproductive tourism

Because ART laws are not integrated international forum shopping, a 'tourisme juridique et procreatique' (Revillard, 1985) has become a common feature of the international ART market (Knoppers and LeBris, 1991) and has been defined as 'the movement of citizens to another state or jurisdiction to obtain specific types of medical assistance in reproduction that they cannot receive at home' (Pennings, 2004). Reproductive tourism can arise where treatment is prohibited in one country but is ethically acceptable in another. Examples include: availability of sex selection for non-medical reasons; denial of access on the basis of marital status or sexual orientation; restrictions on particular techniques, such as cryo-preservation; long waiting lists for gametes; or high costs (Spar, 2005). 'Procreational tourists' now have the ability to avoid national prohibitions by crossing a border into a less or non-regulated state (Storrow, 2005). Reproductive tourism does not always require the tourist to go to the less regulated jurisdiction but may involve a third party coming into a country to assist in the fertility treatment (Pennings, 2002: 337).

Sweden provides an illustration of reproductive tourism. Regulations abolished anonymity of donors with the immediate effect of reducing the availability of gametes, creating a market for reproductive tourists in Denmark (Pennings, 2001). Belgium has one of the least regulated ART regimes and many ART clinics and has a tourist flow, particularly from the restricted jurisdiction of Germany. In fact, a 1999 study showed that 30 percent of patients in ART programs in Belgium were from abroad (Pennings, 2004). In a similar vein, surrogacy is outlawed in most Australian states but not in ACT and this has attracted surrogacy tourists to that jurisdiction. Reproductive tourism extends across the globe, from Californian surrogacy arrangements (Spar, 2005) to French couples obtaining egg donations from fertility clinics in Spain, circumventing French law (McGregor and Dreifuss-Metter, 2007); and to Japanese individuals and couples traveling to access PGD, oocyte donation, and surrogate parenting (Takeshita et al., 2003).

There have been suggestions that the reproductive tourism business cannot and should not be regulated, but left as a trade issue. The internet makes gametes accessible to people who would find access restricted in their country of residence (Chung, 2006). There is a substantial international trade in gametes and strict regulations will probably never work; gametes are regularly frozen and transported between countries. Some countries, like Mexico, have been able to restrict imported semen (Guevara, 2004). The European Union, however, has favoured a restriction in market forces for gametes and has issued a Directive providing that tissues and cells should only be obtained on a non-profit basis with reimbursement for the donor's reasonable expenses; advertising is also restricted under the Directive (EC, 2004).

RESEARCH ON HUMAN EMBRYOS

Research on embryos remains controversial, particularly because of philosophic doubts about the moral status of the embryo (Kennedy, 1985; Lockwood, 1985; Andrews 1986). A failure to differentiate between acceptable research procedures in ART and unacceptable experimental procedures also fuelled debate (Lee and Morgan, 2001: ch. 3). The cloning, somatic cell nuclear transfer (SCNT) and embryonic stem-cell debates revived discussion on the biological and moral definition of a human embryo (Melton et al., 2004).

There is uniform agreement that reproductive cloning is unacceptable internationally but there are substantial differences in stem-cell research regulation around the world, with differing legal and ethical approaches (Isasi et al., 2004: 626). Some countries have maintained their ban on research, such as Austria, Ireland, Canada, Philippines and Germany. Interestingly, the German Embryo Protection [*Embryonenschutzgesetz*] Act 1990) bans embryo research (Gottweis, 2002), although in 2002, the German Parliament allowed embryonic stem-cell research but only on imported lines (Heinemann and Honnefelder, 2002).

Countries that have approved stem-cell research have generally introduced licensing of the research but only on surplus ART embryos (Halliday, 2004: 69). This is the regulatory model in the United Kingdom, Finland, Greece, Israel, the Netherlands, Singapore, South Korea, Australia, and the American States of California and New Jersey (Schenker, 2003; Isasi et al., 2004). In Sweden, the Act Concerning Measures for Research or Treatment Involving Fertilised Human Ova (SFS 1991:115) allows research to be performed within 14 days of fertilisation with the consent of the donors and also prohibits genetic modification of the embryo.

Some other countries, such as China, Spain and Japan have followed the surplus embryos approach but have preferred to use guidelines. Embryonic stem-cell research in Japan is covered by guidelines and the researcher may only use ES cells for basic research and cannot use them in ART (Takeshita et al., 2003). *Law 40* in Italy bans scientific research on embryos, whereas the previous Dulbecco Commission had recommended stem-cell research on surplus embryos. There are stark differences between the regulated countries including Canada and those states 'under regulation' in the USA (Deckha, 2008).

Internationally, legislation and guidelines include broadly similar provisions dealing with embryo research, establishing a generally 'restrictive tilt' (Brownsword, 2004) from the features that only surplus ART embryos may be used; the consent of the parties creating the embryos is required; and the research must be approved by an Ethics Review Committee. Importantly, there is a restrictive tilt because generally the purposes of the research are limited and require careful justification. No country allows undefined research on embryos. The United Kingdom, for example has research purposes for understanding the causes of infertility; miscarriages, genital diseases, contraception and chromosome abnormalities; understanding the development of embryos; increasing knowledge of serious disease; and the treatment of those diseases. The United States has restrictions on the use of public funds for embryo research. Finally, there are some countries that have not introduced specific legislation or guidelines.

SOME CONCLUDING REMARKS

Some concluding remarks can be made in returning to Professor Somerville's tripartite classification of science time, ethics time and law time (Somerville, 2000).

Science time

The science will be refined and continue to develop. A few examples can be given. With the drive towards personalised medicine, greater use of PGD and genetic screening in ART programs may be predicted. However, these scientific advances will be linked inevitably to the discarding of certain embryos with all the attendant ethical concerns (Scott, 2005). Also in the molecular genetics area Yamanaka and colleagues in Japan published the results of induced pluripotent stem cells (iPS) from human fibroblasts (Takahashi and Yamanaka, 2006; Takahashi et al., 2007) without the need either for excess embryos or enucleated human or animal eggs. The leading Wisconsin team (Thomson et al., 1998; Yu. et al., 2007) simultaneously published similar results. This procedure removes much of the moral objection to the use of excess embryos for the production of stem cells. Third, the evidence so far is that there are no major problems arising from ART. However, few countries require long-term data to be kept to enable research on subtle problems that may affect ART children, particularly in adult life (Editorial, 2008).

Ethics time

Apart from PGD and embryo research, significant ethical debate continues in relation to 'reproductive freedom' and 'decisional privacy' (Laing and Oderberg, 2005; Priaulx, 2008) where the question is posed, what is the ethical, juridical, social or factual basis for legislatures to interfere with the freedom of parent(s) to make their own procreative decisions? Some argued that the law should not interfere with reproductive freedom, recognising that the state does generally regulate adoption and other aspects of family law. Liberal democratic societies value the freedom of citizens to act as they choose, provided that their actions do not cause harm to others (Dworkin, 1977; Warnock, 1987; Charlesworth, 1993). If the prospective parent(s) are competent and informed and decide to use ART, their autonomous and private choice should be respected even though others may not agree with that choice.

Second, there are real differences between the requirements for donor anonymity in different countries, and this promotes reproductive tourism. However, more profound research issues arise in relation to the relationships created within ART programs, particularly through the use of donor gametes. The UK Centre for Family Research is conducting longitudinal research on the families involved in gamete donation and surrogacy, addressing questions as to whether disclosure of donor and gamete involvement affects their relationships (http://www.sps.cam.ac.uk/CFR/research/ntf.php). However, this important research is at an early stage. ART centers should provide data to enable effective longitudinal research on ART and outcomes.

Law time

Regulation remains a contested area. As ART has become an established procedure that provides reproductive choices, the question has been asked whether ART should be regulated at all (see Harris and Holm, 1998; Skene, 1999; Jackson, 2002; Savulescu, 2002). The question has been posed as to whether 'the intrusion into the private choices of individuals seeking to have a family can no longer be justified' (HoC, 2005). This fundamental debate is ongoing (Laing and Oderberg, 2005). However, the issue is less about whether to regulate than about what type and level of regulation should be implemented.

Regulation can be justified on a number of grounds. First, regulation provides protection for the parties involved, particularly the children, ensuring proper consent, counselling and record keeping for the offspring. Second, regulation assures the quality of services, including monitoring and audit, the publication of Codes of Practice and licensing of ART providers. Third, regulation can protect the clinicians and scientists involved from potential malpractice complaints as they can refer to compliance to the relevant regulatory standards. Fourth, regulation can address safety issues by specifying procedures that may be undertaken, restricting egg transfer to women of particular ages or specifying procedures to avoid multiple births. Fifth, ART being a worldwide multi-billion dollar industry, regulation can contribute to ensuring proper market forces. Inappropriate market forces work outside basic ethics: surrogacy advertising and sales of gametes that may distort the market and cause exploitation of vulnerable individuals. Finally, regulation can balance public concerns about aspects of ART procedures with the freedom of science and personal autonomy (Deech, 2006; English, 2006).

AN INTERNATIONAL APPROACH

Regulation of ART has international dimensions. The Warnock Committee (1984, para.1.8) recognised '[t] here is a case for an international approach. This approach will be best formulated, however, when individual countries have formed their own views, and are ready to pool knowledge and experience'.

Harmonisation, uniformity or common standards

It is difficult to imagine that the vast diversity of ART regulation around the world could be harmoniously integrated into a unified regulatory system. However, some academics have suggested that it may be possible to harmonise by recognising common international norms, standards and meta-values, such as the inherent dignity of the human person, the security of human genetic material, the quality of services and the inalienability of the sanctity of the human person (Knoppers and LeBris, 1991). Baroness Deech, former Head of the HFEA (United Kingdom), proposed five ethical principles. These were: human dignity; worth and autonomy; the welfare of the potential child; safety of procedures used; respect for the status of the embryo; and saving lives through the use of the procedures (Deech, 2006). However, it is important that harmonisation does not mean pressure for regulations to move from the restrictive to the permissive (McGleenan, 1999). Equally importantly, these norms, standards and meta-values must be expressed to respect and accommodate the cultural and social conditions of individual societies (Fletcher, 1989).

ACKNOWLEDGEMENT

Acknowledgements for support to the Australian Research Council Discovery Grant DP0559760 and Deb Bowring and Lucy DeVries.

REFERENCES

Adamson, D. (2005) 'Regulation of assisted reproductive technologies in the United States', *Family Law Quarterly*, 39: 727–44.

Allahbadia, G. and Kaur, K. (2003) 'Accreditation, supervision, and regulation of ART clinics in India – A distant dream?', *Journal of Assisted Reproduction and Genetics*, 20 (7): 276–80.

Andrews, L. (1986) 'The legal status of the embryo', *Loyola Law Review*, 32 (2): 357–408.

Annas, G. (1980) 'Fathers anonymous: Beyond the best interests of the sperm donor', *Family Law Quarterly*, 14 (1): 1–13.

Arditti, R., Klein, R. and Minden, S. (1984) *Test Tube Women – What Future for Motherhood*. London: Pandora Press.

Atherton, R. (1986) 'Artificially conceived children and inheritance in New South Wales', *Australian Law Journal*, 60: 374–86.

Bennett, B. (1993) 'Gamete donation, reproductive technology and the law', *Law in Context*, 11: 41–57.

Bleiklie, I., Goggin, M. and Rothmayr, C. (2003) *Comparative Biomedical Policy: Governing Assisted Reproductive Technologies*. London: Routledge.

Boggio, A. (2005) 'Italy enacts new law on medically assisted reproduction', *Human Reproduction*, 20:1153–7.

Brazier, M. (1999) 'Regulating the reproduction business', *Medical Law Review*, 7: 166–93.

Brownsword, R. (2004) 'Regulating human genetics: New dilemmas for a new millennium', *Medical Law Review*, 12: 14–39.

Burrell, R. (2005) *Assisted Reproduction in the Nordic Countries – a Comparative Study of Policies and Regulation*. Norden: Nordic Committee on Bioethics.

Carbone, J. and Gottheim, P. (2005) 'Markets, subsidies, regulation and trust: Building ethical understandings into the market for fertility services', *Journal of Gender, Race and Justice*, 9 (3): 509–47.

Chakravarty, B. N. (2001) 'Legislation and regulations regarding the practice of assisted reproduction in India', *Journal of Assisted Reproduction and Genetics*, 18 (1): 10–14.

Chalmers, D. (1996) 'Inheritance rights of embryos', *University of Tasmania Law Review*, 15 (1): 131–5.

Chalmers, D. (2002) 'Professional self-regulation and guidelines in ART', *Journal of Law and Medicine*, 9 (4): 414–28.

Chappell, T. (1997) 'Sex selection for non-medical reasons', *Journal of Medical Ethics*, 23: 120–1.

Charlesworth, M. (1993) *Bioethics in a Liberal Society*. Cambridge: Cambridge University Press.

Chung, L. (2006) 'Free trade in human reproductive cells: A solution to procreative tourism and the unregulated Internet', *Minnesota Journal of International Law*, 15: 263–96.

Corea, G. (1986) *The Mother Machine: Reproductive Technologies from Artificial Insemination to Artificial Wombs*. New York: Harper and Row.

Corea, G., Klein, R.D., Hanmer, J., Holmes, H.B., Hoskins, B., Kishwar, M. et al. (eds) (1985) *Man-made Women: How New Reproductive Technologies Affect Women*. London: Hutchinson.

Cotton, K. and Winn, D. (1985) *Baby Cotton: For Love and Money*. London: Dorling Kindersley.

Cusine, D. (1988) *New Reproductive Techniques: A Legal Perspective*. Aldershot: Gower Press.

Davies, M. (1994) *Asking the Law Question*. Sydney: Law Book Co., pp. 172–204.

Deckha, M. (2008) 'The gendered politics of embryonic stem cell research in the USA and Canada: An American overlap and Canadian disconnect', *Medical Law Review*, 16: 52–84.

Deech, R. (2006) 'Playing God: Who should regulate embryo research?' *Brooklyn Journal of International Law*, 32 (2): 321–41.

Dworkin, R. (1977) *Taking Rights Seriously*. London: Duckworth.

Editorial (2008) 'Editorial', *Nature*, 454 (Jul): 253.

English, V. (2006) 'Autonomy versus protection – Who benefits from the regulation of IVF?', *Human Reproduction*, 21 (12): 3044–9.

European Commission (EC) (2004) Directive 2004/23/EC of the European Parliament and of the Council on *Setting Standards of Quality and Safety for the Donation, Procurement, Testing, Processing, Preservation, Storage and Distribution of Human Tissues and Cells*. Brussels: European Commission.

Fenton, R.A. (2006) 'Catholic doctrine versus women's rights: The new Italian law on assisted reproduction', *Medical Law Review*, 14: 73–107.

Firestone, S. (1970) *The Dialect of Sex*. New York: William Murrow.

Fletcher, J. (1989) 'Where in the world are we going with the new genetics?', *Journal of Contemporary Health Law and Policy*, 5: 33–52.

Freeman, M. (1989) 'Is surrogacy exploitative?', in S. McLean, *Legal Issues in Human Reproduction*. Aldershot: Gower Press.

Galton, F. (1908) *Memories of my Life*. London: Methuen, p. 312.

Gottweis, H. (2002) 'Stem cell policies in the United States and in Germany: Between bioethics and regulation', *Policy Studies Journal*, 30 (4): 444–69.

Guevara, M. (2004) 'Fertile markets', *Latin Trade*, 12 (5): 16.

Gunning, J. (2003) 'Regulation of assisted reproductive technology: A case study of Japan', *Medicine and Law*, 22 (4): 751–61.

Gunning, J. and Szoke, H. (2003) *The Regulation of Assisted Reproductive Technology*. Aldershot: Ashgate.

Haagen, E.C., Hermens, R.P.M.G., Nelen, W.L.D.M., Braat, D.D.M., Grol, R.P.T.M. and Kremer, J.A.M. (2006) 'Subfertility guidelines in Europe: Quantity and quality of intrauterine insemination guidelines', *Human Reproduction*, 21 (8): 2013–109.

Halliday, S. (2004) 'A comparative approach to the regulation of human embryonic stem cell research in Europe', *Medical Law Review*, 12 (1): 40–69.

Harris, J. and Holm, S. (1998) *Rights and Reproductive Choice: The Future of Human Reproduction*. Oxford: Clarendon Press, ch. 5.

Heinemann, T. and Honnefelder, L. (2002) 'Principles of ethical decision making regarding embryonic stem cell research in Germany', *Bioethics*, 16 (6): 530–43.

Heng, B. (2007) 'Legal and ethical issues in the international transaction of donor sperm and eggs', *Journal of Assisted Reproduction and Genetics*, 24 (4): 107–9.

House of Commons (HoC) (2005) Science and Technology Committee Report. *Inquiry into Human Reproductive Technologies and the Law*. London: The Stationery Office, Annex A, p. 6.

Indian Council of Medical Research (ICMR) (2005) Ministry of Health and Family Welfare *National Guidelines for Accreditation, Supervision & Regulation of ART Clinics in India*. New Delhi 110029: National Academy of Medical Sciences.

Isasi, R., Knoppers, B., Singer, P. and Daar, A. (2004) 'Legal and ethical approaches to stem cell and cloning research: A comparative analysis of policies in Latin America, Asia and Africa', *Journal of Law, Medicine and Ethics*, 32 (4): 626–40.

Jackson, E. (2002) 'Conception and the irrelevance of the welfare principle', *Modern Law Review*, 65: 176–203.

Jain, T., Missmer, S.A. and Hornstein, M.D. (2004) 'Trends in embryo-transfer practice and in outcomes of the use of assisted reproductive technology in the United States', *New England Journal of Medicine*, 350 (16): 1639–45.

Johnson, M. and Petersen, K. (2008) 'Public interest or public meddling? Towards an objective framework for the regulation of assisted reproduction technologies', *Human Reproduction*, 23 (3): 716–28.

Kennedy, I. (1985) 'The moral status of the embryo', *King's Counsel*, 37: 21–9

Knoppers, B. and LeBris, S. (1991) 'Recent advances in medically assisted conception: Legal, ethical and social issues', *American Journal of Law and Medicine*, 17 (4): 329–61.

Lag (1991:115) om åtgärder i forsknings- eller behandlingssyfte med befruktade ägg från människa.

Laing, J. and Oderberg, D. (2005) 'Artificial reproduction, the "Welfare Principle", and the common good', *Medical Law Review*, 13: 328–56.

Lee, R. and Morgan, D. (2001) *Human Fertilisation and Embryology: Regulating the Reproductive Revolution*. London: Blackstone Press.

Lockwood, M. (1985) 'The Warnock Report: A philosophical appraisal', in M. Lockwood, (ed), *Moral Dilemmas in Modern Medicine*. Oxford: Oxford University Press.

McGleenan, T. (1999) 'Reproductive technology and the slippery slope argument: A message in blood', in E. Hildt and S. Graumann (eds), *Genetics and Human Reproduction*. Aldershot: Ashgate.

McGregor, J. and Dreifuss-Metter, F. (2007) 'France and the United States: The legal and ethical differences in assisted reproductive technology', *Medicine and Law*, 26 (1): 117–35.

Mackie, L. (1977) *Ethics*. Harmondsworth: Penguin.

McLean, S. (ed.) (1989) *Legal Issues in Human Reproduction*. Aldershot: Gower Press.

Marteau, T., Michie, S., Drake, H. and Bobrow, M. (1995) 'Public attitudes towards the selection of desirable characteristics in children', *Journal of Medical Genetics*, 32 (10): 796–8.

Mason, J.K. (1990) *Medico-legal Aspects of Reproduction and Parenthood*. Aldershot: Dartmouth Publishing.

Melton, D., Daley, G. and Jennings, C. (2004) 'Altered nuclear transfer in stem cell research – A flawed proposal', *New England Journal of Medicine*, 351 (27): 2792.

Morgan, D. (2001) 'Feminisms' accounts of reproductive technology', in *Issues in Medical Law and Ethics*. London: Cavendish Publishing.

Morris, E. (2008) 'Reproductive tourism and the role of the European Union', *Chicago Journal of International Law*, 8 (2): 701–13.

Nelson, E. (2006) 'Comparative perspectives in the regulation of assisted reproductive technologies in the United Kingdom and Canada', *Alberta Law Review*, 43 (1): 1023–48.

Ouellette, A., Caplan, A., Carroll, K., Fossett, J.W., Bjanadottir, D., Shickle, D. et al. (2005) 'Lessons across the pond: Assisted reproductive technology in the United Kingdom and the United States', *American Journal of Law and Medicine*, 31 (1): 419–46.

Pennings, G. (2001) 'The reduction of sperm donor candidates due to the abolition of the anonymity rule: Analysis of an argument', *Journal of Assisted Reproduction and Genetics*, 18 (11): 617–22.

Pennings, G. (2002) 'Reproductive tourism as moral pluralism in motion', *Journal of Medical Ethics*, 28 (6): 337–41.

Pennings, G. (2004) 'Legal harmonisation and reproductive tourism in Europe', *Human Reproduction*, 19 (12): 2689–94.

President's Council on Bioethics (US) (2004) *Reproduction and Responsibility: The Regulation of New Biotechnologies*. Washington, DC: PCB.

Priaulx, N. (2008) 'Rethinking progenitive conflict: Why reproductive autonomy matters', *Medical Law Review*, 16: 169–200.

Revillard, M-L. (1985) 'Fecondation in vitro et congelation d'embryons', in J Stepan, (ed), *Artificial Procreation, Genetics and the Law*. Lausanne: Lausanne Colloquium.

Robertson, J. (2004) 'Reproductive technology in Germany and the United States: An essay in comparative law and bioethics', *Columbia Journal of Transnational Law*, 43 (1): 189–203.

Rothenberg, K. (1996) 'Feminism law and bioethics', *Kennedy Institute of Ethics Journal*, 6 (1): 69–84.

Royal Commission on New Reproductive Technologies (RCNRT) (1994) *Proceed with Care: Final Report of the Royal Commission on New Reproductive Technologies.* Ottawa: RCNRT.

Savulescu, J. (2002) 'Deaf lesbians, "Designer Disability" and the future of medicine', *BMJ*, 32: 771–3.

Schenker, J. (1997) 'Assisted reproduction practice in Europe: Legal and ethical aspects', *Human Reproduction Update*, 3 (2): 173–84.

Schenker, J. (2003) 'Legal aspects of ART practice in Israel', *Journal of Assisted Reproduction and Genetics*, 20 (7): 250–9.

Scott, R. (2005) 'The uncertain scope of reproductive autonomy in preimplantation genetic diagnosis and selective abortion', *Medical Law Review*, 13: 291–327.

SEED (2005) *A Report on the Human Fertilisation & Embryology Authority's review of sperm, egg and embryo donation (SEED) in the United Kingdom.* London: HFEA.

Shenfield, F., Pennings, G., Sureau, C., Cohen, J., Devroey, P. and Tarlatzis, B. (2002) 'ESHRE Task Force on Ethics and Law, Taskforce 3: Gamete and embryo donation', *Human Reproduction*, 17 (5): 1407–08.

Shultz, M.M. (1990) 'Reproductive technology and intent-based parenthood: An opportunity for gender neutrality', *Wisconsin Law Review*, 1990 (2): 297–398.

Skene, L. (1999) 'Why legislate on assisted reproduction?', in I. Freckelton and K. Petersen (eds), *Controversies in Health Law.* Leichhardt, NSW: Federation Press.

Somerville, M. (2000) *The Ethical Canary: Science, Society and the Human Spirit.* Toronto: Viking.

Spar, D. (2005) 'Reproductive tourism and the regulatory map', *New England Journal of Medicine*, 352 (6): 531–4.

Spar, D. (2007) 'The egg trade – Making sense of the market for human oocytes', *New England Journal of Medicine*, 356 (13): 1289–91.

Stanworth, M. (1987) *Reproductive Technologies: Gender, Motherhood and Medicine.* Cambridge: Polity Press.

Stepan, J. (1990) *International Survey Laws on Assisted Procreation* (Publications of the Swiss Institute of Comparative Law). Zurich: Schulthess Polygraphischer Verlag.

Storrow, R. (2005) 'Quests for conception: Fertility tourists, globalization and feminist legal theory', *Hastings Law Journal*, 57 (2): 295–330.

Storrow, R. (2007) 'The bioethics of prospective parenthood: In pursuit of the proper standards for gatekeeping in fertility clinics', *Cardozo Law Review*, 28 (5): 2283–320.

Szoke, H. (1999) 'Regulation of assisted reproductive technology?', in I. Freckelton and K. Petersen (eds), *Controversies in Health Law.* Leichhardt, NSW: Federation Press.

SFS (1988:711) Lag om befruktning utanför kroppen Act on conception outside the body.

Takahashi, K. and Yamanaka, S. (2006) 'Induction of pluripotent stem cells from mouse embryonic and adult fibroblast cultures by defined factors', *Cell*, 126: 663–76. (See also Goldman, B. (2008) 'Embryonic stem cells', *Nature Reports Stem Cells*, published online 1 May 2008.)

Takahashi, K., Tanabe, K., Ohnuki, M., Narita, M., Ichisaka, T., Tomoda, K. et al. (2007) 'Induction of pluripotent stem cells from adult human fibroblasts by defined factors', *Cell*, 131: 861–72.

Takeshita, N., Hanaoka, K., Shibui, Y., Jinnai, H., Abe, Y. and Kubo, H. (2003) 'Regulating assisted reproductive technologies in Japan', *Journal of Assisted Reproduction and Genetics*, 20 (7): 260–4.

Thomson, J.A., Itskovitz-Eldor, J., Shapiro, S.S., Waknitz, M.A., Swiergiel, J.J., Marshall, V.S. et al. (1998) 'Embryonic stem cell lines derived from human blastocysts', *Science* 282: 1145–7.

Thornton, R. (2008) 'European Court of Human Rights: Consent to IVF treatment', *International Journal of Constitutional Law*, 6 (2): 317–30.

Toulmin, S. (1982) 'How medicine saved the life of ethics', *Perspectives in Biology and Medicine*, 25 (4): 736–50.

Triseliotis, J. (1973) *In Search of Origins: The Experience of Adopted People.* London: Routledge and Kegan Paul.

Trounson, A. and Gillam, K. (1999) 'What does cloning offer human medicine?', *Today's Life Science*, 11 (2): 12–14.

Vayena, E., Rowe, P.J. and Griffin, P.D. (eds) (2002) *Medical, Ethical and Social Aspects of Assisted Reproduction: Current Practices and Controversies in Assisted Reproduction,* Report of a WHO meeting. Geneva: World Health Organisation.

Wardle, L. (2007) 'Global perspective on procreation and parentage by assisted reproduction', *Capital University Law Review*, 35 (2): 413–63.

Warnock, M. (1987) 'Morality and the law: Some programmes', *Cambrian Law Review*, 18: 14–24.

Warnock Report (1984) *Report of the Committee of Inquiry into Human Fertilisation and Embryology.* London: Department of Health & Social Security (DHSS).

Wertz, D.C. and Fletcher, J.C. (1989) 'Fatal knowledge? Prenatal diagnosis and sex selection', *Hastings Center Report*, 19 (3): 21–7.

Wikler, N. (1986) 'Societies' response to the new reproductive technologies: The feminist perspectives', *Southern California Law Review*, 59 (5): 1043–57.

Yu, J., Vodyanik, M.A., Smuga-Otto, K., Antosiewicz-Bourget, J., Frane, J.L., Tian, S. et al. (2007) 'Induced pluripotent stem cell lines derived from human somatic cells', *Science*, 318: 1917–20.

15

Reprogenetics

Andrea Kalfoglou

INTRODUCTION

Reproductive genetic technologies fall at the intersection between the development of assisted reproductive technologies and advances in our understanding of human genetics. Genetic testing can now influence reproductive decisions prior to conception, prior to the transfer of embryos into a woman's uterus, and during pregnancy. The original goal of most of this testing was to give couples at risk of passing a serious genetic disease on to their children more reproductive choices, but use has expanded to include screening for risk of adult-onset diseases and the ability to select for socially desirable traits, such as sex.

Use and further development of these technologies have raised a host of ethical questions about safety, the moral status of embryos and fetuses, the appropriate use of these technologies, how the use of technology might change family relationships and women's reproductive experiences, the appropriate role of the state in regulating the use of these technologies, and effects on the future of society. This chapter will briefly review each of these technologies (describing their current and potential uses), discuss the ethical dilemmas that have emerged with advances in the science, and touch on how various countries have attempted to regulate their use.

Reproductive genetic technologies currently available revolve around various ways that genetic tests can provide information that can then be used to make reproductive decisions. These currently available testing technologies and their uses will be discussed first, followed by a discussion of emerging technologies and their possible uses.

REPRODUCTIVE GENETIC TESTING

Reproductive genetic testing refers to those genetic tests and procedures that are used to provide prospective parents with information about their chances of having a child with a specific genetic disorder or characteristic in a current or future pregnancy. It includes: (1) carrier testing; (2) sperm sorting for sex selection; (3) preimplantation genetic diagnosis (PGD) and preimplantation genetic screening (PGS); and (4) prenatal testing.

Carrier testing

Carrier testing is genetic testing to determine whether an individual carries a copy of an altered gene for a dominant or recessive condition. 'Carriers' of these altered genes are usually not affected by the disease. Carrier testing is done because of a family history of a genetic disorder or because a certain racial or ethnic background puts that individual at a higher risk of 'carrying' certain genetic alterations. In the future, population screening for an array of genetic diseases that can be passed on to children could become technologically and financially feasible.

Examples of autosomal recessive disorders that are more frequent in certain populations for which carrier testing can be conducted include cystic fibrosis in Caucasians of Northern European descent; sickle cell disease in African Americans; beta-thalassemia in Asians and individuals of Mediterranean descent; and Tay-Sachs, Canavan and Gaucher disease (among others) in people of Ashkenazi Jewish descent. In autosomal recessive disorders, a child must have two copies of the altered gene (one from each parent) to be affected. When both parents are carriers of one of these autosomal recessive disorders, there is a 1 in 4, or 25 percent risk for each child, of inheriting the alteration from both parents, and thus being affected by the disease or condition.

Autosomal dominant diseases can be passed on to a child when only one parent is a carrier of the disease. An example of an autosomal dominant disease is Huntington's disease. Half of all children born to a carrier of Huntington's disease will be affected by the disease. Some autosomal dominant diseases, like hemophilia and Duchenne Muscular Dystrophy, are linked to the X, or female, chromosome. Women with this genetic alteration are usually unaffected by the disease but have a 50 percent chance of passing it on if they have a son. Daughters have a 50 percent chance of being carriers of the disease.

Carrier testing for genetic disorders is becoming more of a routine part of prenatal care for specific racial/ethnic groups in certain parts of the world. For instance, the American College of Obstetricians and Gynecologists (ACOG) now recommends that in the US, all pregnant women or women planning a pregnancy be given the opportunity to have cystic fibrosis carrier testing (ACOG Committee Opinion, 2005). Cystic fibrosis screening is also routine in Northern European countries where the carrier frequency is much higher than in other parts of the world. Carrier testing for beta-thalassemia, also called 'Mediterranean anemia' or 'Cooley's disease' is routine on the island of Cyprus and other areas in the Mediterranean. Ashkenazi Jewish young adults in the US and Israel are encouraged to have carrier screening for a panel of diseases. Rabbis may even refuse to marry couples who have not been screened. In addition, many sperm and egg donors may be routinely screened for carrier status of certain diseases.

It is up to parents to decide what to do with the information from their carrier test results. People who know they are at risk of conceiving a child with a genetic disease may choose child-free living, gamete or embryo donation, preimplantation genetic diagnosis to avoid affected embryos, or adoption, as alternative paths to parenthood. They can also take their chances with sexual conception because for autosomal recessive diseases, 75 percent of children conceived will be disease free and for dominant diseases, 50 to 75 percent of children conceived will be disease free. Prenatal testing can be conducted on the fetus to give the couple the choice of terminating the pregnancy if the fetus is affected by the disease.

Sperm sorting for sex selection

Sex selection has been attempted for thousands of years. While the effectiveness of most of these technologies is questionable, Microsort™ is an experimental sperm-sorting technique with clinical research showing it is better than chance at selecting sex, particularly when the couple desires a girl (Karabinus, 2009). The sorting process is based on identifying the molecular weight of the sperm because sperm with an X chromosome are heavier. Once the sperm are sorted, the woman is inseminated with the selected sperm, or this sperm is used with IVF to increase the chances of creating embryos of only one sex. If the couple wants additional testing (regardless of whether sperm sorting was used), pre-implantation genetic analysis (described below) can be conducted to confirm the sex of each embryo.

Couples can use Microsort™ for sex selection when they are trying to avoid an X-linked genetic disease or simply because they want to select the sex of their child. This technology, when used with artificial insemination, has limited effectiveness because pregnancy only occurs about 15 percent of the time with each reproductive cycle (Karabinus, 2009). Combining sperm sorting with IVF or IVF/PGD increases the chances of pregnancy (Karabinus, 2009), but also increases the cost of the procedure. Microsort™ is currently under review by the Food and Drug Administration (FDA). A decision is expected in 2010.

Preimplantation genetic diagnosis (PGD)

Preimplantation genetic diagnosis (PGD) is genetic testing on embryos produced through IVF. One or two cells are removed from the embryo when it is at approximately an 8-cell stage (before the cells have begun to differentiate), and these cells are tested for the presence of a particular gene and/or for chromosomal abnormalities. Based on the test results, embryo(s) are selected for transfer into the woman's uterus. For example, parents may want to select only embryos with an absence of a particular genetic disease or chromosomal abnormality, those of a specific sex, or those that have other characteristics like a genetic alteration for deafness (Driscoll, 2002). Thousands of couples carrying chromosomal rearrangements and those at risk of transmitting a single-gene disorder to their offspring have used PGD to avoid having an affected child (Verlinsky et al., 2004).

Carriers of autosomal dominant diseases or couples who both carry a recessive gene for a disease can now use PGD to avoid becoming pregnant with an affected child. PGD genetic laboratories initially focused on genetic diseases that affected children and were terminal or carried significant disease burden; however, laboratories are now testing for genes that increase susceptibility to adult-onset diseases such as breast cancer (Sagi et al., 2009) and early-onset Alzheimer's disease (Verlinsky et al., 2002).

Additionally, PGD can been used to examine the chromosomes of an embryo. This testing may be used for sex selection in order to avoid X-linked diseases or simply because the couple desires a child of a particular sex. Chromosomal analysis of embryos is also useful to avoid genetic disease when there are parental translocations within the embryos' chromosomes, and when the family has a history of chromosomal abnormalities.

Some patients already undergoing IVF are having their embryos screened to weed out aneuploidy embryos (embryos that have more or less than the normal 23 chromosomal pairs) (Munné et al., 1999). This is especially true for women who are over 35 years of age, who have repeat miscarriages, or who have repeat IVF failures. When PGD is used for this purpose, it is referred to as preimplantation genetic screening (PGS).

The goal of PGS is to avoid transferring aneuploidy embryos, because they will usually result in a miscarriage or will simply fail to implant in the woman's uterus. In rarer instances, the child may be born with a chromosomal abnormality such as Down or Klinefelter's syndrome. PGS during infertility treatment is now the number one reason that embryos are biopsied and genetically tested. In theory, this screening should increase IVF success rates, but there is little to no evidence to support this claim. Professional associations including the American Society for Reproductive Medicine (ASRM, 2008) and the British Fertility Society (Anderson and Pickering, 2008) issued practice statements in 2008 that the use of PGS to improve infertility treatment outcomes has not been proven effective in any populations and should be considered experimental.

Finally, PGD (and prenatal genetic testing) can be used to determine whether an embryo or fetus is an HLA tissue-type match to donate stem cells to a sibling who needs a transplant. For example, children suffering with Fanconi Anemia have a 20 percent chance of survival with a stem-cell transplant from an unrelated donor; however, their chances for survival increase to 80 percent when the stem cells come from a matched sibling (Verlinsky et al., 2001). PGD can greatly improve the odds of establishing a pregnancy with an HLA-matched child. Sometimes HLA matching is all that is important to the couple, but other times, the biopsied cell is examined to ensure that it is both a match and is free of the genetic disease that affects the existing child.

Prenatal genetic testing (or prenatal genetic diagnosis)

Genetic testing of fetal cells obtained through procedures such as amniocentesis and chorionic villus sampling (CVS) is collectively referred to as prenatal genetic testing. Prenatal genetic testing frequently follows prenatal screening. Prenatal screening is conducted by evaluating the proteins in a pregnant woman's blood. This screening has become routine in many developed countries, particularly for women over 35 years of age. Protein levels in the woman's blood are used to assess fetal risk for chromosomal and other abnormalities (such as anencephaly and spina bifida), but the test does not provide a definitive diagnosis of an abnormality. In fact, the screening frequently results in a false positive result (Graves et al., 2002). These false positive screening results can cause anxiety for pregnant women and lead to additional, sometimes unnecessary, invasive prenatal genetic testing (Marteau et al., 1992). Prenatal genetic test results are definitive, but, because they are invasive, they carry a small risk of miscarriage (Graves et al., 2002). If prenatal testing confirms that the fetus is affected by a genetic condition, the pregnant woman has two options: terminate the pregnancy or prepare for the birth of a special-needs child.

Currently, standard prenatal genetic testing evaluates the chromosomes of the fetus to look for aneuploidy (an abnormal number of chromosomes). If a couple knows they are at risk for a specific genetic condition like sickle cell disease, the sample can be evaluated for specific genetic diseases. Prenatal genetic testing can also be used to determine paternity and the sex of the fetus.

FUTURISTIC REPRODUCTIVE GENETIC TECHNOLOGIES

Reproductive genetic technologies develop at a breakneck pace. While the technologies discussed below are not clinically available as of 2010, they all are either about to begin clinical trials, have been demonstrated to be feasible in humans in the laboratory, or have already been used successfully in animals.

Karyomapping

Karyomapping is the ability to conduct an array of tests for as many as 15,000 genetic diseases on a single cell biopsied from an embryo. This analysis could provide information about chromosomal and single-gene anomalies. A research team from the US and Britain plan to start clinical trials using this testing technique in the winter of 2009 (Harton et al., 2009). This technology could potentially be used for carrier testing or genetic testing of a fetus. Test results are most reliable when samples of both parents are also available. Along similar lines, laboratories are developing gene chips that could provide carrier screening for hundreds of genetic diseases at a much lower price than traditional carrier testing. Eventually, population screening for carrier status could become the norm.

Artificial gametes

Artificial gametes have been produced in animals from embryonic stem cells and have been used to create offspring (Nayernia et al., 2006). As of 2010, human gametes have been derived from embryonic stem cells, but have not demonstrated an ability to be fertilized or produce offspring (Zhou et al., 2010). Bioethicists have called for more public consultation about the ethical issues on the use of this technology (Mathews et al., 2009). This technology could be used to help infertile men have children, enable two women or two men (with the help of a surrogate womb) to combine their genetic material to create a child, or create embryos for research purposes.

Genetic modification

Genetic modification of human DNA within gametes or embryos has not been attempted as of 2010, but animals, including primates, have had genes introduced at the embryonic stage that have then been expressed in the animal (Chan et al., 2001). Theoretically genetic modification could take place before conception by modifying all the gametes (sperm or eggs) in an adult similar to a 'vaccination' or by modifying individual sperm or ovum in vitro (Green, 2007). Alternatively, embryos could be created through IVF and then altered at a very early stage in development to either correct a disease causing gene or change genes that are responsible for certain phenotypic characteristics. Genetic modification could be used for a wide range of purposes. For instance, the modification might make the future child more resistant to malaria or HIV infection, or 'fix' a gene that would cause hemophilia, or lead to an increased risk of cancer or diabetes. It could make muscles heal faster or grow larger, or alter something about how the brain develops (Gosden, 1999; Silver, 1997; Stock, 2002).

One technique designed to improve success rates for IVF involves taking all or part of the cytoplasm of an oocyte or egg from a fertile woman and combining it with the nucleus of an infertile woman's oocyte. The theory is that conception is more likely if there is younger cytoplasm available. Over 30 children were born around the world using this technique before the FDA stopped the research. These children have the mitochondrial DNA from the cytoplasm donor, and DNA from both parents (Barritt et al., 2001). Research using this technique continued overseas under the direction of US researchers in China (Zhang et al., 2003); however, the Chinese Ministry of Health banned the procedure days after the research was announced (Kaisernetwork.org, 2003). In 2008, scientists from Newcastle University in north-east England announced that they had successfully created embryos using genetic material from three people, but did not transfer these embryos into a woman's uterus (CBS News, 2008).

Reproductive cloning

Reproductive cloning, or creating a child who has the same DNA as another person, is theoretically possible in at least two different ways. First, an embryo created through IVF could be forced to split in half, essentially creating identical twins. Both embryos could be transferred to the woman's uterus at the same time, or one could be transferred while the other is frozen, thawed, and transferred at a later time. Thus, it is possible to have identical twins that are not the same age.

Second, the DNA from somatic cells, or cells that come from the body and have the full set of 46 chromosomes, might be inserted into an oocyte once the nucleus from the oocyte has been removed. The oocyte is then chemically or electrically stimulated to start cell division. The 'embryo' could then be transferred into a woman's uterus. This process has successfully produced animal clones including mice, sheep, rabbits, and even cats (Edwards et al., 2003). Most of the time, these animal embryo clones do not survive. Those that have survived have aged more quickly than normal (Wilmut and Highfield, 2006). While there have been claims of successful human cloning, none have been substantiated.

ETHICAL ISSUES WITH REPRODUCTIVE GENETIC TECHNOLOGIES

Many ethical issues related to the use of reproductive genetic technologies cut across the various technologies. For instance, concerns about the safety and effectiveness of the technology are universal. Concerns about turning children into commodities apply to sex selection, PGD, and genetic modification. In the following sections, the issues have been divided into five broad categories: destruction of embryos and fetuses; avoiding harm to children and mothers; stigma and discrimination; reproductive freedom; and avoiding harm to society.

Destruction of embryos and fetuses

Throughout the world, there is debate about the point at which life begins. For those who believe that life begins when sperm and ovum merge, many of the reproductive genetic technologies that necessitate the destruction of embryos or fetuses may be repugnant and considered unethical. Selective termination of an affected fetus ends the life of that fetus. Additionally, PGD is always used to select one embryo over another. Those embryos diagnosed as being aneuploidy or having a disease causing genetic alteration are usually allowed to die. The PGD biopsy process also results in a certain amount of embryo loss. Some have suggested that embryos that are affected by genetic disease, or simply any embryos leftover from the IVF process ought to be 'adopted' by other couples rather than being used for research or allowed to die. In fact, the US federal government spent tax dollars to develop embryo 'adoption' programs under the Bush administration.

Italy has passed fairly stringent rules regarding the use of IVF designed to ensure that embryos are not destroyed during the process. For instance, there is a limit to the number of oocytes that may be fertilized, and all the resulting embryos have to be transferred into the woman's uterus. Freezing or destroying embryos is not permitted.

Avoiding harm to children and mothers

Harm comes in many forms—these technologies could lead to physical harm if they are not safe or are used to intentionally create disabled children, to financial harm if they are not effective, and to psychological harm even if there was good intent.

Safety and effectiveness

Most reproductive genetic technologies currently in use appear to be reasonably safe; however, there are no or very limited long-term data on the offspring of children created through these technologies. Most of the literature on the safety of techniques such as PGD is reassuring; however, scientists and ethicists have called for national registries of children born after PGD to enable researchers to study large populations of children over time (Baruch et al., 2005). The European Society for Human Reproduction and Endocrinology (ESHRE) has begun a PGD registry. Data collected in 2007 should be available in 2010. There is a lack of data on the error rate of PGD (Baruch et al., 2005) and the accuracy of PGS is under considerable debate (ASRM, 2008).

There are short-term risks for any woman who undergoes oocyte stimulation and retrieval, including hyperstimulation syndrome, which can be a serious complication. Little is known about the long-term effects, particularly of multiple stimulation cycles, on a woman's long-term health (Institute of Medicine, 2007). There is some concern that hormonal stimulation could increase the risk for breast, ovarian, and uterine cancer, but the available data indicate that the increased risk may come from infertility, not exposure to drugs used to stimulate the ovaries (Institute of Medicine, 2007). Experts have called for more and better data including the creation of registries of women exposed to the oocyte retrieval process (Institute of Medicine, 2007).

Any new technology that involves the manipulation of the embryo or the DNA within an embryo intended for use in creating a child will be highly experimental. Research ethics demands that these techniques be proven safe and effective in animal models before they are used with humans. Unfortunately, in the unregulated environment of reproductive genetics in many countries, history has shown that new techniques move very quickly from the laboratory into clinical use without the kind of experimental process that is required for the development of new drugs and devices.

Commodification of children

We may reach the point where it is technologically possible to genetically design our children. Will this ability of one generation to alter the composition of the next change the relationship between parent and child? Will the ability to create children based on our desires or prejudices result in us viewing children as commodities? Will children feel even more compelled to live up to their parents' expectations?

Some ethicists argue that parents have always desired to give their children the best possible advantages. Selecting embryos for certain traits through PGD or genetic modification, according to this view, is no different than private school or musical or athletic training (Silver, 1997). Others argue that there is something fundamentally different about making genetic changes in a child (Murray, 1996). If genetic modification were to become widespread, would we be tempted to redefine parenthood to include choosing particular characteristics in our children as opposed to unconditionally accepting children as a gift? (Kass, 2003)

Still others have argued that children ought to have a 'right to an open future' (Davis, 2001). In other words, they should not have to grow up with the expectations from others that they will enjoy and excel at basketball just because they were engineered to be tall. Are these unproven concerns about potential psychological harm coming to children enough to prevent individuals or couples from reproducing using sex selection, PGD for trait selection, genetic modification, or cloning techniques?

Certain countries, including Germany, Norway, Austria, and Switzerland, as well as a number of US states, have passed laws banning the use of any type of selection based on genetics, including the use of PGD to avoid genetic disease.

Savior siblings

Embryos can be selected through PGD to intentionally create a child who is an HLA match for a sick or dying sibling. Some have argued that this is an unethical use of the technology because a child is created as a means to an end rather than because the child him/herself is desired.

Examined more closely, there are rarely pure motives involved in the conception of a child (Murray, 1996). Children are unintentionally conceived, conceived in an attempt to save troubled relationships, conceived because the parents have a need to receive love, and the list goes on. There is no evidence that children conceived to help save their dying sibling are treated like commodities or are discarded after they have served their purpose.

One concern with the availability of this technology has been that embryos are being subjected to a biopsy procedure for the benefit of someone else, not the benefit of the potential child. In the UK, for example, the Human Fertilisation and Embryonic Authority (HFEA) limited this use of PGD to cases where the embryos were also being screened to avoid a genetic disease. It was only after years of experience with PGD and evidence that the biopsy procedure did not appear to cause harm to the resulting child that the HFEA began allowing PGD for tissue-type matching alone.

One of the factors that limits the ethical concerns about using PGD for HLA matching is that the needed stem cells are collected through the discarded umbilical cord – it is a completely non-invasive procedure. What if the tissue or body part needed to save the sick sibling required an invasive procedure such as the removal of a kidney? Wolf et al. consider this possibility and recommend that the child should not be subjected to more than minimal risk until he/she is able to give informed consent for such procedures. They also suggest guidelines for this use of PGD designed to protect the resulting child (Wolf et al., 2003).

Intentional disability

A number of years ago, a lesbian couple who were both deaf sought out a sperm donor who had five generations of deafness in his family in the hopes that their child would also be born deaf (Driscoll, 2002). For the two women, being deaf was not a disability but a culture they wanted to share with their son. PGD providers have also been asked to participate in helping to select embryos with genetic 'differences' that some might perceive to be disabilities.

Is it ethical to help a couple create a child that has a trait that is a disability or at least a disadvantage in today's society? Should it be up to parents to make this kind of decision about the kind of child they want to have? Based on philosophical arguments put forth by Derek Parfit, John Robertson argues that parents ought to be able to make these decisions because otherwise, they might opt to not have children (Robertson, 1994). In order to put limitations on the choices parents can make about their future children, Robertson argues, one must be able to prove that the child would be better off had he never been born (Robertson, 1994). This argument, referred to as 'the nonidentity problem,' says that the parents do not wrong the child, because if the circumstances were different, the same exact child would not exist. There are many elaborate arguments against the nonidentity problem that claim that parents have a moral obligation not to intentionally cause harm to their children (Roberts and Wasserman, 2009) and that liberty and rights language is not the appropriate framework for issues related to parent–child relationships (Murray, 1996).

Stigma and discrimination

Some of the risks of reproductive genetic testing are psychological. An individual who knows he/she is a carrier of a genetic disorder may feel stigmatized, and some have even experienced discrimination. Within the Orthodox Jewish community, where there may be arranged marriages, being a carrier of a genetic disease or having a genetic disease in the family may reduce an individual's marriage prospects. In other cases, individuals fear discrimination based on their genetics when seeking employment or various types of insurance coverage.

Research with individuals who have genetic illnesses reveals that many have been denied insurance coverage because of their condition, or they fear the loss of their coverage (Billings et al., 1992; Kass et al., 2007). There was so much concern about the potential for genetic discrimination that the US recently passed the Genetic Information Nondiscrimination Act of 2008. Although it does not have the force of law, the UNESCO's 1997 Universal Declaration on the Human Genome and Human Rights 'enshrines the principles of confidentiality of genetic information associated with identifiable persons and the right to "just reparation" for damage sustained as a direct result of intervention affecting an individual's genome' (UNESCO, 2001).

The development of full genome analysis could increase stigma, particularly if the testing is done on an embryo or fetus. Some genetics professional associations in the US, UK, and Australia have recommended that genetic testing only be performed on children when there is a clear benefit for the child (ASHG/ACMG, 1995; McLean, 1995; Otlowski, 2004). If multiplex or full genome analysis were done before a child is even born, a potential wealth of information that currently is very complex and not well understood would be available about that child. While it might be in that child's best interest for his/her parents to stress a nutritional diet and exercise to avoid the risk of heart disease or diabetes, how might the parents' reproductive choices or behavior towards that child change if they were told their son or daughter might have a predisposition towards violence or homosexuality? China has recently begun genetic testing of children to make early decisions about how to develop their specific genetic traits (Chang, 2009).

Reproductive freedom

Eugenic movements in the US and Germany in the mid-twentieth century began as public health campaigns designed to encourage the birth of healthy and strong citizens and limit the birth of the infirm. The introduction of new reproductive genetic technologies has many of the same goals; however, in most parts of the world, they are not being used by governments for social engineering. Instead, it is up to individual couples to decide whether and how to use these technologies under the label of reproductive freedom. Some have questioned whether, in a social world with social and economic pressures, there really can be true autonomous decision making around reproduction (President's Council on Bioethics, 2003).

Ashkenazi Jewish young adults in the US and Israel are expected by their peers and even rabbis to receive carrier testing prior to marriage. The same is true for inhabitants of the island of Cyprus where beta-thalassemia is common. Carrier testing and prenatal screening during pregnancy could easily become routine without women's consent in the name of standards of care or efficiency. Women would only be informed if there was a positive test result. If this happens, will women still be able to make free choices, including the choice to decline genetic testing? Or might women be compelled in some way to use genetic testing? Could insurance coverage policies intentionally or inadvertently coerce people into testing and aborting affected fetuses? Will social and economic pressures create an environment where people feel obligated to avoid the birth of children with special needs?

Avoiding harm to society

Below is a discussion of issues about how reproductive genetic technology might alter society demographically, socially, and politically.

Playing God or messing with Mother Nature

Some have called reproductive genetic testing the next step in preventive medicine. Genes for dread diseases can be weeded out at the source, leading to healthier individuals and improved public health. Is manipulating the reproductive process just the next step in preventive medicine, or are we tampering in an area that should be reserved for God or Mother Nature?

One way of describing this concern is that humans, by seeking to alter human genetics, are being awfully arrogant in thinking that the choices we make will lead to better humans. There is a growing movement called transhumanism that believes we ought to use technology to manipulate human evolution and push it to the next level. Those wary of this view see this as hubris. Michael Sandel puts it this way: 'To believe that our talents and powers are wholly our own doing is to misunderstand our place in creation, to confuse our role with God's' (Sandel, 2007: 85).

Unpredictable or negative population changes

While concerns about widespread population changes are hypothetical at this point, the ability to select for sex has been available for nearly 20 years through prenatal testing and ultrasound. Whether sex selection is performed using prenatal testing and selective abortion, PGD, Microsort™, or a combination of these technologies, many of the ethical issues are the same. From a societies' perspective, there is concern that a preference for one sex over another could lead to sex-ratio imbalances. Some see this as potentially disastrous (Fukuyama, 2003). A sex-ratio imbalance is a potential threat to a stable society, so a number of countries, including India, have made the use of reproductive genetic technologies for the purpose of sex selection illegal. Other countries, such as Germany, believe that sex selection is part of a slippery slope towards eugenic uses of reproductive technology and have also made it illegal.

Some bioethicists and feminist scholars argue that to permit sex selection is to tacitly or overtly support discrimination against women (Davis, 2001) With nearly one million missing women worldwide (George, 2006), there is some merit to this argument. On the other hand, is permitting the use of sex selection technologies discriminatory in countries where daughters are valued just as much as sons? Is it just a logical extension of reproductive rights or a slippery slope towards the commodification of children?

Another concern with making sperm sorting available is that, when it does not work, parents will either abort the fetus or treat the resulting child in such a way that it is psychologically harmed. Yet, the problem is not with the technology. This same couple has the ability to conceive naturally and abort the fetus (at least in many countries) if it is not the desired sex. Those clinics offering sperm sorting may, in fact, prevent the abortion of fetuses that are the undesired sex or the birth of unwanted children.

Additionally, widespread increased use of these technologies could have unforeseen consequences on a population. There are concerns that we might inadvertently select (or alter) our genes in ways that make us genetically weaker. One theory around sickle cell disease is that the alteration survived because it conveyed protection against malaria. Could the elimination of a genetic disease make a group or population more susceptible to something else like an infectious disease?

Loss of compassion/investment for those with disabilities

Although prenatal diagnosis has been routinely offered for nearly 20 years to women at risk of having a baby affected with a disability or disease, some are concerned that as the number of conditions for which testing is available increases, the ability to eliminate potential offspring with genetic conditions through abortion or preimplantation genetic diagnosis may contribute to making society less tolerant of disability. Some have argued that prenatal and preimplantation diagnosis is sometimes driven by economic concerns because the US fails to provide affordable and accessible healthcare to everyone. Thus, prenatal diagnosis and subsequent abortion of affected fetuses or selection of embryos through PGD can save money by preventing the birth of disabled and costly children.

If we are able to select who enters the world based on their DNA, some are concerned that we will lose our compassion for those who are different. There is something uniquely human about confronting and overcoming adversity, including disease/disability. Some have argued that it is through experiencing and observing suffering that we learn compassion for others. How might the loss of genetic diversity adversely affect our society? Might we lose something of our humanity if we do not have people in our midst that struggle with genetic disease?

Justice

Reproductive genetic testing can be very expensive. It is unclear whether, and under what circumstances, health insurance or national health programs will cover testing. For the immediate future, access to this technology may be limited to those with financial means. Could limited access result in a society where only poor families are confronted with the burden of genetic disease? Will differences in access eventually lead to two distinct classes of people – those who have had access to reproductive genetic selection or enhancement and those who have not?

Others are concerned that use of this technology could undermine research and treatment of people living with certain diseases and conditions. For instance, we may see PGD as primary prevention of genetic diseases and stop investing in ways of treating or curing these diseases. Additionally, reductions in the numbers of people living with a particular condition may reduce the political power and advocacy ability of those living with these conditions. Ultimately, could those who were born prior to 'prevention' through genetic testing or manipulation be neglected by society? (Buchanan et al., 2000).

CONCLUSION

Reproductive genetic technologies will likely have a dramatic effect on the way women and couples have children in the future. People who 'carry' genetic alterations that can cause genetic disease in their children will likely be aware of this risk prior to having children. In fact, much of this testing may be done in childhood or even prior to birth and become part of an individual's medical record. Those at risk will have options available to them to have healthy children, but there may be increased pressure to produce disease-free children. Genetic disease that develops during the reproductive process will likely be caught during prenatal screening, and, if current trends continue, most of these affected pregnancies will be terminated. While this may lead to the dramatic reduction in genetic illness, it could have profound affects on those living with disease and disability if society chooses to refocus how resources are allocated. It may also limit the reproductive freedom of couples who would prefer not to use these technologies.

If these technologies are used to alter the characteristics of children, there could be subtle but profound effects on how parents and society view children. If children are more a product of our desires rather than a begotten gift from God, our expectations for our children may change. These changes will be most dramatic if there is disparity in access to these technologies. These disparities might exist within countries, but will more likely exacerbate existing health disparities between developed and developing countries.

While these technologies offer great promise for eliminating disease and suffering, there are also great risks. Governments and the people they govern need to be involved in policy decisions that shape how these technologies are used so that technology contributes to rather than diminishes human flourishing.

REFERENCES

American College of Obstetricians and Gynecologists (ACOG) (2005) Committee Opinion. Number 325, December 2005. 'Update on carrier screening for cystic fibrosis', *Obstetrics & Gynecology*, 106 (6): 1465–8.

American Society for Reproductive Medicine (ASRM) (2008) 'Preimplantation genetic testing: A Practice Committee opinion', *Fertility and Sterility*, 90 (suppl 5): ss. 136–43.

American Society of Human Genetics Board of Directors/American College of Medical Genetics Board of Directors (ASHG/ACMG) (1995) 'Points to consider: Ethical, legal, and psychosocial implications of genetic testing in children and adolescents', *American Journal of Human Genetics*, 57 (5): 1233–41.

Anderson, R. and Pickering, S. (2008) 'The current status of preimplantation genetic screening: British Fertility Society Policy and Practice Guidelines', *Human Fertility*, 11 (2): 71–5.

Barritt, J., Brenner, C., Malter, H. and Cohen, J. (2001) 'Mitochondria in human offspring derived from ooplasmic transplantation', *Human Reproduction*, 16 (3): 513–6.

Baruch, S., Adamson, G., Cohen, J., Gibbons, W., Hughes, M., Kuliev, A. et al. (2005) 'Genetic testing of embryos: A critical need for data', *Reproductive BioMedicine Online*, 11 (6): 667–70.

Billings, P., Kohn, M., de Cuevas, M., Beckwith, J., Alper, J. and Natowicz, M. (1992) 'Discrimination as a consequence of genetic testing', *American Journal of Human Genetics*, 50 (3): 476–82.

Buchanan, A.E., Brock, D.W., Daniels, N. and Wikler, D. (2000) *From Chance to Choice: Genetics and Justice*. New York: Cambridge University Press.

CBS News (2008) http://cbs5.com/health/cloning.science.human.2.646223.html, accessed 12 August 2009.

Chan, A., Chong, K., Martinovich, C., Simerly, C. and Schatten, G. (2001) 'Transgenic monkeys produced by retroviral gene transfer into mature oocytes', *Science*, 291 (5502): 309–12.

Chang, E. (2009) 'In China, DNA tests on kids ID genetic gifts, careers', CNN, 5 August http://www.cnn.com/2009/WORLD/asiapcf/08/03/china.dna.children.ability/index.html?section=cnn_latest, accessed 17 August 2009.

Davis, D.S. (2001) *Genetic Dilemmas: Reproductive Technology, Parental Choices, and Children's Futures*. New York: Routledge.

Driscoll, M. (2002) 'Why we chose deafness for our children', Sunday Times (London), 14 April.

Edwards, J., Schrick, F., McCracken, M., van Amstel, S., Hopkins, F., Welborn, M. et al. (2003) 'Cloning adult farm animals: A review of the possibilities and problems associated with somatic cell nuclear transfer', *American Journal of Reproductive Immunology*, 50 (2): 113–23.

Fukuyama, F. (2003) *Our Posthuman Future: Consequences of the Biotechnology Revolution*. New York: Picador.

George, S. (2006) 'Millions of missing girls: From fetal sexing to high technology sex selection in India', *Prenatal Diagnosis*, 26 (7): 604–9.

Gosden, R.G. (1999) *Designing Babies: The Brave New World of Reproductive Technology*. New York: W.H. Freeman.

Graves, J., Miller, K. and Sellers, A. (2002) 'Maternal serum triple analyte screening in pregnancy', *American Family Physician*, 65 (5): 915–20.

Green, R.M. (2007) *Babies by Design: The Ethics of Genetic Choice*. New Haven, CT: Yale University Press.

Harton, G., Mariani, B., Thornhill, A.R., Griffin, D.K., Affara, N. and Handyside, A.H. (2009) 'Genome-wide karyomapping for pgd of cystic fibrosis combines accurate linkage based testing with 24 chromosome aneuploidy screening', *Human Reproduction*, 24 (suppl 1): i52.

Institute of Medicine/Committee on Assessing the Medical Risks of Human Oocyte Donation for Stem Cell Research/ Board on Health Sciences Policy/National Research Council/Board on Life Sciences/Giudice, L., Santa, E., Pool, R. (eds) (2007) *Assessing the Medical Risks of Human Oocyte Donation for Stem Cell Research: Workshop Report*. Washington, DC: National Academies Press.

Kaisernetwork.org (2003) http://www.kaisernetwork.org/daily_reports/print_report.cfm?DR_ID=20310&dr_cat=2, accessed 12 August 2009.

Karabinus, D. (2009) 'Flow cytometric sorting of human sperm: MicroSort clinical trial update', *Theriogenology*, 71 (1): 74–9.

Kass, L. (2003) *Beyond Therapy: Biotechnology and the Pursuit of Happiness*. Washington, DC: President's Council on Bioethics.

Kass, N., Medley, A., Natowicz, M., Hull, S., Faden, R., Plantinga, L. et al. (2007) 'Access to health insurance: Experiences and attitudes of those with genetic versus non-genetic medical conditions', *American Journal of Medical Genetics Part A*, 143 (7): 707–17.

Marteau, T., Cook, R., Kidd, J., Michie, S., Johnston, M., Slack, J. et al. (1992) 'The psychological effects of false-positive results in prenatal screening for fetal abnormality: a prospective study', *Prenatal Diagnosis*, 12 (3): 205–14.

Mathews, D., Donovan, P., Harris, J., Lovell-Badge, R., Savulescu, J. and Faden, R. (2009) 'Pluripotent stem cell-derived gametes: Truth and (potential) consequences', *Cell Stem Cell*, 5 (1): 11–14.

McLean S. Genetic screening of children: The U.K. position. J Contemp Health Law Policy. 1995;12(1):113–130.

Munné, S., Magli, C., Cohen, J., Morton, P., Sadowy, S., Gianaroli, L. et al. (1999) 'Positive outcome after preimplantation diagnosis of aneuploidy in human embryos', *Human Reproduction*, 14 (9): 2191–99.

Murray, T.H. (1996) *The Worth of a Child*. Berkeley, CA: University of California Press.

Nayernia, K., Nolte, J., Michelmann, H., Lee, J., Rathsack, K., Drusenheimer, N. et al. (2006) 'In vitro-differentiated embryonic stem cells give rise to male gametes that can generate offspring mice', *Developmental Cell*, 11 (1): 125–32.

Otlowski, M. (2004) 'An exploration of the legal and socio-ethical implications of predictive genetic testing of children', *Australian Journal of Family Law*, 18 (2): 147–69.

Roberts, M. and Wasserman, C. (2009) *Harming Future Persons: Ethics, Genetics and the Nonidentity Problem*. New York: Springer.

Robertson, J.A. (1994) *Children of Choice: Freedom and the New Reproductive Technologies*. Princeton, NJ: Princeton University Press.

Sagi, M., Weinberg, N., Eilat, A., Aizenman, E., Werner, M., Girsh, E. et al. (2009) 'Preimplantation genetic diagnosis for BRCA1/2 – A novel clinical experience', *Prenatal Diagnosis*, 29 (5): 508–13.

Sandel, M.J. (2007) *The Case against Perfection: Ethics in the Age of Genetic Engineering.* Cambridge, MA: Belknap Press of Harvard University Press.

Silver, L.M. (1997) *Remaking Eden: Cloning and beyond in a Brave New World.* New York: Avon Books.

Stock, G. (2002) *Redesigning Humans: Our Inevitable Genetic Future.* Boston, MA: Houghton Mifflin.

UNESCO (2001) http://www.unesco.org/bpi/eng/unescopress/2001/01-90e.shtml, accessed 12 August 2009.

Verlinsky, Y., Cohen, J., Munné, S., Gianaroli, L., Simpson, J., Ferraretti, A. et al. (2004) 'Over a decade of experience with preimplantation genetic diagnosis: A multicenter report', *Fertility and Sterility*, 82 (2): 292–4.

Verlinsky, Y., Rechitsky, S., Schoolcraft, W., Strom, C. and Kuliev, A. (2001) 'Preimplantation diagnosis for Fanconi anemia combined with HLA matching', *Journal of the American Medical Association*, 285 (24): 3130–33.

Verlinsky, Y., Rechitsky, S., Verlinsky, O., Masciangelo, C., Lederer, K. and Kuliev, A. (2002) 'Preimplantation diagnosis for early-onset Alzheimer disease caused by V717L mutation', *Journal of the American Medical Association*, 287 (8): 1018–21.

Wilmut, I. and Highfield, R. (2006) *After Dolly: The Uses and Misuses of Human Cloning.* New York: W.W. Norton.

Wolf, S., Kahn, J. and Wagner, J. (2003) 'Using preimplantation genetic diagnosis to create a stem cell donor: Issues, guidelines and limits', *Journal of Law Medicine & Ethics,* 31 (3): 327–39.

Zhang, J., Zhuang, G., Zeng, Y., Acosta, C., Shu, Y. and Grifo, J. (2003) 'Pregnancy derived from human nuclear transfer', *Fertility and Sterility,* 80 (suppl 3): s. 56.

Zhou, B., Meng, Q. and Li, N. (2010) 'In vitro derivation of germ cells from embryonic stem cells in mammals', *Molecular Reproduction & Development*, 77(7): 586–94.

16

Palliative Care Ethics

Pierre Boitte[1] and Jean-Philippe Cobbaut[2]

INTRODUCTION

Over the past 40 years fundamental transformations have taken place in medicine's approach to death. As a consequence of therapeutic innovations and new survival techniques (resuscitation, and artificial respiration and feeding), the end of life is now considered a separate period, during which specific interventions are possible. At the same time, the appearance of new concerns related to patient autonomy, information and rights have contributed to the development of palliative medicine. The emergence of palliative medicine is to a large extent due to the changed relationship with death (Castra, 2003).

Today, the World Health Organisation (WHO) defines palliative care as 'an approach that improves the quality of life of patients and their families facing the problems associated with life-threatening illnesses, through the prevention and relief of suffering by means of early identification and the correct assessment and treatment of pain and other problems, physical, psychosocial and spiritual' (http://www.who.int/cancer/palliative/definition/en/).

Palliative care arose in the late 1960s as a result of the growing indignation over the fact that patients were frequently neglected, or submitted to useless, painful treatments at the end of life, and that they died surrounded by tubes and monitors. The knowledge that death in Western societies (UK, France, Canada, USA, etc.) was often a terrible experience for the people involved (including the patient, his/her family and the healthcare professionals) was the first step in the development of a movement, aimed at improving patient care at the end of life. The supporters of palliative care denounced the real shortcomings of medicine, convinced that it was possible to avoid such suffering at the end of life (Cadoré, 2001; Jacquemin, 2004; Callahan, 2005).

The pioneers of palliative care in the 1970s stated that several changes were necessary to improve this situation:

- questioning the control on patients' end of life by technical medicine, mainly concerned about prolonging life;

- improving the treatment of pain and suffering at the end of life;
- developing a medical practice, focused on patients' needs and wishes (Jennings, 2005).

A specific approach to end of life, referred to as a 'philosophy of palliative care' gradually took shape. It featured the following four determinants (Jacquemin, 2004; ten Have, 2005; Randall and Downie, 2006):

- purposes other than healing and prevention, aimed at a good death, by improving the quality of life;
- a non-interventionist attitude, not focused on prolonging people's lives, without speeding it up either;
- the wish to consider the patient as a whole person, and to focus on the patient rather than on his/her illness, giving him/her multidisciplinary care;
- treat patients as if they were relatives, attaching more value to the partnership with patients and shared decision making.

THE INSTITUTIONALISATION OF PALLIATIVE CARE

From the mid 1970s to the late 1990s, the movement steadily grew, spreading from Europe and North America to the rest of the world, eventually reaching six continents and 87 countries (Jackson, 2001). This expansion took place in medicine by gradually extending the notion of 'end of life' to the diagnosis of 'serious illness'. Moreover, as a consequence of the increased number of chronic diseases (AIDS in particular), palliative care was no longer reserved for oncology patients only. It also found its way into geriatrics and neurology, due to the increased number of neurodegenerative diseases resulting from the ageing population (Boitte, 2005; Olde Rikkert and Rigaux, 2005).

There was an expansion of the organisational structures of palliative care: specific hospices, resulting from the historical structure in England; permanent units in a hospital environment (palliative care units for in-patients), particularly in oncology – the first one in Quebec; mobile equipment for palliative hospital care; day hospitals; home nursing networks, etc. Finally, increasing numbers of palliative care training courses were organised for healthcare professionals (doctors, nurses and psychologists), volunteers and citizen associations (Jennings, 2005).

The institutional changes were accompanied by an ethical reflection on advance directives and substitute decision making with regard to end-of-life care. Depending on the country, this also had consequences on the local laws and legislation.

Therefore, over the last 30 years considerable progress has been made to the benefit of the dying. In only a quarter of a century, our societies have made massive reflective, organisational and financial efforts to enhance the dignity of patients (Callahan, 2005). At the same time, however, international publications show that in reality there are still many unanswered questions concerning end-of-life care practices.

THE COMPLEXITY OF CARE RELATIONSHIPS AT THE END OF LIFE

A 1995 US study (SUPPORT Principal Investigators, 1995) showed that taking care of patients who are facing the end of their existence remains difficult for all persons involved.

The study mentions several problems, e.g. care that patients and their families consider unnecessary and/or they do not wish; the difficulty of giving up aggressive measures aimed at prolonging life; the possibility that certain patients will spend the last days of their lives in severe, non-relieved pain, to the obvious detriment of a high-quality end of life.

Besides the fear of suffering due to the inadequate treatment of pain or other symptoms, this reality also increases patients' fear that they will lose control of their treatment at the end of their lives, be dependent on machines, and be an emotional and financial burden to their families. In this context, the importance given to advance directives and substitute decision making is reappraised: the same survey shows that most patients and families do not want to make any decisions regarding end-of-life care. Of course, it is important to consider people's preferences for their end of life, expressed in advance, but what has to be done when they do not express their preferences? Could this difficulty be due to the fact that only a few people are willing to face the preparation of their own death (Callahan, 2005)? Others put forward the outdated restrictive concept of autonomy as a dominant ethical principle in discussions on the end of life (Burt, 2005).

Another difficulty is that end-of-life situations often involve an increase in conflicts (Dubler, 2005). Disagreement on the decisions taken can exist between doctors, between doctors and the patient, between the family and the patient, between the family and the doctors, between the hospital and the doctors, etc. Today more parties are involved in all kinds of decisions, increasing the possibilities of misunderstandings, incorrect information, disagreements and disputes. Contrary to what happened in the 1970s, increasing numbers of families frequently ask doctors to continue certain treatments that the latter would rather suspend (Goold et al., 2008). The case of Terri Schiavo, the young American woman who fell into a persistent vegetative state, and died in April 2005, dramatically illustrates this situation: she had never filled out any advance directives, and her artificial life support initiated conflicts and impassioned debates (Fins, 2006).

End-of-life patients therefore confront healthcare professionals and their family circle with very complex situations. Over the past 20 years, the development of palliative care has furthered this complexity. Caregivers have compiled a long list of new questions to which they are trying to respond. With regard to the complexity, and attempts to deal with it, the development of palliative care and increased consciousness have raised a number of challenges related to the further development and introduction of palliative care into health practice and care institutions.

ISSUES INVOLVED IN A PALLIATIVE APPROACH

Recognising the complexity of the decision process

The first issue is the evolution of decision-making strategies at the end of life. These strategies must indeed be better prepared before decisions, determined by the application of advanced care planning, and perhaps on the basis of advance directives, are taken. (Tulsky et al., 2008). Although the tendency is to focus on the patient, the idea is to integrate the fact that the end-of-life decision process can no longer be conceived as an individual matter between a doctor and his/her patient. Several studies have shown that the introduction of shared decision making, a process involving patients, family and healthcare professionals, is a real need (SUPPORT Principal Investigators, 1995; Burt, 2005).

Creation of multi-professional teams for the service of the patient's quality of life

The second issue refers to the creation and function of multi-professional teams to meet the multiple needs of the end-of-life patient. These teams are created during a period in which palliative care is in constant transformation. The evolution of end-of-life situations, and particularly of paediatric palliative care, has shown the need to improve communication and coordination between the care services, health institutions and social services. In the context of palliative care, the cooperation between professionals, always situated between conflict and partnership, requires multiple specific and common competences (Firth, 2003). For example, palliative care nurses in the USA today are often expected to educate patients regarding advance directives, initiate families into the end-of-life decision-making process, confirm with patients and their families the treatment plans to be followed or facilitate communication between patients, families and service providers (Furlong, 2005).

Adaptation of the institutions to the ongoing evolution of palliative care

From a wider perspective, palliative care must also take into account significant trends that will have a considerable influence on its evolution. For demographic reasons, contemporary societies are gradually learning to get used to the idea of increasing incapacity and dependence, related to old age. Increasingly populations will feel concerned by palliative care, with ever growing demands. Among those populations, the majority of them will be the chronically ill, and particularly those who suffer from neurodegenerative diseases. Dying will increasingly become a process, rather than an event, with important social consequences (Small et al., 2007). The current organisation of care and health structures is rapidly changing to address these demographic and social transformations. These changes also imply important financial and budgetary consequences.

The essence here is to move from a system, organised from the perspective of individual patient care at the hospital, to a multi-centred system to the benefit of the vast majority of chronically ill patients. Before they come to an end-of-life situation, these patients are, in the first place, very frail and can have recourse to palliative care at anytime. The construction of viable care systems in this context requires the integration of people who may well live for several more years, not only people who are about to pass away.

Such a system will have to be capable of determining population groups with similar needs, and to offer services, adapted to the size and foreseeable needs of this population. Patients then become part of a collective setting of global advance directives that depend on their principal health needs. Adequate care and related decisions are determined by the collective setting, and no longer as individual choices that are either followed or not (Lynn, 2005).

MEETING THE CHALLENGES CREATED BY THESE CHANGES

Taking into account the questions of the people involved

If we want to meet the challenge of developing more adequate palliative care, we will have to take into account caregivers' observations in the further development processes of medicine, and more particularly of palliative care. The palliative care providers question the sense of what they do and their role in it. In this context, the evolution of the ethical approach should probably take into account the opinion of people who work in a care facility, and who are directly involved in the care process. They seem to be looking for changes that offer an answer to the contradictions and inconsistencies of a context undermined by the discovery of new questions and a rapid evolution from the epidemiological and medical point of view. If we want to adjust medicine and palliative care to the real needs of the people involved, then we must act upon the care providers' opinions and the ethical questions that they ask, including the manner in which these questions are asked, in their context.

One of the questions asked in literature refers to the growing involvement of the caregivers, whether they are professionals or not, in what they are doing.

There are also many questions on the position of patients and their families in palliative care. English user associations regret that patients who receive palliative care are far too often considered as incapable of being actively involved in the services offered (Bradburn, 2003). Health professionals ask themselves how they can better integrate patients and their families in the ongoing palliative process by progressively sharing information (Schofield et al., 2006). This concern about the patients' position also means that they try to improve the quality of the care by an increased level of commitment to the people involved (Singer et al., 2008).

Literature on the subject also shows that professionals try to give an account of their experiences. Health professionals wonder how they should react when their patients tell them they refuse to accept treatments or care (Dudzinski and Shannon, 2006; Richard, 2009). Nurses question their experiences with administering palliative sedation (Rietjens et al., 2007). Involvement can refer to the stress and suffering that care providers experience in their work, which is a sign that more attention is being paid to the wellbeing of the professionals who work with patients suffering from chronic or lethal diseases, an issue in the quality of palliative care (Feldman-Desrousseau, 2009). The caregivers' involvement also refers to their perception of patients' wellbeing in the context of empirical quality studies in general (Olthuis and Dekkers, 2005) or specific care needs, e.g. long-term care (Kaasalainen et al., 2007).

This involvement by palliative care providers can result in interactive practices, e.g. patients and natural caregivers participating in interprofessional learning of communication techniques in the care of patients (Davies and Noble, 2003).

This growing involvement of care providers in the essence of what they do seems to be a fruitful approach towards meeting the challenges created by the expansion of palliative care.

Develop the learning abilities of individuals and organisations

An increasing number of publications on palliative care show how practitioners, clinicians, caregivers and others become increasingly reflexive practitioners in situations of uncertainty, instability, singularity or conflict. This way, they become involved in continuous auto-education processes (Schön, 1983). If we want professionals to contribute to increasing patients' and their families' quality of life, then palliative care requires constant training and a growing capacity to face this increasing involvement of patients and their families, both individually and collectively.

One of the ways to move forward on this steep road is to develop training experiences from an interdisciplinary and interprofessional perspective aimed at developing collaborative practice, based on team dynamics. This would allow:

- the roles and the responsibilities of each profession, as well as of the patient and his/her family to be better determined;
- the development of an evaluation that reflects the situation as accurately as possible, based on cross-information;
- provision of more adequate care, respecting patients' expectations (Cobbaut et al., 2006);
- by reinforcing the link between education and professional practice, the possibility of collective reflection on the situation, and better development of the capacity to adapt to unique situations and particular contexts.

On the whole, this evolution has to be seen in the framework of a greater tendency to incorporate learning processes into care and organisational practices. It will be necessary for organisations to facilitate reflexive learning among their members, in order to develop professionals who will be concerned with responding to their actions in an area where the care settings and the healthcare design are undergoing substantial changes (Frankfort and Konrad, 1998; Cobbaut, 2008).

Clinical bioethics (Boitte et al., 2002), the partner of auto-development in collective, reflexive learning can certainly contribute to improvement of the quality of palliative care by acting upon caregivers' difficulties and patients' expectations. Maybe it also contributes towards joining two sides of contemporary medicine that tend to lead separate lives: a clinical practice aimed at relieving pain and suffering, on one hand, and ambitious, fast-growing medical research, focused on postponing as much as possible the moment of death, on the other.

Over the last 30 years, fundamental transformations in medicine's approach to death led to the institutionalisation of the palliative care movement. Such institutional changes have outlined the complexity of end-of-life care practices. Considering this complexity, new questions have arisen, challenging the conditions of palliative care's further development. The improvement of palliative care practices depends on several crucial issues: recognising the complexity of the decision process, creating multi-professional teams to provide the services for patients' quality of life, developing a multi-centred system that offers adapted services. More adequate palliative care will better need to take into account the questions of the people involved and develop the learning abilities of individuals and organisations.

NOTES

1 Associate Professor in Medical Ethics, Faculty of Medicine and Senior Researcher, Center of Medical Ethics at the Catholic University of Lille (France). Fields of research: clinical ethics, research ethics, bioethics education.

2 Director of the Center of Medical Ethics, Catholic University of Lille (France). Lecturer in Law and Ethics at the School of Public Health, Catholic University of Louvain-la-Neuve. Fields of research: clinical ethics, organizational ethics, bioethics theory.

REFERENCES

Boitte, P. (2005) 'Elderly persons with advanced dementia: An opportunity for a palliative culture in medicine', in R.B. Purtilo and H.A.M.J. ten Have (eds), *Ethical Foundations of Palliative Care for Alzheimer Disease*. Baltimore, MD and London: Johns Hopkins University Press, pp. 97–111.

Boitte, P., Cadoré, B., Jacquemin, D. and Zorrilla, S. (2002) *Pour une bioéthique clinique. Médicalisation de la société, questionnement éthique et pratiques de soins*. Lille (France): Presses Universitaires du Septentrion.

Bradburn, J. (2003) 'Developments in user organizations', in B. Monroe and D. Oliviere (eds), *Patient Participation in Palliative Care. A Voice for the Voiceless*. Oxford: Oxford University Press, pp. 23–38.

Burt, R.A. (2005) 'The end of autonomy. Improving end of life care: Why has it been so difficult?', *Hastings Center Report Special Report*, 35 (6): ss. 9–13.

Cadoré, B. (2001) 'Pour recentrer la question éthique', in D. Jacquemin (ed.), *Manuel de soins palliatifs*. Paris: Dunod.

Callahan, D. (2005) 'Death: "The Distinguished Thing". Improving end of life care: Why has it been so difficult?', *Hastings Center Report Special Report*, 35 (6): ss. 5–8.

Castra, M. (2003) *Bien mourir. Sociologie des soins palliatifs*. Paris: Presses Universitaires de France.

Cobbaut, J-Ph. (2008) 'Bioéthique et réflexivité. Analyse de la mise en œuvre d'un "programme éthique" au sein d'une institution de soins'. Doctoral thesis, Faculty of Medicine, University of Louvain-la-Neuve (Belgium).

Cobbaut, J-Ph., Sion, S., Deparis, P., Ponchaux, D., Prestini, M., Pélissier, M-F. et al. (2006) 'Une expérience de formation à la prise en charge interdisciplinaire et interprofessionnelle des personnes âgées à l'hôpital', *Gérontologie et Société*, 118: 101–15.

Davies, E. and Noble, B. (2003) 'Education in palliative care', in B. Monroe and D. Oliviere (eds), *Patient Participation in Palliative Care. A Voice for the Voiceless*. Oxford: Oxford University Press, pp. 62–73.

Dubler, N.N. (2005) 'Conflict and consensus at the end of life. Improving end of life care: Why has it been so difficult?', *Hastings Center Report Special Report*, 35 (6): ss. 19–25.

Dudzinski, D.M. and Shannon, S. (2006) 'Competent patients' refusal of nursing care', *Nursing Ethics*, 13 (6): 608–21.

Feldman-Desrousseau, E. (2009) 'Le stress des soignants', in D. Jacquemin (ed.), *Manuel de soins palliatifs*. Paris: Dunod.

Fins, J.J. (2006) 'Affirming the right to care, preserving the right to die: Disorders of consciousness and neuroethics after Schiavo', *Palliative and Supportive Care*, 4 (2): 169–78.

Firth, P. (2003) 'Multi-professional teamwork', in B. Monroe and D. Oliviere (eds), *Patient Participation in Palliative Care. A Voice for the Voiceless*. Oxford: Oxford University Press, pp. 109–25.

Frankfort, D.M. and Konrad, T.R. (1998) 'Responsive medical professionalism: Integrating education, practice and community in a market-driven era', *Academical Medicine*, 73: 138–45.

Furlong, E. (2005) 'The role of nurses and nursing education in the palliative care of patients and their families', in R.B. Purtilo and H.A.M.J. ten Have (eds), *Ethical Foundations of Palliative Care for Alzheimer Disease*. Baltimore, MD and London: Johns Hopkins University Press, pp. 243–60.

Goold, S.D., Williams, B.C. and Arnold, R. (2008) 'Conflict in health care setting at the end of life', in P.A. Singer and A.M. Viens (eds), *The Cambridge Textbook of Bioethics*. Cambridge: Cambridge University Press, pp.78–84.

Jackson, A. (2001) 'Histoire et rayonnement mondial', in D. Jacquemin (ed.), *Manuel des soins palliatifs*. Paris: Dunod, pp. 21–31.

Jacquemin, D. (2004) *Ethique des soins palliatifs*. Paris: Dunod.

Jennings, B. (2005) 'Preface. Improving end of life care: Why has it been so difficult?', *Hastings Center Report Special Report*, 35 (6): ss. 2–4.

Kaasalainen, S., Brazil, K., Ploeg, J. and Martin, L.S. (2007) 'Nurses'perceptions around providing palliative care for long-term care residents with dementia', *Journal of Palliative Care*, 23 (3): 173–80.

Lynn, J. (2005) 'Living long in a fragile health: The new demographic shapes end of life care. Improving end of life care: Why has it been so difficult?', *Hastings Center Report Special Report*, 35 (6): ss. 14–18.

Olde Rikkert, M.G.M. and Rigaux, A-S. (2005) 'Hospital-based palliative care and dementia, or what do we treat patients for and how do we do it?', in R.B. Purtilo and H.A.M.J. ten Have (eds), *Ethical Foundations of Palliative Care for Alzheimer Disease*. Baltimore, MD and London: Johns Hopkins University Press, pp. 80–96.

Olthuis, G. and Dekkers, W. (2005) 'Quality of life considered as well-being: Views from philosophy and palliative care practice', *Theoretical Medicine and Bioethics*, 26: 307–37.

Randall, F. and Downie, R.S. (2006) *The Philosophy of Palliative Care. Critique and Reconstruction*. Oxford: Oxford University Press.

Richard, J-F. (2009) 'Loi Léonetti et consentement des soignants au refus de traitement des malades', in D. Jacquemin (ed.), *Manuel de soins palliatifs*. Paris: Dunod.

Rietjens, J., Hauser, J., van der Heide, A. and Emanuel, L. (2007) 'Having a difficult time leaving: Experiences and attitudes of nurses with palliative sedation', *Palliative Medicine*, 21: 643–9.

Schofield, P., Carey, M., Love, A., Nehill, C. and Wein, S. (2006) '"Would you like to talk about your future treatment options?" Discussing the transition from curative cancer treatment to palliative care', *Palliative Medicine*, 20: 397–406.

Schön, D.A. (1983) *The Reflective Practitioner: How Professionals Think in Action*. New York: Basic Books.

Singer, P.A., MacDonald, N. and Tulsky, J.A. (2008) 'Quality end of life care', in P.A. Singer and A.M. Viens (eds), *The Cambridge Textbook of Bioethics*. Cambridge: Cambridge University Press, pp.53–7.

Small, N., Froggatt, K. and Downs, M. (2007) *Living and Dying with Dementia. Dialogues about Palliative Care*. Oxford: Oxford University Press.

SUPPORT Principal Investigators (1995) 'A controlled trial to improve care for seriously ill hospitalized patients: The study to understand prognosis and preferences for outcomes and risks of treatments', *Journal of the American Medical Association*, 274: 1591–8.

ten Have, H.A.M.J. (2005) 'Expanding the scope of palliative care', in R.B. Purtilo and H.A.M.J. ten Have (eds), *Ethical Foundations of Palliative Care for Alzheimer Disease*. Baltimore, MD and London: Johns Hopkins University Press, pp. 61–79.

Tulsky, J.A., Emanuel, L.L., Martin, D.K. and Singer, P.A. (2008) 'Advance care planning', in P.A. Singer and A.M. Viens (eds), *The Cambridge Textbook of Bioethics*. Cambridge: Cambridge University Press, pp. 65–71.

17

Medical and Societal Issues in Euthanasia and Assisted Suicide

Georg Bosshard and Lars Johan Materstvedt

INTRODUCTION

In her book *Ending Life. Ethics and the Way We Die*, leading US bioethicist Margaret Battin (Battin, 2005: 329–30) tells a short story that illustrates the current discussion on euthanasia and assisted suicide like no other:

Two friends, old sailing buddies, are planning a sailing trip in the North Sea later in the year, and they are discussing possible dates.

"How about July 21st?" says Willem. "The sea will be calm, the moon bright, and there's a music festival on the southern coast of Denmark we could visit."

"Sounds great," answers Joost, "I'd love to get to the music festival. But I can't be away then; the 21st is the date of my father's death."

"Oh, I'm so sorry, Joost," Willem replies. "I knew your father was ill. Very ill, with cancer. But I didn't realize he had died."

"He hasn't," Joost replies, "That's the day he's going to die. He's made up his mind and picked a date, and we all want to be there with him."

Dying not as something that just happens, but something that you do yourself – is that conceivable? And if it is, would such a change in our attitude to death and dying be something to welcome or be scared of? Or could it be that this shift has already taken place, thanks to the seemingly almost limitless power of modern medicine to sustain and extend life?

In this chapter, we are restricting ourselves to the discussion of assisted suicide and euthanasia. The former usually entails a patient taking a lethal overdose of medicines provided by someone else (a lay person or a doctor), whereas the latter involves a lethal injection by a doctor. In keeping with current terminology, we use "assisted dying" to cover both phenomena (Bosshard et al., 2008), and the term "euthanasia" to mean "voluntary active euthanasia" – something that only takes place when requested by the patient

(Materstvedt and Bosshard, 2010). This interpretation of euthanasia is consistent with Dutch understanding – now the international convention (Griffiths et al., 2008): administration of drugs by a doctor with the explicit intention of ending the patient's life at his/her explicit request (van der Heide et al., 2007). Although not stated in the definition itself, it is here presupposed that the request is a voluntary one. We bring attention to this fact since an individual could explicitly ask for something without doing so freely (Materstvedt and Bosshard, 2010).

Withholding and withdrawing treatment (non-treatment decisions; NTDs), and the medical use of opioids and sedatives with a possible life-shortening effect for the alleviation of pain and other symptoms (APS) will only be touched on – although such decisions are much more important than assisted dying in today's medical practice at the end of life.

The first part of the chapter addresses open regulation as initiated in the Netherlands in the early 1970s, which led to the Dutch model of euthanasia. Developments there have had an unequalled impact on international debate for nearly three decades. We have summarized these developments elsewhere (Materstvedt and Bosshard, 2010), and a recent book describes them in full (Griffiths et al., 2008). In considering the Dutch experience, the 1990 Remmelink study is seen by many as the most important milestone of modern empirical ethics relating to medical end-of-life decisions (van der Maas et al., 1991, van der Maas et al., 1992).

The second part deals with certain present-day questions that the Dutch experience leaves unanswered, especially the appropriate role of doctors in assisted dying and the relationship between palliative care and euthanasia. Here we also look at recent developments, particularly in other places where legislation allowing assisted dying has existed over a significant time period: Belgium, the US state of Oregon, and Switzerland. The chapter closes with some reflections on developments that may be expected in this field in the future.

THE NETHERLANDS: CONTROLLING ASSISTED DYING AS A MEDICAL END-OF-LIFE DECISION

From toleration to legal regulation of physician-assisted dying

In 1973, a regional court in the Netherlands judged the case of a physician who had administered a lethal dose of morphine to her terminally-ill mother, following a serious and persistent request. Case law based on this court's ruling and subsequent judgements allowed the formulation of criteria to constitute a defence against a charge of euthanasia (Legemaate, 1998).

The Royal Dutch Medical Association (the KNMG) entered the discussion in 1984, by attempting to clarify the criteria accepted within the medical profession. Finally, in April 2002, non-penalisation of a doctor who meets the "criteria of due care" in assisted suicide or euthanasia was adopted into the Dutch Penal Code: Termination of Life on Request and Assisted Suicide (Review Procedures) Act, 2002 (Table 17.1, first column).

Table 17.1   Places where legislation allowing assisted dying has existed over a significant time period: overview

	Netherlands[1]	Belgium[1]	Oregon[2]	Switzerland
Year when legal regulation entered into force	2002[3]	2002	1997	AS condoned according to Art. 115 Swiss Penal Code
Regulated end-of-life practice	AS and E	(AS and) E	AS[4]	AS
Restriction to terminal illness	no	no	yes	no
Role for non-doctors allowed	no	no	(yes)[5]	yes

AS = assisted suicide, E = euthanasia

1 In April 2009, a similar legal regulation was adopted in Luxembourg.
2 In November 2008, the US State of Washington enacted a similar regulation. After a landmark court decision in December 2009, the US State of Montana might follow.
3 Assisted dying tolerated by Dutch courts from 1973
4 Terminology: "death with dignity" (Oregon Death with Dignity Act)
5 In practice – however no explicit legal role

Due care requires that the physician must:

a. Be satisfied that the patient's request is voluntary and carefully considered;
b. Be satisfied that the patient's suffering is unbearable, with no prospect of improvement;
c. Inform the patient about his or her situation and prospects;
d. Conclude, together with the patient, that no reasonable alternative exists, given the patient's situation;
e. Consult at least one other independent physician, who must see the patient and give a written opinion on the due care criteria stated in a.-d. above;
f. Terminate the patient's life or provide assistance with suicide with due medical care and attention.

This means that only doctors can take any of the steps to assist dying, accordingly voluntary lethal injections or assisted suicide by others than doctors (e.g., nurses, non-medical staff of right-to-die societies) remains illegal.

Measuring medical end-of-life decisions – the Remmelink study and its successors

In 1990, the Dutch government instructed the Remmelink Commission to conduct a nationwide study of the practice of "euthanasia and other medical decisions concerning the end of life" (van der Maas et al., 1991; van der Maas et al., 1992). Taking a random sample of 7000 deaths in the Netherlands in 1990, a team led by Professor Paul van der Maas questioned a large number of Dutch doctors about decisions they made at the end of their patients' lives. The Remmelink study was the first to provide a comprehensive overview of such decisions throughout an entire country. Van der Maas and his group deserve credit for showing that medical end-of-life decisions, in particular euthanasia and physician-assisted suicide, could be measured and quantified rather than being dealt with only by abstract reasoning. But the importance of this study is not just its design and results: it also established a terminological framework.

At the end of the 1980s, a general consensus in the Netherlands took "euthanasia" to mean "a doctor intentionally taking the life of another person upon his or her request, through the use of a lethal drug". Euthanasia thus became one more "medical end-of-life decision" in addition to withholding/withdrawing treatment (NTDs) and the use of opioids and sedatives with a possible double effect. This narrow definition of euthanasia does not include non-voluntary or involuntary forms of intentional ending of life through the use of drugs, which together are designated as "life-terminating acts without explicit request of the patient"; LAWER (van der Maas et al., 1991). The key results of the Remmelink study (Table 17.2, first column) are:

- 17.9% of all deaths in the Netherlands in 1990 resulted from doctors deciding to withhold or withdraw life-sustaining treatment (NTDs);
- 18.8% of all deaths occurred after the doctor, in order to alleviate pain and other symptoms, administered opioids in doses judged to be sufficient to have a probable life-shortening effect (APS);
- 0.2% of all deaths were caused by patients ingesting a lethal drug prescribed or supplied by their doctors with the explicit intention of enabling them to end their own lives (physician-assisted suicide);
- 1.7% of all deaths were caused by the doctor administering drugs with the intention of ending the patient's life, at the patient's explicit request (euthanasia);
- 0.8% of all deaths were caused by the doctor administering drugs with the intention of ending the patient's life, without the patient's explicit request (non-voluntary and involuntary ending of life).

Early interpretations of the Remmelink study – and what subsequent studies showed

The five simple percentages given above, published in the *Lancet* in 1991 (van der Maas et al., 1991), attracted enormous attention from international experts as well as the general public. By the year 2000, this paper had been cited almost 300 times in publications listed in the International Scientific Index, which does not include many references in law, social sciences, and philosophy journals, not to mention innumerable newspaper articles world-wide. It is however remarkable that neither the terminology nor the results were seriously challenged by the scientific community or the media. On the contrary, these data were immediately used by both opponents and proponents of open regulation of assisted dying, but interpreted very differently.

Opponents of assisted dying claimed these numbers as proof of their worst fears of a slippery slope. US psychiatrist Herbert Hendin wrote: "The Netherlands has moved from assisted suicide to euthanasia, from euthanasia for the terminally ill to euthanasia for the chronically ill, from euthanasia for physical illness to euthanasia for psychological distress and from voluntary euthanasia to involuntary euthanasia." (Hendin, 1995). He criticized what he saw as a "culture of death" developing in the Netherlands:

> If those advocating legalization of assisted suicide prevail, it will be a reflection that as a culture we are turning away from efforts to improve our care of persons who are mentally ill, infirm, and elderly. Instead, we would be licensing the right to abuse and exploit the fears of people who are ill and depressed. We would be accepting the view of those who are engulfed in suicidal despair that death is the preferred solution to the problems of illness, age, and depression. (Hendin, 1994; Hendin, 1997)

And in an editorial in the *British Medical Journal* in 2001, the American oncologist and leading medical ethicist Ezekiel Emanuel asked the obvious question: "Where the

Table 17.2 Frequency of assisted dying and other end-of-life practices investigated according to the Remmelink study design and questionnaire

	NL° 1990	NL 1995	NL 2001	NL 2005	AU+ 1996	BE 1998	BE 2001	BE 2007	DK 2001	IT 2001	SE 2001	CH 2001	UK* 2004
NTD	18	20	20	16	29	16	15	17	14	4	14	28	30
APS	19	19	20	25	31	18	22	27	26	19	21	22	33
DCPS	?§	?§	6	8	?	?	8	15	3	9	3	5	?
Assisted suicide	0.2	0.2	0.2	0.1	0.1	0.1	<0.1	<0.1	<0.1	0	0	0.4	0
Euthanasia	1.7	2.4	2.6	1.7	1.8	1.1	0.3	1.9	<0.1	<0.1	0	0.3	0.2
LAWER	0.8	0.7	0.6	0.4	3.5	3.2	1.5	1.8	0.7	<0.1	0.2	0.4	0.3

Numbers in italics relate to decisions that were illegal in the country concerned at the time

NTD = non-treatment decision

APS = alleviation of pain and other symptoms with possible, non-intended life-shortening (double effect)

DCPS = deep and continuous palliative sedation

LAWER = ending of life through injection of drugs, without an explicit request from the patient

NL = Netherlands, AU = Australia, BE = Belgium (Flanders), DK = Denmark, IT = Italy (four regions of Northern Italy), SE = Sweden, CH = Switzerland (German speaking part), UK = United Kingdom

° Original Remmelink study

* Different study design

+ Different study design and different wording of the questionnaire, comparability therefore limited

§ No data available for these years (no question on DCPS asked)

Netherlands leads will the world follow?" – to which he himself answers: "No. Legislation is a diversion from improving care of the dying." (Emanuel, 2001).

Proponents of open regulation also saw their viewpoint confirmed by the Remmelink data. After conducting a study in Australia in 1996 (Table 17.2), although with different design and formulation of some crucial questions, which may have resulted in a higher estimate of the incidence of euthanasia and drug-induced ending of life without the patient's explicit request (Kuhse et al., 1997; Pollard, 2001), the Australian philosopher and bioethicist Helga Kuhse concluded: "Comparative data from the Netherlands and Australia suggest that a liberal public policy approach which focuses on the patient's consent, rather than on the doctor's intention, is more protective of the rights and interests of patients than a restrictive approach." (Kuhse, 1998).

The Belgian sociologist and end-of-life researcher Luc Deliens put forward a similar argument a few years later after his research group completed the first investigation outside the Netherlands with the same design as the Remmelink study: "Perhaps less attention is given to requirements of careful end-of-life practice in a society with a restrictive approach than in one with an open approach that tolerates and regulates euthanasia and physician-assisted suicide." (Deliens et al., 2000).

And Franco Cavalli, the renowned Swiss oncologist and member of the Swiss Parliament, who in 2001 tried unsuccessfully to introduce a model of assisted dying along Dutch lines in Switzerland (Rosenberg, 2001), wrote: "From my experience I conclude that we are most likely to have the same number of "Remmelink cases" in Switzerland – just that we categorize them mainly as "indirect" euthanasia [or "alleviation of pain and other symptoms, with a double effect"]." (Cavalli, 2001).

Thanks to many subsequent studies, both from the Netherlands (van der Maas et al., 1996; Onwuteaka-Philipsen et al., 2003; van der Heide et al., 2007) and elsewhere (Deliens et al., 2000; Seale, 2006; Bilsen et al., 2009), and in particular to the EURELD study (van der Heide et al., 2003), we now have a much better overview and understanding of the extended data (see Table 17.2), from which it seems safe to conclude that:

- Considering all medical end-of-life decisions either with a potential life-shorting effect or certain to cause death, assisted dying has a numerically marginal incidence. Withholding or withdrawing treatment (NTDs), and alleviation of pain and other symptoms with potential life-shortening side-effects (APS) are much more prevalent – even in the Netherlands where assisted dying is much more frequent than anywhere else. This means that, even excluding the relatively few cases of assisted dying, the exact time when patients die is becoming more a matter of decision rather than just fate.
- The Netherlands is not much different from other countries, at least not within Europe, when it comes to ending life without an explicit request: although rare, this practice seems to exist everywhere whether or not there is a law on assisted suicide and/or euthanasia. Thus there are no signs of a slippery slope from voluntary to non-voluntary and involuntary ending of life by drugs. Additionally, open regulation of assisted dying might not serve to eliminate the latter two. (For more on the slippery slope issue, see Materstvedt and Bosshard, 2010.)
- There is no clear correlation between the incidence of assisted dying and the level of palliative care. The UK, the "home" of the hospice movement, has a low incidence of assisted dying. But countries with open regulation (the Netherlands, Belgium, Switzerland) also offer a comparatively high level of palliative care (Löfmark et al., 2006). The Netherlands in particular made great progress in this field over recent years (Gordijn and Janssens, 2004; Löfmark et al., 2006). So far, therefore, the claim that open regulation of assisted dying is an obstacle to improving palliative care lacks foundation.
- More recent studies have shown that deep and continuous palliative sedation (DCPS; see Materstvedt and Bosshard, 2009, and Table 17.2), also called "terminal sedation", is another important end-of-life decision

largely overlooked by the original Remmelink study. Terminal sedation is more common everywhere than assisted dying (Miccinesi et al., 2006), although ethical discussion of this controversial practice only started recently (Materstvedt and Bosshard, 2009).

Current evidence from the Netherlands suggests that the substantial decrease in the incidence of euthanasia between 2001 und 2004 (Table 17.2) was mainly due to doctors increasingly preferring terminal sedation (Rietjens et al., 2004). These figures reveal that euthanasia is still a dilemma for doctors and far from becoming standard practice even after its legalization. A qualitative study of Dutch general practitioners showed almost half striving to avoid euthanasia or physician-assisted suicide because it is against their personal values or emotionally burdensome (Georges, 2008). If there was an initial fear that once doctors started performing euthanasia they would continue with increasing ease, the opposite now seems to be true. Earlier, qualitative research in which 22 primary care physicians participated displays in an illuminating way just how burdensome carrying out euthanasia is on some of them (van Marwijk et al, 2007).

BEYOND THE PREMISES OF THE DUTCH MODEL

The Dutch model of assisted dying has its normative roots in the 1970s and 80s. Since then, the role of doctors in society and the role and expectations of patients have changed greatly. Such changes are important throughout medicine, but especially for assisted dying, since we know that assisted suicide and euthanasia – much more than withholding or withdrawing treatment, or the use of large doses of opioids and sedatives – are strongly influenced by societal and cultural factors.

The Remmelink study design cannot really capture the context in which these medical decisions are made. It took another study to show that, even within the Netherlands, the motives of individuals asking to die have changed considerably over the last twenty years (Marquet et al., 2003). In 1977, Dutch physicians reported that more than half the requests for euthanasia/physician-assisted suicide were mainly due to pain. The second most important reason was dyspnoea. The situation had changed dramatically by 2001, when fear of deterioration and hopelessness were the main two reasons. The authors note "increasing importance of feelings such as self-esteem" as an obvious reason for these changes. This might be exactly what Johannes van Delden, the Dutch physician and ethicist, described as a "shift to autonomy" – a shift away from euthanasia and physician-assisted suicide being seen as the last medical resort to their being the patient's choice. Van Delden considers this to be a "byproduct of a liberal society with its emphasis on self-government, control and rational choice" (van Delden, 1999).

However, whilst society's acceptance of physician-assisted dying appears to have constantly increased over the last twenty years, at least in Europe (Cohen et al., 2006), doctors' more critical attitudes and reluctance to carry out physician-assisted suicide or euthanasia have been confirmed by many studies (Emanuel, 2002; Vollmann and Hermann, 2002; Müller-Busch, 2004). The different attitudes of doctors and the general public are particularly marked on the question of assisted dying for patients without a serious disease (Rietjens et al., 2005).

What is happening in the Netherlands, with doctors' increasing reluctance to perform euthanasia, can therefore be seen as the Dutch version of the current power struggle over euthanasia occurring between doctors and society as a whole throughout the westernized world (Bosshard et al., 2008). A telling example of this is the argument recently presented by Baroness Finlay, a member of the British House of Lords, and a doctor and professor of palliative medicine, that "if 'society' wants euthanasia – then 'society' must take responsibility for it" rather than dumping it on the medical profession (Finlay et al., 2005). More specifically, she suggests a suicide service outside clinical care, run by a designated interdisciplinary team. This could help clinicians faced with requests for assistance in dying, as their role would be clearly confined to discussing the situation, indicating possible treatment options, and offering appropriate palliative care.

In the light of these developments, it is precisely the issues of the doctor's role in assisted dying and the relationship between palliative care and assisted dying which have been crucial in recent discussions on legal regulation in many countries. The enormous difficulties associated with finding an appropriate legal framework have led to most countries hesitating to take the final step towards open regulation so far. In a few places, regulations different from the Dutch system have evolved, namely Switzerland and Oregon (Table 17.1). Most recently, the US State of Washington followed neighbouring Oregon with a Death with Dignity Act of its own (Washington State Death with Dignity Act, 2008). After a landmark court decision in December 2009, the US State of Montana might have a similar law (Johnson, 2009). Still that ruling has been reported to be likely to be challenged in the legislature and perhaps in a voter referendum (Knickerbocker, 2010). In Europe, Luxembourg has followed the Dutch and Belgian way in April 2009 (Watson, 2009). However, at the time of the writing of the present chapter it is too early to discuss the developments in Washington, Luxembourg and Montana in a satisfactory manner; the data is just too scarce or missing entirely.

Belgium is a special case. Formally speaking, the Belgian euthanasia law is quite similar to the Dutch law (Table 17.1), nothwithstanding the fact that the former contains many more detailed provisions. Yet, the context in which it emerged was very different. Furthermore, Belgium can be seen as a model for the attempt to reconcile assisted dying and palliative care (Bernheim et al., 2008) – on both these issues, see below. In contrast, Oregon and Switzerland independently developed models of assisted suicide (but not euthanasia) in which the doctor's role is more limited than in the Netherlands and Belgium. Non-governmental right-to-die societies become correspondingly more important: their responsibilities are even more extensive and explicit in Switzerland than in Oregon. Finally, we should not forget that illegal does not mean nonexistent – assisted suicide and euthanasia are practiced in other places of the world, although not openly (Magnusson, 2004). These issues will be dealt with in the following sections.

BELGIUM: ASSISTED DYING AS A PART OF "INTEGRAL PALLIATIVE CARE"?

Until the last decade of the 20th century, both assisted suicide and euthanasia were prohibited under Belgian criminal law; there was neither relevant case law nor established or regulated euthanasia practice. But a dramatic change followed the Christian Democratic Party's election defeat in 1999 and by September 2002, Belgium had become the second country to have a euthanasia law (Belgian Euthanasia Act, 2002). As under Dutch law, only doctors can provide assistance in dying (Table 17.1), and provided they comply with the conditions and procedures of the Act they do not commit a criminal offence (Broeckaert, 2001). For a comprehensive treatment of legal developments in Belgium, we refer the reader to Griffiths et al., 2008.

Whereas the euthanasia issue had been settled by the time palliative care came to the fore in the Netherlands and most of the debate had ended, the development of palliative care in Belgium preceded the euthanasia debate (Broeckaert and Janssens, 2005). As a result, palliative care was important in the process of establishing the Belgian regulation on euthanasia.

Palliative care federations achieved recognition of the role of nursing teams, but did not succeed in their main goal, namely the incorporation of a compulsory palliative care consult ("palliative filter") into the new law (Broeckaert and Janssens, 2005). The range of opinions on the new law turned out to be very wide, even within palliative care. In order to avoid a schism between palliative care workers, the Flemish Palliative Care Federation (FPZV) adopted a pluralistic stance but nevertheless managed to agree on the statements that "palliative care and euthanasia are neither alternatives nor antagonistic" and that "euthanasia may be part of palliative care" (FPZV, 2003).

The Belgian oncologist Jan Bernheim describes palliative care and legislation of euthanasia developing together into "integral palliative care" in which "euthanasia is considered as another option at the end of a palliative care pathway" (Bernheim et al, 2008). It is however contested whether the term "integral palliative care" truly reflects the position of the majority of palliative care workers in Belgium, or even of those in Flanders, given that this position was arrived at in the specific context of a country that was about to have a euthanasia law anyway.

In a more recent document, the Flemish federation criticizes the terminology used in both the Dutch and Belgian debates. First, it considers the term "medical end-of-life decisions" inappropriate, as these are first and foremost ethical and not purely medical decisions. Second, the terminology has an unbalanced focus on shortening life ("looking at reality from a euthanasia perspective"), losing sight of other crucial ethical issues such as futile treatment and inadequate pain treatment (Broeckaert, 2006).

OREGON: LIMITING THE DOCTOR'S ROLE

In Oregon, the Death with Dignity Act allows physicians to write a prescription for a lethal substance at the explicit request of a terminally ill patient (defined as a life-expectancy of less than 6 months), provided the physician can confirm the fatal prognosis and the patient's decision-making capacity, and has informed the patient about feasible alternatives such as hospice care or pain-control options. Oregon physicians need not be present at the suicide. Nor are they allowed to administer the lethal drug; the law explicitly prohibits euthanasia. So patients decide independently of the physician where and when they want to die. Additionally, patients can delay their decision as long as they want, and in reality many do up until the point that they die naturally and never take the prescribed lethal medication.

Developments in Oregon must be viewed in the light of the activities of the right-to-die organisation and non-medical NGO Compassion in Dying[1] (Pence, 2000: 98). In 1993-94, Compassion in Dying acted in uncertain legal waters when assisting the suicides of 46 terminally ill patients in neighbouring Washington (Preston and Mero, 1996). In June 1997, the US Supreme Court unanimously ruled that there is neither a constitutional right to, nor a constitutional prohibition of, assisted suicide or euthanasia (Emanuel, 2002). While attempts to legalize physician-assisted suicide failed in several other US states, voters in Oregon approved the Death with Dignity Act in October 1997.

Although their role is not explicitly defined in this Act, evidence from Oregon shows that a right-to-die society was consulted in most cases of assisted suicide (House of Lords, 2005: 310). A recent paper in the *British Medical Journal* describes in detail the various tasks and responsibilities of both doctors and right-to-die societies in Oregon and Switzerland (Ziegler and Bosshard, 2007): see Table 17.3. Compassion and Choices plays a crucial role in Oregon in ensuring access to assisted suicide by discussing the eligibility process with interested parties and by providing information and reassurance to doctors willing to engage in assisted suicide. When a doctor is hesitant and would rather be the consulting physician, the organization suggests that the patient ask to be referred to another doctor willing to act as the prescribing physician. Clients often request that some-one from the organization is present at the time of ingestion of the lethal drugs.

Table 17.3 Services and responsibilities of doctors, right-to-die organizations, and others in assisted dying in the Netherlands, Belgium, Oregon, and Switzerland

	Netherlands, Belgium	Oregon	Switzerland
First contacted – discusses general eligibility	Doctor	Doctor or Organization	Doctor or Organization
Coordinates and supervises overall process	Doctor	Doctor or Organization	Organization
Provides information on diagnosis, prognosis, and treatment options	Doctor	Doctor	Doctor
Refers to counselling or provides information on alternatives (e.g. hospice)	Doctor	Doctor and Organization	Doctor and Organization
Assesses decisional capacity and confirms absence of coercion	Doctor	Doctor	Doctor and Organization
Prescribes lethal drug	Doctor	Doctor	Doctor
Dispenses lethal drug	Pharmacist	Pharmacist	Pharmacist
Is present and offers support during self-administration of lethal drug (assisted suicide)	Doctor	(Doctor or) Organization§	(Doctor or) Organization§
Administers lethal drug (euthanasia)	Doctor	—	—
Reports death to authorities	Doctor	Doctor	Organization

§ Doctor is not excluded from being present, but is unlikely to do so

SWITZERLAND: AN OFFICIAL ROLE FOR RIGHT-TO-DIE SOCIETIES

Even more than in Oregon, openness in assisted suicide in Switzerland is the result of the activities of right-to-die societies, in particular Zurich-based Exit and its French-speaking counterpart Exit ADMD in Geneva.

Article 115 of the Swiss Penal Code, dating from the first half of the 20th century, states "Whosoever incites another person to commit suicide or helps him or her to do so from motives of self-interest, will be liable to a maximum of five years imprisonment if the suicide is carried out or attempted" (Schwarzenegger, 2006). Relying on this implicit exemption from punishment of altruistic assisted suicide, Exit first sent a "suicide manual" to everyone over 18 years old who had been a member of the organization for at least three months. The manual gave precise instructions for committing suicide by placing a plastic bag over the head and/or by taking a particular cocktail of drugs (Bosshard et al., 2002). It consisted of several hypnotics, obtained from different physicians on the pretext of insomnia, for instance. Some Exit members did not find these instructions sufficiently practicable and so, as the initial mutual distrust between Exit and Swiss doctors diminished, use has increasingly been made of a lethal dose (10–15 g) of oral barbiturates prescribed by a physician. During the process of assisted suicide, members suffering from a disease with "poor prognosis, unbearable suffering or unreasonable disability", in accordance with Exit's strict internal guidelines, receive personal assistance and support from an experienced Exit volunteer. This practice, which developed from the early 1990s without any more specific legal regulation than Art. 115 of the Penal Code (Ziegler and Bosshard, 2007), is illustrated in Table 17.3.

Since the late 1990s, the limits of assisted suicide have been established by case law at Cantonal level. In 2006, the Swiss Federal Supreme Court confirmed that assisting in suicide is not incompatible with the rules of medical practice, but that an obligation to ascertain the patient's competence to decide is a prerequisite for the prescription of the lethal drug (Appel, 2007; Bosshard, 2008: 473). A doctor must therefore personally examine the patient and assess the medical condition(s) giving rise to the wish to die.

In recent years, Dignitas, another Swiss right-to-die society, has gained notoriety by offering assisted suicide to people coming to Switzerland for this purpose (Ziegler and Bosshard, 2007; Fischer et al., 2008). Partly in reaction to this "suicide tourism", increasing political efforts are being made to tighten the rules on assisted suicide (Dyer, 2003). Given the crucial role played by right-to-die societies, efforts have mainly focused on these societies, for instance by making their work subject to licensing, registration, and supervision. Interest grew when it became known that Dignitas had used helium instead of barbiturates in a few cases in early 2008, in order to circumvent the regulations on pharmaceutical prescriptions (Ogden et al., 2010). Having previously opposed the above-mentioned initiatives, the Swiss Federal Council recently showed willingness to discuss these (Bosshard, 2008; 480, Vonarburg, 2008). Should Switzerland eventually proceed in this way, it may well become the first country to legally recognize the role of non-medical volunteers specially trained to assist in suicide (Appel, 2007).

ELSEWHERE: GREY AREAS IN RELATION TO ASSISTED DYING

We have pointed to the evidence of deliberate ending of life through the use of drugs also taking place where assisted dying is illegal (Emanuel, 2001; van der Heide et al, 2003; Magnusson, 2004). Table 17.2 shows that a substantial number of these cases belonged to the category "ending of life without an explicit request from the patient" (LAWER) in which morphine or a similar substance is used (van der Heide et al, 2007). Opioids and sedatives are also used in alleviation of pain and other symptoms (APS), including terminal sedation (DCPS) – however the intention is then not to hasten death or end life but to relieve suffering, yet there is the possibility that aggressive symptom control could foreshorten the patient's life somewhat; cf. the doctrine of double effect. Having said that, this is a conceptually and psychologically complex doctrine, as human intention is multilayered, ambiguous, subjective, and often contradictory (Quill et al., 1997).

It might well be that in the unlikely event of criminal prosecution, doctors would not label their intentions in the same way as in a strictly anonymous study setting, and would perhaps say that they had not intended to shorten life even though they realized the possibility of this. Therefore, the line can easily become blurred between the illegal practice of ending life without an explicit request from the patient and the alleviation of pain and other symptoms with a possible double effect, something that is legal in all westernized countries. This might be one reason why "ending of life without an explicit request from the patient" happens everywhere, regardless of whether euthanasia is legal or not in a particular country (Table 17.2).

In most of these cases an explicit request was difficult or impossible to obtain because of conditions such as dementia or coma (Pijnenborg et al., 1993; Rietjens et al., 2007). This means that these cases do not constitute assisted dying as defined previously, and therefore would not have been allowed by law anywhere in the world, as the patient's explicit request is always a precondition for legality or non-penalization. Indeed, in the Netherlands, technically these would be (medical) murder cases under the Penal Code (Griffiths et al., 2008).

Alongside such – legally speaking – grey areas of practice by doctors, there is another phenomenon which, although only rarely subjected to academic scrutiny, might be even more important in some countries. This is assistance in suicide provided by non-medics, be they relatives, community members, sympathizers, or members of right-to die circles (Battin, 1992; Ogden, 2001; Magnusson, 2004). These practices are characterized by the following:

- Assistance in dying does not usually involve a medical doctor and uses means not subject to medical prescription – non-prescription drugs or gases such as helium or carbon monoxide (Ogden and Wooten, 2002; Magnusson, 2004; Ogden et al., 2010);
- The authorities and coroners/forensic experts usually misinterpret these cases as natural deaths or ordinary (non-assisted) suicides (Ogden, 2001; Magnusson, 2004);
- The extent of assistance varies greatly, from just providing general information in books (for instance, Humphry, 1991) or on the Internet about how to commit suicide, to assistance in suicide by trained volunteers (International task force on euthanasia and assisted suicide, 2005);
- The Remmelink study design is unable to document these cases as it gathers data solely from doctors – probably the major reason for the blind spot in this field in much of the research community, particularly in Europe.

Interestingly, recent evidence from the Netherlands suggests that, even within a regulatory framework, the actual restriction of assistance in dying to physicians is largely illusory. Based on interviews with 144 individuals involved in the suicide of a relative or an intimate, it was estimated that 1600 suicides with a combination of non-prescription drugs (1.1% of all deaths) occur every year (Chabot, 2007). Dutch psychiatrist and assisted dying practitioner Boudewijn Chabot concludes that this "auto-euthanasia" does not usually appear in mortality statistics because starvation is mostly reported as natural death and suicide assisted by non-doctors as either "ordinary" suicide or natural death. In the Netherlands, therefore, such hidden cases may be as common as physician-assisted suicide or euthanasia.

EPILOGUE: FUTURE DIRECTIONS

Current debate on assisted dying is shaped by two basic developments in modern westernized countries: by the ever-increasing possibilities of modern medicine to save and prolong life – what we call "the medical shift" – and by the ever-growing importance of autonomy and personal choice within society – what we call "the social shift".

Concerning the medical shift, open regulation of withholding and withdrawing treatment (NTDs), including an extended right to refuse treatment, could in principle be regarded as a sufficient response, as more medical options to prolong life will have to be accompanied by increased rights to refuse such measures.

It therefore seems safe to predict that discussion and more specific regulation of NTDs will continue to gain importance, and will cover the types of treatment and medical circumstances under which they may or may not be withheld or withdrawn. Additionally, the roles of advance directives and of healthcare representatives will become more important. Over the last twenty years, most discussions and regulations were based on the premise that patients have to be protected against over-treatment or "acharnement therapeutique" (therapeutic obstinacy). Consequently, they focussed on patients' rights to be involved in the decision and to refuse unwanted life-prolonging treatment. However, with the growing importance of economic factors in clinical practice, a different pattern of advance directives seems likely, essentially demanding that doctors should not refrain too soon from available diagnostic and therapeutic options. Current shifts in healthcare systems towards a growing competition for limited resources in most westernized countries call for regulation that the allocation of resources for patients at the end of life still be fair and consider the needs of the poorest and most vulnerable members of society.

Concerning the social shift, the question arises whether the current emphasis on autonomy and personal choice in the westernized world will sooner or later include, in some form, a right to die. We can speculate that doctors, on rare occasions, have always used drugs to actively hasten the death of patients, who were in most cases not asked or sought the consent of. Being able to ask their doctor to end their life – or even give instruction to do so – may have been the privilege of better-educated patients. Assuming this is the true picture, we might further speculate that in modern societies, where almost everybody has access to education and relevant sources of information, more people will take advantage of opportunities previously available to only a small number of privileged people. In other words, if something is changing, it is probably not so much the decision itself but, rather, the decision maker – with the patient or his/her relatives taking the place of the doctor (Fischer, 2008).

Following this approach, John Griffiths, professor of sociology of law, who has monitored developments in Dutch practice and regulation of assistance in dying for many years, concludes that the basic result is an increase of society's control over medical practice at the end of life (Griffiths et al., 2008: 520). This finding might be true not only for the Netherlands but for most of the westernized world. Whether or not a tighter regulatory framework must or must not include a law on assisted dying may not be the key question after all. The moral acceptability of deliberately ending one's life has always been a subject of heated debate, and probably always will be. Certainly this question extends far beyond medicine and has not only individual but also societal implications, not least the fear of a shift from a right to die (as claimed by the individual) to a duty to die (as imposed on the individual by society) (Hardwig, 1997). Perhaps each generation must seek the answers which best fit the world as it is – or in which they want to live.

NOTE

1 In 2005, Portland-based Compassion in Dying merged with Denver-based Hemlock Society into a new common organisation called Compassion and Choices.

ACKNOWLEDGEMENTS

The authors are indebted to Dr Meryl Clarke for revising the English language of an earlier version of the manuscript.

REFERENCES

Appel, J.M. (2007) 'A suicide right for the mentally ill? A Swiss case opens a new debate', *Hastings Center Report*, 37: 21–3.

Battin, M.P. (1992) 'Assisted suicide: Can we learn from Germany?', *Hastings Center Report*, 22: 44–51.

Battin, M.P. (2005) *Ending Life. Ethics and the Way We Die.* Oxford: Oxford University Press.

Bernheim, J., Dschepper, R., Distelmans, W., Mullie, A., Bilsen, J. and Deliens, L. (2008) 'Development of palliative care and legislation of euthanasia: Antagonism or synergy?', *British Medical Journal*, 336: 864–7. Full free text: www.bmj.com/cgi/content/full/336/7649/864

Bilsen, J., Cohen, J., Chambaere, K., Pousset, G., Onwuteaka-Philipsen, B.D., Mortier, F. et al (2009) 'Medical end-of-life practices under the euthanasia law in Belgium', *New England Journal of Medicine*, 361: 1119–21. Full free text: http://www.nejm.org/doi/full/10.1056/NEJMc0904292

Bosshard, G. (2008) 'Switzerland', in J. Griffiths, H. Weyers and M. Adams, *Euthanasia and Law in Europe*. Oxford: Hart, pp. 463–82.

Bosshard, G., Fischer, S. and Bär, W. (2002) 'Open regulation and practice in assisted dying. How Switzerland compares with the Netherlands and Oregon', *Swiss Medical Weekly*, 132: 527–34. Full free text: www.smw.ch/docs/pdf200x/2002/37/smw-09794.PDF

Bosshard, G., Broeckaert, B., Clark, D., Materstvedt, L.J., Gordijn, B. and Müller-Busch, H.C. (2008) 'A role for doctors in assisted dying? An analysis of legal regulations and medical professional positions in six European countries', *Journal of Medical Ethics*, 34: 28–32. Full free text: http://jme.bmj.com/content/34/1/28.full

Broeckaert, B. (2001) 'Belgium: Towards a legal recognition of euthanasia', *European Journal of Health Law*, 8: 95–107.

Broeckaert, B. (2006) 'Treatment decisions in advanced disease – a conceptual framework'. Full free text: http://mailsystem.palliatief.be/accounts/15/attachments/Research/conceptual__framework_bb.pdf

Broeckaert, B. and Janssens, R. (2005) 'Palliative care and euthanasia: Belgian and Dutch perspectives', *Ethical Perspectives*, 9: 156–76.

Cavalli, F. (2001) 'Ja, wir brauchen die bedingte Straffreiheit der aktiven Sterbehilfe' [Yes, we need a qualified non-punishment for euthanasia], *Soziale Medizin*, 6: 44–5.

Chabot, B. (2007) *Auto-euthanasie. Verborgen stervenswegen in gesprek met naasten* [Auto-euthanasia: Low-visibility ways to die while in contact with those to whom one is close]. Amsterdam: Bert Bakker.

Cohen, J., Marcoux, I., Bilsen, J., Deboosere, P., van der Wal, G. and Deliens, L. (2006) 'Trends in acceptance of euthanasia among the general public in 12 European countries (1981–1999)', *European Journal of Public Health*, 6: 663–9.

Deliens, L., Mortier, F., Bilsen, J., Cosyns, M., Vander Stichele, R., Vanoverloop, J. et al. (2000) 'End-of-life decisions in medical practice in Flanders, Belgium: A nationwide survey', *Lancet*, 356: 1806–11.

Dyer, C. (2003) 'Swiss parliament may try to ban "suicide tourism"', *British Medical Journal*, 326: 242.

Emanuel, E.J. (2001) 'Where the Netherlands leads will the world follow?', *British Medical Journal*, 322: 1376–7. Full free text: www.bmj.com/cgi/content/full/322/7299/1376

Emanuel, E.J. (2002) 'Euthanasia and physician-assisted suicide. A review of the empirical data from the United States', *Archives of Internal Medicine*, 162: 142–52.

Euthanasia (Belgium) Act, 28 May 2002. Full text of law: www.kuleuven.ac.be/cbmer/viewpic.php?LAN=E&TABLE=DOCS&ID=23

Finlay, I., Wheatley, V., Izdebski, C. (2005) 'House of Lords Select Committee on the Assisted Dying for the Terminally Ill Bill: Implications for specialist palliative care', *Palliative Medicine*, 19: 444–53.

Fischer, S. (2008) *Entscheidungsmacht und Handlungskontrolle am Lebensende. Eine Untersuchung bei Schweizer Ärztinnen und Ärzten zum Informations – und Sterbehilfeverhalten* [Decisional power and control over action at the end of life. An investigation of Swiss doctors]. Wiesbaden: VS Verlag für Sozialwissenschaften.

Fischer, S., Huber, C.A., Imhof, L., Mahrer Imhof, R., Furter, M., Ziegler, S.J. et al. (2008) 'Suicide assisted by two Swiss right-to-die organisations', *Journal of Medical Ethics*, 34: 810–4.

Flemish Palliative Care Federation (FPZV) (2003) *'Euthanasie: standpunt van de Federatie Palliatieve Zorg Vlaanderen'* [Dealing with euthanasia and other kinds of medically assisted dying]. www.palliatief.be/template.asp?f=publicaties_studies_fpzv.htm Go to: Euthanasie: standpunt van de Federatie Palliatieve Zorg Vlaanderen.

Georges, J.J., Onwuteaka-Philipsen, B. and van der Wal, G. (2008) 'Dealing with requests for euthanasia: A qualitative study investigating the experience of general practitioners', *Journal of Medical Ethics*, 34: 150–5.

Gordijn, B. and Janssens, R. (2004) 'Euthanasia and palliative care in the Netherlands: An analysis of the latest developments', *Health Care Analysis*, 12: 195–207.

Griffiths, J., Weyers, H. and Adams, M. (2008) *Euthanasia and Law in Europe*. Oxford: Hart.

Hardwig, J. (1997) 'Is there a duty to die?', *Hastings Center Report*, 27: 34–42.

Hendin, H. (1994) 'Seduced by death: Doctors, patients, and the Dutch cure', *Issues in Law and Medicine*, 10: 123–59.

Hendin, H. (1995) 'Assisted suicide and euthanasia: Oregon tries the Dutch way', *Psychiatric Times*, 12 (4). www.psychiatrictimes.com/display/article/10168/54201

Hendin, H. (1997) *Seduced by Death: Doctors, Patients, and the Dutch Cure*. New York: Norton.

House of Lords Select Committee on Assisted Dying for the Terminally Ill Bill (2005) *Report on Assisted Dying for the Terminally Ill, Vol. 2. Evidence*. London: Stationery Office. Full text: www.parliament.the-stationery-office.com/pa/ld200405/ldselect/ldasdy/86/86ii.pdf

Humphry, D. (1991) *Final Exit. The Practicalities of Self-deliverance and Assisted Suicide for the Dying*. Denver, CO: The Hemlock Society.

International Task Force on Euthanasia and Assisted Suicide (2005) *Facts about Hemlock and Caring Friends*. www.internationaltaskforce.org/hemlockcf.htm

Johnson, K. (2009) 'Montana ruling bolsters doctor-assisted suicide'. *New York Times*, 31 December 2009. www.nytimes.com/2010/01/01/us/01suicide.html

Knickerbocker, B. (2010) 'Montana becomes third state to legalize physician-assisted suicide'. *The Christian Science Monitor*, 2 January 2010. Free full text: www.csmonitor.com/USA/2010/0102/Montana-becomes-third-state-to-legalize-physician-assisted-suicide

Kuhse, H. (1998) 'From intention to consent. Learning from experience with euthanasia', in M.P. Battin, R. Rhodes, A. Silvers and H. Kuhse (eds), *Physician-assisted Suicide: Expanding the Debate*. New York: Routledge, pp. 252–66.

Kuhse, H., Singer, P., Baume, P., Clark, M. and Rickard, M. (1997) 'End-of-life decisions in Australian medical practice', *Medical Journal of Australia*, 166: 191–6.

Legemaate, J. (1998) 'Twenty-five years of Dutch experience and policy on euthanasia and assisted suicide: An overview', in D.C. Thomasma, T. Kimbrough-Kushner, G.K. Kimsma and C. Ciesielsky-Carlucci (eds), *Asking to Die. Inside the Dutch Debate about Euthanasia*. Dortrecht: Kluwer, pp. 19–34.

Löfmark, R., Mortier, F., Nilstun, T., Bosshard, G., Cartwright, C., Van der Heide, A. et al. (2006) 'Palliative care training: A survey of physicians in Australia and Europe', *Journal of Palliative Care*, 22: 105–10.

Magnusson, R.S. (2004) 'Euthanasia: Above ground, below ground', *Journal of Medical Ethics*, 30: 441–6.

Marquet, R., Bartelds, G., Visser, G., Spreeuwenberg, P. and Peters, L. (2003) 'Twenty-five years of requests for euthanasia and physician-assisted suicide in Dutch general practice: Trend analysis', *British Medical Journal*, 327: 201–2.

Materstvedt, L.J. and Bosshard, G. (2009) 'Deep and continuous palliative sedation (terminal sedation): Clinical-ethical and philosophical aspects', *Lancet Oncology*, 10: 622–7. Abstract: http://www.lancet.com/journals/lanonc/article/PIIS1470-2045(09)70032-4/abstract

Materstvedt, L.J. and Bosshard, G. (2010) 'Euthanasia and physician-assisted suicide', in G. Hanks, N. Cherny, N. Christakis, M.T. Fallon, S. Kaasa and R.K. Portenoy (eds), *Oxford Textbook of Palliative Medicine*, 4th ed. Oxford: Oxford University Press.

Miccinesi, G., Rietjens, J.A.C., Deliens, L., Paci, E., Bosshard, G., Nilstun, T. et al. (2006) 'Continuous deep sedation: Physicians' experiences in six European countries', *Journal of Pain and Symptom Management*, 31: 122–9.

Müller-Busch, H.C., Oduncu, F.S., Woskanjan, S. and Klaschik, E. (2004) 'Attitudes on euthanasia, physician-assisted suicide and terminal sedation – A survey of the German Association for Palliative Medicine', *Medicine, Health Care and Philosophy*, 7: 333–9.

Ogden, R.D. (2001) 'Non-physician assisted suicide: The technological imperative of the deathing counterculture', *Death Studies*, 25: 387–401.

Ogden, R.D. and Wooten, R.H. (2002) 'Asphyxial suicide with helium and a plastic bag', *American Journal of Forensic Medicine and Pathology*, 23: 234–7.

Ogden, R.D., Hamilton, W.K., Whitcher, C. (2010) 'Assisted suicide by oxygen deprivation with helium at a Swiss right-to-die organisation'. *Journal of Medical Ethics*, 36:174–9.

Onwuteaka-Philipsen, B.D., van der Heide, A., Koper, D., Keij-Deerenberg, I., Rietjens, J.A.C., Rurup, M.L. et al. (2003) 'Euthanasia and other end-of-life decisions in the Netherlands in 1990, 1995, and 2001', *Lancet*, 362: 395–9.

Oregon Death with Dignity Act (1997). http://oregon.gov/DHS/ph/pas/ors.shtml

Pence, G.E. (2000) *Classic Cases in Medical Ethics*, 3rd ed. Boston, MA: McGraw-Hill.

Pijnenborg, L., van der Maas, P.J., van Delden, J.J.M. and Looman, C.W.N. (1993) 'Life-terminating acts without explicit request of patient', *Lancet*, 341: 1196–9.

Pollard, B. (2001) 'Euthanasia in Europe', *Lancet*, 357: 1039.

Preston, T.A. and Mero, R. (1996) 'Observations concerning terminally ill patients who choose suicide', *Journal of Pharmaceutical Care*, 4: 183–92.

Quill, T.E., Dresser, R. and Brock, D.W. (1997) 'The rule of double effect – A critique of its role in end-of-life decision making', *New England Journal of Medicine*, 337:1768–71.

Rietjens, J.A.C, van der Heide, A., Vrakking, A.M., Onwuteaka-Philipsen, B.D., van der Maas, P.J. and van der Wal, G. (2004) 'Physician reports of terminal sedation without hydration or nutrition for patients nearing death in the Netherlands', *Annals of Internal Medicine*, 141: 178–185.

Rietjens, J.A.C., van der Heide, A, Onwuteaka-Philipsen, B., van der Maas, P. and van der Wal, G (2005) 'A comparison of attitudes towards end-of-life decisions: Survey among the Dutch general public and physicians', *Social Science and Medicine*, 61: 1723–32.

Rietjens, J., Bilsen, J., Fischer, S., van der Heide, A., van der Maas, P., Miccinesi, G. et al. (2007) 'Using drugs to end life without an explicit request of the patient', *Death Studies*, 31: 205–21.

Rosenberg, M. (2001) 'Sterbehilfe soll nicht straffrei werden' [Assistance in dying not to be depenalised], *Neue Zürcher Zeitung*, 12 December.

Schwarzenegger, C. (2006) *Schweizerisches Strafgesetzbuch* [Swiss penal code], 4th ed. Zürich: Liberalis Verlag.

Seale, C. (2006) 'National survey of end-of-life decisions made by UK medical practitioners', *Palliative Medicine*, 20: 3–10.

Termination of Life on Request and Assisted Suicide (Review Procedures) Act (2002) Full text of law: www.healthlaw.nl/wtlovhz_eng.pdf

Van Delden, J.J.M. (1999) 'Slippery slopes in flat countries – A response', *Journal of Medical Ethics*, 25: 22–4.

Van der Heide, A., Deliens, L., Faisst, K., Nilstun, T., Norup, M., Paci, E. et al. (2003) 'End-of-life decision-making in 6 European countries', *Lancet*, 362: 345–50.

Van der Heide, A., Onwuteaka-Philipsen, B.D., Rurup, M.L., Buitig, H.M., van Delden J.J.M., Hanssen-de Wolf J.E. et al. (2007) 'End-of-life practices in the Netherlands under the Euthanasia Act', *New England Journal of Medicine*, 356: 1957–65.

Van der Maas, P.J., van Delden, J.J.M., Pijnenborg, L. and Looman, C.W.N. (1991) 'Euthanasia and other medical decisions concerning the end of life', *Lancet*, 338: 669–74.

Van der Maas, P.J., van Delden, J.J., and Pijnenborg, L. (1992) 'Euthanasia and other medical decisions concerning the end of life. An investigation performed upon request of the commission of Inquiry into the Medical Practice concerning Euthanasia', *Health Policy*, 21:1–262

Van der Maas, P.J., van der Wal, G., Haverkate, I., de Graaff, C.L.M., Kester, J.G.C., Onwuteaka-Philipsen, B.D. et al. (1996) 'Euthanasia, physician-assisted suicide, and other medical practices involving the end of life in the Netherlands, 1990–1995', *New England Journal of Medicine*, 335: 1700–1.

Van Marwijk, H., Haverkate, I., van Royen, P. and The, A.M. (2007) 'Impact of euthanasia on primary care physicians in the Netherlands', *Palliative Medicine*, 21: 609–14.

Vollmann, J. and Hermann, E. (2002) 'Einstellungen von Psychiatern zur ärztlichen Beihilfe zum Suizid' [Attitudes of psychiatrists toward physician-assisted suicide], *Fortschritte in der Neurologie und Psychiatrie*, 70: 601–8.

Vonarburg, V. (2008) 'Parteilose Bundesrätin werde ich nie' [I'll never be a Federal Council outside any political party], *Tages-Anzeiger*, 12 April.

Washington State Death with Dignity Act, Initiative 1000, RCW 70.245 (2008) Full text of law: www.doh.wa.gov/dwda/

Watson, R. (2009) 'Luxembourg is to allow euthanasia from 1 April'. *British Medical Journal* 338: b1248. Full text: www.bmj.com/cgi/content/full/338/mar24_1/b1248

Ziegler, S.J. and Bosshard, G. (2007) 'Role of non-governmental organisations in physician assisted suicide', *British Medical Journal*, 334: 295–8. Full free text: www.bmj.com/cgi/content/full/334/7588/295

18

Advance Directives

Paul Schotsmans

INTRODUCTION

The right to die with dignity is at the time of writing probably one of the most accepted, but at the same time one of the most divergent rights in modern society. Due to the rapid expansion of medical treatments to extend the physical life of patients, many people are concerned about what will happen to them when they are no longer capable of expressing their personal wishes. Therefore, people want to make clear in advance their treatment preferences in the event of them losing decision-making capacity. This may happen for a short period of time due to the trauma of injury, but in more difficult cases, such as patients with severe dementia and the permanently unconscious, they will not be competent to aid decision making for the entire course of their treatment. In recent years the legal and medical professions have recommended advance directives – either a living will or nominating a representative of the patient – as the best way to address this question. In essence, an advance directive attempts to circumvent the question by having the patient, while still competent, determine and state how he/she wants to be treated if and when he/she becomes no longer competent.[1]

Advance directives may allow patients to prevent unwanted and burdensome treatments when struck by terminal illness, permanent unconsciousness or profound mental disability. Advance directives are only one part of a process known as advance care planning, in which patients, ideally in consultation with physicians and loved ones, plan in a thoughtful and reflective manner for medical care in the event of future incapacity.[2] I agree with Nancy King who makes clear in her guiding publication that advance directives should not be treated as an isolated matter. Instead they are often considered as one of the many available means of caring for 'hopelessly ill patients' … or of addressing the problem of 'life-sustaining treatment'.[3] This is the reason why I will focus on good care of the dying patient who is no longer competent. I have divided my contribution into four parts: first, I try to clarify the growing interest in Advance Directives (ADs) in an era of globalization. Second, I will describe the specific function of ADs in countries with legislation on euthanasia

(Belgium and the Netherlands). I do this essentially in order not to repeat several other publications, which consider mostly the whole range of end-of-life decision making, but do not address ADs. Third, I will present my relational view on human existence in order to situate ADs in the general context of the search for a meaningful life. And finally, I will make clear that ADs should therefore be understood as an instrument to realize this relational character of our existence: the nomination of a 'confidant(e)', while giving him/her the necessary instructions, may be the best expression of our search for human dignity.

ADVANCE DIRECTIVES OR HOW TO CONTROL FINITENESS

On several websites about ADs, one may find statements such as:

> A good advance directive describes the kind of treatment you would want depending on how sick you are. For example, the directives would describe what kind of care you want if you have an illness that you are unlikely to recover from, or if you are permanently unconscious. Advance directives usually tell your doctor that you don't want certain kinds of treatment. However, they can also say that you want a certain treatment no matter how ill you are.[4]

It is clear that this presentation refers not only to advance refusals of treatment, but also what 'treatment you want no matter how ill you are'. Although Nancy King provided reassurance to her readers on these request directives ('Although many patients say they would want aggressive treatment in the future and many families request "everything" on behalf of patients incapable of decision making, few patients actually write "request directives"'),[5] it is symbolic of the evolution of our contemporary thinking.

This testifies to an enormous sense of uneasiness within our culture.[6] Even though the normal human biography begins and ends in dependence, we deeply desire independence… There are many reasons for this evolution: therapeutic obstinacy has certainly been the most important one. I am convinced, however, that this is almost fully under control. One of the most important contributions of medical ethics is, in my view, the awareness by medical doctors that therapeutic obstinacy should be limited (see further below) and limiting orders should be set up. I have to admit, however, that one of the main vehicles for controlling medical interventions may indeed have been the writing of ADs.[7]

The growing impact of secularization in a globalized world, whereby the meaning of suffering, finiteness and dependency are seriously questioned, seems to me, increasingly important. Many people have come to view a degenerative dying process as a fate worse than death itself.[8] Due to our emphasis upon self-determination, we no longer accept that others should take over the care of our lives. Therefore we want to extend our autonomy into a future time when we are no longer autonomous.

After all, although significant pain can often be avoided, there will always be exceptions. Even if pain can be medically controlled, much suffering cannot. From the loss of physical control with multiple sclerosis and amyelotropic lateral sclerosis, to the deterioration of mental function with Alzheimer's disease, many experience illness as marked by not just intolerable discomfort, but unacceptable indignities and the loss of self-control: 'if rationality, freedom, dignity, and self-determination distinguish the good life, should they not characterize the good death?', is one of the rhetorical questions of the well-known bioethicist H.T. Engelhardt.[9]

Personally, I doubt that these anxieties about the loss of autonomy would lead to the acceptance of descriptive ADs, prescribing what doctors do or don't do, or even prescribing euthanasia. In part, we deceive ourselves into supposing that we can actually anticipate with precision future medical conditions and possible treatments. I wonder if descriptive ADs are the best answer to this situation. A living will lets others off the hook too easily. Patients who are unable to make decisions for themselves because, for example, they have severe dementia or are permanently unconscious have, in a sense, become 'strangers' to the rest of us. We see in them what we may one day be, they make us uneasy, and we react with ambivalence.[10] Living wills or ADs cannot specify every detail and every contingency. They are open to interpretation, particularly the physician's or family's understanding of what the patient meant.[11]

In my view, this may be the specific reason why we need to reconsider urgently how ADs should be integrated into the care of the dying. It is of course evident that physicians are not bound by so-called positive (demanding, requesting) advance directives. Fortunately, several countries have already developed legislation on this matter (see the Belgian Euthanasia Act, 2002, Art. 14: The request and the advance directive referred to in sections 3 and 4 of this Act are not compulsory in nature). Essentially, we need a broader view on our human existence. Before developing this broader view, I now present the way countries with legislation on euthanasia handle the possible use of ADs, requesting euthanasia.

ADVANCE DIRECTIVES IN THE CONTEXT OF EUTHANASIA LEGISLATION

Several countries have legislation on ADs and in many these are connected to their bills on patients' rights. I will concentrate here on the specific situation of those countries that also have legislation on euthanasia, and where these laws contain regulations on ADs. Belgium and the Netherlands are the first countries in the world to have legalized euthanasia.[12] I was one of the participants in the Belgian debate and will therefore concentrate on these regulations.[13].

Section 4 ss. 1 of the Belgian Act regulates in detail the formal requirements imposed on ADs in cases where a patient is no longer able to express his/her will. The AD may be drafted at any time. It must be set down in writing in the presence of two adult witnesses, at least one of whom has no material interest in the patient's death. It must be dated and signed by the patient making the request, by the witnesses and by the patient's representatives, if any. In the AD, one or more representatives may be appointed, in order of preference, to inform the attending physician of the patient's wishes. In the event of a representative's refusal, hindrance, incapacity or death, he/she will be replaced by another representative as indicated in the AD. The patient's physicians and the members of the nursing team are prohibited from acting as proxy. The AD may be modified or revoked at any time.

If the patient who wishes to draft an AD is permanently physically incapable of doing so, he/she may appoint an adult who has no material interest in his/her death to write down his/her request, in the presence of two adult witnesses, at least one of whom has no material interest in the patient's death. The AD must note that the patient in question is incapable of signing and refer to the reasons why. The AD must be dated and signed by the person who writes it down, by the witnesses and by the representatives, if any. A medical certificate is appended to the AD as proof that the patient is permanently physically incapable of writing and signing the AD.

The Belgian legislature's objective of limiting the validity of the AD to 5 years following its drafting or confirmation cannot be attained with the Euthanasia Act in its current form, since the third last paragraph of section 4 ss. 1 states: an advance directive is only valid 'if it has been drafted or confirmed fewer than 5 years before the moment at which the person in question can no longer express his/her wishes'. This problem could have been avoided by correctly formulating the Euthanasia Bill. In determining the AD's validity, what is crucial is not the moment at which patients can no longer express their wishes, but rather the moment at which the AD's execution is requested. If more than 5 years has elapsed between the drafting or confirmation of the AD and the moment at which its execution is requested, it should no longer be considered valid. That would have been an objective, easily verifiable moment. Herman Nys, one of the most important Belgian experts in Medical Law, made this clear during hearings on the Bill at the Belgian House of Representatives on 27 February 2002. The parliamentary representatives were aware of the problem but did not want to modify the text of the Bill, since this would have had constitutional consequences: had there been the slightest alteration to the text, then the Belgian Senate would have had to vote yet again on the modified version of the text. That would have taken too much time, and the government did not, for political reasons, want this to occur.

Section 2(2) of the Dutch Act stipulates that in cases of an AD, the criteria within section 2(1) apply, which means that the patient must have been capable of making a voluntary, well-considered request at the time the AD was drafted. The Dutch Act does not require the AD to have any specific formal qualities, apart from being drafted in writing.

The patient's situation

The Belgian Act, contains special requirements regarding the patient's state of health when he/she is no longer conscious and where an AD exists. Section 4 ss. 1 stipulates that such a patient must be suffering from a serious, incurable condition caused by accident or illness, and moreover, that the state of unconsciousness must be irreversible according to the state of science's current thinking. The requirement of unbearable suffering is no longer imposed, since the legislature assumed that such patients are no longer capable of suffering. Had this requirement been imposed, the fear was that euthanasia in patients with irreversible unconsciousness would have been impossible. In spite of the Act leaving little room for interpretation as far as this aspect is concerned, most members of Parliament assumed that only patients in a so-called persistent vegetative state (PVS) would meet this criterion. A good deal of discussion nevertheless took place on this point in the Belgian Parliament. One of the members of Parliament who had submitted the legislative bill – the leader of the Dutch-speaking liberal party in the Senate – was of the opinion that, as far as she was concerned, the Act should apply mainly to patients who were comatose, which is broader than a patient who is 'irreversibly unconscious'. This gave rise to questions about the applicability of the Act to older people with dementia, for instance: are they 'irreversibly unconscious' because they no longer possess any real powers of awareness? While most members of Parliament believed that this ought not to be the case, no definitive answer was ever given on this point. As a result, there exists a lack of clarity on this issue.

The Dutch Act, in contrast, states in section 2§2 that an AD can be applied when the patient 'is no longer capable of expressing his/her wishes'. This requirement is clearly broader than the requirement of the Belgian Act (there is no mention of irreversible unconsciousness). The Act places no special requirements on the patient in cases of an AD, but only states, also in section 2§2, that the 'requirements of due care referred to in the first paragraph apply *mutatis mutandis*. In view of what has just been said, we might ask ourselves what this could mean with respect to the requirement of unbearable suffering. For example, can someone who is unconscious suffer unbearably? Because of this, commentators have raised doubts about the feasibility of this provision in practice.

Duties of physicians

In the Belgian Act, there are also specific provisions with respect to the role of the physician in ADs. These are the same as the requirements imposed on the physician when confronted with a conscious patient who requests euthanasia. This implies that the physician in Belgium does not have to consent to a euthanasia request; he/she may refuse to perform euthanasia on grounds of conscience or for medical reasons. In such a case, however, and this is also true for the Netherlands, a duty exists to refer the patient to another physician.

Commentary

Euthanasia as a consequence of an AD occurs very rarely in Belgium and the Netherlands. One reason for this is that before the Act was passed there were already doubts regarding the general ethical and legal validity of such an instrument. This might also explain why very few due care criteria on this issue are to be found in case law and authoritative reports. Even now that there is legislation allowing the use of ADs, few expect that it will be used frequently. The fact that the practice does not follow legal possibilities is in my view very significant. It makes clear that we are confronted with real limitations of autonomy in clinical reality. It is essential, therefore, to clarify from an ethical viewpoint the basic ethical foundation of our human existence.

A RELATIONAL AND COMMUNICATIVE VIEW ON OUR HUMAN EXISTENCE

The interest in the relational structure of humanity finds a very strong foundation in philosophical and anthropological theories concerning the relational structure of the human person.[14] This is linked to some very influential European (and also Jewish) philosophers, such as Emmanuel Levinas[15] and Martin Buber.[16] Rather surprisingly, these philosophers and their relational approach are almost unknown in mainstream medical ethics, although their insights are crucially important for the ethical understanding of human existence in general and the medical profession in particular. Their views present a fundamental criticism on the radicalization of the principle of respect for the autonomy of the patient, as it is now dominant in current Anglo-American bioethics.

This is also clear in the ethical debate concerning the end of life, where the relational approach is unfortunately almost totally absent. As the Dutch author Martien Pijnenburg observes: 'There is too much one-dimensional focus on the human person as an autonomous entity making autonomous choices. Autonomy is an ideal but not an absolute value'.[17] Harry Kuitert, the influential Dutch Protestant theologian who was in favour of the legalization of euthanasia, also makes clear that 'the autonomy of the patient is not, has never been, and cannot be the sole reason for performing euthanasia'.[18] With regard to this disproportional interest in the principle of autonomy, Theo Beemer, a Catholic moral theologian, has accurately spoken of a withdrawal from a common search for the meaning of life. He calls it a movement of retreat because, as experience is teaching us, the difficult common search for insight into what is truly human and good is often broken off prematurely because everyone starts insisting on his or her rights. The question 'who may decide?' thus short circuits the discussion of what is 'the good and human to decide?' The question then becomes one of competency, debating who has the right to decide, rather than being a discussion that is concerned with the fundamental aspects of the matter.[19]

Therefore, I am convinced we should essentially view medical practice in the context of the relational encounter with patients. It is the caring and compassion that makes medicine an art as well a science. It is the capacity for ethical concern for the whole individual that invites patients to share, in total confidence, those intimate aspects of their lives that are shared with few or no others.[20] This should be the context in which medical decisions take place. The dominant interest in the autonomous control of human life should be changed to a more realistic acceptance of the patient–physician relationship as a fully shared decision-making relationship. It leads immediately to a more empathic understanding of medical responsibility.

MEDICAL DECISION MAKING IN A CONTEXT OF RELATIONAL RESPONSIBILITY

This gives a clear indication about the way in which ADs should be formulated: instead of prescribing in detail what one expects the medical doctor to do, when the patient becomes no longer competent, it should concentrate on giving general instructions to a representative, or even better: a confidant(e). This person will be the one who will enter into dialogue with the physician and who will try to fully share decision making. Before clarifying this further, I want to make clear that changes in medical attitudes also make ADs less important than they were in times of therapeutic obstinacy.

The debate on the application of ADs has a counterpart in the way the medical profession tries to avoid therapeutic obstinacy. Decisions on the ethical justification for withholding or withdrawing medical treatment, and treatment limiting orders such as the refusal to admit to the intensive care unit, involve not simply an evaluation of the physical condition of the patient but that of the whole person. Therefore, it is good to be aware of the spectrum of values and norms with regard to life, quality of life and other values. Ethical guidelines seem to be needed essentially for dealing with the problems of the application of excessive medical technology.[21]

The classical distinction between 'ordinary and extraordinary' means has been replaced by a more dynamic distinction between 'proportionate and disproportionate' means.

The classical distinction may have been adequate for a rather static and poor medical environment, but is no longer adequate for coping with the current rapid evolution of medical technology. From a more methodological point of view, we may say that these concepts functioned very well in the context of the ethical model of the so-called act deontology, but lack sufficient dynamic integration of new, evolutionary and changing perspectives. The change started in the 1980s from an unexpected source, namely the Sacred Congregation for the Doctrine of the Faith of the Roman Catholic Church. The Declaration on Euthanasia (May 1980) refers to the proposals of some theologians on proportionate and disproportionate means, and formulates these as follows: in any case, it will be possible to make a correct judgement as to the means by studying the type of treatment to be used, its degree of complexity or risk, its cost and the possibilities of using it, and comparing these elements with the result that can be expected, taking into account the state of the sick person and his or her physical and moral resources (Part IV, Due Proportion in the Use of Remedies). Of importance is the opinion that proportionality is to be decided not only at the beginning of the treatment but also during the course of its application. Treatment can become disproportionate due to factors such as strain or suffering, or by being against the wishes of the patient, or due to the results of the application of the treatment.

It is clear, therefore, that speaking in terms of 'proportionate and disproportionate means' is preferable. Crucially important for us, this approach makes it clear that for every case we have to provide what is most humanely possible.[22] This implies that the best of care must be understood in terms of appropriate care: what is most humanely feasible for the patient at this point? It may imply that limiting orders are decided, or that the patient is transferred to a palliative care unit, or that all possible medical technologies are used in order to prolong the patient's life. Such decisions are of course very delicate and therefore require a careful analysis of the medical condition of the patient, a comprehensive clarification of his/her personal and relational values and an extensive justification for the investment of societal resources.

These end-of-life decisions must be made from the perspective of the well-being of the patient. When the patient is no longer competent, his/her 'confidant(e)' is the privileged partner for the physician. He/she is the patient's spokesperson and he/she enters – as if he/she were the patient – into dialogue with the physician. The point of departure here is the respect for the patient as a person and the process of care as a fully relational event. When a decision must be made concerning medical care, the physician, in communication with the patient's representative and eventually the wider family, has to consider all the various factors including personal and familial as well as medical, and he/she must consider the extent to which a particular treatment might realize human fulfillment. This 'proportionate' judgement needs to be made in each particular case. In collaboration with nurses, colleagues and other healthcare professionals, the physician will discuss with the patient's representative the reasons behind the decisions.

This creates an open atmosphere, avoiding excessive application of medical technology. At the same time it can engender trust among those involved (the representative, the family of the patient, the physician and his/her team). This is an expression of full respect for the relational structure of the medical profession. The physician can only come to a conclusion, when he/she takes the caring and curing relationship with his/her patient seriously. The medical profession is indeed a relational profession. Medicine is one of the best illustrations of the relational structure of human beings: when a physician makes a decision, he/she is not acting in his/her own name, but as an agent by reason of the relational structure of his/her profession.

ADs should best be placed in the context of the full reality of relational encounters. Writing down all possible instructions for physicians is not at all helpful. The relational character of the medical profession and the relational structure of every human being direct us more in the direction of the nomination of a confidant(e). ADs should therefore be developed in such a way that the confidant(e) – by oral and written declarations – has sufficient information to enter into the relational dialogue with physicians.

CONCLUSION

I have tried to place ADs in the relational context of our human existence: not only the medical profession but also we as human beings can only reach the full meaning of our lives, when we take up this relational character of our existence seriously. In such a way, by restricting the function of ADs to the nomination of a representative, while eventually giving him/her the necessary instructions, it is no longer the excessive exercise of autonomy or the dominance of medical authority that is primary, but rather the real well-being of each patient and the promotion of real human dignity.

NOTES

1 Gilbert Meilander (1996 [2005]) *Bioethics. A Primer for Christians*, 2nd ed. (Grand Rapids, MI/Cambridge: William B. Eerdmans) p. 77.

2 Gary S. Fisher, James A. Tulsky and Robert M. Arnold (2004) 'Advance directives and advance care planning', in Stephen G. Post (ed.), *Encyclopedia of Bioethics*, 3rd ed. (New York, Thomson-Gale) vol.1, pp. 74–79.

3 Nancy M.P. King (1996) *Making Sense of Advance Directives*, rev. ed. (Washington, DC: Georgetown University Press) p. 8.

4 Available at http://familydoctor.org.

5 Nancy M P. King, p. 9 (see n. 3).

6 Gilbert Meilander, p. 81 (see n.1).

7 Norman L. Cantor (1993) *Advance Directives and the Pursuit of Death with Dignity* (Bloomington, IN: Indiana University Press). It is symbolic for the early 1990s that the author starts with an introduction under the title: 'On restraining life-preserving medical technology'.

8 Ibid., p. VII.

9 H. Tristram Engelhardt Jr (2000) 'The Foundations of Christian bioethics', *Lisse, Swets & Zeitlinger*, XXIV (414): 312.

10 Gilbert Meilander, p. 80-81 (see n. 1).

11 Edmund D. Pellegrino (1991) 'Trust and distrust in professional ethics', in Edmund D. Pellegrino, Robert M. Veatch and John P. Langan (eds), *Ethics, Trust, and the Professions. Philosophical and Cultural Aspects* (Washington, DC: Georgetown University Press).

12 Maurice Adams and Herman Nys (2005) 'Euthanasia in the Low Countries: Comparative reflections on the Belgian and Dutch Euthanasia Act', in Paul Schotsmans and Tom Meulenbergs (eds), *Euthanasia and Palliative Care in the Low Countries* (Leuven: Peeters Publishers) pp. 5–33. An English translation of the Belgian Act on Euthanasia and the Dutch Termination of Life on Request and Assisted Suicide (Review Procedures) Act may be found in the same publication (pp. 245–64).

13 I follow here the analysis of Adams and Nys, the first from the University of Antwerp and the second from the University of Leuven (Director of the Center for Biomedical Ethics and Law, a center to which I also belong and which I co-founded with him).

14 Paul Schotsmans (2002) 'Palliative care: A relational approach', in Henk ten Have and David Clark (eds), *The Ethics of Palliative Care. European Perspectives* (Buckingham/Philadelphia, PA: Open University Press) pp. 126–40.

See also: Paul Schotsmans (1992) 'When the dying person looks me in the face: An ethics of responsibility for dealing with the problem of the patient in a persistently vegetative state', in Kevin Wm. Wildes, Francesc Abel and John C. Harvey (eds), *Birth, Suffering, and Death. Catholic Perspectives at the End of Life* (Dordrecht: Kluwer) pp. 127–43.

15 Emmanuel Levinas (1974) *Autrement qu'être ou au-delà de l'essence* (The Hague: Martinus Nijhoff).

16 Martin Buber (1923) *Ich und Du* (Leipzig: Insel-Verlag).

17 Martinus Pijnenburg (1998) 'Catholic healthcare and the Dutch national character', in David C. Thomasma, Thomasine Kimbrough-Kushner, Gerrit K. Kimsma and Chris Ciesielski-Carlucci (eds), *Asking to Die: Inside the Dutch Debate about Euthanasia* (Dordrecht: Kluwer) pp. 241–53.

18 Harry Kuitert with Evert Van Leeuwen (1998) 'A religious argument in favor of euthanasia and assisted suicide', in David C. Thomasma et al., op.cit., pp. 221–6.

19 T. Beemer (1984) 'Je leven: in de waagschaal of op de weegschaal?', *Tijdschrift voor Theologie*, 24: 36–55.

20 Richard A. McCormick (1994) 'Beyond principlism is not enough', in Edwin. R. DuBose, Ronald P. Hamel and Laurence J. O'Connell (eds), *A Matter of Principles? Ferment in US Bioethic* (Valley Forge, PA: Trinity Press International) pp. 344–61.

21 Paul Schotsmans (1995) 'Admission to and removal from intensive care: A personalist approach', in Kevin Wm. Wildes (ed.), *Critical Choices and Critical Care. Catholic Perspectives on Allocating Resources in Intensive Care Medicine* (Dordrecht: Kluwer) pp. 127–43.

22 Paul Ricoeur (1975) 'Le problème du fondement de la morale', *Sapienza*, 28: 313–37.

19

Vulnerability: A Futile or Useful Principle in Healthcare Ethics?

Jan Helge Solbakk

INTRODUCTION

On 19 October 2005, the 33rd Session of the General Conference of UNESCO adopted, with acclaim, the *Universal Declaration on Bioethics and Human Rights* (UNESCO, 2005). This Declaration is the first international statement on ethics to deal with the linkage between bioethics and human rights. It provides the international community with global bioethics standards for the first time. It is also the first global policy document on bioethics principles that have been adopted by governments; in total more than 192 Member States of the United Nations have adopted the Declaration.

Among its 15 articles addressing morally binding principles, Article 8 of the Declaration addresses the principles of human vulnerability and personal integrity: 'In applying and advancing scientific knowledge, medical practice and associated technologies, human vulnerability should be taken into account. Individuals and groups of special vulnerability should be protected and the personal integrity of such individuals respected'.

Since it was introduced in 1979 in the so-called *Belmont Report* on the protection of human subjects undergoing research (Belmont Report, 1979), the principle of vulnerability has been given increasing prominence in national and international guidelines, and policy documents applicable to medical research, healthcare or bioethics. The culmination was the integration of this principle into the *Universal Declaration on Bioethics and Human Rights*.

The Declaration does not include an explicit definition of what is meant by 'vulnerability' or by 'human vulnerability'. In this regard the UNESCO Declaration resembles the guidelines of the *Belmont report* as well as the World Medical Association's *Declaration of Helsinki* (World Medical Association, 2008). However, in Article 24 of the UNESCO Declaration it is emphasized that it is not only individuals who may be rendered vulnerable but also families, groups and communities. Furthermore, in the preamble to the Declaration reference is made to vulnerable populations. Reference is made to certain circumstances that may render individuals, families, groups, communities and populations vulnerable. Circumstances explicitly mentioned are:

- disease;
- disability;
- other personal conditions;
- environmental conditions;
- limited resources.

Finally, it should be observed that the Declaration operates with an anthropocentric notion of vulnerability, in that the point of reference is human life and 'human vulnerability', not the fragility and precariousness of life – of bioi – in general.

VULNERABILITY: A COMPLEX AND CONFUSING PRINCIPLE

Although the growing prominence of the principle of (human) vulnerability in contemporary guidelines and policy documents applicable to medical research, healthcare or bioethics is an indisputable fact, the academic literature dealing with this principle gives a more conflicting and unsettled impression.

The first serious attempt in contemporary bioethics at a normative justification and consolidation of this principle dates back to a research initiative launched in 1995 by a group of European academics. The aim of this initiative, bearing the programme title *The great principles of bioethics and biolaw*, was to investigate the possibilities provided by continental European philosophy and theology in developing a theoretical and principle-based framework that could challenge the hegemony of the four-principles approach to bioethics developed at Georgetown University in Washington DC (Beauchamp and Childress, 2009). The alternative that was launched included just one of the four principles of the so-called Georgetown University mantra, namely that of autonomy, coupled with the principles of dignity, integrity and vulnerability:

> In the research project we started out with the methodological presupposition that the philosophy of the basic ethical principles, autonomy, dignity, integrity and vulnerability, can provide a normative framework for the protection of the human person in biomedical development …
> The basic ethical principles express the necessary protection of humanity and the human person as guidelines for a future European politics in bioethics and biolaw. (Rendtorff, 2002: 235)

As stated in the report from the research group, this initiative was not only aimed at building a new foundation for bioethics and biolaw; it was also nurtured by the biopolitical ambition of promoting these principles as a basis for a European policy on human rights:

> The subject of the report should be seen as 'ethical politics', rather than 'moral epistemology'. We are … trying to identify the principles as four important ideas or values for a European bioethics and biolaw. We do not conclude that they are universal everlasting ideas or transcendental truths, but rather that they are reflective guidelines and important values in a post-conventional human rights culture. (Rendtorff and Kemp, 2000a: 14)

Of these four principles, vulnerability is claimed to be ontologically prior to the other three, because of its alleged ability to express, in a more persuasive way and in terms of characteristics, the 'finitude of the human condition' (Rendtorff and Kemp, 2000a: 46). Thus, vulnerability should be viewed as an inherent aspect of the being of humans and not as something merely contingent that could be done away with through scientific and medical progress (Rendtorff and Kemp, 2000a: 47). Besides, it is proclaimed as a principle able to bridge the value gap between moral strangers and as a regulative principle able to function as an ear-opener to ethical discourse in a pluralistic society (Solbakk, 1994: 231ff; Botbol-Baum, 2000: 60, 62; Rendtorff and Kemp, 2000a: 46). For these reasons, respect for vulnerability should be viewed as a biopolitical core principle in the modern welfare state (Rendtorff and Kemp, 2000a: 375).

The scope is wider, however, than promoting vulnerability as the most fundamental and universal expression of the human condition; it appeals to protection of life – of bioi – in general and of 'the teleological auto-organisation of the world' (Rendtorff and Kemp, 2000a: 375; Rendtorff, 2002: 237). Therefore respect for vulnerability should be acknowledged not only as the most essential principle of bioethics but as the foundation of *all* ethics (Rendtorff, 2002: 237).

In a policy proposal sent to the European Commission in November 1998, the 22 partners behind this research initiative summarized their shared view of vulnerability in the following way:

> Vulnerability expresses two basic ideas. (a) It expresses the finitude and fragility of life which, in those capable of autonomy, grounds the possibility and necessity for all morality. (b) Vulnerability is the object of a moral principle requiring care for the vulnerable. The vulnerable are those whose autonomy or dignity or integrity are capable of being threatened. As such all beings who have dignity are protected by this principle. But the principle also specifically requires not merely non interference with the autonomy, dignity or integrity of beings, but also that they receive assistance to enable them to realise their potential. (Rendtorff and Kemp, 2000a: 398)

It is fair to say that this particular research initiative has been given a mixed reception by academics, likewise the growing prominence of vulnerability in contemporary guidelines and policy documents applicable to medical research, healthcare or bioethics. One type of critique levelled against the emergence of this bioethical principle is that it is too vague to provide any clear moral guidance: 'Although various protective guidelines stipulate special protections for vulnerable populations, the concept of vulnerability and consequently the criteria designating vulnerable populations remain vague' (Ruof, 2004: 411).

A similar critique charges the principle of being over broad, something which leads to the depletion of moral force: 'So many groups are now considered to be vulnerable in the context of research, particularly international research, that the concept has lost force' (Levine et al., 2004: 44).

On the other hand, it has also been criticized for being too narrow, with the risk of paying insufficient attention to characteristics not related to the groups labelled vulnerable but to 'features of the research itself, the institutional environment, or the social and economic context that can put participants in harm's way' (Levine et al., 2004: 46). To this, add the lack of any sort of seemingly purposeful categorization (Morawa, 2003: 150) or a specific set of criteria or operational terms to determine which individuals or groups or populations should count as vulnerable and what forms of intervention should count as exploitation (Alwang et al., 2002; Macklin, 2003: 473). Furthermore, there is the problem of stereotyping: '… the concept of vulnerability stereotypes whole categories of individuals, without distinguishing between individuals in the group who indeed might have special characteristics that need to be taken into account and those who do not' (Levine et al., 2004: 47).

The metaphor of label has been introduced to describe this problem: '... one of the shortcomings of current conceptions of vulnerability ... is that they conceive "being vulnerable" as a fixed label on a particular subpopulation' (Luna, 2009: 122).

A more fundamental critique levelled against the proclamation of vulnerability as a bioethical principle has also been formulated. Although welcoming the European research initiative as a much needed 'enrichment of principlist bioethics', this critique draws attention to the need for further scholarly labour before viable bioethical principles may be derived from anthropological descriptions of the human condition:

> When principles describe conditions or characteristic features – vulnerability, integrity, dignity – they are employing an assertive language that slips into the deontic and purports to represent moral requirements rather than the anthropological hallmarks they really are ...
>
> By stating that humans are vulnerable and that this constitutes an ethical principle, a naturalistic fallacy is being committed. Vulnerability is an essential and universal mode of being human, it is not an ethical dimension in itself, but of course it does have a legitimate and strong claim to inspire a bioethical principle of protection. (Kottow, 2004: 284)

COMPETING CONCEPTIONS OF VULNERABILITY

In the previous section the focus was on one particular research initiative that suggested a broad conception of vulnerability; the present section will provide a systematic account of alternative conceptions of vulnerability within the bioethics literature and in contemporary guidelines and policy documents applicable to medical research, healthcare or bioethics. This brings us first to the opposite end of the spectrum, to conceptions of vulnerability of a restrictive or minimalist kind. Differentiation between three subgroups of such conceptions, i.e. between consent-based, harm-based and comprehensive conceptions, has been proposed (Hurst, 2008: 192). A characteristic of the first subgroup is that protection is justified with explicit reference to individuals who for reasons of coercion, lack of capability or undue influence are unable to give their free and informed consent. This is the conception of vulnerability reflected in the *Belmont Report* and also in the latest version of the *Declaration of Helsinki*. In these two normative documents an explicit definition of the principle of vulnerability is lacking, but the vulnerable (be it an individual, a particular research population or a community) are labelled as such because of 'their dependent status and their frequently compromised capacity for free consent' (Belmont Report, 1979) or because they 'cannot give or refuse consent for themselves' for reasons of coercion, incapacity or undue influence (WMA, 2008).

A consent-based conception of vulnerability is, however, too narrow in terms of protection to cover the entire terrain of vulnerability in medical research and clinical practice. For this reason the notions of harm (Kottow, 2003 and 2004), of fairness (Nickel, 2006), of power (Zion et al., 2000) and of wrong (Hurst, 2008) have been introduced to address situations where additional safeguards to consent are necessary to meet the requirements of ethical conduct. According to one of the proponents of embracing such notions '... vulnerability as a claim to special protection should be understood as an identifiably *increased likelihood of incurring additional or greater wrong*' (Hurst, 2008: 196). In spite of these inclusions, such understandings of vulnerability remain of a restrictive or minimalist kind when compared to the human-condition-based conception suggested by the European group, because they do not reflect the human condition per se as vulnerable.

A prominent example of the third subgroup of minimalist conceptions of vulnerability is found in the *International Ethical Guidelines for Biomedical Research Involving Human Subjects* of the Council for International Organizations of Medical Sciences (CIOMS), where it is stated:

> Differences in distribution of burdens and benefits are justifiable only if they are based on morally relevant distinctions between persons; one such distinction is vulnerability. 'Vulnerability' refers to a substantial incapacity to protect one's own interests owing to such impediments as lack of capability to give informed consent, lack of alternative means of obtaining medical care or other expensive necessities, or being a junior or subordinate member of a hierarchical group. (CIOMS, 2002: 11)

In the Commentary on Guideline 13, *Research involving vulnerable persons*, this conception of vulnerability is further elaborated by the introduction of the notion of power: 'Vulnerable persons are those who are relatively (or absolutely) incapable of protecting their own interests. More formally, they may have insufficient power, intelligence, education, resources, strength, or other needed attributes to protect their own interests' (CIOMS, 2002: 44).

A common characteristic of the different versions of the restrictive conceptions of vulnerability, featuring in the literature as well as in contemporary guidelines and policy documents applicable to medical research, healthcare or bioethics, is that much attention is paid to identifying particular groups of individuals or sub-populations that may be rendered vulnerable in biomedical research and clinical practice (Flaskerud and Winslow, 1998; Reeder, 1999; Weijer, 1999; Backlar, 2000; Flanigan, 2000; Reeder, 2000; Zion et al., 2000; Aday, 2001, DeBruin, 2001; Blacksher and Stone, 2002; Danis and Patrick 2002; Stone, 2002; Leight, 2003; Macklin, 2003; Nickel, 2006). For example, in the *Belmont Report* and in the *Declaration of Helsinki* four especially vulnerable subgroups are mentioned, while in the CIOMS guidelines a total of 19 examples of such subgroups are listed (see Table 19.1).

Although lists of individuals and subgroups may provide useful guidance to researchers and health professionals with regard to identifying possible 'groups that share the category of vulnerability' (Luna, 2009: 122), such attempts at homogenously categorizing or labelling subgroups as vulnerable tend to overlook the need for differentiation within a group – the different kinds of vulnerabilities that individuals of the same subgroup may be susceptible to and from which they need protection.

These observations may help explain the emergence of the last category of conceptions of vulnerability, i.e. less rigid and more sensitive conceptions with regard to contextual considerations. Two such conceptions will here be analyzed, one focusing on the need for a layered understanding of vulnerability (Luna, 2009) and a second introducing a distinction between being persistently vulnerable, where vulnerability is conceived of as an essential feature of being human, and *contingent* or *variable* forms of vulnerability, that is to say susceptibility (O'Neill, 1996; Kottow, 2003 and 2004, Schramm, 2008).

The layered understanding of vulnerability emphasizes the importance of paying greater attention to *micro-contextual* considerations, of analyzing relations between particular persons or groups and particular circumstances and contexts. The second understanding, in contrast, advocates the need for a distinction between *macro-contextual* considerations due to persistent forms of vulnerability and lower level considerations due to contingent or variable forms of vulnerability.

Table 19.1   Examples of individuals, populations or communities deemed particularly vulnerable

Belmont Report	Declaration of Helsinki	CIOMS
Racial minorities	Individuals unable to give or refuse consent	Persons who are unable to consent
The economically disadvantaged	Individuals susceptible to coercion or undue influence	Children
The very sick	Populations or communities who will not derive direct benefits from participation	Junior or subordinate members of a hierarchical group (for example, medical and nursing students, subordinate hospital and laboratory personnel, employees of pharmaceutical companies and members of the armed forces or police)
The institutionalized	Patients undergoing medical research in combination with medical care	Elderly persons
		Residents of nursing homes
		People receiving welfare benefits or social assistance
		Poor people
		The unemployed
		Patients in emergency rooms
		Some ethnic and racial minority groups
		Homeless persons
		Nomads
		Refugees or displaced persons
		Prisoners
		Patients with incurable disease
		Individuals who are politically powerless
		Members of communities unfamiliar with modern medical concepts

The metaphor of layer has been introduced as a rhetorical device to rescue the moral force of this principle while at the same time avoiding some of the pitfalls of fixity, categorization and stereotyping typical of previous conceptions:

> The metaphor of a layer gives the idea of something 'softer', something that may be multiple and different, and that may be removed layer by layer. It is not 'a solid and unique vulnerability' that exhausts the category; there might be different vulnerabilities, different layers operating. These layers may overlap: some of them may be related to problems with informed consent, others to social circumstances. The idea of layers of vulnerability gives flexibility to the concept of vulnerability. (Luna, 2009: 127)

Flexibility is here meant in a double sense. Firstly, it is not necessary the case that all members of a particular subgroup that have been labelled vulnerable, as a consequence of applying a restrictive notion of vulnerability, are in fact vulnerable – or vulnerable in the same sense – and therefore indiscriminately in the need of (the same sort of) protection. Besides, there is a need for flexibility with regard to the opacity, diversity and multiplicity of contextual variables. These are variables that need to be carefully analyzed and sifted through – layer by layer, so to speak – in order to identify forms of protection that may prove adequate to the particularities presented by the actual situation. A layered approach to vulnerability may thus represent a sufficiently fine-tuned tool to deal with the 'micro-cosmos' of contingent vulnerabilities that humans may be subjected to in medical research and healthcare settings.

A characteristic feature of the notion of vulnerability operating with a distinction between persistent and variable forms of vulnerability is that it points to the need for a differentiation between at least two distinct regimes of protection. Firstly, a human rights-based regime aimed at protecting persistent or universal vulnerability. This regime requires *negative* action on the part of the State, in the sense that its responsibility is to guarantee 'basic liberties by securing a just social order that gives equal protection to the vulnerability of each citizen' (Kottow, 2003: 463). These protective measures are, however, in need of being supplemented by additional measures of protection – of *affirmative* action – to cope with accidental states and situations when human vulnerability is no longer intact. 'Fallen vulnerability' is a metaphor that has been suggested to label such situations (Kottow, 2004: 281), where individuals and populations are destitute. These are individuals or populations who have never been subjected to protection of their basic liberties, or they are no longer under such protection. They are not 'in command of their fundamental human rights'; they have become victims of 'injured integrity' and thus been deprived of their 'status of unharmed vulnerability' (Kottow, 2004: 281, 284). To cope with such accidental situations of susceptibility, it is not sufficient to rely on measures aimed at protecting basic liberties, as these liberties are no longer in place. What is needed are affirmative and context-sensitive actions of a social and remedial kind aimed at repairing the wounds of the susceptible thus bringing him/her/them back to a baseline state of *intact* vulnerability.

VULNERABILITY APPLIED

'The proof of the pudding is in the eating'. This old proverb might serve as a symbolic entrance to the last section of this chapter, where some practical implications of applying different conceptions of vulnerability in medical research and healthcare settings will be addressed. This brings us back to Article 8 of the *Universal Declaration on Bioethics and Human Rights*. This article on close reading unveils the combination of two different understandings of vulnerability: on the one hand, a stream of thought taking its inspiration from European philosophy – mainly continental philosophy (Mirandola, 1486 [1997]; Hobbes, 1651 [1978]; Herder, 1772 [1966]; Levinas, 1961; Jonas, 1979 and Habermas, 1991) – and developed by the European group of scholars previously mentioned, where vulnerability is conceived of as the human condition par excellence, something persistent and indelible, evoking respect; on the other hand, an understanding of vulnerability prevalent in guidelines and policy documents applicable to medical research, healthcare or bioethics and promoted by Anglo-American scholars in bioethics who imply a particular and relative classification of persons and populations in need of additional protection. Thus, the formulations in Article 8 of the Declaration may rightly be seen as an attempt to bring together two competing concepts of vulnerability (Patrão Neves, 2009: 161–2) and consequently, also two distinct moral regimes of protection. The first one is a human rights-based regime aimed at protecting persistent or universal vulnerability. This is the kind of vulnerability alluded to in the first sentence of the article: 'In applying and advancing scientific knowledge, medical practice and associated technologies, human vulnerability should be taken into account'.

The second regime aims at handling accidental states and situations of 'fallen' vulnerability: those forms of vulnerability that require additional measures of protection and identification of the particular persons and populations in need of protection against forms of harms and wrongs not covered by human rights-based regimes of protection. This is the kind of vulnerability alluded to in the second sentence of Article 8: 'Individuals and groups of special vulnerability should be protected and the personal integrity of such individuals respected'.

As observed by several authors (Kottow, 2003 and 2004; Patrão Neves, 2009), the broad conception of vulnerability proclaimed by the European group of scholars – and echoed in the first sentence of Article 8 of the *Universal Declaration on Bioethics and Human Rights* – lacks in itself prescriptive power. However, together with dignity (Article 3 of the same Declaration) and integrity (included in Article 8), vulnerability addresses 'essential features of human existence' (Kottow, 2004: 286) and may therefore, indirectly, 'inspire' the development of 'bioethical requirements of protection and respect for human rights in the wake of social justice' (Kottow, 2004: 281). In this respect, Article 8 of the Declaration may be viewed as the first bold step at global level towards developing a morally sustainable language of vulnerability:

> first [it] states the obligation of taking into consideration the vulnerability inherent to all human beings. That is to say, it is important to gain awareness of the fact that a person is vulnerable, is exposed to being 'touched' by the other, subject to diverse and often subtle forms of exploitation or abuse, irrespective of his/her level of autonomy.
>
> Secondly, it gives priority to individuals and groups classified as vulnerable, for whom it demands not only protection against being 'touched' but also respect for their integrity, so that they are not reduced to merely a part of themselves and so considered abstractly. (Patrão Neves, 2008: 161)

What are then the practical implications of such a broad and seemingly all-embracing conception of vulnerability, when comparing it with the minimalist candidates previously addressed as well as with the two conceptions mentioned above of less rigidity and higher sensitivity with regard to contextual considerations? The short answer to this question is that all these conceptions may be of use when it comes to identifying vulnerability in concrete situations:

- *Who* may potentially be exposed to additional forms of harm and wrong?
- *What* forms of susceptibility and layers of vulnerability need to be taken into particular consideration?
- *What* contextual variables require special attention?
- *What* kind of additional forms of harm and wrong may potentially be at play?
- *What* additional measures of protection – of *affirmative* action – need to be installed?
- *Whose* obligation is it to install such additional measures in situations of 'fallen' vulnerability?

Thus, such conceptions may also prove instrumental in relation to the implementation and practical application of the second part of Article 8 of the *Universal Declaration on Bioethics and Human Rights*. Alternatively, there are strong reasons against applying these conceptions – including the layered conception of vulnerability – in research or healthcare settings – lacking the kind of base-line protection of persistent fragility alluded to in the first sentence of Article 8. For this may lead to a conflation of alterable forms of vulnerability – and therefore susceptibility – with persistent fragility. If *alterable* forms of vulnerability are perceived as *unalterable* – as being part of the realm of persistent vulnerability which falls under the protective power and responsibility of states, a conflation of protective responsibilities may be the result. This is a problem that has been particularly discussed in international health research (Attaran, 1999; Angell 2000; Kottow, 2000 and 2003, Solbakk, 2004a and b; London 2005; Garrafa and Lorenzo, 2008), giving rise to concerns and charges that researchers from affluent countries and sponsor nations of clinical trials in low-income countries are inclined to abuse the notion of vulnerability to justify the application of double standards in research for health:

> The undiscriminating talk about vulnerable populations has triggered the kind of reactions that smuggle the susceptible under the category of the vulnerable and forgets to give them special consideration, based on the assumption that vulnerability is a human given that elicits no individual responsibilities or obligations beyond the state's protection ...
>
> Defenders of double standards in research ethics are regarding subjects of host countries as vulnerable, immersed in a state of frailty that may be deplorable but requires no outside effort to improve care and protection beyond what is locally available. Were they to be considered as susceptible individuals, it would become clear that sponsor countries are showing indifference to harm and neglect, ignoring the deprivations they confront and failing to exercise the social virtues of palliating destitution of their research subjects. (Kottow, 2003: 466, 467)

Such concerns illustrate not only the potential pitfalls of minimalist notions of vulnerability (London, 2005: 27–8), but also the protective power embedded in a conception of vulnerability of a dual nature. Thus, paradoxically speaking, for the principle of vulnerability not to lose its moral force it needs to be embedded in the human condition of unalterable vulnerability. Only in this way will it be possible to proclaim vulnerability as a universal principle and protect it from becoming an instrument of abuse and exploitation in the hands of moral relativists.

CONCLUSIONS

During the last 20 years or so the principle of vulnerability has been attributed with a steadily increasing role and prominence in national and international guidelines and policy documents applicable to medical research, healthcare or bioethics. The culmination in this regard was marked in 2005 by the integration of this principle into the *Universal Declaration on Bioethics and Human Rights*. Also in the scholarly literature in bioethics and healthcare ethics the principle of vulnerability has been the focus of vivid attention and scrutiny. Looking back at these debates it is possible to trace the emergence of two seemingly conflicting orientations. On the one hand, the emergence of a whole range of restrictive or minimalist conceptions of vulnerability aimed at identifying and categorizing individuals, groups and populations as vulnerable and tracing the different forms of vulnerability that needs to be overcome. On the other hand, a human rights-based approach to vulnerability, differentiating between inalterable forms of vulnerability that require state protection and accidental forms of vulnerability, that is to say susceptibility, that need to be handled by additional measures of protection. Article 8 of the *Universal Declaration on Bioethics and Human Rights* represents the first bold step at the global level towards promoting a conception of vulnerability of a dual nature. In this way, it has also become possible to proclaim vulnerability as a universal principle, while at the same time acknowledging the need for developing a language of vulnerability capable of prescribing context-sensitive measures of protection.

REFERENCES

Aday, L.A. (2001) *At Risk in America: The Health and Health Care Needs of Vulnerable Populations in the United States*. San Francisco, LA: Jossey-Bass.

Alwang, J., Siegel, P.B. and Jorgensen, S.L. (2002) 'Vulnerability as viewed from different disciplines', paper presented at International Symposium Sustaining Food Security and Managing Natural Resources in Southeast Asia: Challenges for the 21st Century. Chiang Mai, Thailand, 8–11 January.

Angell, M. (2000) 'Investigator's responsibilities for human subjects in developing countries', *New England Journal of Medicine*, 342: 967–9.

Attaran, A. (1999) 'Human rights and biomedical research funding for the developing world: Discovering state obligations under the right to health', *Health and Human Rights,* 4 (1): 27–58.

Backlar, P. (2000) 'Human Subjects Research, Ethics, Research on Vulnerable Populations', in T.H. Murray and M.J. Mehlman (eds), *Encyclopedia of Ethical, Legal, and Policy Issues in Biotechnology*. New York: John Wiley & Sons, pp. 641–50.

Beauchamp, T.L. and Childress, J.F. (2009) *Principles of Biomedical Ethics*. Oxford: Oxford University Press.

Belmont Report (1979) National Commission for the Protection of Human Subjects of Biomedical and Behavioral Research. The Belmont Report: *Ethical Principles and Guidelines for the Protection of Human Subjects*.

Blacksher, E. and Stone, J.R. (2002) 'Introduction to "vulnerability" issues of theoretical medicine and bioethics', *Theoretical Medicine and Bioethics*, 23 (6): 421–4.

Botbol-Baum, M. (2000) 'The necessary articulation of autonomy and vulnerability', in J.D. Rendtorff and P. Kemp (eds), *Basic Ethical Principles in Bioethics and Biolaw, Vol. II: Partners Research*. Copenhagen and Barcelona: Centre for Ethics and Law, and Institut Borja de Bioètica, pp. 57–64.

Council for International Organizations of Medical Sciences (CIOMS) (2002) *International Ethical Guidelines for Biomedical Research Involving Human Subjects*.

Danis, M. and Patrick, D.L. (2002) 'Vulnerability, and vulnerable populations', in L.R. Churchill (ed.), *Ethical Dimensions of Health Policy*. New York: Oxford University Press, pp. 310–34.

DeBruin, D. (2001) 'Reflections on "Vulnerability"', *Bioethics Examiner*, 5 (2): 1,4,7.

Della Mirandola, P. (1486 [1997]) Oratio de hominis dignitate / Rede über die Würde des Menschen, bilingual Latin/German edition. Stuttgart: Reclam.

Flanigan, R. (2000) 'Vulnerability and the bioethics movement', *Bioethics Forum* 16 (2): 13–18.

Flaskerud, J.H. and Winslow, B.J. (1998) 'Conceptualizing vulnerable populations: Health related research', *Nursing Research*, 47 (2): 69–78.

Garrafa, V. and Lorenzo, C. (2008) 'Moral imperialism and multi-centric clinical trials in peripheral countries', *Cadernos de Saúde Pública*, 24 (10): 219–26.

Habermas, J. (1991) *Erläuterungen zur Diskursethik*. Frankfurt am Main: Suhrkamp.

Herder, J.G. (1772 [1966]) *Abhandlung über den Ursprung der Sprache*. Stuttgart: Reclam.

Hobbes, T. (1651 [1978]) *Leviathan*. Glasgow: Collins/Fontana.

Hurst, S.A. (2008) 'Vulnerability in research and health care: Describing the elephant in the room?', *Bioethics*, 22 (4): 191–202.

Jonas, H. (1979) *Das Prinzip Verantwortung: Versuch einer Ethik für die technologische Zivilisation*. Frankfurt am Main: Suhrkamp.

Kottow, M.H. (2000) 'Who is my brother's keeper?', *Journal of Medical Ethics*, 28: 24–7.

Kottow, M.H. (2003) 'The vulnerable and the susceptible', *Bioethics*, 17 (5–6): 460–71.

Kottow, M.H. (2004) 'Vulnerability: What kind of principle is it?', *Medicine, Health Care and Philosophy*, 7: 281–7.

Leight, S.B. (2003) 'The application of a vulnerable population's conceptual model to rural health', *Public Health Nursing*, 20 (6): 440–8.

Levinas, E. (1961) *Totalité et infini*. Den Haag: Phenomenologica.

Levine, C., Faden, R., Grady, C. et al. (2004) 'The limitations of 'vulnerability' as a protection for human research participants', *American Journal of Bioethics*, (4) 3: 44–9.

London, A.J. (2005) 'Justice and the human development approach to international research', *Hastings Center Report*, 35 (1): 24–37.

Luna, F. (2009) 'Elucidating the concept of vulnerability. Layers not labels', *International Journal of Feminist Approaches to Bioethics* (IJFAB), 2 (1): 120–38.

Macklin, R. (2003) 'Bioethics, vulnerability, and protection', *Bioethics*, 17: 472–86.

Morawa, A.H.E. (2003) 'Vulnerability as a concept in international human rights law', *Journal of International Relations and Development*, 6 (2): 139–55.

Nickel, P.J. (2006) 'Vulnerable populations in research: The case of the seriously ill', *Theoretical Medicine and Bioethics*, 27: 245–64.

O'Neill, O. (1996) *Towards Justice and Virtue*. Cambridge: Cambridge University Press, pp. 192–93.

Patrão Neves, M. (2009) 'Respect for human vulnerability and personal integrity', in H.A.M. ten Have and M.S. Jean (eds), *The UNESCO Universal Declaration on Bioethics and Human Rights. Background, Principles and Application* [Ethics Series]. Paris: UNESCO, pp. 155–64.

Reeder, R. (1999) 'Special issue on vulnerable populations', *Bioethics Forum*, 15 (2).

Reeder, R. (2000) 'Special issue on vulnerability and the bioethics movement', *Bioethics Forum*, 16 (2).

Rendtorff, J.D. (2002) 'Basic ethical principles in European bioethics and biolaw: Autonomy, dignity, integrity and vulnerability – Towards a foundation of bioethics and biolaw', *Medicine, Health Care and Philosophy*, 5: 235–44.

Rendtorff, J.D. and Kemp, P. (2000a) *Basic Ethical Principles in European Bioethics and Biolaw Autonomy, Vol. I, Dignity, Integrity and Vulnerability*. Copenhagen and Barcelona: Centre for Ethics and Law, and Institut Borja de Bioètica.

Rendtorff, J.D. and Kemp, P. (2000b) *Basic Ethical Principles in European Bioethics and Biolaw Autonomy, Vol. II, Partners' Research*. Copenhagen and Barcelona: Centre for Ethics and Law, and Institut Borja de Bioètica, pp. 57–64.

Ruof, M.C. (2004) 'Vulnerability, vulnerable populations, and policy', *Kennedy Institute of Ethics Journal*, 14 (4): 411–25.

Schramm, F.R. (2008) 'Bioethics of protection: A proposal for the moral problems of developing countries?', *Journal international de bioéthique* [International Journal of Bioethics], 19: 73–86.

Solbakk, J.H. (1994) 'Towards a conceptual framework for an ethics of diversity', in Z. Bankowski and J. Bryant (eds), *Vulnerability, the Value of Human life, and the Emergence of Bioethics: Highlights and papers* of the XXVIIIth CIOMS Conference, Ixtapa, Mexico, 17–20 April. Geneva: WHO, pp. 231–3.

Solbakk, J.H. (2004a) 'Use and abuse of empirical knowledge in contemporary bioethics. A critical analysis of empirical arguments employed in the controversy surrounding studies of maternal-fetal HIV-transmission and HIV-prevention in developing countries', *Medicine, Health Care and Philosophy*, 7: 5–16.

Solbakk, J.H. (2004b) 'Uses and abuses of biomedical research', in *Ethical Eye: Biomedical Research*. Strasbourg Cedex: Council of Europe, pp. 35–50.

Stone, J.R. (2002) 'Race and healthcare disparities: Overcoming vulnerability', *Theoretical Medicine and Bioethics*, 23 (6): 499–518.

UNESCO (2005) *Universal Declaration of Bioethics and Human Rights*. Accessible at http://portal.unesco.org/shs/en/ev.php-URL_ID=1883&URL_DO=DO_TOPIC&URL_SECTION=201.html.

Weijer, C. (1999) 'Research involving the vulnerable sick', *Accountability in Research*, 7 (1): 21–36.

World Medical Association (WMA) (2008) *Declaration of Helsinki*. Accessible at http://www.wma.net/e/ethicsunit/helsinki.htm.

Zion, D., Gillam, L. and Loff, B. (2000) 'The Declaration of Helsinki, CIOMS and the ethics of research on vulnerable populations', *Nature Medicine*, 6: 615–17.

20

Vulnerability in Healthcare and Research Ethics

Agomoni Ganguli-Mitra and
Nikola Biller-Andorno

VULNERABILITY AS ENCOUNTERED IN THE BIOETHICS LITERATURE

Commonly encountered mechanisms to protect the interests of patients and research participants include standard practices such as securing consent, risk–benefit assessments, the protection of confidentiality and an ethics review. However, certain individuals considered particularly 'vulnerable' are normally afforded special attention within bioethical frameworks. With the changing face of healthcare and biomedical research in a globalized world, the term 'vulnerable' as well as its adequate definition and scope have increasingly come under close scrutiny.

Some scholars have proposed moving away from a narrow – and often unclear – use of the term in favour of a comprehensive understanding of vulnerability, reflecting human finitude and fragility (Rendtorff, 2002). However, many insist that the only useful understanding of vulnerability within the bioethical discourse is one that indicates an increased susceptibility to harm or exploitation. They argue that a characteristic of human beings *qua* human cannot be extended as a protective principle or special category (Kottow, 2004).

Indeed, the normative language encountered in the bioethics literature as well as in relevant guidelines and declarations usually reflects a use of the term in this narrower sense: a variable and selective vulnerability, distinct from the 'species vulnerabilities' (O'Neill, 1996: 192) that is characteristic of human beings.

In the current discourse, individuals are considered vulnerable if they are susceptible to being harmed, wronged, exploited, mistreated, discriminated against or taken advantage of in the context of healthcare and research. Being designated 'vulnerable' usually warrants special protection in these contexts since vulnerability is understood as 'an identifiably increased likelihood of incurring additional or greater wrong' (Hurst, 2008: 191). As such, the concept and use of the term has an important impact not only in the bioethical discourse but is also particularly relevant to policy, ethical frameworks, guidelines as well as legal provisions in research and medical care.

Historically, the definition of vulnerability has usually revolved around autonomy (or the lack of it) but the use of the term today has become increasingly inclusive of other characteristics, leading to diverse categories and different ethical approaches. Categories of vulnerable groups have traditionally included children, pregnant women, minorities, prisoners, and people with mental and physical disabilities. Unfortunately, this categorization has often led to paternalistic and exclusionary practices, especially in the context of research. Today the designation of vulnerability has come to be better understood as a matter of degree that varies with the social, cultural, or economic context the individual finds her/himself in, rather than a stringent categorization to be measured against the ability to give consent or to make an autonomous choice. However, while a more flexible or comprehensive account adds to the richness of the ethical debate, it also adds to the complexity of policy-making, which usually makes use of distinct categories and specific definitions for reasons of efficiency and precision.

Over the last decade or so, the concept of vulnerability has further expanded to include larger and more heterogeneous groups, adding characteristics such as poverty, lack of education and other socio-economic factors to the discussion. Macklin (2003: 474), for example, talks about the vulnerability of groups within emerging and developing countries, in relation to researchers and sponsors from a powerful industrial country or a giant pharmaceutical company. In fact, the use of vulnerability has now become so widespread in the bioethical literature that some commentators question its strength and adequacy. Levine and colleagues (2004) have argued that 'so many categories of people are now considered vulnerable that virtually all potential human subjects are included' and that as a result the concept has become 'too nebulous to be meaningful'.

Many commentators agree on the inadequacy of the concept and yet it continues to have a strong pull within the bioethical discourse, similar to notions such as human dignity. The trouble with vulnerability is that while it can, like dignity, be applied to all human beings by virtue of our inbuilt finitude and fragility, it must also account for the special protection afforded to the 'more' vulnerable. For example, individuals who lack basic rights and freedoms are in many ways more vulnerable than the rest of the population (Zion et al., 2000: 615), but it remains unclear how this type of vulnerability may play out in the particular contexts of healthcare and research. It is not clear that doing away with the term would be appropriate, however. In reply to Levine's article, it has been argued that vulnerability, although nebulous, is a 'precautionary principle of human research protection (Grinnell, 2004: 72) and remains a 'needed moral safeguard' (DeMarco, 2004: 83).

Efforts have been made in recent years to further elucidate the meaning and proper use of the concept. In contrast to the traditional autonomy-based understanding of vulnerability, Kipnis (2001) offers a context-sensitive approach, which includes the following six categories:

- cognitive and communicative vulnerability (including cognitive impairment, language difficulties, stressful and emergency situations);
- institutional vulnerability (with the examples of students and prisoners);
- deferential vulnerability (where hierarchy exists but is not formal, such as class, gender, race or trust in one's physician);
- medical vulnerability (for example when seriously ill persons are drawn to research because of unrealistic expectations);

- economic vulnerability (which may lead to undue inducement);
- social vulnerability (when participants belong to an undervalued social group).

Kipnis's categorization goes a long way towards correcting the inadequacy of a purely autonomy-based understanding of vulnerability. In particular, it illustrates that vulnerability is not necessarily intrinsic to the individual, but rather sometimes a mismatch between a characteristic of the individual and the context in which she/he finds her/himself. However, any such categorization is bound to contain gaps and as Kipnis points out, many overlaps. A look at the details of the context must also take into account one of the root causes of such vulnerability: a reflection of an existing unfair state of affairs. Such an assessment would also need to be sensitive to the fact that individuals are vulnerable in certain contexts where they are interrelated with others. For example, participants with few economic resources may be vulnerable in relation to sponsors from the industrialized countries but not necessarily by default, nor for that matter, in relation to each other. Nickel (2006) partly addresses this problem when he proposes that there are consent-based and fairness-based reasons – as opposed to categories – to call individuals or groups vulnerable.

It seems appropriate to use a broad approach – encompassing fairness-based and consent-based reasons – in an effort to capture vulnerability within a global picture of bioethics. We have chosen here to separate the competence and voluntary components of consent, dividing the concept into three broad groups: competence, voluntariness and fairness.

According to this distinction a competence-based understanding of vulnerability would essentially include limited or diminished cognitive capacities. This is best illustrated by the incapability or diminished capability of giving consent or refusing to either being treated or to participating in research, a category that is also most easily recognized by law. Competence-based vulnerability would include children, those suffering from acute mental or behavioural disorder or a critical illness that renders them incapable of giving informed consent. Such a characteristic may also express itself in certain forms of acute but temporary depression, or in certain situations of emergency. Keeping in mind that there is no 'gold standard' for measuring competence (Karlawish, 2007: 614), even such a restricted characteristic might prove difficult to distinguish.

It is important to distinguish between competence and voluntariness, however. Failing to do so results in apparently counter-intuitive if not unduly paternalistic categorization, by for example, putting those cognitively impaired and those who are otherwise prone to undue inducement into the same category. A voluntariness-based approach would include those who have full cognitive capacity but are still susceptible to coercion, manipulation, inducement, misconception or exploitation. This category is broader and less stringent than the first one and might include extrinsic and context-based characteristics that can render individuals less able to look after their own interests, or that might render them susceptible to being influenced by another (more powerful) party. Such vulnerability might be exacerbated by poverty, illness, education and other socially variable factors, many of which cannot be countered solely by elaborate informed consent processes.

The third approach to vulnerability is a fairness-based one and also one to be understood as a broad category. Vulnerability arising from injustice has a range of causes, including poverty, lack of freedom and access to opportunity. This type of vulnerability, however, is not necessarily expressed in terms of lack of power or voluntariness in decision-making processes and goes beyond the idea of protection through informed consent. It is rather pervasive to the context in which persons access medical care or participate in research. For example, in discussing healthcare and discrimination, Francis describes vulnerability as a 'call to remedy injustice' (Francis, 2007: 164). This type of vulnerability would affect poorer sections of society, minorities and marginalized groups as well as groups who, due to injustice and discrimination in history, are inherently suspicious of the healthcare system. In the context of research these would include those who have been especially targeted for research because of their availability. But increasingly, such a label may fit those who have been systematically excluded from research, either because they do not fit the research agenda or because they have been avoided due to exclusionary and paternalistic protective mechanisms, and therefore can never enjoy the benefits of medical progress.

Taking the example of risk to physical and psychological harm, vulnerability from the perspective of competence would mean an inability to adequately assess risk. Vulnerability expressed in the voluntariness category would be illustrated in a situation where a person is prepared to take on risks that may otherwise be unreasonable, because of her/his relative lack of power, the incentives offered or because she/he has few other choices. From the fairness perspective, vulnerability could be expressed by a propensity to be systematically recruited for (or excluded from) research. These perspectives are not mutually exclusive but may in fact co-exist and influence each other. For example, contexts can be so unfair that voluntariness may be questioned, making participants vulnerable at two different levels. Protective mechanisms are structured in the same multi-layered way: When participants or patients have 'passed the test' of competence and of 'voluntariness' they may still be 'caught' in the safety net of a fairness-based mechanism.

VULNERABILITY IN HEALTHCARE

Whereas the use of the term 'vulnerable populations' has been criticized from a health policy perspective as representing an unduly essentialist concept inviting resentment from and discrimination of those who find themselves categorized this way (Danis and Donald, 2002), the hermeneutic value of perceiving the individual patient as a vulnerable 'other' has been emphasized for the clinical encounter (Reeder, 2000; Zaner, 2000). Onora O'Neill suggests that, 'a person who is ill or injured is highly vulnerable to others, and highly dependent on their action and competence' (2002: 38). However, even in the context of illness, respecting the autonomous wishes and choice of a patient remains a central tenet of medical ethics. Medical care involves putting one's interest in the hands of health professionals, but in most cases it does not involve surrendering our decision making and preferences entirely to others.

The most commonly encountered standard to measure vulnerability in healthcare revolves around competence and capacity to give informed consent. A 'settled principle of medical ethics, the law, and medical practice is that physicians may not render medical care to competent patients without their informed consent' (Brock, 2007: 128). Brock identifies three main pillars of autonomous decision making: it must be informed, voluntary and competent. Vulnerability in this context can be seen as lacking the information or capacity to make a competent choice or as a disposition to give in to another person's influence. In these cases, additional protective mechanisms, such as surrogate decision making or best interest standards, come into play (see other chapters on mental health and on children in this volume).

Competence aside, vulnerability is also an inherent characteristic of various other clinical contexts. It is clear that illness – accompanied by diagnosis, treatment and care in institutional or interpersonal settings – can affect voluntariness. Beauchamp and Childress define voluntariness as willing an action without being under the control of another's influence (2001: 93). Such a criterion may be difficult to meet, especially in the context of severe illness, which frequently brings with it situations of significant dependence on physicians, nurses or relatives. Influences that ordinarily are resistible can become controlling: 'What a health professional intends as rational persuasion can irrationally influence the patient by attacking his or her vulnerabilities' (Beauchamp and Childress, 2001: 97). But even healthy persons can be vulnerable in this regard, as the case of living organ donation illustrates: social pressure, the concern for a loved one, the opportunity to gain status within the family system and many other factors may compromise voluntariness (Biller-Andorno and Schauenburg, 2001). When concentrating on competence alone, it is easy to miss or ignore other forms of susceptibilities, resulting in a failure to afford adequate protection to the vulnerable. At the same time, perceived vulnerability when actual vulnerability is absent can also lead to unethical actions. There have been cases where residents of nursing homes, because of their limited mobility and other age-related characteristics, have been overridden in their decision making on account of their perceived lack of capacity (Beauchamp and Childress, 2001: 97). Such situations not only compound existing vulnerabilities but can lead to ethically unacceptable practices.

Upholding the *telos* of healthcare as inextricably linked to the interests and preferences of patients remains one of the best protective measures for vulnerable patients. Meeting the requirements of autonomy and protection and finding the right balance when best interests and preferences of vulnerable patients seem to conflict is an especially challenging task. The problem becomes even more complex when we try to approach vulnerability from the perspective of fairness and justice. However, such an approach is necessary to give a full picture of vulnerability.

For example, vulnerability can result from having inadequate or no access to healthcare in the first place. Such situations are commonly encountered by immigrants, certain marginalized populations and ethnic minorities (Reeder, 1999). Another example concerns certain rationing choices made by healthcare providers, even where the resulting discrimination is not intentional. In age-based rationing, defending a prognosis can be highly unfair, for example to those who have already suffered life-long injustices. Moreover, such an approach may result from a misjudgement regarding prognosis, wronging those who are already medically vulnerable: 'For many years, patients with Alzheimer's dementia were routinely rejected for physical therapy, or mental health visits, by Medicare carriers in the United States, on the misjudgement that they could not benefit from the care' (Francis, 2007: 171).

This brings us back to O'Neill who questions whether the concept of autonomy and more importantly the procedure of informed consent is sufficient to uphold the interest of patients (2002: 40). The prohibition of paying for live organ donation, for instance, has been criticized as pure paternalism and an intolerable infringement on the few choices of the poor, whereas rich people were at more liberty to take risks for more trivial matters than trying to make a living (Radcliffe-Richards et al., 1998). Although it is worth remaining cautious of excessive protectionism vis-à-vis certain groups who are deemed vulnerable, the argument misses the point. It focuses on the competence level of vulnerability only, ascertaining the decision-making capacity of the poor and requiring potential educational efforts. It does not, however, address the voluntariness and fairness levels. A study from Iran (Zargooshi, 2001), so far the only country with a regulated kidney market, has shown that many vendors make their decisions under conditions that can hardly be described by terms such as 'voluntariness' or 'free choice'. Another study from India (Goyal et al., 2002) has shown that people who have sold a kidney within a non-regulated market setting fared worse than previously in terms of their health and economic status, showing the structural vulnerability for exploitation and coercion that comes with poverty. Recognizing vulnerability related to justice and fairness will become increasingly relevant in an era of globalization and healthcare systems that are characterized by institutionalization, commercialization and a move away from the traditional focus on the doctor–patient dynamic.

VULNERABILITY IN RESEARCH

Unlike medical care, the main purpose of biomedical research is to produce generalizable knowledge for the benefit of current and future patients. While in healthcare, the central focus remains the interests of the patients, the paradigmatic research situation must reconcile two competing interests, that of society, which might benefit from successful research and that of participants who volunteer to take part. In most cases other additional interests come into play, such as profit for sponsors and professional advancement for researchers.

Because of this shift in focus, stringent and elaborate mechanisms are usually in place to protect participants from harm and exploitation. Such mechanisms usually divide the responsibilities amongst participants, researchers, sponsors and review committees and never rely solely on the autonomous choice of those who volunteer to take part. Most regulatory frameworks have arisen as a result of abuses carried out by researchers on vulnerable individuals such as prisoners, children and ethnic minorities and guidelines are in place to avoid coercive measures, undue inducement, exploitation and harm.

With regard to participants who are considered to be vulnerable from the point of view of *competence* (children and adults with serious mental disorders, for example), strict guidelines are in place to protect them from abuse. In such cases, research is usually considered permissible only when the research contains minimal risk; it cannot be carried out on a 'non-vulnerable' population, if it holds potential for direct benefit to the group. Unfortunately, because competence, voluntariness and other factors contributing to vulnerability are not always clearly defined, the boundary between protection and paternalistic exclusion is often unclear.

The *Declaration of Helsinki* (WMA, 2004), for example, has specific guidelines for children and individuals considered legally incompetent (2004: para. 25–6), those who are in a dependent relationship with a physician or may consent under duress (2004: para. 23). The Declaration also addresses vulnerability as an umbrella concept, stating that

> [s]ome research populations are vulnerable and need special protection. The particular needs of the economically and medically disadvantaged must be recognized. Special attention is also required for those who cannot give or refuse consent for themselves, for those who may be subject to giving consent under duress, for those who will not benefit personally from the research and for those for whom the research is combined with care. (World Medical Association, 2004: para. 8)

The Declaration addresses both intrinsic reasons (competence) and context-dependent factors (economic disadvantage) and concerns of fairness (participation without personal benefit). The different sources of vulnerability (competence, voluntariness and fairness) are combined and there is no clear indication as to the scope of the special protection required.

In the US, the Federal Policy for the Protection of Human Subjects, informally known as the 'Common Rule', included in 45 Code of Federal Regulations (CFR, 2005), part 46, remains a particularly controversial framework in this regard, referring to vulnerable groups as including children, prisoners, pregnant women, handicapped or mentally disabled persons, and fetuses. Additional requirements of protection include the restriction to participate in research with minimal risk unless there is potential direct benefit to the mother or the fetus. Characterizing pregnant women as vulnerable has been criticized as paternalistic and many guidelines today avoid this terminology, while affording special protection to pregnant women.

The Council of Europe's Convention on Human Rights and Biomedicine makes no reference to vulnerability in particular. It has, however, specific, restrictive guidelines for those unable to give informed consent, whose participation in research is only allowed when it entails 'minimal risk and minimal burden' (Art. 17, II, ii) (Council of Europe, 1997).

Finally, one of the most widely used international research guidelines, the CIOMS *International Ethical Guidelines for Biomedical Research Involving Human Subjects*, approaches the topic of vulnerability from different angles (CIOMS, 2002). Guideline 9 is restricted to individuals who are not capable of giving informed consent. This includes those with limited cognitive capacity and prisoners, combining the competence and voluntariness-based understanding of vulnerability. Such participants are afforded the equivalent of the minimal risk criteria. In contrast to the *Declaration of Helsinki*, the CIOMS document has a specific guideline for research in populations with 'limited resources', which, for that reason, are vulnerable to exploitation (Guideline 10). Such research must address the health needs of the population and successful products of research must be made 'reasonably available'. Guideline 13, entitled 'Research involving vulnerable persons', sets up a general principle according to which 'special justification is required for inviting vulnerable individuals to serve as research subjects and, if they are selected, the means of protecting their rights and welfare must be strictly applied'.

The Commentary on this Guideline explains that 'vulnerable persons are those who are relatively (or absolutely) incapable of protecting their own interests. More formally, they may have insufficient power, intelligence, education, resources, strength, or other needed attributes to protect their own interests'. Guidelines 14 and 15 deal more specifically with different categories of persons regarded as vulnerable such as children, individuals with mental and behavioural disorders, women and pregnant women. Moreover, CIOMS specifies 'other vulnerable groups' as including hierarchical subordinates (medical students, for example), elderly persons and those institutionalized, residents of nursing homes, people receiving welfare benefits, the poor and the unemployed, some ethnic and racial minorities, homeless persons, nomads, refugees, or displaced persons, prisoners, patients with incurable disease, individual who are politically powerless, and members of communities unfamiliar with modern medical concepts (see also Chapter 19, Table 19.1).

While CIOMS begins with a category similar to those found in earlier guidelines, its inclusion of 'other vulnerable groups' and those who have 'attributes resembling those classes identified as vulnerable' is a perfect case to illustrate the difficulty in pinpointing the intuitively powerful concept of vulnerability. This gives strength to the criticism by Levine et al. of the concept being 'too broad and too narrow' but also reiterates the importance of taking into account factors that are far more subtle and complex than competence and cognitive abilities. Moreover, in terms of normative guidelines, CIOMS fails where other guidelines have failed. In cases of clear vulnerability, such as incompetence, it offers clear procedures of protection and restriction, however, as the classes of vulnerability become broader and less clearly defined, CIOMS also collapses into unclear recommendations, stating that 'the need for special protection of their rights and welfare should be reviewed and applied, where relevant'. Without clear guidance as to what special protections may entail or how to detect relevance, review bodies and protective mechanisms may fail miserably in addressing such vulnerabilities or may resort to inadequate and paternalistic protective measures.

Protection becomes even more delicate when we address vulnerability from the perspective of *voluntariness*. What may appear to be voluntary consent to participate may in fact be the result of various influencing factors, such as dependence on authority or poverty. At the same time, categorizing all poor communities or ethnic minorities as vulnerable can be unduly paternalistic, leading to harm in the long term because benefits do not accrue to them as they do to other groups (Nickel, 2006: 248). Women, especially pregnant women, have historically been excluded from research and as a result also from the successful products of research (Dresser, 1992: 24), a situation which, in the long term increases the vulnerability of the group, depriving them of the benefits of research and exposing them to inadequate therapy and preventive methods.

Vulnerability from the point of view of *power relations* can be more or less obvious. In the case of prisoners, for example, the effect of authority over voluntariness can perhaps be more easily addressed, given the obvious dependency and lack of freedom. Other forms of authority act more subtly and yet perhaps as potently. Research in the clinical context is perhaps a good example of this problem. The trust involved in the patient–physician relationship may act as a powerful inducement to participate in research, especially if this takes place within a 'care' setting. There have been reports that physicians offering participation in research are often also interpreted as endorsing participation (Kass et al., 1996).

Although the topic of financial compensation for participation often arises in the discussion on voluntariness, it remains unclear as to what type of payment would be adequate compensation for participation and would not be considered undue inducement, especially to those considered vulnerable. Much of the discourse has centred on participants with limited economic resources, such as populations from developing countries, where the effects of both power and inducement can be highly exacerbated, especially because in such contexts economic disadvantage is often on a par with lower levels of education and understanding and as a result the suitability of informed consent might be highly question-able (Luna, 2007: 626). It is often argued that in such circumstances, participants are more likely to enrol in high-risk research if there are benefits, especially financial benefits. However, some scholars have reported on studies showing that financial compensation does not necessary lead participants with limited economic resources to disregard study risks (Denny and Grady, 2007: 383).

This debate is also closely related to fairness in research. Participants in this situation may be induced into enrolling into exploitative research that offers benefits because they are in a situation of disadvantage. In response to this concern, Denny and Grady (2007) suggest that benefits offered in a study should be considered fair both from the point of view of those who are economically disadvantaged and those who are not. However, in such situations, vulnerability may go well beyond financial factors. For example, a lack of infrastructure for a rigorous local review or even lax legislation may render participants vulnerable to exploitative research whether or not consent is voluntary and adequate. In this case, fair benefits would certainly not be adequate in addressing vulnerability. Nor would fair benefits automatically make an unfair research setting fairer; for example, while there has been an over 400 percent increase in international research (Benatar, 2007: 10), the health needs of the economically and educationally vulnerable are still not being adequately addressed. Against this background of a global research agenda, vulnerability from the perspective of fairness still requires a reasonable amount of attention.

VULNERABILITY AT THE INTERSECTION BETWEEN RESEARCH AND HEALTHCARE

There are two ways in which research and healthcare may intersect, and both have an effect on the vulnerability discourse. Although they have been mentioned earlier in this chapter, it is worth looking at them more explicitly. The first is a genuine combination of healthcare and research, that is, research undertaken using participants already suffering from an illness, and the second is a perceived combination, more commonly known as the therapeutic misconception.

In the first case, there may be an 'inherent conflict in the physician-investigator role' (Henderson et al., 2004: 50): that of the carer for her/his patients, and that of the researcher contributing to the generation of useful knowledge. There is no clear agreement as to whether patients, in general, should be considered vulnerable because of the trust they have in their physician or whether they are so only in certain cases, for example, if they suffer from an incurable illness. According to Nickel, such individuals are particularly vulnerable when it comes to deciding to participate in research: 'Seriously ill persons are, by virtue of their special vulnerability, less able to evaluate rationally whether they ought to participate' (Nickel, 2006: 256). While this is related to consent, it might sometimes be expressed as vulnerability due to lack of voluntariness and at other times, due to lack of competence. Another such example is the case of research within emergency situations, where 'planned risky but important emergency research that has been independently reviewed and approved but for which truly meaningful informed consent cannot be obtained' (Brody, 1998: 34). Again, guidelines have conflicting recommendations, some only allowing minimal risk in the context of emergency research, others allowing risky research when it is intended for the direct health benefit of the patient (Brody, 1998: 33–34). Brody further points out the need to consider several factors: the vulnerability of the subjects, the possible benefits to them, the need to protect them from the risks of the research, the possibility of getting some degree of consent beforehand and the possibility of finding other participants for this research.

Consideration related to the fairness of the social context in which research takes place is also relevant here. In research conducted in emerging and developing countries, research is often not only mixed with healthcare but often constitutes the only access to healthcare. Whether this type of situation always leads to exploitative research is a matter of disagreement (Denny and Grady, 2006: 384), but that a certain amount of vulnerability exists in this situation is fairly obvious.

Finally, the therapeutic misconception, itself subject to much current discussion and debate, is an illustration of vulnerability often encountered in the research setting. One of the keys to the protection of research subjects is that they must clearly understand they are taking part in research and not therapy, unless there is a clear indication that an experimental treatment may have therapeutic benefits. In many randomized, placebo-controlled trials, however, patients need to clearly understand that they will not or are unlikely to benefit from participation. Nevertheless, many participants may enrol under the false belief that they would somehow benefit from research; this is known as the therapeutic misconception. It may lead to an 'overestimation of benefit, underestimation of risk of harm, or of existing alternatives to participation' (Henderson et al., 2007). Current research suggests that up to 70 per cent of participants may suffer from therapeutic misconception (Appelbaum, 2002). This phenomenon may be even more prevalent in the international context, where participants with lower economic and educational resources may more easily fall prey to such misconceptions.

CONCLUSION

Reasons for vulnerability are heterogeneous: limited capacities, or competence, are just one factor, which can be appropriately addressed by surrogate decision making or by acting according to the patient's presumed preferences or, if those are unknown, in what is judged to be his/her best interest. The other main reasons – lack of voluntariness and lack of fairness – need to be dealt with through other mechanisms, which aim at interpersonal relationships, and, even more intricate, the social fabric of an institution or community.

The vulnerability of an 'other' imposes certain moral obligations on us: the negative obligation not to exploit the situation, and possibly also a positive obligation to protect the vulnerable other, but at the same time to help him/her overcome this state, if at all possible. Integrating protection and empowerment is a formidable challenge, as is identifying the border between necessary protection and excessive and potentially harmful protectionism.

Long-standing discussions in clinical and research ethics, for example on child assent or on the inclusion of pregnant women in research trials, illustrate these difficulties.

Vulnerability is a useful concept in bioethics. Certainly not as a simple black or white category but as a gradual, dynamic, multifaceted concept that can inspire the search for the right moral response. 'Who' has 'what' responsibility in the face of 'whose' vulnerability is becoming an increasingly complex question in an era of globalization, as illustrated by the intense discussion on sponsors' responsibilities in international clinical trials, including in emerging and developing countries. In order to approach these questions in a more systematic way, further research is needed on: the evolution of vulnerability from a mismatch between an individual's capacities and his/her environment; the perspective of groups and individuals deemed 'vulnerable'; the special moral obligations that vulnerability entails; and ways to reduce the structural or contextual causes of vulnerability.

REFERENCES

Appelbaum, P.S. (2002) 'Clarifying the ethics of clinical research: A path toward avoiding the therapeutic misconception', *American Journal of Bioethics*, 2 (2): 22–3.

Beauchamp, T.L. and Childress, J.F. (2001) *Principles of Biomedical Ethics*, 5th ed. Oxford and New York: Oxford University Press.

Benatar, S.R. (2007) 'New perspectives on international research ethics', in T.T. Matti Häyry and P. Herissone-Kelly (eds), *Ethics in Biomedical Research*. Amsterdam and New York: Rodopi, pp. 10–19.

Biller-Andorno, N. and Schauenburg, H. (2001) 'It's only love? Some pitfalls in emotionally related organ donation', *Journal of Medical Ethics*, 27 (3): 162–4.

Brock, D.W. (2007) 'Patient competence and surrogate decision-making', in L.P.F. Rosamond Rhodes and A. Silvers (eds), *Blackwell Guide to Medical Ethics*. Oxford and Malden, MA: Blackwell, pp 128–41.

Brody, B.A. (1998) 'Research on the vulnerable sick', in A.C.M. Jeffrey, P. Kahn and J. Sugarman, (eds), *Beyond Consent: Seeking Justice in Research*. Oxford and New York: Oxford University Press, pp. 32–46.

Council of Europe (1997) *Convention for the Protection of Human Rights and Dignity of the Human Being with regard to the Application of Biology and Medicine*. Convention on Human Rights and Biomedicine.

Council for International Organisations of Medical Sciences (CIOMS) (2002) *International Ethical Guidelines for Biomedical Research Involving Human Subjects*. CIOMS.

Danis M. and Donald, L. (2002) 'Health policy, vulnerability, and vulnerable populations', in M. Danis, C. Clancy and L.R. Churchill, (eds), *Ethical Dimensions on Health Policy*. New York: Oxford University Press, pp. 310–34.

DeMarco, J.P. (2004) 'Vulnerability: A needed moral safeguard', *American Journal of Bioethics*, 4 (3): 82–4.

Denny, C.C. and Grady C. (2007) 'Clinical research with economically disadvantaged populations', *Journal of Medical Ethics*, 33: 382–85.

Dresser, R. (1992) 'Wanted: Single, white male for medical research', *Hastings Center Report*, 22: 24–29.

Francis, L.P. (2007) 'Discrimination in medical practice', in L.P.F. Rosamond Rhodes and A. Silvers (eds), *Blackwell Guide to Medical Ethics*. Oxford and Malden, MA: Blackwell, pp. 162–79.

Goyal, M., Mehta, R.L., Schneiderman, L.J. and Sehgal, A.R. (2002) 'Economic and health consequences of selling a kidney in India', *Journal of the American Medical Association*, 288 (13):1589–93.

Grinnell, F. (2004) 'Subject vulnerability: The precautionary principle of human research', *American Journal of Bioethics*, 4 (3): 72–4.

Henderson, G.E., Davis, A. M. and King, N.M.P. (2004) 'Vulnerability to influence: A two-way street', *American Journal of Bioethics*, 4 (3): 52–3.

Henderson, G.E., Churchill, L.R., Davis, A.M., Easter, M.M., Grady, C., Joffe, S. et al. (2007) 'Clinical trials and medical care: Defining the therapeutic misconception', *PLoS Medicine*, 4 (11): e324.

Hurst, S.A. (2008) 'Vulnerability in research and health care: Describing the elephant in the room?', *Bioethics*, 22 (4): 191–202.

Karlawish, J. (2007) 'Research on cognitively impaired adults', in B. Steinbock, (ed), *Oxford Handbook of Bioethics.* Oxford and New York: Oxford University Press, pp. 595–620.

Kass, N.E., Sugarman, J., Faden, R. and Schoch-Spana, M. (1996) ''Trust: The fragile foundation of contemporary biomedical research', *Hastings Centre Report,* 26: 25–9.

Kipnis, K. (2001) *Vulnerability in Research Subjects: A Bioethical Taxonomy.* Bathesda, MD: National Bioethics Advisory Committee, G-1–G-13.

Kottow, M.H. (2004) 'Vulnerability: What kind of principle is it?', *Medicine, Health Care and Philosophy,* 7: 281–7.

Levine, C., Faden, R., Grady, C., Hammerschmidt, D., Eckenwiler, L. and Sugarman, J. (2004) 'The limitations of "vulnerability" as a protection for human research participants', *American Journal of Bioethics,* 4 (3): 44–9.

Luna, F. (2007) 'Research in developing countries', in B. Steinbock, (ed), *Oxford Handbook of Bioethics.* Oxford and New York: Oxford University Press, pp. 621–47.

Macklin, R. (2003) 'Bioethics, vulnerability and protection', *Bioethics,* 17 (5–6): 472–86.

Nickel, P.J. (2006) 'Vulnerable populations in research: The case of the seriously ill', *Theoretical Medicine and Bioethics,* 27: 245–64.

O'Neill, O. (1996) *Towards Justice and Virtue: A Constructive Account of Practical Reasoning.* Cambridge, New York and Melbourne: Cambridge University Press.

O'Neill, O. (2002) *Autonomy and Trust in Bioethics.* Cambridge: Cambridge University Press.

Radcliffe-Richards, J., Daar, A.S., Guttmann, R.D., Hoffenberg, R., Kennedy, I., Lock, M. et al. (1998) 'The case for allowing kidney sales', *The Lancet,* 351: 1950–2.

Reeder, R. (ed.) (1999) 'Special issue on vulnerable populations', *Bioethics Forum,* 15 (2).

Reeder, R. (ed.) (2000) 'Special issue on vulnerability and the bioethics movement', *Bioethics Forum,* 16 (2).

Rendtorff, J.D. (2002) 'Basic ethical principles in European bioethics and biolaw: Autonomy, dignity, integrity and vulnerability – Towards a foundation of bioethics and biolaw', *Medicine, Health Care and Philosophy,* 5: 235–44.

US Code of Federal Regulations (CFR) (2005) *Title 45, Public Welfare; Part 46, Protection of Human Subjects.* Washington, DC: DHHS.

World Medical Association (WMA) (2004) *Declaration of Helsinki. Ethical Principles for Medical Research Involving Human Subjects.* WMA.

Zaner, R.M. (2000) 'Power and hope in the clinical encounter: A meditation on vulnerability', *Medicine, Health Care and Philosophy,* 3 (3): 265–75.

Zargooshi, J. (2001) 'Iranian kidney donors: Motivations and relations with recipients', *Journal of Urology,* 165 (2): 386–92.

Zion, D., Gillam, L. and Loff, B. (2000) 'The Declaration of Helsinki, CIOMS and the ethics of research on vulnerable populations', *Nature,* 6 (6): 615–7.

21

Mental Health and Disorder

Rachel Cooper

INTRODUCTION

Debates about the nature of mental health and disorder are essentially problematic, for they quickly lead us to questions about the necessary frailty of human rationality, the nature of the good life, and the distinction between evil and illness. While these issues are all clearly important, they are also, unfortunately, very difficult, and none will be tackled here. My aims in this chapter are modest. I will sketch an overview of current debates regarding the nature of mental health and disorder and show how these link with broader problems.

THE NATURE OF MENTAL DISORDER

Those who dispute the nature of mental disorder can usefully be split into two camps – conservative and radical. Conservatives assume that mental disorders are real, and seek to understand their nature. Radicals contest the very existence of mental illness. Within the literature the terms 'disorder', 'disease', and 'illness' are used interchangeably.

The conservative debate

The most influential of the conservative accounts of mental disorder is that included in the *Diagnostic and Statistical Manual of Mental Disorders* (DSM), a classification of mental disorders published by the American Psychiatric Association (APA), but increasingly used worldwide. The DSM has included a definition of mental disorder since the publication of the DSM-III in 1980:

each of the mental disorders is conceptualized as a clinically significant behavioral or psychological syndrome or pattern that occurs in an individual and that is typically associated with either a painful symptom (distress) or impairment in one or more areas of functioning (disability). In addition there is an inference that there is a behavioral, psychological, or biological dysfunction, and that the disturbance is not only in the relationship between the individual and society. (APA, 1980: 6)

With minor revisions this definition has also been included in later editions of the DSM. The definition of 'mental disorder' included in the DSM is a direct descendent of definitions developed within the American Psychiatric Association in the 1970s (Spitzer, 1973; 1981), and bears traces of the historical context within with it originated. During the 1970s, the APA was under heavy attack from 'antipsychiatrists' who challenged the legitimacy of psychiatry as a branch of medicine, and also from gay activists who protested at homosexuality being classified as a mental disorder. Defining 'mental disorder' was rhetorically useful for the APA in both these battles (Kutchins and Kirk, 1997; Cooper, 2005). Armed with the 'right' definition, it hoped to argue that mental disorders are a subset of medical disorders, and to settle the question of whether homosexuality is pathological.

In the 1960s and 70s, a number of theorists had claimed that whether a condition is a disease is purely a matter of biological fact (for an example applying this idea to psychiatry, see Kendell, 1975). The most developed account is that of Christopher Boorse (1975; 1976; 1977; 1997), who claims that diseases are biological dysfunctions of some subsystem of the body or mind. In such accounts the status of homosexuality is problematic, as in the current state of knowledge no-one can be sure whether homosexuality is a biological dysfunction. Notably, the DSM definition sidesteps this issue. For a condition to be considered a disorder, the DSM requires there to be both a behavioural or psychological syndrome (that is assumed to be caused by a dysfunction) *and* for it to be the case that this syndrome generally causes distress or impairment (meaning it has to be a bad thing). This ensures that homosexuality will not be classed as a disorder. In the case of homosexuality there may or may not be some biological dysfunction, but even if there is a dysfunction, this need not be harmful, and so homosexuality will not be a disorder.

The core idea behind the DSM definition is that a condition that is a harmful dysfunction is a disorder. In a series of influential articles, Jerome Wakefield endorses this approach and attempts to flesh out the details of how such an account might work (1992a; 1992b; 1993). Wakefield adopts an evolutionary account of normal function, and claims that the function of a bodily or psychological sub-system is whatever it has been naturally selected to do. When a sub-system fails to do whatever it has been naturally selected to do there is thus a dysfunction. In Wakefield's account 'harmful' is taken to be a 'value-term based on social norms' (1992a: 373).

It is worth noting that Wakefield's claim that an evolutionary account can be given of normal functions is problematic. Selective pressures will frequently shift over time, as environments change, and sub-systems come to serve new needs. According to one hypothesis, for example, flies originally used their wings as heat regulating organs, and only later came to use them for flying. As such shifts can occur, an evolution-based account of function must specify the time period in which selection pressures are going to be taken to be important for determining the functions of sub-systems (that is it must specify whether the function of a sub-system is what it was selected for originally, or what it is selected for in the present, or in the recent past). The complications induced by this in itself may lead one to entertain doubts about evolutionary accounts of normal function.

Even if such worries could be overcome, there are other difficulties. Most importantly, the claim that diseases are harmful evolutionary dysfunctions is problematic: it does not seem to be necessary for a condition to be an evolutionary dysfunction for us to consider it to be a disease. Evolutionary psychologists have been struck by many mental disorders appearing to have a genetic basis and yet occurring at prevalence rates that are too high to be solely the result of mutations. Examples include manic-depression, sociopathy, obsessive-compulsivity, anxiety disorders, drug abuse and some personality disorders (Wilson, 1993). This means that the genetic bases of these conditions must be promoted by natural selection, which implies that the genes are adaptive in some way or other. In such cases, from an evolutionary point of view, there may be no dysfunction when such conditions occur. We are thus left with an alternative. Either one can adhere to Wakefield's account and claim that if manic-depression, sociopathy, and so on are evolutionarily advantageous then this just shows that they are not disorders. Or, if one thinks that it is conceptually possible that there might be evolutionarily advantageous disorders one must abandon Wakefield's account.

If Wakefield's account is abandoned, one of several alternatives might be adopted instead: Aristotelian accounts claim that diseases are dysfunctions, but adopt an Aristotelian, as opposed to evolutionary account of normal function (Megone, 1998; 2000). For the Aristotelian, a healthy human is one in which physical and mental sub-systems function in ways that facilitate the living of a flourishing life. In such accounts the distinction between diseases and vices (which the Aristotelian also sees as traits that diminish one's chances of flourishing) is diminished. Aristotelians see this as an attractive feature of their account. Others, who are more committed to the idea that there is a distinction between those who are evil and those who are ill, may perceive it as a difficulty. Another possible problem with adopting an Aristotelian approach to illness is that it commits one to Aristotelianism elsewhere. At the very least, one will need to adopt an Aristotelian approach to human flourishing and human biology. This will commit one, for example, to the rejection of a fact–value distinction, and to the endorsement of teleological explanation as an irreducible form of explanation. In modern times, Aristotelian approaches to science have been underdeveloped and the full implications of adopting such views are unclear. The risk is that buying into the Aristotelian world view may lead to problems elsewhere even if it permits an attractive account of disorder.

Alternatively, one might adopt one of several accounts that seek to provide a number of criteria that are jointly considered to be necessary and sufficient for a condition to be a disorder. Characteristically, some combination of criteria such as being abnormal, being statistically infrequent, being harmful, having a biological basis, and being medically treatable is considered to be jointly necessary and sufficient for a condition to be a disease. For example, Lawrie Reznek has argued that a condition is pathological if and only if it is an abnormal bodily/mental condition which requires medical intervention and which harms standard members of the species in standard conditions (1987: 163–4). He takes it that we decide what we will count as abnormal ('abnormal' functions as a call to action stating that we consider dealing with the harmful condition to be a priority), and that 'medical interventions' can be defined by enumeration, via a list of possible pharmacological and surgical interventions (1987: 94). Along similar lines I have argued that by 'disease' we mean a condition that it is a bad thing to have, such that we consider the afflicted person to be unlucky, and that can potentially be appropriately medically treated (Cooper, 2002). As I see it, the fundamental difficulty with such multi-criterion accounts is that to date they have only been sketched, but their intrinsic complexity means that in order to be fully evaluated they will need to be developed in some detail.

Finally, one might claim that it is impossible, in principle, to give a set of necessary and sufficient conditions for something being a 'mental disorder' (Lilienfeld and Marino, 1995). Scott Lilienfeld and Lori Marino claim that 'mental disorder' is what they call a 'Roschian concept' (by which they mean something very close to a Wittgensteinian family resemblance concept) (Rosch, 1978; Wittgenstein, 1953: §66, 67). On such an account, whether a condition counts as a mental disorder depends on how similar it is to prototypical cases, such as psychotic depression and schizophrenia. Conditions that seem like these central cases are counted as disorders, but there are no general rules that determine what it takes for something to be a disorder.

Lilienfeld and Marino's main reason for thinking that mental disorder is a Roschian concept is that they think that attempts to provide necessary and sufficient conditions for the concept have repeatedly failed. Such reasoning ties in with Wittgenstein's approach in *Philosophical Investigations*. Wittgenstein asks his reader to 'look and see whether there is anything common to all [games]' (1953: §66). It is because games can be seen to have nothing in common that he concludes that game is a family resemblance concept. I suggest that whether this is the case with 'mental disorder' remains to be established. As we have seen, a number of people are attempting to produce accounts that would provide necessary and sufficient conditions for something to be a disease. It is too early to conclude that these accounts will all fail. As such, in my view, it would be premature to follow Lilienfeld and Marino and to claim that mental disorder is a Roschian concept.

As this brief review indicates, at present there are several competing accounts of disease being developed, and it is not clear which, if any, will eventually prove satisfactory. It might thus be tempting to conclude that it is too early to attempt to apply any such accounts to practical matters. I suggest, however, that this would be the wrong conclusion to draw. Although there is much work still to be done with developing an account of disease, a consensus is emerging with respect to some key issues: First, and most importantly, there is a general consensus that diseases are necessarily harmful conditions. The prospects for purely descriptive accounts of disease (such as Boorse's) look bleak. The second point that can be noted is that most of the accounts of disease being developed treat physical and mental disorders together. While this does not imply that no distinction can be drawn between mental and physical disorders, it looks likely that any such distinction will not simply emerge naturally out of a satisfactory account of disease. Rather, even if a satisfactory account of disease is developed, the problem of working out how mental and physical disorders can be distinguished will likely remain as a separate task.

Before moving onto the more radical critics of psychiatry, it is worth reviewing the views of a theorist who lies midway between the conservative and radical camps. In *What is Mental Disorder?*, Derek Bolton (2008) argues that the term 'mental disorder' is best discarded, both because attempts to define the concept have failed, and because the term carries unhelpful historical baggage. However, Bolton believes that psychiatry has a justifiable role in the treatment of patients. His starting point is that patients come, or are brought, to the clinic in distress, and that mental health professionals treat them in a way that is recognisably medical, as opposed, to, say, political or educational. Deciding when such interventions are appropriate is a matter for negotiation, and depends on diverse factors, such as whether the patient's particular problem is most effectively dealt with by medical or other means, and also ethical and political decisions regarding the sort of lives we wish to lead. To illustrate, in Bolton's view, in so far as depression is justifiably treated, this will be because antidepressants work and we consider their use ethically justifiable, rather than because depression is a 'mental disorder'. If Bolton is right, philosophical debates about the nature of mental disorder will turn out to be merely a distraction.

The radical debate – What became of antipsychiatry?

While the conservative debate assumes that mental disorders exist, more radical thinkers question this, and tend to see mental disorder and physical disorder as radically different types of state. Such views are most strongly associated with the 1960s 'antipsychiatrists'. Antipsychiatry was never a unified movement and different writers had quite different reasons for their suspicion of psychiatry. Thomas Szasz (1960) claimed that psychiatrists act to label and control those whom society finds problematic. R.D. Laing and A. Esterson (1964) argued that schizophrenics are not sick individuals but are treated as scapegoats by their families. Michel Foucault argued that 'mental illness' is an historically contingent category (1967). David Rosenhan (1973) sent fake patients to hospital, and on finding that psychiatrists were fooled into considering them insane, claimed that psychiatrists are char-latans. Although these thinkers had different reasons for rejecting the category of mental illness each can be seen as claiming that judgements of mental illness are radically unsta-ble (varying with perceiver, or historical period, or social context) and that this should lead us to question the reality of mental illness.

Few thinkers would nowadays call themselves antipsychiatrists, but somewhat similar ideas can still be found amongst those who belong to the 'critical-' or 'post-' psychiatry movement and in the more radical wings of the patient/user/survivor movement (Inglby, 1981; Bracken and Thomas, 2005). Like the antipsychiatry movement that preceded them, these movements are not unified, but include thinkers who are critical of psychiatry for diverse reasons. Some thinkers restrict themselves to critiquing the contemporary treat-ment of psychiatric patients – they protest against the compulsory use of electroconvulsive therapy, for example, or argue that various drugs may not be as effective or safe as their manufacturers claim (for example, Moncrieff et al., 2005). Others go further and argue that if we wish to understand mental distress, the voices of patients rather than doctors should be considered authoritative. Most radically of all, some authors have sought to tie in a critique of contemporary psychiatry with a postmodern account of truth. Patrick Bracken and Philip Thomas (2005) argue that on a postmodern understanding a psychiatrist has no greater access to 'The Truth' than a 'delusional' patient, and so both are forced to enter into an equal negotiation with each other.

Positive mental health

Compared to mental illness, positive mental health is rarely discussed. Indeed it is unclear whether any content can be given to positive mental health whereby it would be something distinct from simply not being mentally ill. When there are debates about the nature of mental health they bring out very clearly the strength of connection between the good life and mental health. Descriptions of the mentally healthy person are suspiciously similar to descriptions of the flourishing human. Unsurprisingly, such descriptions are deeply contested and also run the risk of being culturally shaped. Descriptions offered by past theorists can now appear quaint and parochial (see, for example, Marie Jahoda's (1958) *Current Concepts of Positive Mental Health*, where great emphasis is placed on the masculine American ideals of independence and autonomy).

With the rise of user/survivor/patient groups, notions of positive mental health have become contested in previously unimaginable ways. It is now commonplace for those with a wide variety of conditions to claim that they are not sick, but merely atypical. Thus there exist groups that argue that conditions ranging from Asperger syndrome (http://www.aspiesforfreedom.com/) to attention-deficit hyperactivity disorder (ADHD) (http://addeddimensions.info/) to asexuality (http://www.asexuality.org/home/) are all compatible with leading a flourishing life and should be regarded as normal variations rather than as disorders.

VALUES AND SPECIFIC DIAGNOSES

Moving away from general questions about the nature of mental disorder, there are also specific and ethically-charged issues about particular psychiatric diagnoses. Many diagnoses are disproportionately likely to be attached to persons of a particular sex or race. Thus, hysteria, depression and borderline personality disorder are stereotypically female diagnoses, while those who are diagnosed as suffering from schizophrenia or antisocial personality disorder are likely to be men.

It is difficult to determine the reasons why it is that a particular race or sex appears to be diagnosed in a particular way (see, for example, McKenzie and Murray, 1999; Piccinelli and Wilkinson, 2000). Some claim that biological differences account for the diagnostic rates (for example, depression in women may be linked to hormonal fluctuations linked with pregnancy and childbirth). Some suggest that social pressures affect distinct groups differently and lead to different rates of breakdown (for example, racism may explain why black men are more likely to develop paranoid delusions). Some think that differential rates of diagnosis are caused by racism and sexism within psychiatry itself. This might come about in a variety of ways. Perhaps psychiatrists perceive the behaviour of their patients in stereotyped ways – thus black men may be perceived as violent, and women as sexually manipulative (Loring and Powell, 1988). Alternatively, the diagnostic criteria that are used to make diagnoses may themselves be shaped by sexist and racist assumptions (Lunbeck, 1994; Busfield, 1996).

Many diagnoses appear to have built into them notions of the normal or ideal human life that are highly contestable. Everyone accepts that emotions that may be normal to feel under certain circumstances may be pathological in other circumstances. For example, grieving often resembles depression, but grief is normal. In recognition of this, the DSM diagnosis of Major Depressive Episode can only be given when a grieving person continues to manifest depressive symptoms two months after a death. Such criteria raise hard questions (Horwitz and Wakefield, 2007). If my child dies, who is to say how long I should grieve? If I grieve for a year rather than two months, am I ill or just out of step with my community? Other emotions apart from grief raise similar issues: How nervous should I get when I meet strangers? (Lane, 2007) What level of insult should make me angry? How long should a bored school child be able to concentrate? How much should someone desire sex? Addressing such questions requires us to make judgements regarding the sorts of people that we want to be. Not only are such questions hard to answer, notions of what is normal, or acceptable, are highly culturally specific.

The DSM is now used around the world and there is a concern that North American norms are now imposed on non-American peoples; Icelanders and Indonesians are now expected to act as the American Psychiatric Association thinks people should act.

A further concern is that the assessment of what is normal may be shaped by the needs of industry and commerce (Elliott, 2003: chs. 6, 10). Certain types of personality are easier to govern and more productive than others. A child who can sit still for an hour is cheaper to teach than one who needs constant stimulation. An impulsive personality, which leads someone to flit from job to job, is problematic in an advanced capitalist society. This can lead to pressures for fidgety children and unreliable adults to be treated. Moreover the possibilities for treatment are greater than ever before. Psychoactive drugs open up the promise of the direct chemical shaping of personality in previously unimaginable ways. While people have always used substances such as alcohol and coffee to make themselves more productive or socially acceptable, drugs such as Prozac offer new possibilities for shaping selves (Kramer, 1993). Once again, we see that determining who is ill, and who should be treated, is inextricably linked to deciding what types of people we want to be.

THE ETHICS OF DIAGNOSIS

Treatment and diagnosis

The diagnoses that patients receive determine the ways in which they are treated. The costs associated with certain diagnoses are so great that, in certain circumstances, a psychiatrist may feel the diagnosis should not be given. All diagnoses of mental disorders are stigmatising, and many mental health professionals thus seek to treat their patients without explicitly labelling them as mentally ill. Certain diagnoses – such as personality disorders or schizophrenia – are additionally problematic. Within psychiatry, some diagnoses carry with them the possibility not only that someone can be appropriately treated if they so wish, but also that they should be treated against their will, if necessary. Certain disorders are taken to imply that an individual cannot be expected to know their own best interests. When such diagnoses are made this thus exposes the patient to the benefits and costs of treatment and also undermines their autonomy.

Narratives and diagnosis

The narratives that structure people's lives are important. Some go so far as to link such narratives with a person's identity, but at the very least such narratives help to shape what an individual thinks they might do and how they come to understand how they have acted in the past (Elliott, 1999: ch. 7). In so far as diagnostic labels enter into the narratives by which people understand themselves and others, they can have welcome and also less welcome consequences.

Some thinkers claim that the act of diagnosis is inextricably linked to the objectification of people (Bracken and Thomas, 2005). The risk is that, with diagnosis, a patient shifts from being an individual with her or his own distinctive life history, problems, and ways of coping, and becomes just another case. With diagnosis a pattern of behaviour becomes a 'symptom'. This tends to mean the problem becomes an issue for the medical profession, rather than one individuals and their friends and family might seek to deal with themselves.

Receiving a diagnosis affects how people see themselves. Sometimes the effect of being diagnosed may be minimal, and arguably diagnosis may enable someone to practice reasonable planning and thus gain control over their life. So, suppose I come to think of myself as having depressive tendencies. This may structure my actions in certain ways – I may avoid drugs that have been found to trigger depression in those who are susceptible – I avoid ecstasy, the contraceptive pill, and so on. Such actions may be reasonable and helpful for me.

However, other diagnoses, such as being diagnosed with schizophrenia, restrict options for action. A patient's dreams can no longer appear simply as dreams but are now potentially delusory hopes. Even when a patient resists traditional views of the psychiatric patient and joins the survivor/user/patient movement the narratives associated with resistance and recovery tend to take limited forms. In extreme cases, it may be utterly unclear how a person who has accepted a particular diagnosis can continue to think of themselves as a rational human being who can be responsive to moral demands and make plans for the future. If one self-defines as a psychopath then one's options for telling a good story about oneself are practically closed off rather than simply curtailed. Such diagnoses have built into them the idea that one is essentially evil and untreatable. As such examples illustrate, diagnosis can act to solidify a set of practices in such a way that they come to seem essential to a person's identity (Elliott, 1999: ch. 2); psychopaths are not just people who sometimes do bad things, they are bad people.

The ways in which the narratives associated with particular diagnoses can shape how people live have been explored at depth by Ian Hacking. In his work, Hacking describes looping that occurs between diagnoses and behaviour (Hacking, 1986; 1988; 1992; 1995a; 1995b). A diagnosis of Multiple Personality Disorder (MPD), for example, is first introduced to describe a set of behaviours. The people thus diagnosed, however, do not remain unaffected by their diagnosis as knowing they are classified as suffering from MPD shapes their activities. Those with MPD may embrace the idea that they are multiples, and start to manifest more numerous and more varied personalities than they otherwise would have done. Alternatively, they may resist their classification. In any event, people's behaviour is shaped by their knowledge of their diagnoses. This leads to looping. Over time, the behaviour of people with MPD shifts from what it would otherwise have been. Thus, people with MPD used to typically have only two or three personalities, but by the late 1980s they frequently had scores or hundreds. Via such effects MPD becomes a moving target – the behaviours emerge and develop alongside the descriptions associated with the diagnosis.

Hacking stresses that the ways in which patients respond to being diagnosed are not determined or entirely outside their control. Patient groups can respond to diagnoses in creative and surprising ways – thus homosexuality can start as a medical diagnosis, and through the actions of gay activists, shift into a label that some may embrace (Hacking, 1995b). Nevertheless, although people in groups can change the implications of the labels that are applied to them, the opportunities for individual creativity remain limited.

When a set of behaviours is diagnosed this alters our moral understanding of the situation (Conrad and Schneider, 1980; Martin, 2006). Some diagnoses turn vices into illnesses – thus drunkards become alcoholics, and fidgety children come to be seen as suffering from ADHD. However, even though medicalisation is often claimed to reduce the sphere of moral responsibility, this is not entirely true. Medicalisation certainly *alters* the sphere of moral concern, but it is not clear that it reduces it. In a medicalized society, each individual is considered to be responsible for monitoring his or her health. As such, actions that used to be morally innocent now come under suspicion. Thus, while our grandparents could get merry every weekend without this being a moral issue, we are expected to count the units of alcohol we drink. As these examples illustrate, it is not only the diagnosed who are affected by their knowledge of diagnoses; "normal" people also come to think of their actions in medically structured ways. The ways in which we come to think of mental health and illness thus affect us all.

REFERENCES

American Psychiatric Association (APA) (1980) *Diagnostic and Statistical Manual of Mental Disorders (DSM)*, 3rd ed. Washington, DC: American Psychiatric Association.
Bolton, D. (2008) *What is Mental Disorder?* Oxford: Oxford University Press.
Boorse, C. (1975) 'On the distinction between disease and illness', *Philosophy and Public Affairs*, 5: 49–68.
Boorse, C. (1976) 'What a theory of mental health should be', reprinted in R. Edwards (ed.) (1982), *Psychiatry and Ethics*. Buffalo, NY: Prometheus Books, pp. 29–48.
Boorse, C. (1977) 'Health as a theoretical concept', *Philosophy of Science*, 44: 542–73.
Boorse, C. (1997) 'A rebuttal on health', in J. Hunter and R. Almeder (eds), *What is disease?* Totowa, NJ: Humana Press, pp. 1–134.
Bracken, P. and Thomas, P. (2005) *Postpsychiatry: Mental Health in a Postmodern World*. Oxford: Oxford University Press.
Busfield, J. (1996) *Men, Woman and Madness*. Houndmills, Basingstoke: Macmillan Press.
Conrad, P. and Schneider, J. (1980) *Deviance and Medicalization: From Badness to Sickness*. St Louis, MO: CV Mosby.
Cooper, R. (2002) 'Disease', *Studies in History and Philosophy of Biological and Biomedical Sciences*, 33: 263–82.
Cooper, R. (2005) *Classifying Madness: A Philosophical Examination of the Diagnostic and Statistical Manual of Mental Disorders*. Dordrecht: Springer.
Elliott, C. (1999) *A Philosophical Disease: Bioethics, Culture and Identity*. New York: Routledge.
Elliott, C. (2003) *Better Than Well*. New York: W.W.Norton and Co.
Foucault, M. (1967) *Madness and Civilisation*. London: Routledge.
Hacking, I. (1986) 'Making up people', in T. Heller, M. Sosna and D. Wellbery (eds), *Reconstructing Individualism*. Stanford, CA: Stanford University Press, pp. 222–36.
Hacking, I. (1988) 'The sociology of knowledge about child abuse', *Nous*, 22: 53–63.
Hacking, I. (1992) 'World-making by kind-making: Child abuse for example', in M. Douglas and D. Hull (eds), *How Classification Works*. Edinburgh: Edinburgh University Press, pp. 180–238.
Hacking, I. (1995a) *Rewriting the Soul*. Princeton, NJ: Princeton University Press.

Hacking, I. (1995b) 'The looping effects of human kinds', in D. Sperber and A. Premark (eds), *Causal Cognition*. Oxford: Clarendon Press, pp. 351–94.

Horwitz, A. and Wakefield, J. (2007) *The Loss of Sadness: How Psychiatry Transformed Normal Sadness into Depressive Disorder*. Oxford: Oxford University Press.

Ingleby, D. (ed.) (1981) *Critical Psychiatry*. Harmondsworth: Penguin.

Jahoda, M. (1958) *Current Concepts of Positive Mental Health*. New York: Basic Books.

Kendell, R. (1975) 'The concept of disease and its implications for psychiatry', *British Journal of Psychiatry*, 127: 305–15.

Kramer, P. (1993) *Listening to Prozac*. New York: Penguin.

Kutchins, H. and Kirk, S. (1997) *Making Us Crazy*. New York: The Free Press.

Laing, R.D. and Esterson, A. (1964) *Sanity, Madness and the Family*. Harmondsworth: Penguin.

Lane, C. (2007) *Shyness: How Normal Behaviour became a Sickness*. New Haven, CT: Yale University Press.

Lilienfeld, S. and Marino, L. (1995) 'Mental disorder as a Roschian concept: A critique of Wakefield's "Harmful Dysfunction" analysis', *Journal of Abnormal Psychology*, 104: 411–20.

Loring, M. and Powell, B. (1988) 'Gender, Race, and DSM-III: A study of the objectivity of psychiatric diagnostic behaviour', *Journal of Health and Social Behaviour*, 29: 1–22.

Lunbeck, E. (1994) *The Psychiatric Persuasion: Knowledge, Gender and Power in Modern America*. Princeton, NJ: Princeton University Press.

Martin, M. (2006) *From Morality to Mental Health: Virtue and Vice in a Therapeutic Culture*. Oxford: Oxford University Press.

McKenzie, K. and Murray, R. (1999) 'Risk factors for psychosis in the UK African-Caribbean population', in D. Bhugra and V. Bahl (eds), *Ethnicity: An Agenda for Mental Health*. London: Gaskell, pp. 48–59.

Megone, C. (1998) 'Aristotle's function argument and the concept of mental illness', *Philosophy, Psychiatry and Psychology*, 5: 187–201.

Megone, C. (2000) 'Mental illness, human function and values', *Philosophy, Psychiatry and Psychology*, 7: 45–65.

Moncrieff, J., Hopker, S. and Thomas, P. (2005) 'Psychiatry and the pharmaceutical industry: Who pays the piper? A perspective from the Critical Psychiatry Network', *Psychiatric Bulletin*, 29: 84–5.

Piccinelli, M. and Wilkinson, G. (2000) 'Gender differences in depression', *British Journal of Psychiatry*, 177: 486–92.

Reznek, L. (1987) *The Nature of Disease*. London: Routledge and Kegan Paul.

Rosch, E. (1978) 'Principles of categorization', in E. Rosch and B. Lloyd (eds), *Cognition and Categorization*. Hillsdale, NJ: Lawrence Erlbaum Associates, pp. 27–48.

Rosenhan, D. (1973) 'On being sane in insane places', *Science*, 179: 250–8.

Spitzer, R. (1973) 'A proposal about homosexuality and the APA nomenclature: Homosexuality as an irregular form of sexual behaviour and sexual orientation disturbance as a psychiatric disorder', *American Journal of Psychiatry*, 130: 1214–16.

Spitzer, R. (1981) 'The diagnostic status of homosexuality in D.S.M-III: A reformulation of the issues', *American Journal of Psychiatry*, 138: 210–15.

Szasz, T. (1960) 'The myth of mental illness', *American Psychologist*, 15: 113–18.

Wakefield, J. (1992a) 'The concept of mental disorder – On the boundary between biological facts and social value', *American Psychologist*, 47: 373–88.

Wakefield, J. (1992b) 'Disorder as harmful dysfunction: A conceptual critique of D.S.M-III-R's definition of mental disorder', *Psychological Review*, 99: 232–47.

Wakefield, J. (1993) 'Limits of operationalization: A critique of Spitzer and Endicott's (1978) proposed operational criteria for mental disorder', *Journal of Abnormal Psychology*, 102: 160–72.

Wilson, D. (1993) 'Evolutionary epidemiology: Darwinian theory in the service of medicine and psychiatry', reprinted in S. Baron-Cohen (ed.) (1997) *The Maladapted Mind*. Hove: Psychology Press, pp.39–55.

Wittgenstein, L. (1953) *Philosophical Investigations*. Oxford: Basil Blackwell.

22

Medical Research Involving Children: A Review of International Policy Statements

Julie Samuël, Bartha Maria Knoppers
and Denise Avard

INTRODUCTION

The participation of children in research is of great importance to child health and well-being, but has always been a source of controversy. Because of their incapacity to give informed consent, children have been either under- or over-protected in clinical research. History in the nineteenth and twentieth centuries is illustrative of the abuse of children in research (Grodin and Glantz, 1994). As a result, the protection of children has been equated by most researchers with their exclusion from research (Kodish, 2005). In spite of their vulnerability, research involving children is essential since physiologically and psychologically they differ from adults. They are not small adults and some diseases are unique to them (e.g. type I insulin dependent diabetes). It goes without saying that all research involving their participation must be subject to rigorous evaluation, monitoring and governance.

International norms governing the involvement of children in research acknowledge the importance of conducting paediatric research and provide a framework for protecting them. In particular, parental consent or that of the legal representative is required as well as the assent of the child when appropriate, and the evaluation of the risks and benefits.

The present chapter will review the international norms governing research involving children by considering these issues. The first part examines the evolution of paediatric research and analyzes the international norms concerning the inclusion of children in research. The second part outlines the international norms governing such research and critically assesses the issues of consent, assent and potential risks and benefits.

INCLUSION OF CHILDREN IN RESEARCH

Research involving vulnerable persons such as children has a tragic past, since they have often been exploited (Grodin and Glantz, 1994). Retracing the evolution of medical research involving children, we identify some of the ethical concerns raised by paediatric research and highlight international guidelines specific to this field.

Evolution of research involving children

The history of research shows that children have often been victims of unethical research practices. In the eighteenth century, researchers used their slaves, servants, and even their own children as test subjects (Field and Behrman, 2004). Researchers also used institution-alized children to conduct trials of new vaccines. The smallpox vaccine, for example, was first tested on the children of researchers and then on children living in an almshouse (Grodin and Glantz, 1994). In order to study diseases such as syphilis, gonorrhea and tuberculosis, children were deliberately infected with the disease (Beecher, 1966). During this period, researchers performed spinal punctures on hospitalized children to determine if this procedure was harmless (Grodin and Glantz, 1994).

Research involving institutionalized children continued to be conducted well into the nineteenth and twentieth centuries. A Swedish researcher even said that experimentation on institutionalized children was 'cheaper than [on] calves' (Grodin and Glantz, 1994). Infants, newborns and healthy children were also involved in medical research. One example of such clinical research involved tests of the utility and efficacy of X-rays, which were performed on both sick and healthy children to study their development (Grodin and Glantz, 1994). The inclusion of children is explained in part by the lack of appropriate animal models for testing new drugs during this period (Friedman Ross, 2006).

After World War II, experiments involving children continued to be conducted even in the wake of the *Nuremberg Code*. At the end of the 1950s, a hepatitis study was conducted on healthy institutionalized children at Willowbrook State School in New York (Beecher, 1966). Researchers intentionally infected children with hepatitis to better understand the course of the disease and to develop a vaccine (Friedman Ross, 2006). This research was not intended for their direct benefit; indeed, the children were harmed (Beecher, 1966). Moreover, the consent provided by the children's parents was coerced and uninformed (Breslow, 2003). This study did not respect the ethical guidelines provided by the 1949 *International Code of Medical Ethics* of the World Medical Association (Friedman Ross, 2006).

This Willowbrook case created worldwide controversy. Strong disapproval from the ethics and scientific communities led to the elaboration of norms on the protection of human subjects in research (Grodin and Glantz, 1994). In an attempt to protect them from harmful experiments, children were excluded from clinical trials (Kodish, 2005). Denied the opportunity to participate in research, children became 'therapeutic orphans': they were not treated as a distinct category of patients, nor were their particular therapeutic concerns addressed (Kodish, 2005). This situation was exacerbated by the general lack of data regarding children, as well as the lack of appropriate medical treatments for them (Kodish, 2005).

Indeed, forty years later, a survey conducted in the United States in 1991 revealed that 80 percent of the drugs listed in a pharmaceutical guide frequently used by physicians contained no information on children (Field and Behrman, 2004). In Europe, studies in 2000 showed that most of the drugs provided to children were prescribed off label due to the fact that they had never been tested in the paediatric population (Saint Raymond and Brasseur, 2005). As a result, physicians continued to extrapolate paediatric dosage from adult pharmacological data (Truong, 2005). In fact, the lack of available data on the efficacy or toxicity of these drugs in the paediatric population continues to expose them to serious harms.

Perhaps the most important reason to include children in research is because some disorders belong to them and are not found in adults, or will have progressed beyond efficient treatment by adulthood (e.g. juvenile diabetes). Moreover, the development of children can influence the efficacy or dosage of drugs (Truong, 2005). Confronted with these important issues, governments have recognized the need to include children in research. The challenge then is to develop policies that protect children and yet ensure they are not excluded from research precisely because of their vulnerable status.

International norms governing the inclusion of children in research

Following the atrocities committed during World War II, international organizations took the lead in the preparation of norms for the governance of human research. These norms provide important guidance on the inclusion of persons incapable of giving their consent, such as children. Inspired by these norms, as well as the lack of adequate scientific evidence on children, some professional organizations and non-governmental organizations have taken the initiative to encourage paediatric research by making it obligatory. The *Belmont Report*, the work of the World Medical Association (WMA), the Council for International Organizations of Medical Sciences (CIOMS) and of the Council of Europe are illustrative of this approach.

International norms justifying the inclusion of children in research

The principle of justice requires a fair distribution of the burdens and the benefits of research (*Belmont Report*, 1979). A distinction has been made between individual justice and social justice (*Belmont Report*, 1979). Individual justice requires researchers to be fair in the choice of participants in research (Beauchamp and Childress, 2001), whereas social justice requires that a distinction be made between persons who should be able to participate in research and those who should not be involved (*Belmont Report*, 1979). The *Belmont Report* indicates that the protection of vulnerable persons from exploitation in research must prevail. It maintains that in some circumstances it may be fair to give preference to the participation of adults rather than conducting research on children. Nevertheless, the Report leaves the door open to the involvement of children in research. Indeed, the Report recognizes that research involving children may be justified to cure childhood disease and to improve the health and well-being of children. The Report therefore acknowledges that the principle of beneficence may be invoked to justify the participation of children in research.

The *Declaration of Helsinki* (WMA, 1964, with amendments of 2008) builds on the *Belmont Report* and addresses the issue of research involving children with more specificity. It attempts to balance the duty to protect vulnerable persons with the need to include them in sometimes risky research, an important policy shift from the original Declaration. Following the *Declaration of Helsinki,* two conditions must be met before vulnerable persons, such as children, may be involved in research: (1) the research must be indispensable to promote the health of the paediatric population; and (2) it cannot be conducted on persons capable of providing consent (WMA, 1964, with amendments of 2008, art. 27).

Following the footsteps of the *Declaration of Helsinki*, the CIOMS holds that if the proposed research cannot be carried out with adults, children can participate if 'the purpose of the research is to obtain relevant knowledge to the health needs of children' (CIOMS, 2002, Guideline 14; CIOMS, 2008, Guideline 14). This CIOMS goes further than the *Declaration of Helsinki*. It endorses the participation of children in clinical trials as essential research for understanding diseases unique to them. It emphasizes that the absence of knowledge on the safety and efficacy of medical treatments for children may compromise their health by exposing them to serious harm (CIOMS, 2002, Guideline 14; CIOMS, 2008, Guideline 14). CIOMS cites the dangerous consequences of administering new drugs that have been tested only on adults (CIOMS, 2002, Guideline 14; CIOMS, 2008, Guideline 14). In contrast to the *Belmont Report* and the *Declaration of Helsinki*, CIOMS explicitly takes a proactive stand in favour of research that includes children.

Finally, in its 1997 *Convention on Human Rights and Biomedicine*, the Council of Europe encourages research involving vulnerable persons, and has set out requirements concerning their participation (Council of Europe, 1997, art. 17). The Council reiterates these requirements in its 2005 *Additional Protocol to the Convention on Human Rights and Biomedicine*. It is interesting to note that the Council of Europe repeats the requirements stated by the *Declaration of Helsinki* without further expanding on the desirability of research involving children.

Recognition of the vulnerability of children is not a recent concept. However, with the exception of CIOMS, international organizations do not take a clear position regarding the need to include children in research. In contrast, guidelines from the European Union and the United States for example adopt a stronger position by positing that the participation of children in research be made mandatory.

Europe

The European Union also reacted strongly to the findings of the surveys conducted in 2000 that medications provided to children were not adequately evaluated. The European Forum for Good Clinical Practice highlighted the urgent need for legislation promoting research involving children. Indeed, in 2001, the European Parliament and the Council of Europe adopted the *Directive 2001/20/EC on the approximation of the laws, regulations and administrative provisions of the Member States relating to the implementation of good clinical practice in the conduct of clinical trials on medicinal products for human use*

(OJ L 121/34, 1.5.2001). The Directive recognized that children have physiological differences from adults, and emphasized the need to include them in research in order to improve treatments offered before the widespread use of such treatments (European Parliament, 2001, par. 3). It also provided guidance on clinical trials involving children, such as informed consent from parents and legal guardians, assent of child participants and expectations of direct benefit.

These guidelines, however, were general and in the wake of the problems regarding the implementation of this Directive, the European Commission formed an ad hoc group to examine the ethical issues related to clinical trials involving children. In February 2008, the European Commission published the *Ethical Considerations for Clinical Trials on Medicinal Products Conducted with the Paediatric Population: Recommendations of the Ad Hoc Group for the Development of Implementing Guidelines for Directive 2001/20/EC Relating to Good Clinical Practice in the Conduct of Clinical Trials on Medicinal Products for Human Use*. The main objectives of these guidelines are: to contribute to the protection of children involved in clinical trials; to facilitate the conduct of paediatric clinical trials in the European Union; and to harmonize the conduct of these trials. The recommendations assert that because most children cannot consent to their participation in clinical research programs, they should nevertheless be involved in research but only when they benefit from specific protections, hence the need to establish more specific norms.

United States

In 1994, 'six of the ten drugs most commonly prescribed to children [in United States] had no pediatric labeling' (Breslow, 2003). These alarming findings brought the National Institutes of Health (NIH) to require the inclusion of children in research. In 1998, NIH prepared a policy document entitled the *NIH Policy and Guidelines on the Inclusion of Children as Participants in Research Involving Human Subjects* (NIH, 1998). In the introduction, NIH clearly specified that the primary goal of its policy was to increase the participation of children in research in order to improve the treatments available.

NIH denounced the lack of resources allocated to research involving children and encouraged paediatric research. In NIH's opinion, 'children ... must be included in all human subjects research ... unless there are scientific and ethical reasons not to include them' (NIH, 1998). This effectively shifted the burden of proof since previously researchers were required to demonstrate why children should be included in research. This approach transformed policy on the involvement of children in research by evaluating the rationale for excluding them from research. The NIH stated that if children are to be excluded from the research, researchers 'must present an acceptable justification for the exclusion' (NIH, 1998). NIH policy thus creates an obligation and now 'it is expected that children will be included in all research involving human subjects' (NIH, 1998).

The Food and Drug Administration (FDA) also took important initiatives to reinforce research involving children. In 1997, the Congress adopted the Food and Drug Administration Modernization Act of 1997 (FDAMA). FDAMA offered incentives to manufacturers to encourage clinical testing of drugs in the paediatric population. The FDA granted six-month extensions on pre-existing patents to medical product manufacturers who were conducting drug research involving children (FDAMA, 1997). This was not enough, however, to convince manufacturers to do so (Breslow, 2003). To remedy this situation, Congress then adopted the Best Pharmaceuticals for Children Act of 2002 (BPCA). Again, the main objective of this initiative was to increase the number of drug trials involving children (Breslow, 2003). To that end, the BPCA provided that the NIH and FDA should establish an annual list of off-patent drugs that need 'additional studies to assess the safety and effectiveness of the use of the drug in the pediatric population' (BPCA, 2002, sec. 409 a) (1) B). If manufacturers chose not to conduct research with children on one of these drugs, the FDA published requests for proposals to third parties, such as universities and laboratories (BPCA, 2002, sec. 409 c). By proceeding this way, the FDA sought to ensure that medical products administered to children would be tested beforehand on the paediatric population.

INTERNATIONAL NORMS GOVERNING RESEARCH INVOLVING CHILDREN

Children are vulnerable and their inclusion must be balanced with the need to protect them from potential harm, making the issues of consent of parents or legal representatives, the assent of the child and the assessment of the risks and benefits particularly important.

Informed consent

Since children themselves cannot consent to participation in research, international norms provide protection mechanisms, such as requiring the informed consent of the parents or legal representative. In 1949, the *Nuremberg Code* restricted participation in research to individuals who could give free and informed consent. This meant that only research conducted on adults capable of giving their consent was allowed. In 1964, the *Declaration of Helsinki* addressed the exclusion of children by requiring researchers to obtain the informed consent of the minor's legal representative, where research involved legally incompetent minors (WMA, 1964, with amendments of 2008, art. 27). CIOMS also maintained that researchers should obtain the informed consent of parents and legal representative (CIOMS, 2002, Guideline 4; CIOMS, 2008, Guideline 4). However, CIOMS did not use the term 'consent', but rather 'permission', in specifying that where the participation of a minor is sought, the permission of a parent or legal representative must be given (CIOMS, 2002, Guideline 14; CIOMS, 2008, Guideline 14). Technically speaking only the individual concerned (whether competent or not) can consent. Thus, parents or legal representatives are 'authorized' by law to act on their behalf (Knoppers, 1978).

According to the *Universal Declaration on the Human Genome and Human Rights* (UNESCO, 1997) as well as the *Universal Declaration on Bioethics and Human Rights* (UNESCO, 2005), authorization should be obtained not only in accordance with applicable law, but also with the best interest of the research participant in mind. In its *Universal Declaration on Bioethics and Human Rights*, UNESCO underlined the importance of making a decision based on the best interests of the child (UNESCO, 2005). It refers to an 'authorization' in lieu of 'permission' or 'informed consent' (UNESCO, 2005, art. 7). The *Convention on Human Rights and Biomedicine* uses the vocabulary of the UNESCO declarations, and requires the authorization of the child's representative (Council of Europe, 1997, art. 6). The *Additional Protocol to the Convention on Human Rights and Biomedicine* reiterates the requirements contained in the previous Convention (Council of Europe, 2005, art. 15). This difference in terminology could be due to the fact that the term 'consent' should be used only when an individual becomes or is competent (Knoppers et al., 2002).

At present, obtaining the authorization of parents or legal representatives must meet a number of requirements set out in the international norms governing research. These requirements focus on its voluntary and informed character.

Consent should be voluntary, meaning that it is obtained without manipulation, coercion or undue influence. It should also be informed, meaning that the researchers should provide the parents or legal representative with the required information in an understandable language and adapted to their abilities. In particular, the information should describe: (1) the goal and nature of the research, the research methods and the length of time the child's participation; (2) the risks and benefits; and (3) the right to withdraw at any time, without any negative consequences to the child (WMA, 1964, with amendments of 2008, art. 24). Their consent should be obtained in writing before enrolment of the child.

Consent is a continuing process to be maintained throughout the research project. It should be renewed if there are significant changes to the research project. In some very exceptional circumstances, the obtaining of consent may be waived subject to the approval of a research ethics committee (CIOMS, 2002, Guideline 4; CIOMS, 2008, Guideline 4). Exceptional situations that could give rise to such exemptions are cases in which the child involved in research is the victim of abuse or neglect.

Finally, it should be noted that genetic research can reveal very sensitive information concerning not only the child but also the family. Thus, it is important to define the parameters of parental consent. For example, when parents are consenting to the collection of biological samples, the issue of a broad consent allowing for unrestricted future use of these samples may arise (Gurwitz et al., 2009; Samuël et al., 2009a). In the context of genetic testing, the parental consent for testing for adult-onset diseases also raises important issues (Friedman Ross, 2008).

Informed consent is not the only requirement. Indeed, international norms insist on the importance of obtaining the assent of the child in order to respect the child as an individual.

Assent

Assent may be defined as the will of the child to participate in proposed research (European Commission, 2008). Assent derives from the principle of respect for the person and makes it possible for children to express their wishes within the limits of their capacity to do so. Indeed, the *Belmont Report* states that respect for the person demands that legally incompetent persons be given 'the opportunity to choose, to the extent they are able, whether or not to participate in research' (*Belmont Report*, 1979). It adds that objections should be respected unless the research proposed is the only therapy available (*Belmont Report*, 1979).

The *Declaration of Helsinki* explicitly states that, when a child is able to give assent, researchers should obtain it (WMA, 1964, with amendments of 2008, art. 28). This is in addition to the consent given by the parents or legal representative. It also adds that dissent should be respected with no further guidance.

In accordance with the *Declaration of Helsinki*, CIOMS also requires that assent must be obtained 'to the extent of the child's capabilities' (CIOMS, 2002, Guideline 14; CIOMS, 2008, Guideline 14). However, it provides more details about the scope of the assent of the child. It specifies that researchers shall seek for the willing cooperation of the child by informing him/her to the extent that his/her 'maturity and intelligence permit' (CIOMS, 2002, Guideline 14; CIOMS, 2008, Guideline 14). Once the child has understood the objectives of the research and the procedures that will be performed, he/she may give his/her assent to participate in research. CIOMS underlines that some children may be too immature to give an assent.

CIOMS specifies that the objection of the child should always be respected, except when: (1) the child needs a treatment that cannot be offered in another context; (2) the research is expected to provide therapeutic benefit to the child; and (3) there is no other treatment available (CIOMS, 2002, Guideline 14; CIOMS, 2008, Guideline 14). The guidelines add that when the child is too young or immature, his/her objections can be overridden by a parent or legal representative (CIOMS, 2002, Guideline 14). CIOMS holds that if the child becomes capable of giving an informed consent, researchers must obtain his/her informed consent before continuing to participate (CIOMS, 2002, Guideline 14; CIOMS, 2008, Guideline 14).

While not mentioning children per se, according to the *Universal Declaration on Bioethics and Human Rights*, vulnerable persons should be involved to the greatest extent possible in decision making regarding their participation in research (UNESCO, 2005, art. 7a). UNESCO also recommends that a vulnerable person's refusal to participate in research should be respected (UNESCO, 2005, art. 7 b). Both the *Convention on Human Rights and Biomedicine* (Council of Europe, 1997) and the *Additional Protocol to the Convention on Human Rights and Biomedicine* (Council of Europe, 2005), agree with the previous norms, and state that the minor's opinion should be taken into consideration 'as an increasingly determining factor in proportion to his or her age and degree of maturity' (Council of Europe, 1997, art. 6 (2); Council of Europe, 2005, 15 (1) iv). It also specifies that the research subject should take part in the authorization procedure as far as possible and should not object to participation (Council of Europe, 1997, art. 6 (3) and 17 (1) viii; Council of Europe, 2005, 15 (1) iv and v).

International norms show the importance of involving the child in the decision-making process by obtaining assent to participation in research. However, in practice, the involvement of children presents important dilemmas for researchers. There are many reasons for this including: (a) the lack of specifications in the international norms on how to obtain a child's assent (Friedman Ross, 2006; Wendler, 2006; Sénécal et al., 2009); (b) the lack of standardized guidance on the age or criteria of assent; (c) the absence of guidance on recognizing the child's decision-making capacity; and (d) on what should be communicated before participation in research.

The European Commission has recently proposed to divide children into three age groups as concerning the assent process: (1) children from birth to 3 years of age;

(2) children from 3 years of age onwards; and (3) adolescents (European Commission, 2008, art. 7.1). In the first group, it is impossible to obtain the assent of the child. In the second group, there are children that may understand the notion of altruism (e.g. 3-4 year-olds) and some may be able to understand the risks and benefits of the research (e.g. 9 years old). This age group is very broad and there is not much guidance for researchers. Finally, the third age group concerns adolescents, who may have the capacity to make independent decisions in certain areas of their life. The European Commission does not specify however when adolescence starts. Nevertheless, it seems that there is a consensus in the literature on the age of 14 (Wendler, 2006; Sénécal et al., 2009). This example from the European Commission shows that it is difficult to categorize children into fixed age groups for assent purposes.

Moreover, international norms, while silent on the issue of the age of assent, state that researchers should obtain the assent of the child based on capabilities, degree of maturity, and intelligence. This means that researchers should take into account the ability of the child to understand what participation in research involves. In order to do so, researchers will have to inform the child about the method, the procedure, the risks and benefits resulting from participation and the right of withdrawal. This information should be provided in language appropriate to the age of the child and to his/her level of understanding and stage of development. The difficulty is that there is considerable variation from one child to another, even among children of the same age. When the child's illness severely affects comprehension, it may be impossible to involve the child in the decision-making process and obtain assent. This may also be the case when the child is too young. Moreover, children's intellectual and emotional capacities do not necessarily develop at the same rate (Field and Behrman, 2004). Numerous factors influence their development. For example, a sick child, because of having lived through the experience of their illness, could be more mature and thus more able to understand compared to a healthy child of the same age (Kodish, 2005).

Because of these variations among children in their capabilities and degree of maturity, researchers should intervene on a case by case basis. There are currently two ways of proceeding. An informed consent form can provide a specific space for assent, to allow the child to express the will to participate in research. Alternatively, assent may be addressed on different information leaflets for the parents and children as well as on the separate assent and consent forms (European Commission, 2008). Under this second approach, researchers will have to adapt the information sheet and assent form to the age and level of understanding and maturity of each child (European Commission, 2008). This is challenging on a practical level and could create unrealistic and additional burdens for researchers (to say nothing of more bureaucracy). It would be more realistic to have a single information sheet and assent form, and to adapt verbally the information to be provided according to each child's level of understanding and maturity (Sénécal et al., 2009).

The process for obtaining assent raises particular issues in the context of genetic research that involves biobanking. One of these issues concerns the renewal of consent when the child reaches majority. For example, should the child when of the age of consent be asked to allow for the use of samples collected in a longitudinal study (Ries, 2009)? According to some ethical norms, children should ratify such a use (MRC, 1997), while another states that samples should not be shared before the child reaches such an age

(Gurwitz et al., 2009). Another issue related to longitudinal studies is the withdrawal of the child (Ries, 2007). As the child's autonomy increases over time, participation in research may be continued. Alternatively, if the child has reached majority, withdrawal is an option. This may, however, compromise the quality of the research and, therefore, the future data to be collected. Finally, understanding genetic research is difficult since it refers to scientific terms that children may not be familiar with. This fact needs to be taken into consideration when explaining research to a child. Also, children might not be able to understand concepts, such as the objectives of the research (INVOLVE, 2004). Thus, the information given must be communicated at a level of language that children can understand.

In short, informed consent and assent constitute two very important means of protecting children involved in research. The approval of research is further guided by the evaluation of its potential risks and benefits.

Evaluation of the risks and benefits

The principle of beneficence imposes two obligations on researchers: (1) do not harm; and (2) maximize possible benefits while minimizing the possible harms (*Belmont Report*, 1979). The second obligation, also called the principle of non-maleficence, is derived from the Hippocratic oath, that physicians must 'do no harm' and also prevent harm (Beauchamp and Childress, 2001). Beneficence requires researchers to act in the best interest of the person subject to treatment, as well as to promote his/her well-being and quality of life wherever possible (Beauchamp and Childress, 2001). Non-maleficence requires the concrete application of this principle in the evaluation of risks and benefits. It must be determined 'when it is justifiable to seek certain benefits despite the risks involved, and when the benefits should be foregone because of the risks' (*Belmont Report*, 1979). Prevention of harm is equally important as doing no harm.

Benefit is defined as 'something of positive value related to health or welfare' (*Belmont Report*, 1979). Expected benefits should be sufficient to justify possible risks. As discussed previously, the possibility of finding effective treatments to treat or cure childhood diseases and to contribute to the healthy development of children constitutes a benefit that justifies children's inclusion in research (*Belmont Report*, 1979).

In the context of research, risk may be defined as a potential harm to the person participating in research and also to his/her family or community (*Belmont Report*, 1979). Harm can be physical, psychological, legal, social or financial (*Belmont Report*, 1979). It is important, however, to underline that when research involves children, potential harms should be evaluated from a child's perspective and not from that of an adult. This is because children often entertain fears that adults do not have, such as the fear of separation from their parents (Field and Behrman, 2004).

Risks and benefits should also be balanced before involving individuals in research. The *Belmont Report* suggests some elements to take into consideration in evaluating risks and benefits when involving children in research, such as 'the nature and degree of risk, the condition of the particular population involved, and the nature and level of the anticipated benefits'. The *Belmont Report* states that beneficence may play a justifying role in allowing research involving children in some circumstances. This principle, however, does not provide more guidance on how to proceed when evaluating risks and benefits from the research. Despite this, international norms rely on this principle to provide more specific guidelines.

The *Declaration of Helsinki* requires that every research project be preceded by a 'careful assessment of predictable risks and burdens ... in comparison with foreseeable benefits to the [individuals] or to other individuals or communities' (WMA, 1964, with amendments of 2008, art. 18). Taking up the principle of beneficence, the Declaration specifies that research is only justified when there is a 'reasonable likelihood that this population or community stands to benefit from the results of the research' (WMA, 1964, with amendments of 2008, art. 17). Moreover, if risks outweigh the benefits during the research, the Declaration provides that researchers should stop the research (WMA, 1964, with amendments of 2008, art. 20). It also adds that researchers should be confident that possible risks have been adequately assessed and can be managed (WMA, 1964, with amendments of 2008, art. 20).

CIOMS provides more detailed guidelines on the evaluation of risks and benefits. It specifies that researchers must ensure both an equilibrium between the potential risks and benefits of the research, and that risks have been minimized (CIOMS, 2002, Guideline 8; CIOMS, 2008, Guideline 8). CIOMS differentiates between interventions that do and do not hold out the prospect of direct benefit to participants (CIOMS, 2002, Guideline 8; CIOMS, 2008, Guideline 8). It states that when the intervention offers hope for direct benefits for the research subject, the risks must be justified in light of these expected benefits (CIOMS, 2002, Guideline 9; CIOMS, 2008, Guideline 9).

When a research-based intervention offers only hope for indirect benefits, risks must be reasonable considering the significance of the knowledge obtained, and research subjects cannot be exposed to anything beyond a minimal risk or risk comparable to that of a routine medical procedure (CIOMS, 2002, Guideline 9; CIOMS, 2008, Guideline 9). This acceptable level of risk may be slightly increased when there is a scientific or medical insight of major significance to be gained, or where there is research ethics committee approval (CIOMS, 2002, Guideline 9; CIOMS, 2008, Guideline 9). The research ethics committee should therefore ensure

(1) that the research is designed to be responsive to the disease affecting the prospective subjects or to conditions to which they are particularly susceptible; (2) that the risks of the research interventions are only slightly greater that those associated with routine medical or psychological examination of such persons for the condition or set of clinical circumstances under investigation; (3) that the objective of the research is sufficiently important to justify exposure of the subjects to the increased risk; and (4) that the interventions are reasonably commensurate with clinical interventions that the subjects have experienced or may be expected to experience in relation to the condition under investigation. (CIOMS, 2002, Guideline 9)

The general conditions given above, applicable to every research project involving humans, are subject to further CIOMS limitations when the research involving vulnerable persons does not 'hold out the prospect of direct benefit' (CIOMS, 2002, Guideline 9; CIOMS, 2008, Guideline 9). In such a situation, the risk 'should be no more likely and not greater than the risk attached to routine medical or psychological examination of such persons' (CIOMS, 2002, Guideline 9; CIOMS, 2008, Guideline 9). CIOMS, however, allows slight or minor increases above such risk if there is an overriding scientific or medical reason and an approval from a research ethics committee (CIOMS, 2002, Guideline 9; CIOMS, 2008, Guideline 9).

The *Universal Declaration on the Human Genome and Human Rights* (UNESCO, 1997) as well as the *Universal Declaration on Bioethics and Human Rights* (UNESCO, 2005) both state that research involving vulnerable persons should only be carried out if there is a direct health benefit for the person concerned (UNESCO, 1997, art. 5(e); UNESCO, 2005, art. 7 b). If the research does not hold out such benefit, UNESCO provides that it may still be carried out only if the person concerned is exposed to minimal risk and if the research is 'intended to contribute to the health benefit of other persons in the same age category or with the same genetic conditions' (UNESCO, 1997, art. 5 (e). Likewise, the *Convention on Human Rights and Biomedicine* also states that research involving vulnerable persons may only be carried out for the direct benefit of the specific vulnerable research subject (Council of Europe, 1997, art. 6 and 17 (1) ii). It specifies that in situations in which the research will generate no direct benefit, such research may still be allowed in those exceptional cases where the research: (1) is expected to contribute significantly to the person's disease and the results will confer benefits to other persons in the same age category or suffering from the same disease; and (2) entails only minimal risk and minimal burden for the person concerned (Council of Europe, 1997, art. 17 (2). The 2005 *Additional Protocol to the Convention on Human Rights and Biomedicine* maintains the same position as the *Convention* (Council of Europe, 2005, art. 15 (2).

These norms make important distinctions based on whether research will or will not confer direct benefits to the child. It seems clear that when research is expected to directly benefit the child, greater risks may be taken if they are justified in light of the expected benefits. It is interesting to note how expected benefits can justify serious potential risks. In England, in the case of *Simms v. Simms*, a 16-year-old and an 18-year-old were suffering from an incurable variant of Creutzfeldt-Jakob disease for which no treatment exists (*Simms v. Simms*, [2003] 1 All ER 669). Acknowledging the particularities of this situation, the judge authorized a highly experimental treatment, even though the treatment had never been tested on humans before. According to the judge,

[w]here there is no alternative treatment available and the disease is progressive and fatal, it seems to me to be reasonable to consider experimental treatment with unknown benefits and risks, but without significant risks of increased suffering to the patient, in cases where there is some chance of benefit to the patient. (*Simms v. Simms*, [2003] 1 All ER 669:682)

When the research does not entail any prospect of direct benefit, however, international norms agree that children should not be exposed to more than minimal risk. The difficulty is that these same norms do not provide a definition of what constitutes minimal risk. Some national norms give a definition of this concept. The United States Department of Health and Human Services (DHHS) states that minimal risk means 'that the probability and magnitude of harm or discomfort anticipated in the research are not greater in and of themselves than those ordinarily encountered in daily life or during the performance of routine physical or psychological examinations or test' (45 CFR 46.102 (i)). In Canada, the *Tri Council Policy Statement* refers essentially to the same definition as that provided by the DHHS (Canadian Institutes of Health Research, Natural Sciences and Engineering Research Council of Canada, Social Sciences and Humanities Research Council of Canada, 1998, with 2000, 2002 and 2005 amendments, rule C.1); the European Commission has also adopted this definition (European Commission, 2008, art. 11.1). In Canada, the *Tri-Council Policy Statement* is currently under revision. The *Draft 2nd Edition of the Tri-Council Policy Statement* gives essentially the same definition of this concept (Interagency Advisory Panel on Research Ethics, 2008, p. 14).

Even if there is consensus regarding this definition, it still raises important questions. For example, what risks entailed in research are ordinarily encountered in daily life (Friedman Ross, 2006)? Do the norms refer to risks that might occur when a child plays a sport, has ear piercing or crosses a street? Is it referring to 'all people' or 'ordinary people' (Friedman Ross, 2006)? In order to try to help researchers to determine minimal risk, the Royal College of Paediatrics and Child Health in the UK provides some examples of minimal-risk procedures (such as having the child complete a questionnaire, observation and the collection of urine and/or blood samples) (RCPCH, 2000).

Another concept difficult to apply in practice is that of risk that does not exceed those conventionally associated with routine medical interventions. The application of this concept requires a case by case analysis of each child approached to participate in the research project. Indeed, a child suffering from a disease is subject to medical interventions that are very different from those encountered by a healthy child. In fact, children with disease are subject to medical procedures that might include, for example, blood drawing, injections, chemotherapy and scans. By comparison, a healthy child might only see a physician once a year and may not be subject to any invasive medical procedures. If children are healthy, does that mean that they cannot participate in research that necessarily does not hold the prospect of direct benefit to them?

Finally, the concept of slightly increased risk or minor increase over minimal risk also raises several questions. No definition of this concept is provided by international norms. CIOMS recognizes that no precise definition currently exists (CIOMS, 2002, Guideline 9). It follows that the scope of this concept is left to the judgement of research ethics committees. CIOMS provides few examples of which procedures could constitute a slight or minor increase: additional lumbar punctures or bone-marrow aspirations (CIOMS, 2002, Guideline 9). However, CIOMS emphasizes that the meaning of this concept is 'inferred from what various ethical review committees have reported as having met the standard' (CIOMS, 2002, Guideline 9).

The decisions of the research ethics committees do not set out standards to determine what constitutes 'slightly increased risk'. Also, the elements to take into consideration can change from one research ethics committee to another. In 2002, in its document *Clarifying Specific Portion of 45 CFR 46 Subpart D That Governs Children's Research*, the National Human Research Protections Advisory Committee (NHRPAC) defines 'minor increase over minimal risk' as risk that is 'a little more than minimal' (NHRPAC, 2002). The difficulty of applying this concept lies, on one hand, on the absence of definition of what constitutes a minor or slight increase, and on the other hand, on the lack of precision of the definition of minimal risk. It is difficult to find any consensus regarding this definition.

In the context of genetic research, risk assessment may be frustrated by the fact that the information collected is sensitive. Genetic research may involve psychosocial and possibly eventual socioeconomic risks. Children may perceive themselves differently after learning the results of their genetic testing (Kodish, 2005). They may also experience negative emotions, witness distress in parents or family or distance themselves from family members

(Duncan et al., 2008). In the category of economic risks, a breach of confidentiality could have important implications for employment or insurance (Duncan et al., 2008).

CONCLUSION

The examination of the history of research involving children helps us understand why children require special protection. The exploitation of children during the nineteenth and twentieth centuries led to their exclusion from clinical research, thereby making them 'therapeutic orphans'. Confronted by the lack of information regarding the efficacy and safety of medical therapies in children, and acknowledging that the inclusion of children in research was essential, various international, governmental and non-governmental organizations responsible for the governance of clinical research elaborated ethical and legal norms for the protection of children as research participants. In light of our review, we conclude that the international norms tend to balance the protection of children with the need to include them in research.

Several concerns were discussed. First, there was the common recognition of the need for an informed and free consent. As we have seen, international norms state that the consent of the parents or legal representative shall be informed and voluntary. The discussion of the second concern stressed the problem of obtaining assent. The lack of specifications in international norms on the definition of assent or on how to obtain the assent of the child raises important dilemmas for researchers. In practice, they have to take into consideration different factors, such as the degree of maturity, capabilities, degree of comprehension and level of language of the child. The difficulty lies in the fact that these factors can vary considerably from one child to another, which forces researchers to intervene on a case by case basis. A third concern addressed the need to analyze carefully the potential risks and benefits for the children involved in research. As we have demonstrated, it is very difficult to apply this concept in practice because some terms, such as minimal risk and slightly increased risk, are not defined by international norms. Although some countries have tried to define these terms, the definitions that they provide are still unclear.

There are important concerns that still remain in the realm of paediatric research. In the context of paediatric biobanks, the use of parental broad consent challenges the ethical principle of respect for persons. It questions the ability of the growing child to make autonomous decisions regarding the use of data and samples as well as the right to withdraw from the research (Samuël et al., 2009a). It also illustrates how difficult it is to really involve the child in the decision-making process. Another important issue is the confidentiality of the child's information. Paediatric research creates a particular tri-partite relationship between the researcher, the parents and the child. Therefore, it is difficult to ensure privacy and confidentiality (Samuël et al., 2009b). Finally, the return of results is an emerging issue that raises many questions. International norms do not provide guidance on how, when, to whom and by whom results should be returned (Knoppers et al., 2006). The disclosure of incidental findings also raises the same questions (Wilfond and Carpenter, 2008). Since the parents are the most likely ones to receive the results, it can be asked if they have a parental duty to disclose such results to the child (Samuël et al., 2009b).

These important issues will have to be clarified as research expands to encompass childhood diseases as well as studying the interaction between genes and genes and environment via longitudinal paediatric studies. Moreover, the participation of children in research is currently increasing. Indeed, children are more and more included in biobanking projects, longitudinal studies, palliative care research and pharmaceutical trials (Avard et al., 2009). Consequently, ethical guidelines governing research with children should be clarified to ensure that researchers respect the rights of parents and children in the context of research.

REFERENCES

Avard, D., Samuël, J. and Knoppers, B.M. (2009) *Paediatric Research in Canada*. Montreal: Les Éditions Thémis.

Beauchamp, T.L. and Childress, J.F. (2001) *Principles of Biomedical Ethics*, 5th ed. New York: Oxford University Press.

Beecher, H.K. (1966) 'Ethics and clinical research', *New England Journal of Medicine*, 274 (24): 1354–60.

Belmont Report (1979) *Ethical Principles and Guidelines for the Protection of Human Subjects of Research*. National Commission for the Protection of Human Subjects of Biomedical and Behavioral Research.

Best Pharmaceuticals for Children Act 2002 (BPCA), Pub. L. No. 107–109, 115 Stat. 1408.

Breslow, L.H. (2003) 'The Best Pharmaceuticals for Children Act of 2002: The rise of the voluntary incentive structure and congressional refusal to require pediatric testing', *Harvard Journal on Legislation*, 40: 132–92.

Canadian Institutes of Health Research, Natural Sciences and Engineering Research Council of Canada, Social Sciences and Humanities Research Council of Canada (1998, with 2000, 2002 and 2005 amendments) *Tri-Council Policy Statement: Ethical Conduct for Research Involving Humans*. Ottawa.

Council of Europe (1997) *Convention for the Protection of Human Rights and Dignity of the Human Being with Regard to the Application of Biology and Medicine: Convention on Human Rights and Biomedicine*, no. 164. Oviedo: Council of Europe.

Council of Europe (2005) *Additional Protocol to the Convention on Human Rights and Biomedicine, Concerning Biomedical Research*. Strasbourg: Council of Europe.

Council for International Organization of Medical Sciences (CIOMS) (2002) *International Ethical Guidelines for Biomedical Research Involving Human Subjects*. Geneva: CIOMS.

Council for International Organization of Medical Sciences (CIOMS) (2008) *International Ethical Guidelines for Epidemiological Studies*. Geneva: CIOMS.

Duncan, R.E., Gillam, L., Savulescu, J., Williamson, R., Rogers, J.G. and Delatycki, M.B. (2008) '"You're one of us now": Young people describe their experiences of predictive genetic testing for Huntington disease (HD) and familial adenomatous polyposis (FAP)', *American Journal of Medical Genetics*, 148 (C): 47–55.

European Commission (2008) *Ethical Considerations for Clinical Trials on Medicinal Products Conducted with the Paediatric Population: Recommendations of the Ad Hoc Group for the Development of Implementing Guidelines for Directive 2001/20/EC Relating to Good Clinical Practice in the Conduct of Clinical Trials on Medicinal Products for Human Use*. Brussels: European Commission, available on line at: http://ec.europa.eu/enterprise/pharmaceuticals/eudralex/vol-10/ethical_considerations.pdf.

European Parliament and the Council of Europe (2001) *Directive 2001/20/EC on the Approximation of the Laws, Regulations and Administrative Provisions of the Member States Relating to the Implementation of Good Clinical Practice in the Conduct of Clinical Trials on Medicinal Products for Human Use*. Brussels: EP/CoE, OJ L 121/34, 1.5.2001.

Field, M.J. and Behrman, R.E. (2004) *Ethical Conduct of Clinical Research Involving Children*. Washington, DC: National Academies Press.

Food and Drug Administration Modernization Act 1997 (FDAMA), Pub. L. No. 105–115 § 111, 111 Stat. 2296, 2305–09.

Friedman Ross, L. (2006) *Children in Medical Research: Access versus Protection*. New York: Clarendon Press.

Friedman Ross, L. (2008) 'Ethical and policy issues in pediatric genetics', *American Journal of Medical Genetics,* 148 (C): 1–7.

Grodin, M.A. and Glantz, L.H. (1994) *Children as Research Subjects: Science, Ethics, and Law*. New York: Oxford University Press.

Gurwitz, D., Fortier, I., Lunshof, J.E. and Knoppers, B.M. (2009) 'Children and population biobanks', *Science,* 325: 818–19.

Interagency Advisory Panel on Research Ethics (2008) *Draft 2nd Edition of the Tri-Council Policy Statement: Ethical Conduct for Research Involving Humans*. Ottawa: IAPRE.

INVOLVE (2004) *Involving Marginalised and Vulnerable People in Research: A Consultation Document*. Eastleigh, Hampshire: NHS, Involve.

Knoppers, B.M. (1978) 'Les notions d'autorisation et de consentement dans le contrat médical', *Cahiers de Droit,* 19: 893–902.

Knoppers, B.M., Avard, D., Cardinal, G. and Cranley Glass, K. (2002) 'Children and incompetent adults in genetic research: Consent and safeguards', *Nature Reviews Genetics,* 3: 221–4.

Knoppers, B.M., Joly, Y., Simard, J. and Durocher, F. (2006) 'The emergence of an ethical duty to disclose genetic research results: International perspectives', *European Journal of Human Genetics,* 14: 1170–8.

Kodish, E. (2005) *Ethics and Research with Children: A Case-based Approach*. New York: Oxford University Press.

Medical Research Council (MRC) (1997) *Human Tissue and Biological Samples for Use in Research*. London: MRC.

National Human Research Protections Advisory Committee (NHRPAC) (2002) *Clarifying Specific Portion of 45 CFR 46 Subpart D that Governs Children's Research*. Washington, DC: US Government Printing Office.

National Institutes of Health (1998) *NIH Policy and Guidelines on the Inclusion of Children as Participants in Research Involving Human Subjects*. Bethesda, MD: NIH.

Nuremberg Code (1949) National Institutes of Health, s. 1, reprinted from *Trials of War Criminals before the Nuremberg Military Tribunals under Control Council Law No. 10, Vol. 2*. Washington, DC: US Government Printing Office, 181–2, online: http://ohsr.od.nih.gov/guidelines/nuremberg.html; World Medical Association (WMA), *Code of Ethics of the World Medical Association* (1964) online: http://www.pubmedcentral.nih.gov/picrender.fcgi?artid=1816102&blobtype=pdf.

Ries, N.M. (2007) 'Growing up as a research subject: Ethical and legal issues in birth cohort studies involving genetic research', *Health Law Journal,* 15: 1–41.

Ries, N.M. (2009) 'Longitudinal studies involving children and adolescents', in D. Avard, J. Samuël and B.M. Knoppers (eds), *Paediatric Research in Canada*. Montreal: Les Éditions Thémis.

Royal College of Paediatrics and Child Health (RCPCH): Ethics Advisory Committee (2000) *Guidelines for the Ethical Conduct of Medical Research Involving Children*. London: RCPCH.

Saint Raymond, A. and Brasseur, D. (2005) 'Development of medicines for children in Europe: Ethical implications', *Paediatric Respiratory Reviews,* 6: 45–51.

Samuël, J., Ries, N.M., Malkin, D. and Knoppers, B.M. (2009a) 'Biobanks and children: Comparative international policies', in D. Avard, J. Samuël and B.M. Knoppers *Paediatric Research in Canada*. Montreal: Les Éditions Thémis.

Samuël, J., Black, L., Avard, D. and Knoppers, B.M. (2009b) *Best Practices for Research Involving Children and Adolescents: Genetic, Pharmaceutical, Longitudinal Studies and Palliative Care Research*. Working Document. Montreal.

Sénécal, K., Samuël, J., and Avard, D. (2009) 'Research and the assent of the child: Towards harmonization?', in D. Avard, J. Samuël, and B.M. Knoppers (eds), *Paediatric Research in Canada*. Montreal: Les Éditions Thémis.

Simms v Simms [2003] 1 All ER 669.

Truong, R.D. (2005) 'Increasing the participation of children in clinical research', *Journal of Intensive Care Medicine,* 31: 760–1.

United Nations Educational Scientific and Cultural Organization (UNESCO) (1997) *Universal Declaration on the Human Genome and Human Rights*. Paris: UNESCO.

United Nations Educational Scientific and Cultural Organization (UNESCO) (2005) *Universal Declaration on Bioethics and Human Rights*. Paris: UNESCO.

Wendler, D.S. (2006) 'Assent in paediatric research: Theoretical and practical considerations', *Journal of Medical Ethics*, 32: 229–34.

Wilfond, B.S. and Carpenter, K.J. (2008) 'Incidental findings in pediatric research', *Journal of Law Medicine and Ethics*, 36: 332–40.

World Medical Association (WMA) (1949) *International Code of Medical Ethics*. London: WMA.

World Medical Association (WMA) (2008) *Declaration of Helsinki*. Seoul: WMA.

23

Orphan Diseases

Ruth Chadwick and Paul McCarthy

DEFINING ORPHAN DISEASES: RARE VS NEGLECTED

While the term 'orphan diseases' is a technical one defined in health policy literature, it is worth reminding ourselves in the context of healthcare ethics of the common uses of the term 'orphan'. The primary meaning, derived from the Greek term *orphanos* is one bereft of a parent or parents. This is important in healthcare terms, because of the high numbers of orphans in some, especially war-torn, countries, whose healthcare needs may not even be identified let alone met. To this primary meaning, the secondary meaning 'bereft of protection' is clearly related. Again, however, in the context of healthcare ethics it is important to remember there may be significant healthcare issues and needs that are not appropriately identified as orphan *diseases,* or indeed recognised, and so it is necessary to think about orphan healthcare issues and populations as well as diseases per se.

Turning to orphan diseases, however, by their very nature they have something missing or absent, analogous to the lack of a protector on the part of an orphan, and until recently at least have arguably been missing sufficient recognition within strategic approaches to health research and healthcare policy. This has particularly been the case within the UK and more generally across the EU. Internationally, the situation in the US has been more organised in terms of a systematic approach to rare diseases, a point we discuss in more detail in our examination of policy responses to orphan diseases, but sporadic interventions into particular orphan diseases would seem to be the rule. These trends for the most part can be explained by the observation that most orphan diseases have a low visibility in policy and scientific arenas, have low public interest (although specific orphan diseases are often the subject of special media coverage for various reasons), are of less economic interest for medical industry actors, and suffer from a general obscurity in terms of their impact, knowledge and awareness (Gericke, 2005). These trends are not only present for those who might be on the outside 'looking in' but for sufferers and relatives of those afflicted by orphan diseases; similar fragmentations of knowledge and awareness are often to be found as well.

The problematic conceptualisation of what an orphan disease is extends into the very definition of what constitutes such a disease. In reviewing the literature, both medical and policy, it is clear that various definitions exist. In the broadest sense, two types of orphan diseases are most often referred to, these being:

1. neglected diseases, or diseases of poverty, which are usually prevalent in the developing world;
2. rare disorders afflicting a small number of individuals, often with a genetic basis, which can be either simple or complex.

While the two categories may represent different issues, for the most part the commonalities in why these might be called orphan diseases more generally are easily outlined. First, there is an obvious sense in which a rare disease may be neglected, even if it is not a disease associated with poverty in that the strongest link between the two types is that both are groups of diseases for which there is little financial incentive or interest in the commercial development of cures, treatments or diagnostics. In other words, they are indeed 'neglected' in terms of investment. Other links include a lack or neglect by scientific interests (though this is less pronounced in certain neglected diseases where various initiatives have been supported) as well as a lack of clear support or patient group mobilisation, which often characterise other non-orphan diseases.

The difficulty in beginning an analysis of *rare* diseases also starts at the very outset in terms of how a rare disease is defined. Here we are immediately faced with the fact that what constitutes a rare disorder varies from country to country. In the US, for example a rare disease is one which has fewer than 200,000 individuals with the condition. The WHO suggests a rare disease is one where 0.65-1 per 1000 are afflicted with it, while the EU defines it as 1 per 2000. While what is 'rare' may differ between contexts, there then remains the question of what counts as rare in the context of global health ethics. The issue of borderline cases of diseases is likewise not addressed within these numerical categories (other than in the WHO classification, which allows for some variation); the fact that these limits are now often associated with specific types of incentivised legislation suggests a particular framing of rare diseases in order to objectively set policy criteria for such things as preferential regulations in terms of patenting and research (Huyard, 2009).

Ethics, strategies and opportunity costs

Orphan diseases raise a number of difficult challenges in terms of their ethical impact, their social aspects and the economic responses for health policy required to deal with them. This is true both for those orphan diseases which fall into the rare category and those which do not. While each rare disease is generally unique in terms of its epidemiology and effects, we would argue that there is a potential commonality in terms of approaches through the importance to which knowledge and practice can be ascribed to providing potential cures, therapies and diagnostics for a large number of rare and neglected diseases.

In healthcare ethics in general, the rival merits of different strategies for combating disease have long been discussed – for example the benefits of public health measures such as clean water and sanitation, versus the technical fix. Investing heavily in high-tech solutions not only sets a particular course from which it may prove difficult if not impossible to deviate for political reasons, but also has opportunity costs. The commitment to providing genomic solutions to healthcare needs is a case in point.

What has to be considered, from an ethical point of view, is what genomic solutions have to offer to neglected and rare diseases. On the one hand, it might be hypothesised that the greater precision offered by genomics might benefit rare diseases – indeed, the promise of more accurate disease classification may redefine the very boundaries of what counts as rare. On the other hand, in so far as 'neglected' diseases can be alleviated by low-tech, non-genomic solutions, it might at the same time be hypothesised that these may be an opportunity cost of the post-genomic era.

In the aftermath of the Human Genome Project, following the production of the first map and sequence at the beginning of the twenty-first century in particular, the relevance of genomics to tackling orphan (and other) diseases has moved centre stage. Before discussing the specific issues related to genomics and orphan diseases, it is worth remembering that as we progress further down this road to what many have seen as the post-genomic era, a number of realities and limitations continue to characterise research and clinical practice within the field. On the one hand, the discourse of promise which for long has been intimately connected with genomics has to date delivered few major meaningful related healthcare benefits in the manner in which many believed they would (Hjorleifsson, 2008). The majority of the promises of translation have yet to be realised. The completion of the Human Genome Project, which took a shorter time than anticipated, has not yet radically transformed clinical practice or the manner in which societies have conceptualised the potential impacts of genomic knowledge.

The heady days of human genome mapping and sequencing were characterised by a number of problematic elements related to the surrounding hype. These included misleading reporting on the part of the media, a playing up of expectations; reports on the discovery of 'genes for x' on a regular basis, reflecting an unrealistic and flawed set of assumptions of the degree of the role of genetics in a variety of diseases and behavioural patterns. Both social scientists and geneticists (of the cautious variety) argued consistently against such genetic *determinism* and on reflection a genetic *expectation*, but many, particularly within policy settings, explicitly picked up on the *promise* of genomics to be a revolution in knowledge with the potential to be as dramatic as the shift from agriculture to industrialisation. The lure of genomic promises can be seen clearly in agendas set out by the UK government in reports such as *Our Inheritance, Our Future* (Department of Health, 2003).

What is significant about the way in which those promises were framed in *Our Inheritance, Our Future*, however, was the predominant individualism informing policy. It was envisaged that genomics knowledge would lead to a situation in which both lifestyle advice and treatment could be 'tailored' to the individual. An obvious difficulty with such a vision of the future, however, is the infrastructure required. This individualistic model of health care has been described as the 'boutique' model by Abdallah Daar and Peter Singer, and as inappropriate for the developing world (Daar and Singer, 2005). The individualisation of health has another side also: a greater responsibility on the part of citizens to ensure their health. The language of responsibility has increased the discourses of burden associated with genetic diseases in an environment characterised by the necessity to further rationalise already scarce health resources through the prevention of genetic diseases and abnormality.

Genomics, diet and neglected healthcare issues

While Daar and Singer discuss this in relation to pharmaceuticals, discussed elsewhere in this volume, we will illustrate it by a discussion of genomics and food. It is noticeable that the 'tailoring' promised in *Our Inheritance, Our Future*, applies to lifestyle, and not only to treatment. In other words, what is at issue here includes diet. To what extent might nutrigenomics, the science of the relationship between genetic factors and response to diet, have relevance to orphan diseases, especially to those neglected diseases and healthcare issues that are concomitants of poverty? A focus on personalised nutrition is arguably not a strategy most likely to further nutrition-related public health goals. An additional point might be whether the results of nutrigenomics research from one culture, with one specific set of standard staple foods, can be transferred to other cultures with completely different sets of foods, or whether gene-environment interactions are sufficiently complicated to undermine transferability. There might be a risk of providing harmful advice.

Public health goals may need, rather, to focus on prevention and management of nutrition-related diseases, through identifying susceptible populations or subpopulations and focusing on their needs. Identification of potential impacts of issues related to global food security, for example, would be an important prerequisite. In so far as nutrigenomics requires large amounts of investment, 'personalised diet' seems likely to be implemented primarily in richer countries, where it would not directly be a threat to food security, but indirectly, nevertheless, poorer countries may still be liable to domination by the companies involved.

A focus on population groups, then, might be more helpful than an emphasis on personalised nutrition, whether these populations are defined in terms of geographical ancestry or in some other way – e.g. groups who are undernourished, or who are suffering from eating disorders. Here, the relationship between nutrigenomics and taste may become relevant. Given individual differences in perceptions of bitterness, which may have a genetic basis as well as being due to differences in age and ethnicity, the identification of these factors may facilitate the development of food products specifically suited to particular population groups. Populations may also, however, be categorised according to nutritional status, for example, undernourished or not; overeating (and who may still be undernourished) or not; or according to specific needs of other sorts. This may be useful in designing food products for particular population groups: elderly persons, for example, may have specific needs in this regard. Public health strategies should also involve environmental strategies including sustainable food production (i.e. not overemphasising genetic aspects, while giving them their due), as well as investigation of other technological possibilities such as functional foods.

Population-based genomic research

In so far as genomics has the potential to make a significant contribution here, a secure evidence base is needed, establishing the associations between genetic factors and dietary response. This is true not only to facilitate nutrigenomics, but also to make possible the development of pharmacogenomics and a greater understanding of population variation and of the genetic factors underlying complex diseases. To secure such an evidence base, however, requires large-scale investment in population-wide research. The late 1990s and the first decade of the twenty-first century have seen a massive explosion in biobanking initiatives, to establish the genetic factors underlying disease, which may be minor variations between individuals. At the time of writing, there are increasing moves to link up these initiatives internationally, both in Europe, through endeavours such as the Biological and Biomolecular Resource Infrastructure (BBMRI) and beyond – for example, through the P3G project (Public Population Projects in Genomics). The rationale for linking such initiatives is the greater statistical power that will ensue to provide the secure evidence base. Clearly, where rare diseases are at stake, the issue of statistical power becomes more acute.

The ethical discussion surrounding biobanking has tended to focus on issues of consent to sample donation (e.g. whether it should be broad or narrow); the right of participants to withdraw; provision of feedback; access by third parties to samples for research or other purposes; commercialisation and benefit-sharing. Clearly in the case of some underserved population groups, whether or not they have rare diseases, these issues are highly likely to be challenging to address, and there are questions about whose interests are served by research into the genetic make-up of those groups. This is a key ethical issue for orphan diseases and groups in particular.

Whole genome sequencing

It is not the aim of this chapter to suggest that pursuing genomic goals is not a laudable endeavour, but rather to show that how the goals are defined may obscure some less prominent areas where arguably genomics may indeed deliver meaningful results in the near to medium term. Within the science at the time of writing, the increasing focus is on whole genome sequencing of individuals, a field energised by continual reductions in computing time with increased processing power (the $1000 dollar genome) and the expansion of the 'book of life' to the notion of a library capable of mapping and analysing variation between individuals and population groups. Indeed, with such a library and more whole genomes sequenced, there has even been a resurgence in the notion that these will provide a platform for more comprehensive and sophisticated analysis of gene-environment as well as gene–gene interactions. Whether this represents a re-articulation of the genomic promise rather than a change of emphasis, and to what extent the greater promised precision will reinvigorate genetic determinism, are not clear. The prospect of genetic profiling of individuals, perhaps at birth, however, once again reinforces an individual-based approach. As long as this is the holy grail, we see this positioning as emblematic of why particular diseases continue to have low prominence within the genomic enterprise, despite being of high relevance in terms of genomic knowledge and potential genomic clinically derived practice.

The concomitant pressures of reconciling reality with future promissory advances continue to be strong discourses that frame the workings of the genomic enterprise at national and international levels. However, discussions of ethical, legal and social issues within the post-genomic era have similarly continued to shift and realign with the new visions that are being promulgated. The language of rights and responsibilities has increasingly become associated with actual and potential therapies, not solely for those related to genomics, it must be said; but diseases with genomic causal factors lend themselves to particular forms of *screening* which can be said to be visibly 'cost-effective', using measures that frame healthcare policy decisions.

GENOMICS AND RARE DISEASES

The relevance of genomic knowledge to orphan and rare diseases specifically has been identified in a number of documents. It is, for example, estimated by the European Union that some 80 per cent of rare diseases have genetic causal factors. Unlike other common diseases which are often *multi-factorial*, rare genetic diseases, having potential genetic and environmental causal factors, are often relatively *simple* in terms of the number of genes deemed to play a role in the expression of the disease. Some have thus termed such diseases as being *complex simple*, the complexity referring partly to the difficulties in comprehension in terms of a genetic framework, but more so, through a lack of dedicated research into the field itself, to difficulties in being able to detect and screen for the particular genes responsible for such diseases. However, it must also be stressed that there are a number of *complex* rare diseases that are complicated in respect of the difficulties that are inherent in trying to understand not only causal factors but also expression being polygenic. One such example here would be diseases caused by defects in the mitochondrial genome, which are variably expressed, difficult to predict, with no known effective therapies for sufferers (besides those aimed pre-natally at prevention).

Mitochondrial genomics

When the 'human genome' is discussed it is normally the nuclear genome that is at issue, rather than the mitochondrial genome, which was sequenced much earlier, without the publicity that accompanied the Human Genome Project of the 1990s. Debates about genetic reductionism and the relationship between genes and identity also tend to be carried out in relation to the nuclear genome rather than the mitochondrial. So it is perhaps not inappropriate to describe the mitochondrial genome as the 'orphan genome'. The mitochondrial genome is particularly significant because if a woman suffers from a disorder caused by mitochondrial DNA, all her children will inherit it (although severity can differ markedly); mitochondrial DNA is passed down the maternal line, while nuclear DNA is inherited from both parents. From the start, then, the mitochondrial genome gives rise to issues of gender, and provides a focal point for discussion in the context of ancestry tracing. While it might be argued that the nuclear genome is primarily responsible for the genetic influences that make an individual who he or she is, diseases caused by a variant on the mitochondrial genome can be among the most devastating.

Given the critical role that genetics demonstrably plays in the incidence, prevalence and occurrence of many rare diseases, it is pertinent to question why such diseases continue to suffer from poor diagnostics, a dearth in applicable treatments and therapies, and indeed a lack of cohesive knowledge frameworks in terms of comprehension and understanding.

A number of reasons for this can be suggested. First, there is the question of familiarity; most rare diseases are never encountered by most clinicians and when they are, clinicians are faced with the immediate difficulty of having little to no knowledge available on the disease unless they are able to access some network or other individuals who have encountered the disease. This in turn translates into the observation that many rare diseases may not be represented within standard text books and hence may not be taught about or find their way into research journals unless those who encounter said diseases are able to combine clinical practice with research. This is the case for mitochondrial diseases, for example, where most research teams working in the field in the UK and internationally are derived from clinical centres directly engaged with sufferers.

Policy responses

While our discussion so far has perhaps highlighted a particularly negative view of how rare and orphan diseases have been dealt with in relation to genomics, it is not the case that policy actors have likewise completely rejected the field. For example, where pharmaceutical treatments are appropriate for rare diseases, orphan drug policy responses can make possible variations in requirements for clinical trials (e.g. where it is not possible to recruit large numbers of participants because the disease is rare) or provide incentives for development of products which otherwise would not for economic reasons be produced. However, policy responses such as they have been thus far have not been without problems or their detractors and critics. In this chapter, we examine two of the main areas where responses have been formulated: the US and the EU; and in the latter examine how EU regulation has impacted on the UK as a member state responding to EU legislation. A number of countries however, such as Canada and Australia, have seen renewed calls to develop a national plan on rare diseases (Jaffe, 2010).

US

The US can be characterised as having a relatively established legislative framework for dealing with orphan diseases. The passing of the 1983 Orphan Drugs Act and the linked establishment of the National Organisation for Rare Diseases have indeed arguably been the template and model followed by other jurisdictions in approaching the issues involved in orphan diseases. Both developments are linked in that it was because of the coming together of a coalition of various support groups for rare disorders that made it possible to lobby successfully for the introduction of the Act.

The Act targets explicitly one of the critical issues in orphan diseases, namely the lack of commercial interest in the development of therapies and treatments. This is therefore framed in terms of the pharmaceutical industry and the development of drug based treatments. The Act provides for a range of incentives and benefits for companies who engage in the development of drugs for orphan diseases. These include:

- tax reliefs on the conducting of clinical research;
- exemptions from some Federal Drug Agency fees;
- market exclusivity for 7 years;
- other grants and concessions, such as Congressional aid.

The introduction of the Act, at least in terms of the development of drugs, has been seen by most as a success. It is estimated that in the decade prior to the Act some 10 treatments for orphan diseases had been developed, in contrast to over 500 in the decade following its introduction, including ones for AIDS (Arno et al., 1995). However, criticisms have been levelled against the Act on a number of grounds, such as abuse of the regulations (Amgen's use of the exclusivity protections to safeguard its investment in erythropoietin (EPO)) (Maeder, 2003). Likewise, market exclusivity presupposes that a drug will still remain profitable and it is unclear how many orphan diseases would generate enough of a profit to recoup the ever increasing costs associated with drug development, clinical trials and drug discovery (Drummond et al., 2007).

The Act aside, the National Organization for Rare Disorders (NORD) presents a model and template for patient advocacy that is likewise being copied in other settings. National Organization for Rare Disorders NORD follows the US definition of a rare disorder in setting out its agenda in representing the 25 million Americans suffering from the 6000 disorders affecting fewer than 200,000 people. NORD seeks to perform a number of functions, supporting sufferers and their families, and promoting research on rare diseases. These include providing networking opportunities for those afflicted with rare disorders to meet others and clinicians, sponsorship programmes for access to treatments and a resource guide detailing reports on roughly 1200 disorders.

The US system of health care has an obvious bearing on the positioning of both NORD and the framing of the Orphan Drug Act. This reflects the overwhelming focus of the US healthcare system on private insurance and commercial interests within health (although the Obama healthcare reforms represent a significant reshaping of these). The positioning of NORD as an alliance or umbrella group representing those suffering from rare disorders may therefore be seen as a relatively successful attempt to portray rare diseases as a sizeable issue through reference to the 25 million Americans thought to be afflicted with a rare disease. However, this approach is we argue problematic, albeit one which is being followed elsewhere. It is unclear how successful this approach has been in attracting the specific interest of genomics, given its key role in various rare disorders. EU responses however are notable in this regard for specifically highlighting this aspect of rare diseases.

European Union

EU approaches in terms of respective member states have been widely divergent in tackling orphan diseases. Difficulties may be further compounded as a result of the varied ethical frameworks within with health care, genomic research and orphan diseases, are contextualised throughout Europe. For a start there are few pan-European medical support groups equivalent to NORD in the US, which could be seen to be playing the advocacy role. However, as with the US, the EU has regulated on the issue of orphan drugs.

The Regulation of the European Parliament and the European Council on Orphan Medicinal Products (EC 141/2000) sets out the European approach to the issue. It provides for a number of incentives to aid in the development of treatments for orphan diseases, these include:

- ten-year market exclusivity (where drugs exist, exclusivity will be granted only on the basis that the new treatment is proved to be clinically superior);
- assistance in various areas of the development of drugs, guidance on regulations and assistance with the running of clinical trials, for example;
- discretionary measures, such as the waiving of various regulatory fees.

Although enacted some 17 years after the US Act, the parallels are quite clear in terms of providing economic and regulatory incentives for companies to pursue developments related to orphan diseases. The specific assistance of the EU in terms of the running of clinical trials is a response to the fact that while as a whole the population of the EU is comparable to the US (and hence the numbers needed to run trials effectively easier to recruit) taking member states individually this is not the case. It is not only a question of numbers, however, as the regulations governing clinical trials within different member states may differ as well as issues with the sharing of medical data between member states. Furthermore, arguments have been raised questioning whether the drug route should be the favoured route in legislation where support in other ways would be much more beneficial to sufferers and their families (Haffner, 2008).

Recently, the EU has mapped out a potential new policy framework for orphan diseases in the Communication on Rare Diseases (formally adopted by the European Council on 9 June 2009). The Communication frames rare diseases as a specific public health issue and an area where community action can be uniquely beneficial (Chatzimarkakis, 2009). The Communication makes a number of recommendations and observations and, most pertinent for this article, explicitly identifies genomics, in terms of research and potential therapies, as a key pillar of future healthcare policy dealing with orphan diseases.

As with NORD's positioning of rare diseases, the Communication defines rare diseases as those with a prevalence of not more than 5 per 10,000 persons, but stresses that across the EU this translates into an estimated 29 million people. It is perhaps not surprising that attempting to frame orphan diseases as an issue in respective healthcare settings requires such aggregation of the numbers of sufferers. This could be seen to be a result of the observation that questions of scale appear to be increasingly important in determining future allocations of scarce healthcare resources. However, aggregation brings with it, or suggests, other problems that we discuss later.

In relation to genomics, the Communication both frames a number of problems related to orphan diseases where the science can help, and sets out a number of objectives to be achieved through coordinated action in genomics across Europe. These include for example:

- improving visibility and recognition of rare diseases;

This is not solely a recommendation targeting increased public knowledge about rare diseases but about increasing clinical and research knowledge about rare diseases (Budde, 2009). The recommendation is for a complete review and revamping of coding and classificatory systems dealing with rare diseases, with a specific role for genomics in achieving this.

- supporting policies in member states;

In respecting the principles of subsidiarity enshrined in the EU the Communication proposes supporting member states in developing coherent and cohesive policies on rare diseases. These include assistance in the classification and detection of rare diseases, harmonising research between member states and allowing for the sharing of expertise between actors in different member states.

- developing a European approach;

The Communication continually refers to the problems of fragmentation (of knowledge and of sufferers) and the need to link and coordinate in order to negate these issues.

In terms of recommendations, the Communication calls for a number of specific actions, of which some are listed and described here.

- redefining rare diseases;

The Communication calls for a better and more nuanced definition of a rare disease (as well as one which is harmonised internationally).

- better coding and classification;

Through the framework, Europe will lead for the Communication refining of the International Classification for Disease and its entries dealing with rare diseases. This will allow for better codification of rare diseases.

- dissemination of information and knowledge and the creation of disease information networks;

The Communication suggests that where a disease is rare then expertise and knowledge will similarly be rare. In response to this it suggests that mechanism and networks of excellence be created in order to bring disparate knowledge together and to disseminate it effectively across Europe.

- screening practices, registries and databases, and research and development (R&D).

The Communication explicitly suggests that the costs of screening and testing for disorders will continue to fall and that EU-wide strategies should be developed through research on the most effective means. Linked to the developments in biobanks we discussed previously, there is also the call for more effective data collection and sharing on rare disorders across member states through the creation of databases and registries in order to aid in the study of the epidemiology of rare diseases. The Communication likewise recommends that R&D in therapies and diagnostics be coordinated across Europe in order to deal with the issues of scarcity, lack of commercial interest and lack of clinical and research knowledge in dealing with rare diseases.

Evaluating policy responses

The EU Communication provides an interesting reference point in analysing frameworks dealing with rare diseases by virtue of the comprehensive set of objectives and recommendations it makes in dealing with the issues. It must be stressed, however, that the Communication (as other Communications) does not represent actual policy. If it is adopted then regulations will be derived from it, but at the time of writing it marks out a particular vision and agenda for orphan diseases in the EU. What it does set out as a framework can be subjected to a number of criticisms as well as a number of endorsements in terms of strong and beneficial policy goals.

We argue that a reliance solely on the pharmaceutical industry in developing these drugs may not in the long term be a feasible policy. Already for other neglected diseases, such as those associated with poverty, new models of public–private partnership have been and need to continue to be considered; but also the genomic issues highlighted above need to be addressed. Implicit in many, but not all, of the diseases where genes play a major role is debate concerning the dictum that prevention is always better than cure. It is beyond the scope of this chapter to deal in any sustained manner with the wide variety of arguments that have been deployed within these contexts, but ongoing controversies over genomic prevention (e.g. screening and selection methods) in addition to treatment methods, are clearly relevant.

CONCLUSION

We have tried to identify the ways in which diseases and populations become characterisable as 'orphan', and the strategies that have been adopted to address this. The ways in which different strategies become prioritised remains an issue for politics, economics and ethics. While policy continues to a large extent to focus on pharmaceuticals, strategies for prevention, both of a traditional public health variety, and using genomic technologies, need further consideration – as do genomic-informed treatment possibilities for diseases, whether their orphan status is 'neglected' or 'rare'.

REFERENCES

Arno, P., Bonuck K., and Davis M. (1995) 'Rare diseases, drug development, and AIDS: The impact of the Orphan Drug Act', *Milbank Quarterly*, 73 (2): 231–52.

Budde, W. (2009) 'Healthcare funding: Rare diseases, a priority? AIM's proposals', *Pharmaceuticals Policy & Law*, 11 (4): 335–41.

Chatzimarkakis, J. (2009) 'The rare diseases agenda of the European Parliament', *Pharmaceuticals Policy & Law*, 11 (4): 319–21.

Daar, A.S. and Singer, P.A. (2005) 'Pharmacogenetics and geographical ancestry: Implications for drug development and global health', *Nature Reviews Genetics*, 6: 241–6.

Department of Health (2003) *Our Inheritance, Our Future: Realising the Potential of Genetics in the NHS.* London: Department of Health.

Drummond, M.F., Wilson, D.A., Kanavos, P., Ubel, P. and Rovira, J. (2007) 'Assessing the economic challenges posed by orphan drugs', *International Journal of Technology Assessment in Health Care*, 23 (1): 36–42.

Gericke, C.A. (2005) 'Ethical issues in funding orphan drug research and development', *Journal of Medical Ethics*, 31 (3): 164–8.

Haffner, M.E. (2008) 'Does orphan drug legislation really answer the needs of patients?' *The Lancet*, 371 (9629): 2041–4.

Hjorleifsson, S. (2008) 'Decoding the genetics debate: Hype and hope in Icelandic news media in 2000 and 2004', *New Genetics and Society*, 25 (3): 234–47.

Huyard, C. (2009) 'How did uncommon disorders become "rare diseases"? History of a boundary object', *Sociology of Health & Illness*, 31 (4): 463–77.

Jaffe, A. (2010) 'Call for a national plan for rare diseases', *Journal of Paediatrics & Child Health*, 46 (1/2): 2–4.

Maeder, T. (2003) 'The orphan drug backlash', *Scientific American*, 288 (5): 80.

24

Poverty and Indigenous Peoples

Leonardo D. de Castro, Peter A. Sy and Teoh Chin Leong

Vulnerability easily comes across as the characteristic that makes poor people and indigenous populations the common subject of this chapter. However, bioethical issues arising in connection with healthcare for indigenous peoples should not have to be seen in the context of poverty. Insofar as their health and well-being are concerned, people could independently be rendered vulnerable by their poverty or by their being members of certain indigenous groups. While indigenous peoples are likely to be less well off economically compared to the general population in which they are situated, the factors affecting their health and well-being have to be understood independently of this fact in order to arrive at an accurate picture of their situation. Vulnerabilities relating to poverty and indigenous peoples generate distinct ethical issues. Insofar as certain indigenous persons are poor, they share 'poverty' issues, but the added dimension of ethnicity deserves separate treatment.

While poor populations and indigenous peoples do share the description of being 'less able than others to safeguard their own needs and interests adequately' (AHRQ, 1998), it is a mistake to regard this as their defining characteristic. Nevertheless, there is no universally accepted approach to defining poverty and indigenous peoples. These are polycontextual phenomena, and the vulnerabilities of indigenous peoples and the poor (even those relating only to health matters) are multidimensional and complex.

Definitions of poverty have been variable and it is important to see where the differences lie because poverty has been seen as a critical factor that determines to whom responsibilities are owed and by whom.

DEFINITIONS

Poverty

Poverty is a polycontextual phenomenon in that different people may be categorized as poor on account of the lack of different baskets of things or of different capabilities.

Thus, while there may be a universal recognition of the importance of reducing poverty as a global goal (see MDG), there is hardly universal agreement as to what particular criteria should be used and who may be considered 'poor'. Varying measures of poverty have varying significance for different populations, including indigenous peoples. Thus, the ethical implications of adopting particular measures could be diverse and far-reaching. It makes sense to distinguish carefully between varying conceptions and measurements of poverty. These conceptions are ultimately tied to concerns to reduce inequality and promote social justice.

There are various challenges to the conception and measurement of poverty and to questions regarding the adequacy of income as a defining variable (Sen, 2006). In assessing equity and social justice, the goal is to understand how the 'capability to function' with respect to a certain quality of life and basic freedoms is impeded, for instance by poverty. Poverty will thus be understood in terms of failures relating to basic capabilities rather than in terms of having low income per se (Sen, 2006: 34). This follows from the understanding of development as involving the 'enhancement of human living and the freedom to live the kind of life that we have reason to value' (Sen, 2006: 35). In this regard, Sen's list of capabilities includes, but is not limited to, good health, education and social capacities, e.g. taking part in 'the life of the community' (Sen, 2006: 35).

Another view puts emphasis on the need for a basic level of social justice and human rights that revolve around 'minimally adequate shares of basic freedoms and (socio-political) participation, of food, drink, clothing, shelter, education, and health care', even if this is (rightfully) developed with a low level of substantive specificity (Pogge, 2008b: 57). If one accepts and starts from the existential as well as 'personal and ethical value of human life', one can outline the sociopolitical context and environment within which such human flourishing and a 'minimally worthwhile life' must take place. This would constitute 'an internationally acceptable core criterion of basic justice' (Pogge, 2008b: 54) that determines the standards all nations should strive to uphold. Although the interrelations of cause and effect may be complex, both national and international sociopolitical institutions and accompanying appointment holders are implicated in and accountable for lapses and the 'underfulfillment of human rights' (Pogge, 2008b: 55) where they occur, precisely because they have been allowed to prevail.

The amount of reformation that takes place either in the form of correcting and redesigning inadequate institutions, conditions and practices or protecting the vulnerable should be proportionate to the harms and benefits the respective institutional members have inflicted or enjoyed. Pogge's (2008b) definition of the inadequacies in healthcare provision and poverty prevention is thus meant to be normative and not merely descriptive. The remaining challenge is to negotiate between internationally warranted and locally specified expressions of social justice as they pertain to poverty and healthcare provision.

Adam Smith's focus on the idea of relative deprivation has also been cited (Sen, 2006). The idea is that the standards of the community determine if one has reached a certain level of acceptable 'social functioning', irrespective of whether those standards are comparatively better than absolute deprivation levels elsewhere: 'relative deprivation in terms of income can … lead to absolute deprivation in terms of (social) capabilities' (Sen, 2006: 36). Thus, some of the current economic measures of poverty or income inequality are deficient precisely because of a lack of theorizing about the nature of social relations and '(e)conomic data cannot be interpreted without the necessary sociological understanding' (Sen, 2006: 45). The implication of this line of reasoning for healthcare appears to be that relative deprivation in healthcare is as much a cause for concern as not meeting requirements of justice for a minimal level of healthcare (for example, as defined by Pogge).

Indigenous peoples

There is no universally accepted definition of 'indigenous peoples'. Nevertheless, this lack has not been an obstacle to well-organized advocacies for this group, including those of global organizations. Notwithstanding the institutional advocacies, structural injustices have continued. For instance, a Pan American Health Organization (PAHO) study of indigenous health across the Americas leads to the observation that 'indigenous peoples are more likely than non-indigenous people to die from malaria, diarrhoea and other treatable conditions, and that the maternal mortality rate is far higher in areas where indigenous peoples are concentrated' (Hall et al., 2006: 17). In Columbia, life expectancy for almost one million indigenous peoples was '10–15 years less than the national average', while indigenous areas of Mexico 'have three times the rate of death from intestinal infections' (Hall et al., 2006: 17–18).

Part of the problem includes the lack of access to health services and the low rate of insurance protection. Hall and Patrinos argue that failure of proper policy formulation and inadequate service implementation account for much of the problem and assert that

indigenous peoples have yet to benefit from the many poverty reduction initiatives that have been implemented in the region over the past decade, either because the programmes have failed to reach them, are of poor quality or inadequately address the composite causes of their poverty. (Hall and Patrinos, 2006: 221)

They further note that '(i)n virtually every basic health indicator (from maternal mortality and hospital births to vaccination coverage) indigenous peoples have worse health outcomes' in Bolivia, Ecuador, Guatemala, Mexico and Peru. Hall and Patrinos also note the 'extremely high malnutrition rate among indigenous children' in these countries, which can lead not only to health issues like 'high infant and child mortality rates (and) vulnerability to disease' but also to 'lower educational attainment', which in turn exacerbates their condition of poverty (Hall and Patrinos, 2006: 228, 235).

The situation calls for health policies that are tailored specifically for the needs of indigenous populations; but determining which policies are responsive and how they can truly address unjust imbalances in access to healthcare is not an easy matter. Various steps have been suggested in order to deal with structural forms of discrimination, including (1) the recognition, financing or certification of traditional medicine; (2) adapting Western practices to indigenous values and traditions; (3) making effective indigenous healthcare practices available in the national health system; (4) recruiting indigenous peoples as healthcare practitioners or training health providers to properly relate to indigenous peoples; and (5) ensuring equal opportunities for indigenous peoples, and particularly mothers and children (Hall and Patrinos, 2006).

Issues of social, economic and political marginalization also permeate debates about the inequality in health status of indigenous peoples in developed countries. Larger questions about the social genealogy of indigenous health inequalities revolve around the historical fact of colonization and the dispossession of indigenous peoples from their own land, with similar negative health outcomes reported in Canada and New Zealand (Gray and Saggers, 2002: 119). Where past (and present) sociocultural structures and practices have contributed to indigenous health inequalities, debates about what society now owes to these marginalized groups persist, including those relating to the nature and extent of affirmative action policies and the 'critical assessment of the impact of welfare policies on Indigenous people' (Gray and Saggers, 2002: 122).

The issues recall the 'capability to function' criterion with respect to definitions of poverty and, by extension, the ability to lead healthy lives. Also highlighted are contested notions of social justice and egalitarianism. One challenge pertains to the 'common-sense' ideology of liberalism that has a tendency to minimize structural inequalities by holding on to the presumption that individuals are responsible for their successes and failures. In also proclaiming that all should be treated equally, the view mitigates against solutions by perpetuating inequality through the equal treatment of unequal individuals (Gray and Saggers, 2002: 128).

THE CASE OF THE 'GLOBAL POOR' AND GLOBAL MORAL RESPONSIBILITY

The situation of the 'global poor' has seen plenty of elaboration in recent documents and publications. A critical component of discussions concerning poverty and health pertains to the moral responsibility that is thought to accrue to certain parties in relation to the need to address the condition. For instance, questions arise about the scope of such responsibility. On one account, responsibility is acquired broadly, transcending the seemingly natural limits set by national boundaries. Thus, a corporation's responsibility to address the health needs of the poor extends beyond the country in which it directly operates. It has to be concerned with the global implications of its operations and not merely be preoccupied with the limited impact at the national or community level. Thus, cosmopolitanism contends that distributive justice applies globally, not simply nationally or locally; therefore, there are moral obligations to address the plight of the poor of the world as a whole.

This characterization of cosmopolitanism naturally lends itself to a *positive claim* to the duty to promote justice globally, and such a claim has been associated with the works of people like Charles Beitz (1999) and Henry Shue (1980). A *negative claim* is also possible under cosmopolitanism. For instance, Thomas Pogge states that ' we are behaving unjustly towards the global poor by imposing on them the lasting effects of historical crimes, or by holding them below any credible state-of-nature baseline'. We could be violating a negative duty not to impose a global order that systematically violates poor people's rights (Pogge, 2005b). By 'we', Pogge refers to adult citizens of the USA, EU, Canada, Australia, New Zealand – 'at least those who share the economic security and basic Western values of these countries' (Pogge, 2008b).

A second account holds that the scope of responsibility must be defined along the lines of traditional geopolitical boundaries. Thus, communitarianism is claimed to have denied cosmopolitanism on various grounds, including the following: that distributive justice is a special duty limited only to fellow-nationals (nationalist); that global distributive justice is violative of the independence of states; and that global distributive justice is unrealistically utopian.

Part of this debate can be seen in the area of healthcare when we consider the duties and obligations of pharmaceutical companies in the development of drugs for developing countries. There is argument about the nature and scope of such obligations and how they should be derived, with related debates about the supporting policies, structures and conditions needed so that both can be helped in fulfilling their (presumed) obligations.

It has been argued that global pharmaceutical companies have a social and moral responsibility towards developing nations to develop affordable drugs that cater to the specific needs of such nations (Resnik, 2001). While the moral obligation of pharmaceutical companies resides in the principles of beneficence and justice, Resnik believes there are limits to such responsibilities, which depend on the companies being able to obtain a 'reasonable profit' from their endeavours within a conducive business environment. Emphasizing the importance of reciprocity and a 'cooperative approach', Resnik argues that developing nations have a significant role to play in ensuring that pharmaceutical companies are able to meet their socio-moral obligations by removing the limits to responsibility outlined above. Some ways of doing this include respecting product patents, incorporating international frameworks protecting intellectual property rights and promoting the rule of law, open markets and democracy.

A contrary view holds that it has not been established that corporations, like individual moral agents, have moral obligations to begin with. Furthermore, it would seem that the principle of beneficence is an imperfect obligation and one where, without special relations, we have no absolute obligation to pursue. Since we cannot help everyone, pharmaceutical companies would have fulfilled their obligation in relation to the principle of beneficence by focusing their efforts exclusively on the developed, instead of developing, world. Resnik also needs a more developed account of the nature of justice as an obligation that applies to corporations, given that companies and moral individuals may only be incompletely identical qua moral agents. Finally, the existence of large income inequalities between the developed and developing world make the principle of reciprocity difficult to uphold. As Brock argues, '(w)hen developing countries choose not to respect product patents as their only effective means of making available pharmaceuticals necessary to save lives and protect the health of their citizens, doing so is arguably a step towards greater justice between the developed and developing world' (Brock, 2001: 37).

It has also been argued that the existence of private corporations in a particular society does not necessarily entail specific corporate obligations and responsibilities specified by the values deemed important by that society (Daniels, 2001). Clarity and specificity about social responsibilities assigned to corporations can only be achieved when appropriate negotiation has been undertaken in the context of the appropriate social or inter-societal contract. The fact that corporate actions have consequences for other people does not specify the nature of obligations they do have. Deliberation is crucial to the specification of responsibilities. The mere fact of moral agency and the consequences that flow from it do not suffice to elicit the required specificity. Moreover, the reciprocity that Resnik argues for is especially absent in international treaties requiring developing countries to honour intellectual property rights unless they also demand that corporations honour their social obligations to developing countries. In addition, if there is no enforcement mechanism to ensure social responsibilities are met, and in the absence of some form of regulation that assists corporations in meeting their obligations, corporations (under the pressure of competition) can feel justified in not meeting obligations to conduct research into and produce affordable drugs for the developing world. The solution has to be found in the institutionalization of responsibilities through open social deliberation and negotiation (Daniels, 2001).

Another side to the debate concerns the rights of developing nations compared to patent holders in relation to access to healthcare. What is the justification for patents? Are there limits to these rights, or conditions under which they do not apply? Will better patent laws and enforcement of laws by themselves lead to 'incentives for innovation'? The WTO-TRIPS agreement of 1994 gave rise to intense debate about the potential conflict between intellectual property rights implementation and ensuring access to healthcare, particularly as it pertains to patent protection in developing countries.

Reviewing the moral justification of patents on the basis of natural rights, distributive justice and utilitarianism, Sterckx critically examines the utilitarian (economic) position, which many consider the 'most convincing' argument in favour of the current regime. In particular, it has been argued that patents provide both an 'incentive-to-invent-and-innovate' and an 'incentive-to-disclose' details of one's research and innovations, which can benefit developing nations.

However, Sterckx argues that these arguments 'do not necessarily apply to developing countries'. For instance, while it is assumed that the WTO-TRIPS agreement will spur drug research that caters especially to the health and disease profile of developing nations, the lack of research and drug production in these countries is due more to economic considerations such as infrastructure and technology capacities than to the absence of patent laws. Furthermore, the (ultimately) economic objective of patents will mean that pharmaceutical corporations will view developing nations as unprofitable centres of research and development, given the latter's limited purchasing power. Sterckx then notes the significance of the Doha Declaration on the TRIPS Agreement and Public Health in 2001, which attempts to balance commercial interests with patient interests. In particular, the Declaration acknowledges that WTO member states have a right to 'protect public health and … promote access to medicines for all' (Sterckx, 2004: 70) via the provision of compulsory licenses for local use and the determination of what constitutes a national public health emergency. While this can provide a better balance between a patent holder's rights and obligations, much remains to be done at the level of international negotiation and accommodation to achieve that balance (Sterckx, 2004).

On the other hand, there is the view that some medical patents, the TRIPS agreement and supporting bilateral treaties, count as human rights violations when pharmaceuticals lobby for their own rights without regard for the plight of the poor in developing countries (Pogge, 2005a). The latter are knowingly denied life-saving drugs because of unjust systemic and institutional arrangements. Shareholders of pharmaceutical companies are implicated in such violations when they choose profits over ethical conduct. In effect, patents allow for overly high monopoly pricing of essential drugs over extended periods of time, thus depriving the poor of access to life-changing medication. By widening the moral circle of responsibility, Pogge (2008a) holds that even ordinary citizens of rich countries are implicated in such human rights violations insofar as they are aware of and yet do not seek to remedy the injustices inherent in the dominant global economic order of which they are authors and which perpetuate and sustain poverty in developing countries.

Part of the problem appears to be the unwillingness of the establishment to explore solutions that tend to undermine the monopoly-pricing model. There are those who feel a differential pricing strategy would work, and suggest a global drug development reform plan based on a 'public-good strategy' (Pogge, 2005a). Results of 'essential drug' development by pharmaceutical companies would be seen as a public good which all other drug companies can make use of at no cost, thereby lowering the overall price of drugs through competition – hopefully to their marginal cost of production. Additionally, in order to preserve the incentives for drug research, inventor firms 'should be rewarded, out of public funds, in proportion to the impact of their invention on the global disease burden' (Pogge, 2005a: 188–9).

Thus, pharmaceutical firms would be incentivised to work with and improve the local medical system of developing countries and cooperate with other stakeholders because the criteria of evaluation of their work comes from how well, and to what extent, their medications help to alleviate the global disease burden. This emphasis on impact (measured in terms of market share of drug use and its level of effectiveness) would also help refocus the attention of drug companies on research into neglected developing-world diseases and medical conditions. The intent is to

> align and harmonize the interests of inventor firms with those of patients and the generic drug producers … The reform would also align the moral and prudential interests of the inventor firms who, under the present regime, are forced to choose between recouping their investments in the search for essential drugs and preventing avoidable suffering and deaths (Pogge, 2005a: 189).

A related concern (Sen, 2004) when talking about rights and obligations is the question of how human rights should be promoted in society and when legislation ought to be considered in its promotion. There are times when recognition, advocacy and informational monitoring may be more appropriate as a means of human rights promotion as opposed to turning that right into a legal right. It remains to be seen if rights related to healthcare ought to fall under the former or latter category, even if it is recognized that human rights should be extended to include social rights such as medical care.

STANDARD OF CARE IN HEALTH RESEARCH

The Standard of Care debate in connection with the conduct of international health research has raged on, although the main parameters have remained basically the same. The inadequacy of healthcare resources in poverty stricken countries has provided the context for global debate regarding the standard of care for participants in biomedical research. Initial debates were fuelled in 1997 by the publication of an article by Lurie and Wolfe in the *New England Journal of Medicine* criticizing the use of placebo controls in zidovudine trials in poor countries. The authors claimed that most of the trials were unethical and would have led to hundreds of preventable HIV infections in infants (Lurie and Wolfe, 1997). Stressing that researchers assume greater ethical responsibilities when they enrol human subjects in clinical studies, they pointed out that people from economically poor countries need to be protected from potential exploitation. They also warned against using the low level of healthcare in such countries as a reason to conduct research that could not be ethically justified in sponsoring countries (Lurie and Wolfe, 1997).

The presumption behind the criticism was that potentially vulnerable research partici-pants had to be protected from harm resulting from being deprived of standard medical treatment while enrolled as subjects of human experiments. Placebo controls were regarded as unacceptable when there was a proven efficacious treatment for the condition being investigated. The subjects who were randomized to use them were put in a disadvantaged position because they were then deprived of a course of treatment that was already proven to be efficacious. Critics of the trials cited the provision of the Declaration of Helsinki that '[i]n research on man, the interest of science and society should never take precedence over considerations related to the well-being of the subject' (WMA, 1996). Moreover, even in the name of scientific advancement, patients who are randomized to control arms of biomedical research should be provided an alternative form of proven efficacious treatment, when this is available.

Other criticisms noted the double standards applied in approving studies in poor countries that would not have been allowed to take place in wealthy ones (Lurie and Wolfe, 1997). The ACTG 076 protocol was available in the wealthy world, making placebo controlled studies of a shorter course of treatment unacceptable. Approval of the placebo controls thus constituted an injustice characterized by the application of different standards for the poor and wealthy countries.

The other side of the debate was taken up by those who cited 'standard treatment' as practised in poverty stricken countries where treatment was not ordinarily available for the prevention of vertical transmission of HIV. The argument was that the participants who ended up in the control arm were not actually being deprived of a form of treatment that would have been otherwise available to them. There was no way they could have availed themselves of the expensive drugs in their usual setting. On the contrary, the research subjects in the control arm were expected to gain more knowledge about their condition through the counselling that was being provided. Hence, they stood to gain benefits and very low prospects of actual additional harm.

This argument favouring double standards did not appeal to those who pointed out that what typically emerges as standard treatment in impoverished contexts is something that is determined more by economic and political conditions than by medical knowledge or medical indications. It would be ironic to justify the use of placebo controls in such environments because the pricing structures for drugs set by the sponsors of many trials are themselves responsible for the unavailability of what should be ideal comparator drugs. By lowering standards of care requirements, one effectively supports those pricing structures, whereas maintaining a single standard of care could put pressure on drug manufacturers to revise pricing structures to suit the needs of poor countries.

As the debate progressed, the World Medical Association engaged in consultations resulting in several changes to the Declaration of Helsinki until the current version was adopted, providing that 'the benefits, risks, burdens and effectiveness of a new intervention must be tested against those of the best current proven intervention', but allowing for exceptions where placebo (or no treatment) may be used because no current proven intervention exists; or where there are compelling and scientifically sound methodological reasons to use them in order to determine the efficacy or safety of an intervention. The provision further states that this may only be allowed when patients will not be subjected to any risk of serious or irreversible harm (WMA, 2008).

The current wording of this section of the Declaration does not totally support the three conditions that many have regarded as essential to any exceptions to providing research subjects the best worldwide standard of care: (1) that there must be a valid scientific reason for using a lower standard of care than that available elsewhere; (2) that the research must provide a sufficient level of benefit for the host community; and (3) that there must be an acceptable balance of risks and potential benefits for the individual participants in the trial (Lie et al., 2004). (R.K. Lie and colleagues arrived at this 'international consensus opinion' by comparing opinions expressed by various bioethics bodies regarding the care of trial participants [see Table 1 in Article quoted]; but see also Schuklenk's reply (Schuklenk, 2004).

ORGAN TRADING

The debate concerning organ transplantation relating to poverty has tended to focus on the issue of compensation or incentives. On the one hand, massive poverty in developing country communities has provided the backdrop for debates regarding compensation for organ donors. In some communities, organ selling has reached wholesale proportions, making organ trading a literal reality. In addition, patients from affluent foreign countries have exploited the opportunities that are ably facilitated by clandestine brokers, thus setting in motion a practice that has straddled the boundary between transplant tourism and organ trafficking.

From one extreme perspective, organs such as kidneys and livers must be regarded as sacrosanct and outside the realm of commerce. On this basis, many hold that organ donation must always be motivated only by altruism. Monetary considerations demean human donors and transform their bodies into commodities that can be reduced to a monetary or material equivalent. Thus, the Declaration of Istanbul on Transplant Tourism and Organ Trafficking rejects 'transplant commercialism' as 'a practice in which an organ is treated as a commodity, including by being bought or sold or used for material gain' (Steering Committee of the Istanbul Summit, 2008).

An opposite extreme view regards human organs as having nothing more than a conditional value that depends on their being indispensable for healthy and viable human lives. Hence, it would not be wrong for organ donors to receive compensation, especially if it serves as an incentive that encourages donation and thereby increases the number of lives that may be saved or enhanced through the practice. On the contrary, it would even be negligent of health authorities not to institutionalize the use of incentives that could go a long way in narrowing the gap between supply and demand and possibly even eliminate waiting lists for transplantable human organs.

Extreme positions such as the above could be difficult to maintain, especially in view of exceptional circumstances that lead to untenable consequences. For instance, the idea that money should never be exchanged in an arrangement involving organ donation ignores the fact that organ transplantation involves costs to organ donors that they would otherwise not have to bear. Organ donors not only have to assume the risks pertinent to the medical procedure – they have to forego normal life for a significant period, miss opportunities to earn a living, and make other material sacrifices. These factors serve as a disincentive for organ donors, thus punishing them and not merely failing to reward them. The situation leads to fewer volunteers and a decrease in the number of saved or enhanced lives.

On the other hand, the use of material incentives to promote organ donation could lead to uncontrolled commerce and expose donors to the financial exploitation, coercion and manipulation by unscrupulous agents usually associated with transplant tourism. Thus, the Istanbul Declaration has been touted to inspire regional and global efforts to stop transplant commercialism, organ trafficking and transplant tourism, as these tend to diminish the value of transplantation as a gift and a symbol of human solidarity (Participants in the International Summit on Transplant Tourism and Organ Trafficking convened by The Transplantation Society and International Society of Nephrology, 2008). While the Declaration rejects the idea of financial compensation, it sees the need to allow reimbursement of actual expenses incurred in order to remove socioeconomic disincentives that serve as a barrier to altruistic giving. In the same vein, the World Health Organization's Guiding Principles on Human Cell, Tissue and Organ Transplantation permit reimbursement for actual costs as specifically documented (WHO, 2010).

While justice-based approaches to organ donation appear to be incompatible with proposals to increase the supply of organs for transplant by offering financial payments or other material incentives, free-market advocates have endorsed payments on a scale determined by supply and demand (Williams, 1984; Peters, 1991). Others have argued for a regulated market with various mechanisms for providing protection to organ donors (Harris and Erin, 2002: 114–15; Matas, 2004: 2007–17, 2006: 1129–32; Hippen, 2005: 593–626; Daar, 2006: 600–1).

Arguments based on respect for individual freedom have led to contrasting positions regarding offers of material compensation or incentives. On one account, offers of payment are exploitative of people with extreme economic vulnerabilities. They are also seen as coercive in the context of extreme economic need. On the other hand, a case is put forward for compensation by those who cite the options that are opened up for poor donors, thereby giving them a window to deal with the effects of poverty. The point is that the poor already have very limited opportunities to overcome poverty, and prohibiting material compensation for organ donors deprives them of a rare chance that they might never have otherwise. Rather than accepting the argument from coercion as a valid criticism founded on enhancing the value of individual freedom, this view turns the argument around and uses the value of individual freedom to justify the use of compensation or incentives. Even in a wealthy country like the United States, Veatch observes that people living in pockets of poverty are still being forced to live below intolerable standards of living and some of them are so desperate to provide the most basic necessities for themselves and their families that they might make one kidney available for transplant in exchange for an economic payment (Veatch, 2003: 31–2).

The point is that a society that deliberately and systematically neglects the basic needs of the poor is being indifferent to the plight of this population and cannot be justified in prohibiting the means the poor have to address the problems themselves. Thus, Veatch referred to the 'strange twist [that] the very same reason that made a market in organs unethical 20 years ago, today makes it a moral necessity, at least if we continue to live in a society in which desperate poverty is tolerated amidst affluence' (Veatch, 2003: 32).

In response to the above argument, one could point out that the option to sell an organ has not been shown to be an effective means to address the poor's economic concerns. Many organ vendors have been coerced to sell not only through monetary offers they find irresistible, but through deceptive and exploitative mechanisms. Perpetrated by unscrupulous characters or organized syndicates, most transactions have not truly enabled the poor to transcend their economic desperation.

In order to avoid the exploitation and coercion that tend to characterize organ trading, some writers have proposed a regulated market (cf. de Castro, 2003; Erin and Harris, 2003; Matas, 2004; Friedman and Friedman, 2006). A system established in Iran with the blessing of the government has also often been cited as a viable alternative (Ghods, 2004). Supporters claim that the Iranian system has successfully eliminated a renal transplant waiting list and provided hope for end-stage renal disease patients in other countries. The pragmatic approach has also been claimed to have removed an opportunity for the exploitation of the poor local population by foreigners coming from affluent countries, because it only allows transplants to patients of the same nationality as the organ donors. However, critics have raised concerns about the effectiveness of the program's implementation, citing the futility of measures intended to prevent unauthorized commercial transactions running parallel to (and thereby subverting) the officially recognized system of incentives.

MIGRATION OF HEALTH PROFESSIONALS

The migration of health professionals is a phenomenon that has posed difficult questions with deep ethical undertones to policymakers in health and economics. Although there has long been an awareness that developing countries have been losing huge numbers of their healthcare workers (HCWs) to developed countries, there is also a realization that the migration of health professionals across national boundaries has followed a pattern of globalization that is an inevitable outcome of the breaking down of barriers to trade and the exchange of services among countries. It may also be seen as a glaring illustration of the need for safety nets to ensure that global developments do not result in the exploitation of the poor and vulnerable. The movement has followed a clearly established trend away from developing countries with inadequate physician densities (about 17 per 100,000 population) to developed countries with much higher physician densities (about 300 per 100,000 population) (Buchan and Calman, 2004). Hence, migration has been thought to reflect an injustice that needs to be urgently addressed.

The nature of the injustice, as well as the identification of those responsible, has been the subject of discussion and disagreement. In the first place, not all are agreed that an injustice is truly being perpetrated. However, it cannot be denied that countries in most need of healthcare professionals are getting the least and those that have the most are getting even more. The impact of the disparity could be severe. Health services have deteriorated and source countries with inadequate numbers of physicians can see their health services suffer seriously as a result of the loss of even a few physicians. (Martineau and Decker, 2002). As one may expect, those who come from the poverty stricken areas are the worst affected, with health services (and their users) in the remoter rural areas being the ultimate losers because they come lowest in the order of people's preferences for working locations (Martineau and Decker, 2002).

The fact that poor countries spend their resources for medical education in order to meet their health needs and rich countries divert the human resources produced to their own communities through their recruitment programs can be seen as a form of unjust exploitation. Nevertheless, alternative perspectives exist. Governments of source countries have themselves encouraged the migration, either directly or indirectly. Some governments have provided direct encouragement by aiding in the recruitment process, anticipating that remittances from the migrant healthcare professionals would offset the losses resulting from the cost of medical or related education. These governments have established infrastructures for the training of health professionals needed abroad, for their placement in overseas communities, and for the inward remittance of money earned from their jobs. Countries such as India, the Philippines, and Nigeria – highly populated countries that train large numbers of health professionals and have a long-standing remittance culture, in which professionals working outside the country send money back home to relatives – have produced doctors and nurses for 'export' (Dovlo, 2004).

Unfortunately, by facilitating the external migration of health workers, these poor countries have contributed to worse health outcomes for their people. Low health worker density in some countries has had a damaging impact on maternal and child mortality, whereas an increase in the number of health workers has been associated with a reduction of maternal mortality, so that 'a 10 per cent increase in the density of the health workforce is correlated with about a 5 per cent decline in maternal mortality' (Joint Learning Initiative, 2004: 26).

One of the first options that come to mind in dealing with the loss of health resources is a direct prohibition or limitation on the outward migration of individual workers. However, severe restrictions on personal travel could violate a basic human right for people to live where they choose. While the provision of state subsidy for education may justify the imposition of conditions like required return service, such conditions can only be enforced to the extent that they do not compromise a person's freedom of movement.

There are other ways in which required return service could raise ethical issues. For example, physicians from wealthy families may be able to buy off their debt while those with no means for payment are forced to a period of servitude. Some may also illegally break their contract while invoking human rights considerations pertaining to freedom of movement, career choices or changes, educational opportunities or family issues. Freedom-based arguments may have a valid basis, especially in cases where those concerned are below the age of majority when they start their healthcare education, and so lack the maturity required to commit themselves legally to adopt, many years afterwards, a particular profession or even place of practice.

Mindful of the large impact of health resource migration and considering the complicated interplay of various factors involved, one cannot rely heavily on individualist notions of responsibility to understand the resulting injustices. By focusing on the agency of individuals, one tends to overlook the large-scale social patterns surrounding HCW migration. If we take these social patterns into account, we could see that the proper role of governments is not to impose restrictions on individual movement but 'to motivate and organize people to achieve their collective best interests and to implement systems for solving large-scale social coordination problems such as this one' (Crozier, 2009: 9). And considering the resources at their command, countries with a greater ability to rectify systemic injustices have a greater responsibility to do so. Hence, developed countries may have greater responsibilities than developing ones in addressing the ethical problems arising from the migration of healthcare professionals (Crozier, 2009).

COMMON THEMES AND CHALLENGES; NEGLECTED AREAS

While policies to help the poorest countries and the poor within countries have been drawn up over the years, more can be done to address the issue of health inequalities in particular (Leon and Walt, 2001). Such inequalities are a dynamic phenomenon around the world, 'driven by multiple factors including biology, social organization, and health systems' (Leon and Walt, 2001: 14). Given that it is ultimately an ethical issue that health inequalities ought to be reduced, problems remain about understanding the causal factors of such inequalities, the conceptual, methodological and logistical issues of measurement and the method of tracking the effectiveness of specific public policy provisions. Emerging and developing countries face the challenge of collecting reliable surveys of inequalities in socioeconomic health profiles and mapping the distributional aspects of health data to reflect the needs of the poorest in their country.

With different priorities, solutions and perceptions of what the problems are, there are nevertheless some common themes that have emerged. There appears to be a more concerted effort at recognizing the plight of the poor within individual countries. The recognition has led to (economic) suggestions that improvements in the health of the poor can help lead to the alleviation of poverty. Another theme is the attempt to identify the nature of such inequalities – whether they are primarily a problem of unequal access to healthcare (a problem given prominence in low- to middle-income nations) or whether they should be viewed as socioeconomic in nature (an issue that many developed countries are concerned with). Furthermore, globalization and the privatization of health services have contributed to inequalities in healthcare access and there is a need to examine whether the healthcare system is itself exacerbating social inequities. There is room for improvement in sharing ideas in relation to the measurement of inequalities in health status between countries (Leon and Walt, 2001).

Other areas that have been relatively neglected include health inequalities concerning or generated by age, gender, ethnicity, mental health, injuries and advances in genetics (Leon and Walt, 2001). Both international and local initiatives are important in reducing health inequalities and it is a challenge to determine on whose shoulders the ethical responsibilities fall. Examples of international initiatives include aid to the poorest within poor developing nations and coming up with better data collection and measurement models for intra-country comparisons. At the national level, public health policies need to encompass fiscal, economic and social policy initiatives as well if they are to be effective.

Mental health

Mental health is a crucial concern in dealing with 'health problems arising out of inequality' (Patel, 2001: 247). It is also a contributory factor to the preponderance of inequality in developing countries. There is evidence of the 'high prevalence' of Common Mental Disorders (CMDs) of up to 40 per cent of 'adult primary care populations' in low income countries ranging from Lesotho and Uganda to India and Chile (Patel, 2001: 248). Alcohol abuse has also been an under-treated condition despite the fact that it has been the most common form of addiction in developing countries with severe physical, mental and social repercussions, including traffic accidents and domestic violence. Mental health concerns were also shown to constitute half of the top ten causes of disability in *Global Burden of Disease*, a study published in the mid-1990s (Murray and Lopez, 1996), while incidences of greater mortality have been noted in suicides linked to depression and substance abuse.

The stressful life conditions of the poor in developing countries contribute to the high prevalence of CMDs. In just one of many examples, 82 per cent of suicides in the Indian state of Maharashtra came from the disadvantaged Dalit minority, which comprised only 12 per cent of the state's inhabitants (Patel, 2001: 251). Studies of developing countries such as Indonesia, Zimbabwe, Brazil, Chile and India pointed to a strong link between indicators of poverty (for example debt, experiencing hunger, low education) and CMD. While the prevalence of CMDs appears tied to poverty levels, Patel suggests that the policy objective for developing countries is not only to raise people out of absolute poverty but also to control relative poverty, given that income inequalities in developed countries have been associated with CMDs as well. Preventive measures include better education (at least until secondary level) so families can break out of the poverty cycle and banking systems that would reduce reliance on traditional moneylenders who bring much stress to the poor. Policymakers should also do more to make mental wellness a priority in public health, especially with regard to CMDs and alcohol abuse.

Injuries

Intentional and unintentional injuries, which make up a large percentage of the disability adjusted life years (DALYs) lost, affect the poorest members of a society the most (Zwi, 2001). At the same time, the latter have the 'least access to the mechanisms for altering their exposure to risk' (Zwi, 2001: 263). Reducing 'inequalities in injury occurrence' and violence would help reduce the 'differential burden of ill-health between rich and poor' (Zwi, 2001: 263). While few studies have been conducted in developing countries connecting injuries with poverty, these typically mirror the results of studies done in North America, Australia and Europe, which show higher injury rates among the less well off.

Zwi emphasizes that effective injury interventions and injury control are possible and that it is imperative that developing countries and poorer communities learn to take preventive safety measures, for example in relation to reducing traffic injuries, fire prevention, accidental poisoning and drowning. One challenge is that poorer communities tend not to have the social and political influence to affect public policymaking. As a result, they may suffer the most but yet their voices remain unheard. Another challenge is that specific injuries are not perceived as a matter of public health but as the concern of the transport department (in the case of traffic injuries), police (in the case of homicides) or a matter of private concern (in the case of family violence, for instance). Better collaboration between different sectors of society is needed if such (mis)perception is not to continue.

Suggested as an important part of the solution is the provision of more research-based evidence of the trends, patterns, extent and costs of injury inequalities, so that the data itself forces injury control onto the policy agenda, aided by calls for attention from civil society groups and the media (Zwi, 2001). This can also have the effect of helping marginalized groups regain their voice in society. Policy formulation and implementation is also crucial and involves a myriad of activities, including engaging different stakeholders, providing for needed resources, putting in place and transferring good practices across different domains, setting public targets and constructing a framework of systems and procedures to carry the policy process to completion and review. The theme of safety and security should also permeate other sectors of society so that industry leaders and the community at large start to view their activities through the lens of injury control and prevention. Finally, donors who provide developmental assistance to various countries and regions also have an influential role to play in ensuring that development imperatives are carried out with safety measures and standards firmly in mind.

Gender bias

Gender bias and gender blindness in research into health inequalities should not be overlooked. This can take the form of assuming that both sexes are similar enough so that research that applies to one gender will apply to the other, even when the latter was not part of the research. The uniqueness of each gender is thus discounted. Gender biased research may also assume that both sexes are different in important ways, so that different 'outcome measures' are prescribed or else not enough attention is given to compare how each gender may be similar in relation to the health issue being studied. This is made worse when it is assumed that certain problems are predominantly 'female' (or 'male'). Even when there are good reasons for research that surveys just one gender, there is not the consciousness that this is in fact being done. Yet such research observations are erroneously seen as generalizable to all (Macintyre, 2001).

The idea is that important socioeconomic and gender inequalities in health point to exposure and vulnerability factors related to socioeconomic and cultural processes (and hence may vary depending on prevailing conditions) rather than any essentialist difference between men and women. What is needed is greater study of the mechanisms that generate such inequalities, given the basic difference in the biology of each gender, so that we can redress these inequalities in health (Macintyre, 2001).

There is thus a need to be more conscious of the impact of gender bias, injuries and CMDs on the poor and on indigenous peoples in future research, and the methodological or policy solutions that have been proposed to resolve them.

REFERENCES

Agency for Healthcare Research and Quality (AHRQ) (1998) *Request for Applications on Measures of Quality of Care for Vulnerable Populations. Rockville, MD: AHRQ* (RFA: HS-99-001, released 22 December 1998). Available at: http://grants.nih.gov/grants/guide/rfa-files/RFA-HS-99-001.html, accessed 28 February 2008.

Beitz, C. (1999) 'International liberalism and distributive justice: A survey of recent thought', *World Politics*, 51 (2): 269–96.

Brock, D. (2001) 'Some questions about the moral responsibilities of drug companies in developing countries', *Developing World Bioethics*, 1 (1): 33–7.

Buchan, J. and Calman, L. (2004) *The Global Shortage of Registered Nurses: An Overview of Issues and Actions.* Available at http://www.icn.ch/global/shortage.pdf, accessed 13 February 2009.

Crozier, G.K.D. (2009) 'Agency and responsibility in health care worker migration', *American Journal of Bioethics*, 9 (3): 8–9.

Daar, A.S. (2006) 'The case for a regulated system of living kidney sales', *National Clinical Practice of Nephrology*, 2 (11): 600–1.

Daniels, N. (2001) 'Social responsibility and global pharmaceutical companies', *Developing World Bioethics*, 1 (1): 38–41.

de Castro, L.D. (2003) 'Commodification and exploitation: Arguments in favour of compensated organ donation', *Journal of Medical Ethics*, 29: 142–6.

Dovlo, D. (2004) Human resources for health, 2: 7; doi:10.1186/1478-4491-2-7. Available at http://www.human-resources-health.com/content/2/1/7 2, accessed 13 February 2009.

Erin, C.A. and Harris, J. (2003) 'An ethical market in human organs', *Journal of Medical Ethics*, 29: 137–8; doi: 10.1136/jme.29.3.137.

Friedman E.A. and Friedman A.L. (2006) 'Payment for donor kidneys: Pros and cons', *Kidney International*, 69: 960–2.

Ghods, A.J. (2004) 'Governed financial incentives as an alternative to altruistic organ donation', *Experimental and Clinical Transplantation*, Dec 2 (2): 221–8.

Gray, D. and Saggers, S. (2002) 'Indigenous health: The perpetuation of inequality', in L Germov, (ed.), *Second Opinion: An Introduction to Health Sociology*, 2nd ed. Oxford: Oxford University Press, pp. 112–31.

Hall, G. and Patrinos, H.A. (2006) 'Key messages and an agenda for action', in G. Hall and H.A. Patrinos (eds), *Indigenous Peoples, Poverty and Human Development in Latin America.* Basingstoke: Palgrave Macmillan, pp. 221–40.

Hall, G., Layton, H.M. and Shapiro, J. (2006) 'Introduction: The indigenous peoples' decade in Latin America', in G. Hall and H.A. Patrinos (eds), *Indigenous Peoples, Poverty and Human Development in Latin America.* Basingstoke: Palgrave Macmillan, pp. 1–24.

Harris, J. and Erin, C. (2002) 'An ethically defensible market in organs' (editorial), *British Medical Journal*, 325: 114–15.

Hippen, B.E. (2005) 'In defense of a regulated market in kidneys from living vendors', *Journal of Medicine and Philosophy*, 30: 593–626.

Joint Learning Initiative (2004) *Human Resources for Health: Overcoming the Crisis.* Global Equity Initiative, Harvard University. Available at: http://www.healthgap.org/camp/hcw_docs/JLi_Human_Resources_for_Health.pdf, accessed 20 February 2009.

Leon, D. and Walt, G. (2001) 'Poverty, inequality, and health in international perspective: A divided world?', in D. Leon and G. Walt (eds), *Poverty, Inequality and Health: An International Perspective.* Oxford: Oxford University Press, pp. 1–16.

Lie, R.K., Emanuel, E., Grady, C. and Wendler, D. (2004) 'The standard of care debate: The Declaration of Helsinki versus the international consensus opinion', *Journal of Medical Ethics*, 30: 190–93; doi: 10.1136/jme.2003.006031.

Lurie, P. and Wolfe, S.M. (1997) 'Unethical trials of interventions to reduce perinatal transmission of the human immunodeficiency virus in developing countries', *New England Journal of Medicine*, 337: 853–6.

Macintyre, S. (2001) 'Inequalities in health: Is research gender blind?', in D. Leon and G. Walt (eds), *Poverty, Inequality and Health: An International Perspective.* Oxford: Oxford University Press, pp. 283–93.

Martineau, T., Decker, K. and Bundred, P. (2002) Briefing note on international migration of health professionals: Levelling the playing field for developing country health systems. Available at http://www.liv.ac.uk/lstm/research/documents/InternationalMigrationBriefNote.pdf, accessed 13 February 2009.

Matas, A.J. (2004) 'The case for living kidney sales: Rationale, objections, and concerns,' *American Journal of Transplantation*, 4: 2007–17.

Matas, A.J. (2006) 'Why we should develop a regulated system of kidney sales: A call for action!', *Clinical Journal of the American Society of Nephrology*, 1: 1129–32.

Murray, C.L. and Lopez, A.D. (eds) (1996) *The Global Burden of Disease*. Boston, MA: Harvard School of Public Health.

Participants in the International Summit on Transplant Tourism and Organ Trafficking convened by The Transplantation Society and International Society of Nephrology in Istanbul, Turkey, April 30–May 2, 2008, 'The declaration of Istanbul on organ trafficking and transplant tourism', *Transplantation*, 86 (8, October): 1013–18.

Patel, V. (2001) 'Poverty, inequality, and mental health in developing countries', in D. Leon and G. Walt (eds), *Poverty, Inequality and Health: An International Perspective*. Oxford: Oxford University Press, pp. 247–62.

Peters, T.G. (1991) 'Life or death: The issue of payment in cadaveric organ donation', *Journal of the American Medical Association*, 265: 1302–5.

Pogge, T. (2005a) 'Human rights and global health', *Metaphilosophy*, 36 (1/2): 182–209.

Pogge, T. (2005b) 'World poverty and human rights ethics', *International Affairs* 19 (1): 1–7.

Pogge, T. (2008a) 'Testing our drugs on the poor abroad', in J. Hawkins and E. Ezekiel (eds), *Exploitation and Developing Countries: The Ethics of Clinical Research*. Princeton, NJ: Princeton University Press, pp. 105–41.

Pogge, T. (2008b) *World Poverty and Human Rights: Cosmopolitan Responsibilities and Reforms*, 2nd ed. Cambridge: Polity Press.

Resnik, D. (2001) 'Developing drugs for the developing world: An economic, legal, moral, and political dilemma', *Developing World Bioethics*, 1 (1): 11–32.

Schuklenk, U. (2004) 'The standard of care debate: Against the myth of an "international consensus opinion"', *Journal of Medical Ethics*, 30: 194–7.

Sen, A. (2004) 'Elements of a theory of human rights', *Philosophy & Public Affairs*, 32 (4): 315–56.

Sen, A. (2006) 'Conceptualizing and measuring poverty', in D. Grusky and R. Kanbur (eds), *Poverty and Inequality*. Palo Alto, CA: Stanford University Press, pp. 30–46.

Shue, H. (1980) *Basic Rights: Subsistence, Affluence, and US Foreign Policy*. Princeton. NJ: Princeton University Press.

Steering Committee of the Istanbul Summit (2008) 'Organ trafficking and transplant tourism and commercialism: The declaration of Istanbul', *Lancet*, 372: 5–6.

Sterckx, S. (2004) 'Patents and access to drugs in developing countries: An ethical analysis', *Developing World Bioethics*, 4 (1): 58–75.

Veatch, R.M. (2003) 'Why liberals should accept financial incentives for organ procurement', *Kennedy Institute of Ethics Journal*, 13 (1): 19–36.

Williams, W. (1984) 'Vital organs—let the market decide', *Washington Times,* 19 April, p. C1.

World Health Organization (WHO) (2008) *WHO Guiding Principles on Human Cell, Tissue and Organ Transplantation*. Revised 6 May. Available at http://www.who.int/transplantation/TxGP08-en.pdf, accessed 23 March 2009.

World Medical Association Declaration of Helsinki (1996) *Recommendations Guiding Medical Doctors in Biomedical Research Involving Human Subjects*, Version III.4. Available at http://www1.va.gov/oro/apps/compendium/Files/Helsinki96.htm, accessed 19 March 2009.

World Medical Association Declaration of Helsinki (2008) *Ethical Principles for Medical Research Involving Human Subjects*. Available at http://www.wma.net/e/policy/b3.htm, accessed 15 March 2009.

Zwi, A. (2001) 'Injuries, inequalities, and health: From policy vacuum to policy action', in D. Leon and G. Walt (eds), *Poverty, Inequality and Health: An International Perspective*. Oxford: Oxford University Press, pp. 263–82.

25

Research Ethics

Paul Ndebele

INTRODUCTION

Advanced knowledge and practices related to disease prevention and control are a direct result of biomedical research conducted in past decades using humans as subjects. Today, it is common to hear people talk about medications for heart and kidney problems, organ donation, heart transplants, human clones, eradication of waterborne diseases and other technologies that are aimed at lengthening human lives. In the past century, however, society has become increasingly sensitive to the ethical issues associated with such research, especially the risks that research participants were exposed to during the conduct of the research. Society has also become very sensitive to the potential exploitation of research volunteers who make sacrifices by being placed at the risk of harm for the good of society. Ethical requirements have therefore been developed to ensure the minimization of the possibility of exploitation and harm by ensuring that research participants are not merely used as a means to an end but are treated with respect while they contribute to the social good. There are several events in history that have led to the development of these ethical requirements as well as the current drive towards the conduct of ethical research in general.

When one talks about the ethical requirements that have been developed, especially during the past century, one is automatically delving into the discipline of research ethics. The intensive development of the discipline of research ethics can be traced back to the twentieth century – a period that witnessed a sudden surge in the amount of human research being conducted globally. Research ethics is a special branch of the subject of ethics and is now recognized as a stand-alone discipline, which is taught at tertiary level. Research ethics can be defined as the subject that deals with standards and ethical dilemmas and issues in research (Brody, 1998). Research ethics is about the rights and wrongs in research, values of science and expected standards of conduct in science. Without an understanding of the historical context, it would be very difficult for one to understand the sense and need for research ethics, more so its development into a fully fledged discipline.

For this reason, the chapter begins with a brief history of research ethics, then looks at its current status, the areas of controversy and debate, and ends with a telescopic view into its future.

HISTORICAL DEVELOPMENT OF RESEARCH ETHICS

Early work in the area of research ethics can be traced back to the writings of Thomas Percival, William Beaumont and Claude Bernard (see Figure 25.1). Thomas Percival in 1803 developed a code of medical ethics, emphasizing that physicians should use good scientific methods and be competent; he did not stress the importance of informed consent (Beauchamp and Childress, 2001). William Beaumont in 1833 argued that experimentation is needed, that without experimentation new information cannot be obtained, but also that voluntary consent is needed (Lefor, 2005). A strong proponent of experimentation was Claude Bernard who in 1865 wrote that experimentation was permissible if it could save, cure or gain personal benefit for the subject.

Before Percival, uncontrolled, unscientific human experiments were common. For example Edward Jenner in 1776 inoculated his own child as well as other children with cowpox material in an experiment that created new knowledge on vaccinations as a way of protecting humans against specific diseases (Lakhani, 1992). During this time, research standards were mainly up to the discretion of the individual researcher and in academic institutions individuals had only to secure the support and cooperation of peers and superiors in their departments for them to conduct research. Some researchers even conducted some risky experiments using themselves as subjects and some died during the course of their experiments (Altman, 1998).

One of the earliest regulations on medical research was the Prussian Directive of 1900 in response to the case of Dr Neisser who studied the immunization of healthy persons against syphilis by inoculating them with serum from syphilitic patients (Vollmann and Winau, 1996). In 1931, the Reich Health Council Regulations were adopted after 75 children died in experiments with tuberculosis vaccinations. The regulations demanded complete responsibility of the medical profession for carrying out human experimentation. Among other things, the regulations emphasized the necessity of informed consent, documentation of justification of protocol deviation, risk benefit requirements, justification for research involving vulnerable populations and the necessity for written records.

The phenomenal growth of research ethics into a discipline in recent times is rooted in responses to abuses of research participants involved in human research, mostly during the twentieth century. An important chapter in the history of research ethics began during the Second World War. In December 1946, 23 physicians and administrators, many of them leading members of the German medical hierarchy, were indicted before the war crimes tribunal at Nuremberg for their willing participation in the systematic torture, mutilation, and killing of prisoners in experiments. Despite the arguments of the German physicians that the experiments were medically justified, the Nuremberg military tribunals in August 1947 condemned the experiments as crimes against humanity; 16 of the 23 physicians were found guilty and imprisoned, and 7 were sentenced to death (McGuire et al., 1999). The Nuremberg judgment included a list of precautionary measures that scientists were supposed to take when conducting research with human beings, including informed consent and minimizing risk (Nuremberg code, 1947). After the lessons learned during the Nuremberg trials, the World Medical Assembly (WMA) decided to come up with a code of ethics to guide medical doctors in their research activities involving their patients. This decision culminated in the Declaration of Helsinki (WMA, 1964). The Council of International Organisations in the Medical Sciences (CIOMS) in collaboration with the World Health Organization (WHO) came up with guidelines on epidemiological research involving human subjects in 1982 as a way of filling the gaps left by the Declaration of Helsinki (CIOMS, 1982). The CIOMS guidelines were meant to cover all kinds of biomedical research and also to address the growth in research funded by rich countries and conducted in poor countries. The Declaration of Helsinki, CIOMS guidelines and other useful guidance documents are described in detail in a separate section.

Before the experiments by the Nazi scientists, researchers from the US Health Services Department began a study in 1932 examining the effects of untreated syphilis in black men in Macon County Alabama, the so-called Tuskegee study. The study involved a total of 399 men including some who already were in the late stages of syphilis. About 201 acted as negative controls. The men were poor and illiterate and most had never seen a doctor before. They were promised free physical exams and free rides to the clinic, hot meals on exam days, free treatment for minor ailments as well as a burial stipend if any of them were to die during the study. The men were misled into believing that they were receiving treatment for 'bad blood' when in reality they were simply being observed. During the 1950s when antibiotics were already available, the men were denied access to penicillin and several of them died as a result of complications related to syphilis. This study was only exposed in 1972 after it had been running for about 40 years and the press later labelled it 'racial medicine'. The Tuskegee study led to the development of various ethical requirements in research in the United States. In 1974, the National Research Act made it a requirement for IRB review and approval of all research involving human subjects. The Act also established the National Commission for the Protection of Human Subjects of Biomedical and Behavioral Research, which was tasked with the responsibility of looking at research involving human subjects. The Commission came up with the Belmont Report in 1979. In the Belmont Report, the Commission highlighted the ethical principles of respect for persons, beneficence and justice. The principles are discussed in detail in a separate part of this chapter.

Another milestone in research ethics was the thalidomide tragedy. Thalidomide, a drug approved as a sedative in Europe in the 1950s, resulted in the birth of deformed babies in Europe, Canada and the USA after pregnant mothers had taken it for minor complaints such as nausea. The thalidomide disaster led to the adoption of the 'Kefauver-Harris Amendments' to the Food, Drug and Cosmetic Act in 1962, requiring drug manufacturers to prove to the FDA the effectiveness of their products before marketing them. The amendment also made it mandatory for researchers to obtain informed consent of all research volunteers receiving experimental drugs.

Another important milestone in the development of research ethics was the publication of Henry Beecher in 1966, criticizing the lack of sincerity in implementing the basic concepts of informed consent in about 50 studies published in peer reviewed journals. As a result of his publication, the National Institutes of Health in the USA, which is one of the major funders of research today, in that same year, required that Institutional Review Boards (IRBs) be established for institutions receiving government funds for medical research. The NIH directed that the IRBs should include members from the medical disciplines as well as lay-members and that the role of the IRB would be that of reviewing and approving research protocols prior to conducting research. Today, IRBs which are also commonly known as Research Ethics Committees have been established throughout the world and it is now difficult for researchers to conduct research without IRB approval, as journal editors now require proof of IRB approval.

Trigger events	*Research Ethics Milestones*
	1803 – Thomas Percival in Britain wrote the first code of medical ethics to include requirements concerning research
	1833 – William Beaumont in United States wrote an ethical code specifically focused on human experimentation
	1865 – Claude Bernard in France published a book titled 'Introduction to the study of clinical medicine'
Experiments by Dr Neisser during the 1890s performed without consent on poor and vulnerable people including abandoned children and prostitutes. This raised a lot of public debate	1900 – Research regulations in Prussia introduced demanding complete responsibility of the medical profession for carrying out human experimentation. The regulations emphasized the necessity of informed consent, documentation of justification of protocol deviation, risk benefit requirements, justification for research involving vulnerable populations and the necessity for written records.
75 children die in Germany during the 1920s in experiments with tuberculosis vaccinations	1931 – Directive from the Home Secretary of the German Reich forbids innovative therapy unless the subject or his legal representative has unambiguously consented to the procedure in light of relevant information provided in advance
1940–45 – Unethical Experiments by Nazi doctors on prisoners of war	1947 – The Nuremberg Trial and Nuremberg Code was published
1950s – Thalidomide Tragedy	1962 – Kefauver-Harris amendments – need for data to support drug registrations and informed consent for all subjects receiving test drugs.
World Medical Association learned lessons from the Nuremberg Trial and decided to come up with a code to guide members	1964 – World Medical Associations Declaration of Helsinki to replace the Nuremberg Code.
1966 – Article by Henry Beecher in *New England Journal of Medicine*	NIH requires all government funded studies to be reviewed by an IRB before initiation.
1970s – Increase in research sponsored by Developed Countries and conducted in Developing countries.	1982 – CIOMS International Ethical Guidelines for Biomedical Research Involving Human
1972 – Tuskegee study exposed	Research Act makes ethical review mandatory and establishes the Commission on Behavioural Research involving human subjects, which came up with Belmont report.
1980s & 1990s – Increase in multi-centre trials leads to the need of standards aimed at ensuring data that is acceptable to regulatory authorities in different countries	1996 – ICH Tripartite Guidelines on Good Clinical Practice in Clinical Trials issued.
Debates during the 1990s – on various issues in international research	Emanuel and others propose a framework to complement the ethical guidelines (2000).
Emphasis on human rights in research and health care.	2005 – UNESCO Declaration on Bioethics and Human Rights

Figure 25.1 Development of the discipline of research ethics

INTERNATIONAL ETHICAL CODES IN HUMAN SUBJECTS PROTECTION

The important codes that are available at present in the area of research ethics are a direct response to abuses of research participants by researchers. This section highlights the important codes and documents. The above incidences (and others that have not been described here) serve as important milestones in bioethics in as much as they have raised the awareness of the world to the bad that scientists can do to unsuspecting subjects in the name of science. During the past 50 years the main sources of guidance on the ethical conduct of research have been the Nuremberg Code (1947), the Declaration of Helsinki (1964, 1975, 1983, 1989, 1996, 2000, 2002, 2004, 2008), the Belmont Report (1979), the CIOMS International Guidelines for Biomedical Research Involving Human Subjects (1982), and the International Conference on Harmonisation Good Clinical Practice Guidelines (1997). It is evident that most of these documents were written in direct response to specific issues or events in order to avoid future similar scandals. By focusing on the instigating issues, the guidelines have tended to emphasize different ethical requirements. It is however important to note that although the events highlighted above occurred in different countries, settings and times, they have all contributed significantly in the development of different international, national and institutional codes and regulations as they are today.

The *Nuremberg Code* served as the first set of principles outlining professional ethics for medical researchers. It was a part of the judicial decision condemning the atrocities committed by the Nazi physicians. The ten points decision included the statement that 'voluntary consent of the human subject is absolutely essential' and further established that animal experimentation should precede human experimentation; all unnecessary physical and mental suffering and injury should be avoided; the degree of risk to the participants should never exceed the 'humanitarian importance of the problem' and should be minimized through 'proper preparations'; and that the participants should always be at liberty to withdraw from the experiments. This set of points established the basic principles that must be observed in order to satisfy moral, ethical and legal requirements in the conduct of human participant research. It has been the model for many professional and governmental codes since the 1950s, and has, in effect, served as the first international standard for the conduct of research.

The *Declaration of Helsinki* is the code developed by the World Medical Association (WMA) for the medical community in response to the Nuremberg trials. The new declaration was supposed to deal with the shortcomings of the Nuremberg code and especially the issue of physicians who conduct research using their patients. After the Nuremberg trials, the WMA saw it fit to come out with a code to guide its own members as a way of avoiding the recurrence of the atrocities committed by the Nazi scientists some of whom were physicians. The declaration made an important distinction between therapeutic and non-therapeutic research and, like the Nuremberg code, it made informed consent a central requirement for ethical research, but allowing for surrogate consent when the research participant is incompetent, physically or mentally incapable of giving consent, or a minor. The declaration states that research with these groups should be conducted only when the research is necessary to promote the health of the population represented, and when this research cannot be performed on legally competent persons. The Declaration of

Helsinki has been revised several times including at the 29th WMA General Assembly in Tokyo in 1975, the 35th WMA General Assembly in Venice in 1983, the 41st WMA General Assembly in Hong Kong in 1989, the 48th WMA General Assembly in South Africa in 1996, the 52nd WMA General Assembly in Edinburgh, Scotland in 2000 and the 59th WMA General Assembly, Seoul, October 2008.

Another important document is the *Belmont Report* of 1979, written by the National Commission for the Protection of Human Subjects of Biomedical and Behavioral Research. This Commission was established by the US Congress in 1974 to identify the basic ethical principles that should underlie the conduct of biomedical and behavioural research involving human subjects and to develop guidelines that should be followed to ensure that such research is conducted in accordance with those principles. The Belmont Report highlights and describes the basic ethical principles of respect for persons, beneficence and justice that underlie the ethical conduct of research. While the Belmont Report is a national document, it is important internationally as it is binding for international collaborative research that is conducted using funds provided by some US agencies.

The *Council for International Organizations of Medical Sciences (CIOMS) Guidelines,* which were proposed in 1982 were an attempt to adapt the Declaration of Helsinki to developing country situations especially in view of the rise in the number of researches conducted in emerging and developing countries and were sponsored by developed countries and it includes a section on the compensation of subjects.

The CIOMS guidelines were revised in 1993 and 2002 so as to reflect the changing research landscape as well as to address controversies that have emerged since 1982 when the guidelines were proposed. The guidelines continue to reflect the conditions and the needs of low-resource countries, and the implications for multinational or transnational research in which they may be partners. The 2002 version specifically discusses the following issues from a justice point of view: research in populations and communities with limited resources; choice of control in clinical trials; equitable distribution of burdens and benefits in the selection of groups of subjects in research; research involving vulnerable persons; research involving children; research involving individuals who by reason of mental or behavioural disorders are not capable of giving adequately informed consent; women as research participants; pregnant women as research participants; ethical obligation of external sponsors to provide healthcare services as well as other issues.

Integration of human rights issues in biomedical research has been recognized by the international community. UNESCO in 2005 adopted the *Universal Declaration on Bioethics and Human Rights* (UNESCO, 2005). This declaration addresses ethical issues related to medicine, life sciences and associated technologies as applied to human beings, taking into account their social, legal and environmental dimensions. The aims of the declaration include amongst others, to promote respect for human dignity and protect human rights, to guide the actions of individuals, groups, communities institutions and corporations (public and private), to recognize the importance of freedom of scientific research and the benefits derived from scientific and technological developments, and to provide a universal framework of principles and procedures to guide states in the formulation of their legislation, policies or other instruments in the field of bioethics. The declaration calls on member states to adhere to the following principles, among others: human dignity and human rights; maximizing benefits and minimizing any possible harm to patients, research participants and other affected individuals in applying and advancing scientific knowledge, medical practice and associated technologies; respect for autonomy and individual responsibility even for people who are not capable of exercising autonomy where for such people special measures are to be taken to protect their rights and interests; respect for privacy and confidentiality; promoting equality, justice and equity; and promoting non-discrimination and non-stigmatization.

Good Clinical Practice (GCP) guidelines have assumed great importance in clinical trials. GCP is an international quality standard that was provided by the International Conference on Harmonisation (ICH), an international body that defines standards, which governments can transpose into regulations for clinical trials involving human subjects. Good Clinical Practice guidelines include standards on how clinical trials should be conducted; define the roles and responsibilities of clinical trial sponsors, clinical research investigators and monitors. The ICH started its work in 1990 and was a joint effort to develop a single set of GCP guidelines to ensure that data generated from clinical trials are mutually acceptable to regulatory authorities in the USA, European Union and Japan. The harmonization of standards was aimed at enabling efficient licensing of new drugs in all participating countries. GCP is now accepted internationally as a standard for the protection of safety and welfare of research participants as well as assurance of the quality and credibility of data (Emmanuel et al., 2000). Some governments have since adopted GCP into their legislation as a way of ensuring that the requirements of GCP are binding on the researchers. While the title 'Good Clinical Practice' suggests that these guidelines have something to do with clinical practice, GCP is about clinical trials and some have suggested that it should be renamed 'Good Research Practice' or at least 'Good Clinical Trial Practice'. There are also other useful guidance documents such as Good Laboratory Practice (GLP) guidelines, which guide the laboratory aspects of clinical trials.

FROM CODES OF ETHICS TO A FORMAL DISCIPLINE

Research ethics has moved over the years to become a strong discipline that is offered at various levels in tertiary educational institutions. The growth in research ethics has been driven by the expansion of international research during the later part of the twentieth century. There are various agencies that are now involved in promoting the growth of research ethics. For example, in the USA the NIH through the Fogarty International Center has made funds available for the strengthening of research ethics worldwide. Other agencies such as the World Health Organization (WHO), the Wellcome Trust, and the European Developing Countries Clinical Trial Partnership (EDCTP) are also playing an important role in the strengthening of the discipline. Research ethics courses are now available online and some institutions offer higher degrees in research ethics. In several universities, research ethics is now a stand-alone course or part of the research methodology courses. Professional qualifications also exist for those working for research ethics committees. For example, in the USA people working in IRBs may become Certified IRB Professionals (CIP). Persons involved in IRBs, researchers and persons working for national drug regulatory agencies are some of the categories who need to be conversant with research ethics as they are involved in promoting ethical research in one way or other.

CURRENT ISSUES, DEBATES AND CONTROVERSIES

The past few decades have witnessed several debates and controversies in the area of research ethics. While some of these relate to the application of ethical principles in different situations, most have been generated by the increase in international research in the past few decades. As the number of studies being sponsored by agencies from rich countries and conducted in poor nations and communities have increased, questions concerning fairness have dominated the realm of research ethics. With the movement of researchers across cultures questions have been asked about the acceptability of certain practices among other cultures. In this section, past and present debates and controversies in the area of research ethics are summarized.

Are ethical principles universal?

With the internationalization of human health research, some scholars have questioned whether the three (or four) ethical principles can be applied across all countries and cultures (Beauchamp and Walters, 1999; Macklin, 1999). Concerns have been expressed concerning the validity of applying ethical principles and international guidelines that have primarily been drafted in response to the way that medical research was and is being conducted in developed countries. From the debates it appears that most people agree on the four basic ethical principles at the most abstract level, but usually have some differences on how these ethical principles ought to be operationalized in any specific context (Tangwa, 2000). A close look at the four basic principles would suggest that they are over-arching and can be further broken down into lower-level ethical principles.

Controversies around the issue of informed consent

There has been considerable debate amongst ethicists and members of the legal and scientific communities as to what constitutes valid consent in different circumstances. Several authors have reported difficulties researchers are facing in describing and explaining the concepts of randomization, placebo use and double blinding to research subjects. Most consent documents do not address adequately the purpose and justification of the trial procedures in use as well as the implications of those procedures (Featherstone and Donovan, 1998; Bhutta, 2004; Pace et al., 2005). Consent documents and study materials mainly explain the study procedures involved as a way of promoting adherence. This may be due to an assumption that lay people do not understand science and scientific procedures. Several studies have confirmed that there is a tendency among trial participants to confuse research with routine care (Appelbaum et al., 1987; Kerr et al., 2004). This aspect mainly relates to a very important component of research protection, that of disclosure of information to research participants. Whilst disclosure may not necessarily reduce the risks associated with participation, it ensures that each person is responsible for what happens to their body and is therefore an important aspect of respect for persons.

In recent times, debates have also taken place concerning a number of procedural issues that usually arise during the process of obtaining informed consent. They include, for example, determining when it is necessary to obtain written consent and when oral consent should be permitted; when, if ever, it is appropriate to withhold important and relevant information from potential participants; the need in some cultures to obtain a community leader's or a family member's permission before seeking an individual's consent; and standards of disclosure for research participants in communities in which people lack basic information about modern science or have different explanations for disease emanating from traditional and non-scientific beliefs. It is important to distinguish procedural challenges from those that reflect substantive differences in ethical views.

Regulations in some countries as well as Good Clinical Practice guidelines have often been criticized for focusing primarily on the informed consent document and requiring written consent. This is difficult to implement among illiterate individuals and such documents may be viewed in a different way in certain communities. There is however general agreement that informed consent needs to be viewed as an ongoing process throughout the research and not merely as an initial documentation of willingness to participate in the research. It is also agreed that informed consent needs to be focused on the process, rather than on the documentation (Ijsselmuiden and Faden, 1992).

The issue of deception or concealment of information to research participants has also taken centre stage in research ethics. Deception or concealment of information are often used by social scientists or behavioural researchers as part of their methods after observing that research participants often change their behaviours if they observe that they are being studied. As a general principle, the deception of identifiable participants, concealment of the purposes of research or covert observation are not considered ethical because they are contrary to the principle of respect for persons and the obtaining of informed consent.

The above discussion regarding issues in informed consent illustrates that informed consent involves complex interactions between moral, cultural and political values. Informed consent processes and procedures therefore need to be formed on the basis of personal and cultural appropriateness and acceptability. Upholding the principle of respect for autonomy does not only entail respecting the individual person, but should even go as far as respecting their convictions, culture and traditions. The above has also illustrated that informed consent is a complex process involving negotiation between the researcher and the research participants (and their significant others) and that this process varies from individual to individual, from society to society and from culture to culture. The discussion suggests the need for researchers to be trained in skills to make sensitive judgments according to the demands of the situation.

Controversies in international research

Recent years have seen growing international debate about the ethics of conducting medical research in developing countries. Concerns are being expressed about the exploitation of research participants from poor countries in research that cannot be conducted in developed countries as a result of their stringent legislation. Some of the concerns are also partly fuelled by fears of medical-ethical imperialism and fears about the use of double standards especially in international collaborative research. Typically, developed countries sponsor or conduct research in developing countries for some combination of the following four reasons: (1) the host country might desire information about effective and affordable interventions for an indigenous health problem; (2) in order to be marketed in some developing countries, drugs and biologicals, even if already tested and approved in other countries, must be approved by national regulatory authorities; (3) it is more efficient to conduct research in a country in which the condition being studied is more prevalent; and (4) it might be less expensive and faster to conduct research in emerging and developing countries.

Aspects of research that have proved particularly controversial in poor countries include the relevance of the research to the research participants as well as their communities and nations. At present, many emerging and developing countries have a limited capacity to determine national health and research priorities, or to conduct relevant research. As a result, they become dependent on the interests of external sponsors. In such circumstances developing countries may find it difficult to refuse offers to sponsor research, even if it is unlikely to benefit their populations, because of the accompanying incentives, such as improved healthcare facilities and other benefits to individual researchers, their institutions and even policymakers and politicians.

Conducting research in poor countries often poses special challenges and these mainly arise from the combined effects of distinctive histories, cultures, politics, judicial systems and economic situations. There is extreme poverty that afflicts so many, and primary healthcare services are generally inadequate due to many factors, and the high prices of drugs often places them out of reach of both individuals and developing country governments. Some justification is therefore necessary for conducting research in developing countries other than their less stringent or less complex regulatory or ethical requirements. Whatever the reason or combination of reasons, sponsors and researchers must ensure that these activities are conducted ethically and that they are responsive to the health needs of the country or community and that they do not exploit either the participants or the populations of the host country (NBAC, 2001).

A report by the Commission on Health Research for Development (COHRED) in 1990 has concluded that about 90 per cent of the resources availed for research throughout the world is being used to address the health needs of 10 per cent of the world's population (COHRED, 1990). Diseases affecting poor nations are receiving less attention as attention is being turned to diseases affecting the populations of developed nations. The statistics point to the need to strike a balance in the way that resources are used in research between the developed countries and developing countries. With improvements in travel and communication technologies, the world has become a single village. The movement of disease has become even easier. Diseases such as ebola, HIV/AIDS, SARS and bird flu have shown the need for all countries to cooperate in the eradication of diseases, as diseases have no boundary. Discussions continue to be held at the international level regarding how developed countries can assist in addressing the health problems of poor countries and to date various strategies have been adopted aimed at ensuring that resources are available to address the research needs of poor nations.

Equivalent protection in multi centre trials

Besides all the above challenges related to the application of ethical guidelines and principles, there are also challenges that relate to ethical review, in particular in poor countries (Rugemalila and Kilama, 2001). For example, a significant proportion of the institutions in Africa do not have ethics committees. In some institutions, ethics committees were established to meet the requirements of the sponsoring agents and these as such merely serve as rubber stamping authorities. Some ethics committees have inadequate ethical review processes and mechanisms and their reviewers and members are poorly equipped for ethical review. The problem of ethics committee shopping is still rampant since the review systems are still in their infancy in most developing countries (when a proposal is rejected by one ethics committee, the researchers resubmit it to another ethics committee).

Some research ethics committees are poorly grounded and hence are not recognized by the researchers and also by the institutions and some are under-resourced even to the extent that they do not have office space and stationery. Other problems bedevilling ethics committees relate to the abuse of expedited review processes, interference from outsiders, researchers, politicians, etc. (lack of independence), gender imbalance as well as the non-involvement of lay persons. Currently, there are discussions centred on the principle of equivalent protection. According to this principle, research participants whether in an African, American, Asian or a European country should all be protected at the same level. This principle recognizes the equality of research participants in contributing data, which is useful in answering a research question regardless of country of origin.

The use of placebos in clinical trials

Placebo controls are commonly used in clinical trials of investigational treatments because they have important advantages. Supporters of placebo controlled trials (PCTs) point to the interpretive problems inherent in the use of active controls in equivalence trials to establish the efficacy of a new treatment (Senn, 1997). In recent years some bioethicists have criticized the use of placebos in controlled trials especially where alternative therapy exists in favour of standard treatment controlled trials (Crouch, 1998). The use of placebos was also widely debated during the revision of the Declaration of Helsinki in 2000. In 1999, the World Medical Assembly circulated a draft version of the declaration, which restricted the use of placebos. There were arguments that this provision would discourage the development of new drugs. Some bioethicists were concerned that the use of placebos may deny adequate care to participants on the placebo arm and may even lead to a deterioration of their health status.

On the other hand, those who justified the use of placebos were justifying their use as ethical in instances where delaying or omitting available treatment has no permanent adverse consequences for the patient and for as long as patients are fully informed about their alternatives (Ellenberg and Temple, 2000). Some sponsors of clinical trials in emerging and developing countries have argued that the use of a placebo is acceptable if treatment of established efficacy exists but, for economic reasons, is not readily available in that developing country. Most, if not all, commentaries on this proposal from an ethical perspective have rejected the argument. Subsequent debates on this and other issues finally led to revisions of the Declaration of Helsinki in 2004 to allow the use of placebos under certain conditions such as where no proven alternative therapy exists and where delayed treatment does not result in serious harm to the patient. Generally, where no proven alternative exists, as in the case with HIV microbicides or HIV vaccines, the use of placebos is routine and generally less controversial. Regardless of all the arguments against the use of placebos in research, placebos will remain in use in clinical research in future because of their advantages. Placebo-controlled trials are regarded as the gold standard by most regulatory agencies and funding agencies because of their advantages such as the conclusive nature of the results they yield within a short period of time thereby saving on costs.

Debates on standard of care

Having debated the use of placebos and coming up with some position that placebos can be used only under special circumstances, the clinical trials community then moved into another contentious issue – that of the standard of care that should be provided to participants in the control group of clinical trials. The issue raised by this principle is that not all subjects are equal: some will have access to better healthcare than others. This is purely an ethical issue as it relates to fairness and has been magnified by the fact that some studies are now being conducted in populations so radically different that participants in one locality will have access to healthcare far superior than those in another locality during and after the same research. In most cases, research provides access to superior treatment than is otherwise available in the health delivery system. Those with access to treatment equivalent to that in the research will not experience discrimination but those from poor settings will. For some, the answer is that everyone should be given the most effective treatment, regardless of cost. Many developing countries are wrestling with issues of poverty, basic healthcare and sanitation, and are unable to provide every sick person with cutting-edge or even effective treatments.

The standard of care debate has led to three questions: (1) Is it fair for participants from limited resource settings to receive a lower standard of care simply because they are from a poor country or simply because their country has a lower standard? The question has even been extended to situations in which there is no local standard and yet a standard is available in rich countries; (2) Some have asked whether no standard is a standard at all; (3) Is it fair to subjects that they be included in a research project that will offer superior treatment than is otherwise available, but only for the duration of the research, after which they will return to a lower standard?

Guidance in the earlier versions of the Declaration of Helsinki was agreeable to the use of placebos in countries where no standard of care existed and this was very worrisome to proponents of egalitarian access to care because of its implication that if no treatment is available, as is the case in many developing countries, then doing nothing for a control group would satisfy the declaration's principle. The Declaration of Helsinki has since been revised so as to clarify on this issue. Globally there is a general understanding that researchers and pharmaceutical companies from richer countries should not take advantage of the lower standards in poor countries and that the best standard available should be used wherever and whenever possible depending on various factors.

Post trial access debates

Historically, concern for justice in research involving human subjects has focused on whether research subjects were treated fairly: were they overburdened relative to the direct benefits they received from their participation in research? Contemporary concerns with justice in research have broadened: are the overall benefits and burdens of research distributed fairly, and have disadvantaged individuals and groups received a fair share of the benefits of research? The above concerns form the basis of the principle of distributive justice: members of society should neither bear an unfair share of the direct burdens of participating in research, nor should they be unfairly excluded from the potential benefits of research participation. Another question that is now receiving an increasing amount of attention is what should happen once a research project in a developing country is completed. Concerns include:

- ensuring that the intervention if found successful can be availed to the whole community (and or country);.
- ensuring that researchers receive appropriate recognition of, and where appropriate a share of the financial rewards for their endeavours;
- how to sustain improvements to healthcare systems made during research; and
- in the HIV vaccine and microbicide arena what happens to those who are infected during the trial?

It is now recognized that the benefits of research should be made available to the participants and communities that bear the burden of that research. Without this principle, participants could be exploited for the purposes of the research while its benefits go wholly elsewhere – for example, back to developed world patients who can afford to pay the high price of the treatment. Thus, the application of the principle prevents researchers, in testing an unproven treatment, from recruiting their research subjects solely on the basis that they do not have access to the best existing treatment for the disease for which the new treatment is being tested. This is ethically unacceptable because it may involve exploitation in the selection of research subjects. Participation in research should not deprive subjects of the optimal available standard of healthcare.

Vulnerable persons and over protection of groups

The majority of international and national guidelines and legislations deal with the issue of vulnerable populations. The CIOMS guidelines have defined vulnerable populations as those groups who are not in a position to defend their interests due to their economic or social circumstances. In the past, research has always tended to rely on the weak, the poor and the defenceless from the prisoners of war during Nazi times to poor communities in developing countries, hence the discussions in recent times about undue inducements and coercion.

The problem of coercion becomes even more serious when a physician is involved in the recruitment of his/her patients or members from the communities they serve. The problem of undue inducements is created by the poor economies of developing countries and people are forced to consider the benefits and ignore the risks associated with a particular study. In some cases, the remuneration offered to participants as compensation appears reasonable to the sponsors and other participants in developed countries, and yet it is irresistible in developing countries. It is generally agreed that researchers need to justify the selection of communities for their research, and research ethics committees need to ensure that the justifications are acceptable. In the interest of protecting the poor from undue inducements as a result of irresistible incentives, some of the benefits may have to be converted into community benefits such as supporting clinics or engaging in other community projects that promote good health. At least in that way researchers can ensure that they are dealing with the 10/90 gap in an ethical manner.

Some have also argued that the emphasis on protection against harm is overly protective in some cases as it may negate a person's right to participate in studies that may benefit an individual in their own way if they so desire. In the majority of guidelines, pregnant women and children are considered vulnerable populations. For pregnant women the reason is that the test product may harm the unborn baby who would not in any way consent to participate in research. For the children, the reasoning relates to the fears concerning their bodies' ability to absorb the products under study as a result of the fact that their body systems are still in their formative stages. Some have argued that this over-protection of pregnant women and children excludes them from research that might benefit them or which may benefit other children and women in the future. As a result, it is common to find a statement on the package inserts accompanying many medications indicating that the medicine has not been tested in pregnant women and children and as such the side-effects on these groups are unknown (Sherwin, 1994).

From individuals to communities

Over time, the questions in research ethics have been extending beyond the individual research participants to include the communities at large. In clinical trials, while the focus of the trial is on the individuals who are directly participating, considerations also have to be made regarding the communities. It has been argued that the care that is offered to trial participants from poor areas through research often serves as an undue inducement to other members of the communities and hence the need to consider benefits for communities. The focus on communities also has to do with the distinction between rich and poor countries. Poor countries need to ensure that they are benefiting from the research in which their citizens and communities participate. Recent decades have witnessed some serious discussions on how poor communities can be assured of access to drugs whose trials their citizens would have participated in. The focus on communities has also been a result of the importance that some cultures place on communities. The discussions on research benefits have culminated in the ancillary care debate. Proponents of access to healthcare have argued that researchers need to provide ancillary care to research participants. Ancillary care is care that is over and beyond the problem being investigated in a particular study. Debates have been held with funding agencies on the need for them to support ancillary care. Some were arguing that ancillary care was not the role of researchers and funding agencies, as the role of researchers was simply to conduct research. They argued that to provide ancillary care is to take away the role of governments. As a result of these debates there is now a general understanding that research plays an important role in guaranteeing access to care for the less privileged. Ancillary care also serves as a kind of token of appreciation for the poor who volunteer as research participants.

Ethical issues related to human genetic research

Genetic research involving humans raises many ethical issues that need consideration. Some genetic research may address socially contentious issues such as the nature of intelligence or personality traits, or have the potential to lead to results that may be used in a culturally or socially harmful manner in relation to specific ethnic or racial groups. Genetic research also raises special issues concerning privacy and confidentiality. At times obtaining informed consent may be difficult because of the complexity of the issues involved. In some studies, the information that is obtained from one specific individual can be applied to a whole family, clan or nation. Issues may also arise related to the storage and future use of genetic materials and information. Such issues could relate to the provision of research participants with the results of research. Some genetic studies may produce information of significance to the future health of specific participants. There is general agreement that all these issues need to be identified before research commences and participants should be informed of such a possibility prior to giving consent. In addition, the mechanism for feedback of research results should be defined (Glass, 2003).

Research involving stem cells, gene therapy or cloning

Gene therapy refers to innovative techniques that involve the modification of genetic material for the purposes of overcoming an inherited or acquired genetic abnormality. Cloning refers to a range of techniques directed at asexual reproduction, or copying of cells and organisms, including the possibility of manufacturing human beings. Both techniques are the subject of vigorous public debate about scientific, social, legal and ethical implications. At present, it is generally agreed that gene alteration involving human germline cells or human embryos, and cloning directed towards the production of new human individuals, should not be carried out (Ryan, 2003). In stem cell research, there are debates concerning the source of stem cells that are used. Some of the stem cells are obtained from embryos. Religious groups have argued against the use of such stem cells as they are obtained after the destruction of a human zygote. Therefore, at present, applications to consider research involving human participants employing such innovative techniques should be considered with extreme caution and individuals with appropriate expertize should be consulted.

Storage of tissue and future use of stored material

Tissue banks are now a booming business in research. Researchers are involved in the collection of specimens that they store for future research work. There are several questions that come to mind regarding stored specimens including the following:

- What will the specimens be used for?
- Who will have access to the specimens?
- Will they have identifiers?
- What if the researchers find out about something that directly impacts on the donor?

It is generally agreed that if a participant's tissue is to be stored after the completion of a research project, they should be informed of this beforehand.

Where they have not been informed beforehand, it is agreed that the researchers need to approach the ethics committee for permission to use those samples for other studies. For tissue collected within the context of medical treatment, consent procedures usually relate to diagnostic tests and routine archiving, with any surplus tissue being discarded. If researchers wish to make other use of the stored or surplus tissue, in order for consent to be informed or genuine, the patient must have been informed of the possibility of either type of tissue being used in future research, and also have been given the opportunity to object to this, or even to opt for disposal of all tissue (Merz et al., 1997).

Over-researched communities

The concept of over-researched communities has been introduced to refer to those communities that are said to be bearing the burdens of research more than others. In several countries, there are research centres that are internationally known. These centres of excellence are mostly situated in poor rural areas and lots of studies are conducted in these centres as well as their surrounding areas. In some situations this phenomenon has resulted in the stigmatization of the communities as a result of the findings from the various studies that would have been conducted in those areas. Some communities also suffer from research fatigue and their members would refuse to participate in any future research because of the fact that they would have been exposed to too many burdens from research that could have been taken to other communities. The communities in these areas serve as 'human laboratories' and end up bearing all the burdens of research. Researchers need to ask themselves the reason why they have chosen a particular area for their study. Is it because the people are too receptive or is it to take advantage of the existing infrastructure? Certainly burdens and benefits from research need to be shared out equally among all communities.

Ethics in research using animals and hazardous materials

The realm of research ethics has not only been limited to human research. Over the years, considerations have been extended to research using animals. Animals play a very important role in research as they are used to understand more about test products before research can be conducted in humans. In recent times, animal rights activists have become very active internationally in fighting for the rights of animals. Concerns have been raised regarding the ways in which animals have been treated in research including the excessive use of research animals in some situations. There is, however, general agreement that researchers need to handle research animals humanely, minimize their suffering, use other means of obtaining data wherever possible and try to come up with models that can be used instead of animals. Concerns continue to be raised over the use of harmful materials, including biological organisms, in research. Concerns are raised about the possible effects of such materials on staff working in the research programmes, research participants and the public as well as on the environment. Hazardous materials need to be handled and used appropriately so that they do not cause harm. Some institutions have since set committees responsible for looking at the care and use of animals in research and those responsible for providing oversight for research involving hazardous substances.

Issues of key silence or omissions

A close look at the literature on research ethics, including the ethical guidelines, would suggest that there are some areas of omission that need to be addressed as the discipline continues to grow. One of the important observations is that the majority of literature on informed consent emphasizes the elements that need to be included in informed consent documents. The literature assumes that illiterate or ordinary people cannot understand information about science and clinical trial procedures. It is important to emphasize the need to come up with interventions aimed at ensuring that potential participants understand the research studies being proposed to them so that they become more responsible for what happens to them as individuals.

The majority of ethical guidelines and legislations address issues that are common in biomedical research. This is understandable as these were developed in response to specific cases involving abuse of research participants in biomedical research. Ethical issues in behavioural research have not been adequately addressed and more often research ethics committee members are not very conversant with the issues in behavioural research. In some institutions, separate ethics committees have been formed to review behavioural research as a result of the realization that some of the ethical issues involved are unique.

The development of the current international guidelines was dominated by persons from rich countries. Poor countries have always been inadequately represented in their discussion. As a result the voice of the pharmaceutical companies is beginning to dominate discussions on ethical codes. The debates on issues such as the use of placebos, standard of care and ancillary care have been very protracted as the private companies had to make sure that they do not reduce their profit margin as a result of demands from those who are interested in addressing the inequalities between rich and poor nations and those who are interested in ensuring access to care for the poor.

The international ethical codes emphasize so much the relationship between the researcher and the research participant that they do not view the community as playing an important role in research and hence fail to address the issue of community research. While there are some differences in interpreting the term 'community', for our purposes, we will use the term to refer to a group that share a particular characteristic or set of characteristics that may set them apart as a unique group. This definition caters for both geographical boundaries and social and political groups. The major international guidelines also give much emphasis on medical research and ignore the many other types of research that are conducted by researchers.

The majority of current guidelines emphasize the direct benefits for individuals. On the other hand, some would argue that the benefits for participants should not be such that they lead the participant to forget about the risks posed by the study. In the interest of closing the 10/90 gap and also ensuring that research is recognized as one of the enterprises, it may be useful to avail some community benefits to communities participating in research as a way of ensuring that undue inducement on the individual is avoided.

With the increase in international research, there are examples of researchers who have gone against other cultures intentionally as well as unintentionally in some cases. Cases abound of researchers who have gone against some cultural taboos, in some cases leading to other scholars calling for an additional principle – respect for culture. It is very important to stress that one may not respect another person adequately if one does not respect their culture. A person may only be fully respected if their culture is also respected. To respect someone's culture is to ultimately respect him or her as it shows that the person is being treated as a complete being who is part of a particular culture.

FUTURE DIRECTIONS

Research ethics as a discipline is still growing as it seeks to address current concerns in human research. There is a lot of genetic research being conducted after the completion of the human genome project. Yet the genetic studies will present more and more ethical challenges. A lot of the information that is generated by research projects ends up being stored in electronic databases. Researchers and information technology experts need to consider the best ways of ensuring confidentiality – the cabinet, lock and key are no longer adequate. There are also issues of involving communities in genetic research as the data to be obtained would apply to a specific community or group. In the testing of some public health intervention, communities also need to be involved especially in those interventions in which it may be difficult to single out some individuals.

While the individual research participant remains very important in research, other new stakeholders continue to come on to the scene. History has shown that informed consent by itself cannot serve as an automatic guarantee that a study is ethical or that participants are truly informed. Emphasis in the future will be on ensuring that the public, including trial participants, understands about research and what it entails. The public also needs to become aware of the difference between research and routine care. Ethicists and researchers have to work together to come up with interventions aimed at addressing these shortcomings.

Regarding the issue of protecting vulnerable populations, researchers and ethics committees carefully need to consider reasons why certain groups are being excluded from certain studies. During the 1960s, after the research atrocities, research ethics was focused mainly on individuals and individual informed consent. During the 1990s, research ethics moved to focus on justice issues with emphasis on issues that related to the avoidance of the exploitation of poor communities by rich countries and pharmaceutical companies. Research ethics is now moving its focus again towards the issue of empowering individuals through education so that they can make informed decisions. This is evidence that the research ethics discipline is always evolving so as to respond to current issues.

Society is becoming more and more sensitive to human abuses. There is need for greater balance between scientific advances, the common good and the needs of the individual.

The public are becoming increasingly more informed about human rights and accountability in research. Governments throughout the world are increasingly taking a more active part in ensuring the ethical conduct of research by putting up legislations, structures and additional ethical requirements. In some cases some serious sanctions are being imposed against those who do not adhere to the regulations. With all these developments research ethics will continue to grow in its relevance.

REFERENCES

Altman, L.K. (1998) *Who Goes First? The Story of Human Experimentation in Medicine.* Berkeley, CA: University of California Press.

Appelbaum, P.S., Roth, L.H., Lidz, P. and Winsdale, W. (1987) 'False hopes and best data: Consent to research and the therapeutic misconception', *Hastings Center Report*, 12 (2): 20–4.

Beauchamp, T. and Childress, J. (2001) *Principles of Biomedical Ethics.* New York: Oxford University Press.

Beauchamp, T. and Walters, L. (1999) *Contemporary Issues in Bioethics.* Belmont, CA: Wadsworth Publishers.

Beecher, H.K. (1966) 'Ethics and clinical research', *New England Journal of Medicine*, 274: 1354–60.

Belmont Report (1979) *National Commission for the Protection of Human Subjects of Biomedical and Behavioral Research: The Belmont Report.* Washington, DC: US Government Printing Office.

Bhutta, Z.A. (2004) 'Beyond informed consent', *Bulletin of World Health Organization*, 82 (10): 771–8.

Brody, B.S. (1998) *The Ethics of Biomedical Research.* New York: Oxford University Press.

Council for Health Research and Development (COHRED) (1990) *Commission on Health Research for Development, Health Research: Essential Link to Equity in Development.* Cambridge, MA: Oxford University Press.

Council for International Organizations of Medical Sciences (CIOMS) (1982) *Proposed International Guidelines for Biomedical Research Involving Human Subjects.* Geneva: CIOMS.

Council for International Organizations of Medical Sciences (CIOMS) (1993) *International Ethical Guidelines for Biomedical Research Involving Human Subjects.* Geneva: CIOMS.

Council for International Organizations of Medical Sciences (CIOMS) (2002) *International Guidelines for Biomedical Research Involving Human Subjects.* Geneva: CIOMS.

Crouch, R. (1998) 'AZT trials and tribulations', *Hastings Center Report*, 28: 26–34.

Ellenberg, S. and Temple, R. (2000) 'Placebo controlled trials and active control trials in evaluation of new treatments', *Annals of Internal Medicine*, 133: 464–70.

Emmanuel, E., Wendler, D. and Grady, C. (2000) 'What makes clinical research ethical?' *Journal of the American Medical Association*, 283: 2701–11.

Featherstone, K. and Donovan, J. (1998) 'Random allocation or allocation at random? Patients' perspectives of participation in a randomized controlled trial', *British Medical Journal*, 317: 1177–80.

Glass, K.C. (2003) 'Structuring the review of human genetics protocols: Gene localization and identification studies', in E. Emanuel, R. Crouch, J. Arras, J. Moreno and C. Grady (eds), *Ethical and Regulatory Aspects of Clinical Research: Readings and Commentary.* Baltimore, MD: Johns Hopkins University Press.

Ijsselmuiden, C. and Faden, R. (1992) 'Research and informed consent in Africa – Another look', *New England Journal of Medicine*, 326: 830–4.

International Conference on Harmonization of Technical Requirements for Registration of Pharmaceuticals for Human Use (ICH) (1997) *Good Clinical Practice: Consolidated Guidance.* 62 Federal Register 25692.

Kerr, C., Robinson, E., Stevens, A., Braunholtz, D., Edwards, S. and Lilford, R. (2004) 'Randomisation in trials: Do potential trial participants understand it and find it acceptable?', *Journal of Medical Ethics*, 30: 80–4.

Lakhani, S. (1992) 'Early clinical pathologists: Edward Jenner (1749–1823)', *Journal of Clinical Pathology*, 45: 756–8.

Lefor, A.T. (2005) 'Scientific misconduct and unethical human experimentation: Historic parallels and moral implications', *Nutrition*, 21 (7): 878–82.

Mcguire Dunn, C. and Chadwick, G. (1999) *Protecting Study Volunteers in Research.* Boston, MA: Center Bay Watch.

Macklin, R. (1999) *Against Relativism.* New York: Oxford University Press.

Merz, J.F., Sankar, P., Taube, S.E. and LiVolsi, V.A. (1997) 'Use of human tissues in research: Clarifying clinician and researcher roles and information flows', *Journal of Investigative Medicine,* 45: 252–7.

National Bioethics Advisory Commission (NBAC) (2001) *Ethical and Policy Issues in International Research: Clinical Trials in Developing Countries: Report and Recommendations of the National Bioethics Advisory Commission,* Vol. 1. Rockville, MD: NBAC.

Nuremberg Code (1947) *Reprinted from Trials of War Criminals before the Nuremberg Military Tribunals under Control of Council Law (1949),* No. 10, Vol. 2. Washington, DC: US Government Printing Office, pp 181–2.

Pace, C., Emanuel, E., Chuenyam, T., Duncombe, C., Bebchuk, J.D., Wendler, D. et al. (2005) 'The quality of informed consent in a clinical study in Thailand', *IRB: Ethics and Human Research,* 27 (1): 9–17.

Rugemalila, J.B. and Kilama, W.L. (2001) 'Proceedings of seminar on health research ethics in Africa', *Acta Tropica,* 78: S1–S126.

Ryan, M. (2003) 'Creating embryos for research: Weighing symbolic costs', in E. Emanuel, R. Crouch, J. Arras, J. Moreno and C. Grady (eds), *Ethical and Regulatory Aspects of Clinical Research: Readings and Commentary.* Baltimore, MD: Johns Hopkins University Press.

Senn, S.J. (1997) *Statistical Issues in Drug Development.* Chichester: John Wiley.

Sherwin, S. (1994) 'Women in clinical studies: A feminist view', in A. Mastriani, R. Faden and D. Federman (eds), *Women and Health Research – Ethical and Legal Issues of Including Women in Clinical Studies.* Washington, DC: National Academy Press.

Tangwa, G. (2000) 'The traditional African perception of a person: Some implications for Bioethics', *Hastings Center Report,* 3095: 39–43.

UNESCO (2005) *Universal Declaration on Bioethics and Human Rights.* Paris: UNESCO.

Vollmann, J. and Winau, R. (1996) 'Informed consent in human experimentation before the Nuremberg code', *British Medical Journal,* 313 (7070): 1445.

World Medical Association (WMA) (1964) *Declaration of Helsinki – Ethical Principles for Medical Research Involving Human Subjects.* As adopted by the 18th WMA General Assembly, Helsinki, June.

World Medical Association (WMA) (1975) *Declaration of Helsinki – Ethical Principles for Medical Research Involving Human Subjects.* As amended by the 29th WMA General Assembly, Tokyo, October.

World Medical Association (WMA) (1983) *Declaration of Helsinki – Ethical Principles for Medical Research Involving Human Subjects.* As amended by the 35th WMA General Assembly, Venice, October.

World Medical Association (WMA) (1989) *Declaration of Helsinki – Ethical Principles for Medical Research Involving Human Subjects.* As amended by the 41st WMA General Assembly, Hong Kong, September.

World Medical Association (WMA) (1996) *Declaration of Helsinki – Ethical Principles for Medical Research Involving Human Subjects.* As amended by the 48th WMA General Assembly, Somerset West, Republic of South Africa, October.

World Medical Association (WMA) (2000) *Declaration of Helsinki – Ethical Principles for Medical Research Involving Human Subjects.* As amended by the 52nd WMA General Assembly, Edinburgh, October.

World Medical Association (WMA) (2002) *Declaration of Helsinki – Ethical Principles for Medical Research Involving Human Subjects.* As amended by the 53rd WMA General Assembly, Washington (note of Clarification on paragraph 29 added).

World Medical Association (WMA) (2004) *Declaration of Helsinki – Ethical Principles for Medical Research Involving Human Subjects.* As amended by the 55th WMA General Assembly, Tokyo (note of Clarification on Paragraph 30 added).

World Medical Association (WMA) (2008) *Declaration of Helsinki – Ethical Principles for Medical Research Involving Human Subjects.* As amended by the 59th WMA General Assembly, Seoul, October.

26

Health Research in the Global Context

Michael McDonald and Nina Preto

INTRODUCTION

We begin with three observations. First, conflict of interest is a relatively new topic in healthcare ethics and not one that would likely have been included in a volume of this sort a few years ago. Despite its recent appearance, conflict of interest is an important topic and has significant implications for research practice and its governance. Second, it is a topic that is germane to many of the issues discussed in this volume. While we focus on the ethics of health research, conflict of interest is also important in clinical practice, as well as in population and public health. Third, conflict of interest is an often misunderstood and misused concept.

Briefly, a conflict of interest can be described as 'a set of conditions in which professional judgment concerning a primary interest (such as a patient's welfare or the validity of research) tends to be unduly influenced by a secondary interest (such as financial gain)' (Thompson, 1993; Lemmens and Freedman, 2000; Krimsky, 2006). Conflict of interest has three components – a trust-based relationship, a conflicting interest and an exercise of judgment.[1] The relationship between the parties in question is often trust based, such that one party (the trustor) is entitled to trust that the other (the trustee) will promote or protect their interests in relation to matters within that relationship. The second component is an influence that tends to make the trustee's judgment on a given decision less reliable for promoting or protecting the trustor's interests than it would normally be (Davis, 1998). Third, the trustee must be in a position to make a decision that affects the trustor's interests.

With this provisional definition in mind, we provide in Part 1 a historical context for the current focus on conflicts of interest in health research. We identify precipitating factors and the reactions to them. In Part II, we develop a more detailed analysis of the concept of conflict of interest, differentiating it from other tensions often mistakenly termed 'conflicts of interest'. We also draw on work in law and business ethics to provide insights into conflicts of interest and their management. In Part III, we make suggestions for policy, practice and further research.

Unpacking the context

Key to understanding conflicts of interest in health research is the dynamic relationship between public and private funding for health research. Various factors (e.g. slow commercialisation of research by public research institutions, lack of government support for research, and an increasingly powerful private sector) support a shift away from science as a 'public calling in which research findings should be shared and made publicly accessible' (Lemmens, 2004: 644) to a field dominated by a heavy commercial focus on patents and other intellectual property protections. Many governments have encouraged this as part of a deliberate shift towards a growing, competitive, knowledge-based economy.[2]

The dangers in this shift are widely recognized and discussed in an extensive literature on the commercialization of science (Downie et al., 2002; Krimsky, 2003; Lemmens, 2004; Labonte and Torgerson, 2005; Lemmens and Waring, 2006). Key concerns include the focus on intellectual property protections and the resulting impact on exchange of ideas and research results. Others relate to the erosion of scientific disinterestedness, such that 'science driven by private interest is laden with bias ... (and) therefore ... will take more time with repeated replication of results and critical reviews to reach the truth' (Krimsky, 2003: 78). This happens when researchers focus on questions with commercial relevance and ignore more scientifically significant issues that are more in the public interest (Krimsky, 2003).

A further concern is that the commercial pressures will have pervasive effects on how research studies are designed and conducted, and how results are recorded and analyzed. However, it can be argued that 'commercialization of research harnesses the collective intellectual and creative talents of university faculty, speeds the development of new and improved therapies, stimulates regional economic growth, and contributes to the economic viability of research institutions' (AAMC, 2001: 4). Given these wide-ranging benefits of commercialization, and the fact that even among critics of commercialization few call for researchers to foreswear all interactions with industry, the key question seems to be how to identify, assess and manage the conflicts of interest that arise when the goals and motivations of the private sector conflict with the fiduciary traditions of medical research.

Such concerns about conflicts of interest are far from theoretical, with numerous incidents related to subject safety and the erosion of scientific integrity to point to as examples. We next review key incidents, and responses to them.

CONFLICT OF INTEREST AND HUMAN SUBJECT PROTECTION

It has been stated that 'while there is no definitive evidence that conflict of interest has directly injured a research subject, a number of cases have certainly created the suspicion or appearance of that eventuality' (Blumenthal, 2002; Ferris and Naylor, 2006: 98). Among the most highly publicized of these cases was the death of Jesse Gelsinger. In 1999,

18-year-old Jesse Gelsinger died in a gene transfer study at the Institute for Human Gene Therapy at the University of Pennsylvania. Both the institution and the physician investigators had commercial interests in the outcome of the trial. These interests were not adequately disclosed to trial participants. This case greatly focused attention on the dangers of conflicts of interest in clinical research.

> [The Gelsinger case] is paradigmatic for at least three reasons. First, it occurred notwithstanding the oversight of an experienced IRB, thus exposing serious limitations of the current review system. Second, the investigators and the institution in which the research took place had significant commercial interests in the study's outcome. These interests appear to have influenced how the study was promoted and how the investigators behaved once Jesse was enrolled as a subject. Finally ... this case illustrates the possibility of legal action against researchers and against individual scientists and research institutions. (Lemmens and Waring, 2006: 4, bracketed insertion added)

In addition to changes in University of Pennsylvania policy, the case prompted widespread discussion of both individual and institutional conflicts of interest (e.g. Caulfield, 2001–2; Caulfield and Griener, 2001; Barnes and Florencio, 2002; Blumenthal, 2002; Downie et al., 2002; Bekelman et al., 2003; DeAngelis et al., 2004; Brown, 2006; Emanuel et al., 2006; Ferris and Naylor, 2006). It also prompted the production of influential guidance documents on the part of such key organizations as the Association of American Medical Colleges (AAMC) and the Association of American Universities. Hearings were held by the US Department of Health and Human Services (DHHS) to look into whether and to what extent the financial interests of clinical investigators should be included in informed consent information given to prospective candidates for clinical trials. However, key science and medical associations (including the AAMC) opposed such regulatory guidance suggesting that it would not effectively protect subjects' interests. This concern was echoed by researchers and sponsors who added that such regulations would simply add another impediment to recruiting subjects (Krimsky, 2006). The guidance document that ultimately emerged from the DHHS hearings (T.G. Thompson, 2004)[3] recognizes the 'complexity of the relationship between government, academia, industry and others ..., that these relationships often legitimately include financial relationships' and that 'not all financial interests cause conflicts of interest or affect the rights and welfare of subjects'. It suggests a range of strategies for dealing with conflicts of interest, many of which have been outlined in other guidance documents.[4] These include scrutinizing the financial interests of individuals and institutions involved in the research and determining whether subjects' rights and interests would be best protected by disclosure, or instead by the reduction or elimination of the interest. While there is a brief discussion of the kinds of information that ought to be disclosed, this is essentially left to the IRB's discretion. Steps such as conducting the research elsewhere, separating responsibilities for financial and research decisions, and adding additional third party oversight or monitoring are also suggested as possible approaches to mitigating and eliminating conflicts.

While US cases and resulting guidelines have been influential internationally, there have also been a number of highly relevant international documents. Among the best known is the *Declaration of Helsinki*.[5] While conflict of interest is only explicitly mentioned in one article (Article 22 which calls for disclosure to the subject of possible conflicts of interest and institutional affiliations of the researcher in the consent process), others have noted that this is enhanced by the clear aim of the Declaration to 'place the interests of the subject above all else, including the interests of science and society ... [and that] research done for or influenced by other personal or social goals, such as financial gain, would arguably conflict with the general tone of the entire Declaration' (Caulfield, 2001–2: 39).[6]

CONFLICT OF INTEREST AND EROSION OF SCIENTIFIC INTEGRITY

As mentioned, the other main concern with conflicts of interest in health research is the threat to scientific integrity. The South Korean 'Hwanggate' cloning scandal is a leading case. Dr Hwang had risen to become a national hero and an international scientific celebrity with his 2004 claim to have cloned a human blastocyst and successfully extracted stem cells from it – two highly significant scientific firsts. This was followed in 2005 with the claim that Dr Hwang and colleagues had successfully created patient-specific embryonic stem cells from human blastocysts created through somatic cell nuclear transfer (SCNT). While questions were raised quite early on within the scientific community and from media groups in Korea as to the authenticity and ethical integrity of Dr Hwang's work, these concerns were largely ignored by institutional and governmental authorities. In fact, the Korean government announced in October 2005 that it planned to create a World Stem Cell Hub, based on the work of Dr Hwang. Ultimately, however, Hwang's work was found to be both ethically and scientifically fraudulent. For example, junior researchers were coerced into providing eggs for research, and subsequent investigations demonstrated that much of the data on which the two landmark papers had been based was fabricated (Saunders and Savulescu, 2008). Reflecting on the pressures on Dr Hwang at the peak of his popularity, Saunders and Savulescu comment that:

> Hwang was a symbol of everything that South Korea stood for and desired, his picture was plastered on public transport and posters were released proclaiming that he would change the world. South Koreans viewed Hwang as holding the hopes of the world; to further Hwang's research was to further South Korea (216).

The funding, pride and fame that can result from being first to make a scientific breakthrough affects not only the individual researcher, but also their institution and their nation. The goal of conducting scientifically sound research can be easily eroded or compromised by these other secondary interests.

Other concerns center on the impact funding sources have on the scientific enterprise in terms of what is studied and how, as well as for the sharing and reporting of research results. Several authors have reviewed studies linking funding source to research results, and changes in the likelihood of research publication (Warner and Gluck, 2003; DuVal, 2004; Brown, 2006). Among the frequently cited studies in this regard are studies demonstrating that in comparative drug studies, the results invariably favor the sponsor (Davidson, 1986). A study by Friedberg et al (1999) that explored the association between pharmaceutical industry sponsorship and economic assessment of oncology drugs found that industry sponsored studies were far more likely to have a favorable economic assessment relative to existing treatment than were nonprofit sponsored studies. In another example, a study by Stelfox et al. (1998):

> ... revealed a strong association between researchers' published statements about the safety of calcium-channel antagonists (CCA) and their financial relationships with drug companies ... Authors who recommend

the use of CCAs in 70 published journal articles were much more likely [96 percent] than those who did not recommend their use [37 percent] or who were neutral [60 percent] to have financial relationships with a maker of CCAs. (Warner and Gluck, 2003: 41)

It is also of note that in this study, financial conflicts of interest were only disclosed in two of the 70 articles reviewed (Brown, 2006).

Such reports raise troubling questions about how study results are interpreted and reported. As the International Committee of Medical Journals noted in their statement announcing their trials-registration policy:

Unfortunately, selective reporting of trials does occur, and it distorts the body of evidence available for clinical decision making. Researchers (and journal editors) are generally most enthusiastic about the publication of trials that show either a large effect of a new treatment ... or the equivalence of two approaches to treatment ...Researchers (and journals) typically are less excited about trials that show that a new treatment is inferior to standard treatment ... and even less interested in trials that are neither clearly positive nor clearly negative, since inconclusive trials will not in themselves change practice. Irrespective of their scientific interest, trial results that place financial interests at risk are particularly likely to remain unpublished and hidden from public view .... The case against selective reporting is particularly compelling for research that tests interventions that could enter mainstream clinical practice. (DeAngelis et al., 2004)

Selective reporting (and, it seems, publishing) clearly presents a significant threat to the integrity and robustness of scientific and medical research. Practices such as guest and ghost authorship also threaten to erode scientific integrity. For example, a recent study that looked at these practices in documents that came publicly available through litigation found that 'review manuscripts [of clinical trials] were often prepared by unacknowledged authors and subsequently attributed authorship to academically affiliated investigators who often did not disclose industry financial support' (Ross et al., 2008: 1800).

These and other problems related to 'data misrepresentation, data analysis and selective reporting' (DeAngelis and Fontanarosa, 2008:1834) have prompted responses on the part of various groups including particularly the editors of key international journals. The Uniform Requirements for Manuscripts Submitted to Biomedical Journals, revised by journal editors in 2005 and updated as recently as October 2007 (ICMJE, 2007), discuss in detail procedures for handing conflicts of interest on the part of authors, reviewers and editors. The document outlines (among other issues): rules for authorship; disclosure of financial interests; and the requirement that all authors have access to the full data set. The guidelines also stress that editors and reviewers must avoid conflicts of interest in their roles in the peer review and publication process. While such guidelines will not alone resolve the challenges posed by conflicts of interest (indeed, others such as DeAngelis and Fontanarosa, 2008 would recommend stronger safeguards), the ICMJE guidelines are a good start. One commentator notes that 'if rigorously enforced [the guidelines] should go a long way in helping improve the situation' and states that 'in fact ... the journals have come close to doing everything they can do' (Brown, 2006: 84). Yet, such measures do not address unpublished studies or concerns that areas and questions that are not commercially friendly will get ignored in favor of (potentially) less scientifically interesting questions. Such questions, insightfully termed 'self-censorship' by some (Brown, 2006), are only partially addressed by (for example) clinical trial registries and other such initiatives. Moreover, registration is not a universal requirement. It also requires significant vigilance on regulators, researchers and the public to follow up and make effective use of registry data.

It is worth noting that health research encompasses much more than drug development. However, this has been the main source of concern for conflict of interest. While major benefits have come with significant drug breakthroughs, the pharmaceutical industry is also driven by the huge dollar figures involved – not only for research and development (DiMasi et al., 2003; Dickson and Gagnon, 2004;) but also for very high profit margins.[7] A variety of factors, including increased regulatory requirements, the need for more study subjects, the increasing difficulty of subject recruitment and the chronic nature of many of the diseases being investigated today, all contribute to increasing the time it takes to develop a new drug and get it approved – which in turn increases the cost of the process (Dickson and Gagnon, 2004).

Conflicts and remedies

In Part I, we explored the contemporary context of conflict of interest in health research. In Part II, we go into greater depth on the main features of conflict of interest and its remedies.

DEFINING CONFLICTS OF INTEREST

As noted above, conflicts of interest can be broken down into three elements: a trust-based relationship, a requirement for independent judgment on the part of the trusted decision maker ('trustee') in the best interests of the person placing their trust ('trustor'), and an interest (usually private or personal) that conflicts or appears to conflict with the trustee's exercise of judgment, with the result that the trustee's judgment on a given decision is 'less reliable than it would otherwise normally be' (Davis, 1998: 590). We discuss management strategies later in this part.

There are some common confusions around the concept of conflict of interest. Most common is the confusion with 'competing values or interests'. David Thompson remarks:

> It is a mistake to treat conflicts of interest as just another kind of choice between competing values .... To do so dilutes the concept of a conflict of interest and encourages the attitude that conflicts are so pervasive that they cannot be avoided. In ethical dilemmas, both of the competing interests have a presumptive claim to priority, and the problem is in deciding which to choose. In the case of financial conflicts of interest, only one of the interests has a claim to priority, and the problem is to ensure that the other interest does not dominate. This asymmetry between interests is a distinctive characteristic of conflicts of interest. (D. Thompson, 1993: 573)

That is, 'competing values' exemplify 'a right *vs.* right choice', while conflicts of interest present 'a right *vs.* wrong' choice.

Conflicts of interest are sometimes confused with a variety of judgmental failures that may adversely affect the judgment of trustees. A trustee's ethical judgment and action can be impaired by many other factors: inattention, insensitivity, lack of appropriate expertise, misperception, judgmental error, incompetence and the like. In general, these factors cannot be addressed through conflict of interest management strategies and therefore need to be addressed and guarded against by other means (training, mentoring, monitoring, accreditation, etc.). One further mistaken belief about conflicts of interest is that they are exclusively financial. As shown in the Hwanggate scandal discussed above, other conflict of interest factors, including reputation and concern for one's research team, can be significant.

Stark (2000) divides conflict of interest into three stages: antecedent acts, states of mind and (resulting) behavior of partiality.[8] The first stage includes 'factors that condition an individual's state of mind towards partiality …' (Krimsky, 2006: 66). An example would be where a researcher receives significant payments from a company whose drug they are testing. The second stage, 'states of mind', refers to 'the affected sentiments, dispositions, proclivities, or affinities conditioned by the antecedent acts' (Krimsky, 2006: 66). In this case the researcher who received financial payments would likely be disposed to over-report positive results and understate negative ones. Finally, the behavior of partiality refers to the ways in which the researcher responds to and acts on his 'state of mind affected by the antecedent acts' (Krimsky, 2006: 66). Thus, the researcher in this example might weaken inclusion/exclusion criteria in a study to ensure adequate recruitment.

It is tempting to read the example just given as a case of conscious bias on the part of the researcher (i.e. deliberately interpreting findings in a way that favors the company's interests); however, this need not be so. The bias or predisposition may be unconscious or hidden to the individual though potentially visible to others. It is harder to deal with unconscious biases through such strategies as self-awareness or self-management. Unconsciously biased researchers may feel that they are immune to the effects of having an investment in or research sponsorship from a pharmaceutical company. When questioned, they may offer self-serving rationalization for their biased behaviors. Similarly, conflicted research institutions may show unawareness of institutional biases (e.g. in advancing university investments in drug start-up companies) and set or enforce self-servingly low standards for dealing with institutional and individual conflicts of interests.

Hence, it may be difficult to know when we are in a conflict of interest. Moreover, it can be dangerous to assume that simply because we are aware of the potential for bias that we will be able to guard against it. For such conflicts, McDonald (1999) has suggested 'A good test is the "trust test": would relevant others [my employer, my clients, professional colleagues, or general public] trust my judgment if they knew I was in this situation?'

This test highlights the importance of transparency, in particular for revealing private interests to relevant parties so as to allow them to be on their guard. It also shifts the emphasis from self-assessment by a potentially conflicted party to a more objective gauging of the potential effects of such interests on trustors. This test further suggests the importance of carefully done studies of possible biases in research judgment described in Part I of this article. If, as Stelfox and others have shown, researchers with commercial connections to pharmaceutical sponsors tend view that company's products more favorably than other researchers, then fair-minded researchers would have to seriously entertain the possibility that they too may also be biased by similar commercial connections.

INSTITUTIONAL AND SYSTEMIC CONFLICT OF INTEREST

Like individual researchers, research institutions may find themselves in situations where a secondary interest (such as monetary donation or promise of prestige) threatens to influence institutional decision makers so as to override the proper primary interest (such as academic integrity or subject protection) (Thompson, 1993). In its 2001 Report on Individual and Institutional Conflict of Interest, the Association of American Universities'

Task Force on Research Accountability ('AAU Report') aptly describes the tension faced by research universities.

> ... research universities are concerned about financial conflict of interest because it strikes to the heart of the integrity of the institution and the public's confidence in that integrity ... Transferring university developed knowledge to the private sector fulfills one of the goals of federally funded research, by bringing the fruits of research to the benefit of society. With this important technology transfer come increasingly close relationships between industry and universities, which provide benefits but also increases the risk of academic research being compromised ... through individual and or institutional financial conflicts of interest. (AAU, 2001: i)

The task force then notes that:

> ... institutional financial conflicts of interest ... may occur when the institution, any of its senior management or trustees, or an affiliated foundation or organization has an external relationship or financial interest with in a company that itself has a financial interest in a faculty research project .... The existence (or appearance) of such conflicts can lead to actual bias, or suspicion of possible bias, in the review or conduct of research at the university. If they are not evaluated or managed, they may result in choices or actions that are incongruent with the missions, obligations, or the values of the university. (AAU Report: i)

Three main points emerge from the AAU Report. First, as noted in Part 1, relationships between academia and industry are now an established part of the landscape, at least in certain areas of research, and such relationships will likely only increase in strength and frequency. Second, when actual and perceived institutional conflicts of interest are not forthrightly addressed or appropriately managed, the institution's integrity and the quality of its research are likely to be undermined. This may well erode public trust in the quality of ethical review for research and adversely affect research subject recruitment. Third, such negative consequences can be avoided or at least mitigated by addressing and appropriately managing institutional conflicts of interest. In relation to this last point, the AAU Report concludes that ' ... the problem is rarely a particular conflict itself – rather it is the question about what is done with the conflict. In most cases, problems arise when the conflict is not made apparent, or when it is not assessed or managed' (AAU Report: ii).

Some institutional conflicts of interest are systemic. These include conflicts that arise, for example, when a funding body is also responsible for maintaining standards. In the Canadian context, an illustration of this is in relation to the three major federal research funding agencies who are not only responsible for funding research and facilitating commercialization (CIHR, 2005), but also for establishing standards for ethical research, determining when the standards are not being met and imposing the penalty of withdrawing funding. Several years ago, the United States recognized a similar situation at the National Institutes of Health and dealt with it by moving human research protection outside NIH into an arm's length agency OPRR (now known as OHRP). There have been suggestions by Emmanuel and colleagues that this is still insufficiently arm's length and that IRBs should be moved outside research institutions and become free-standing authorities (Emanuel et al., 2006).

ADDRESSING AND MANAGING CONFLICTS OF INTEREST

This description of conflicts of interest shows that they are complex and occur at various levels. It highlights the importance of adopting appropriate ethical management strategies.

For example, management strategies that target the antecedent acts (such as disclosure, or avoidance) recognize that public trust can be eroded simply by pre-existing situations whether or not they culminate in inappropriate behavior. Such prophylactic or presumptive management strategies arguably represent a more comprehensive approach to conflicts of interest management than a strategy that is primarily 'after the fact' or reactive. Waiting until after the fact and relying, for example, on litigation to address real or perceived wrongs is more likely to decrease public trust in the integrity of research institutions and researchers.

Disclosure and avoidance are important management strategies for conflicts of interest. Appropriate disclosure provides relevant information to those relying on the individual or institution, and allows them to 'adjust their reliance accordingly' (Davis, 1998:593). For example, by requiring authors to disclose their conflicts of interest, journal editors are able to assess for themselves the integrity of the research. Moreover, by making authors' disclosures public, the editors empower readers to make their own assessments.

Nonetheless, disclosure does not resolve the conflict itself. In particular, it may not address the underlying power imbalance between the trustee and trustor. There are other issues with disclosure. For example, when a researcher informs a subject of an actual or potential conflict, the subject may still have no real idea of whether and to what extent the disclosed interest actually influences the researcher. Potential desensitization is another issue with adopting disclosure as a standard policy. Where disclosure is approached as an automatic, formulaic process without intelligent consideration, the resulting disclosure deluge threatens to erode subjects' abilities to determine when conflicts are truly problematic. Moreover, in some cases conflict of interest disclosure may produce the opposite effect of what was intended. Instead of alerting subjects to potentially distorting influences, the disclosure of commercial ties may be seen as a sign of researcher competence.

Thus while disclosure is often an appropriate management strategy, it may need to be supplemented with other approaches. These include third party oversight (e.g. in scientific research, having conflict of interest committees that review both individual and institutional conflicts), and divestiture of private interests to a disinterested third party for the duration of the time one's judgment could be compromised (as occurs, for example, when individuals are elected into public office). In some cases, however, such management strategies are not considered sufficient to ensure the integrity of public trust, and it is therefore deemed necessary to avoid such situations or antecedent acts completely. In other words, the most appropriate strategy sometimes is to have the conflicted party bow out of the picture.

However, as in all prophylactic or presumptive judgments, there is always the possibility that the responses may be inappropriate or disproportionate to the danger or threat being addressed. In health research, there may be a trade-off between knowledge of an area of research and having judgment affecting conflicts in that area. In some cases, it is now difficult to find expert peer reviewers who do not have deemed conflicts of interests. Is a journal editor or a research agency forced to choose between biased experts and unbiased non-experts for peer reviews of journal submissions or research proposals? In particular circumstances, there may be reasonably good hybrid models that provide a mix of biased experts (but whose biases cancel each other out) along with neutral individuals who are somewhat less expert (MacDonald et al., 2002). In other cases, we wonder if the pendulum has swung too far in terms of managing conflicts through the exclusion of interested experts (i.e. experts with some conflicting interests). This seems to have been the case in the establishment of the Stem Cell Oversight Committee in Canada where experts in stem cell research and stem cell ethics have been excluded from serving on the Committee on the grounds that their research is sponsored by the Canadian Stem Cell Network (Ogbogu, 2007).

Because trust can be eroded by apparent as well as actual breaches, there needs to be a strategy for dealing with apparent conflicts of interest. Davis notes that 'apparent conflicts of interest are no more conflicts of interest than counterfeit money is money'(1998: 593). Hence, the remedy for an apparent conflict of interest is to provide information that demonstrates that there is in fact no conflict. Consider, for example, the usual practice of university REBs charging industry sponsors a fee for reviewing their protocols. To the public, this might seem to be an incentive to provide more lenient reviews of industry protocols. These concerns may well be alleviated if universities make it known that the fee is charged whether or not the protocol is favourably or unfavourably reviewed.[9] By providing sufficient information, trust in the process should be restored.

A major issue related to any conflict management strategy is to ensure meaningful and effective compliance. A recent example illustrates that even where management strategies are in place they may not be effective. In recent congressional testimony it was alleged that two prominent Harvard University child psychiatrists (Dr Beiderman and Dr Wilens) failed to disclose at least $3.2 million that they received from pharmaceutical companies between 2000 and 2007. By doing so, they may have violated federal laws and university regulations that are meant to address/manage conflicts of interest and encourage transparency to protect both research integrity and research subject safety. Two points are of particular interest here. First, this is not a case where there were no guidelines in place. In fact, Dr Biederman has explicitly stated that he takes conflicts of interest policies 'very seriously', and both physicians have commented that they thought they were acting in compliance with conflicts of interest policies and rules (Harris and Carey, 2008). This suggests that the guidelines were either unclear, ineffective or both. Second, while most universities have conflict of interest policies in place that require researchers to report their conflicts (Weinfurt et al., 2006), it appears there may not be much emphasis on ensuring the accuracy of such reports. The dean of Yale's medical school revealingly commented that 'it has really been an honor system thing ... if somebody tells us that a pharmaceutical company pays them $80,000 a year, I don't even know how to check on that' (Harris and Carey, 2008). This apparent failure to effectively implement and enforce existing policies highlights a lack of institutional concern towards conflicts of interest that some may find unsurprising. As seen in Part 1, the relationship between industry and academia has become much closer in recent decades, and universities rely heavily on industry support to finance a wide range of activities. Perhaps much of the recent flurry around conflicts of interest has resulted more in window dressings than in effective safeguards for addressing the strong secondary interests that may unduly influence institutional decision makers and individual researchers.

AGENCY THEORY AND CONFLICT OF INTEREST

As a final comment in this section, it is worth stating that the kind of trust-based relationships within which conflicts of interest can and do arise are not unique to research or healthcare, and in fact arise in many areas of public and private life. Such fiduciary type relationships are pervasive (lawyer–client, board of directors and stockholders, parents–children, etc.). It is hard to imagine conducting our daily lives without them. Every time we rely on someone to act in our interests (especially because we lack the time or expertize to do so ourselves), we are faced with the challenge of ensuring that the interests of the person we are trusting (our trustee or agent) are sufficiently aligned with our best interests so that they will fulfill their obligations towards us. These are matters that are much discussed in the voluminous literature in economics and business on the agent–principal relationship. This is a literature that grew substantially with the notorious failures of such companies as Enron, World Com and Tyco and was accompanied by a cascade of reports of misstated earnings and, in several cases, out-and-out accounting fraud. Buchanan usefully reminds us that complex bureaucratic organizations are webs of agent–principal relations and that a major challenge for senior administrators is to ensure that agents act in the best interests of the organization (Buchanan, 1996; McDonald, 2000).

However, it is also worth taking note from the business ethics literature that trustees (agents) can be 'too loyal' from an ethical perspective to the interests of their trustors (principals) and thus wrongfully damage innocent third parties (Westra, 1986; Michalos, 2005). There have been numerous examples where senior and middle managers have relentlessly advanced the corporate agenda and earnings at the expense of workers' safety, the environment and basic human rights. Similar actions have been reported in the public sector as party apparatchiks and loyalists sacrifice the public interest to partisan success. We would argue that the same is true in many cases of institutional conflict of interest in research where overly loyal institutional officials advance their institution's interests at the expense of research subjects or overall scientific integrity. There are, then, moral limits to advancing the interests of trustors. It is within those limits that we have framed our discussion of conflict of interest. There is no conflict of interest when a trustee refuses to act immorally to advance a trustor's interests. In such a case, the trustee serves the public interest.

Observations and recommendations

In creating this article, we read well beyond the standard literature in bioethics and drew on work in law, business ethics, professional ethics and economics (particularly accounting and management theory). We also took a strongly institutional as opposed to mainly individual focus. We took these wider perspectives because both sets of factors are so prominent in contemporary healthcare and health research. Using Buchanan's idea of large-scale institutions as complex webs of agent–principal relations, we can picture international health research as a complex web of webs with multiple potential stress points including conflicts of interest.

Drawing on a wider literature has the advantage of bringing together relevant areas of expertize and avoiding isolationism in bioethics. It is also salutary to remind ourselves that public concern about conflict of interest in health research is part of larger public concern about other fiduciaries (corporate, professional and governmental) abusing trust relationships to serve their own interests. It also allows us to see if management mechanisms effective for dealing with conflict of interest in one area (e.g. protection of minority stockholder rights) are relevant to issues in research ethics (e.g. protection of research subjects).

Attention to this bigger picture helps identify important areas for research into conflict of interest in health research. We need well-designed social science research to determine the extent of conflict of interest in various health research contexts and the actual effectiveness of existing modes of control. Given the major shift in the venue and control of health research from the public to the private sector, there is an urgent need for good research into contract research organizations and other aspects of private sector research endeavours. Such research will likely be much more difficult than research into public sector sponsors (though we remain daunted by how much public sector health research is not open to critical scrutiny). A further challenge lies in the continuing globalization of health research, including the movement of controversial research on humans (or animals) from developed to developing countries and the importation of human subjects from developing countries to developed countries (Lemmens, 2004; Lemmens and Miller, 2006).

As noted above, conflict of interest was until quite recently a fringe topic in bioethics. The general opinion seemed to be that conflict of interest was largely a non-issue for health researchers and patient-centered health professionals who were in the main acting as disinterested seekers of wisdom and patient wellbeing. Where there was an issue, it could be dealt with by appeals to individual vigilance and virtue. This complacency was shattered by a number of incidents and resulting studies (see Part I) that pointed to pervasive conflict issues and the need for organizational and political change. For good reasons the research community is moving away from this self-congratulatory and self-deceptive naive social stance that problems can be handled at the individual level.

As this process continues, we must not either overrate or underrate the importance of conflict of interest. It would be overrated if we thought that it was the sole or main problem in health research ethics. Even if we narrow the target to the responsible conduct of research where many conflict problems reside, it still is the case that other types of ethical issues remain central including such macro issues as how much to invest in health research (as opposed to healthcare or to other social goods such as education and housing), who sets the research agenda and whether there is an equitable distribution of the benefits and burdens of research. There is a further (and quite disturbing) risk that extensive focus on external controls for conflict of interest will not only ignore internal controls (virtue and conscience), but also encourage widespread scepticism and even cynicism about the motives of health researchers, their institutions and sponsors (see Moreno, 2001). Such cynicism could have especially corrosive effects within the health research community and between health researchers and the general public.

There are also risks associated with underrating conflict of interest. Conflicts could become regarded as the subject of *pro forma* bureaucratic regimes (somewhat like consent forms in research subject recruitment). Some may argue that because conflicts are utterly pervasive that nothing needs to be done about them other than filing annual reports. As officials realize that the mere existence of a conflict is not by itself wrongful, they may mistakenly conclude that nothing needs to be done about such conflicts and fail to manage them appropriately.

We need to be clear about the ethical significance of conflict of interests. Fiduciary relationships are one of several ethical modalities for protecting the individual or collective interests. Other non-fiduciary modalities also are interest-protecting. For instance, the general obligation of non-maleficence does not assume a fiduciary relationship between a person who could harm another and the person who could be harmed. Rather, 'do not harm (coerce, intimidate or manipulate)' is a standing ethical order in all human relations. The same is true of respect for persons and general benevolence. These do not require pre-existing fiduciary relations. Fiduciary relationships of the sort discussed in this chapter provide additional individual or group specific protections that go beyond rights to non-maleficence, respect and general beneficence.

We note too that specific fiduciary responsibilities are debatable at individual and policy levels. Which of the interests of this particular research subject is a researcher responsible for and for how long? At a policy level there may be competing public interest reasons for widening or narrowing the extent of fiduciary responsibilities of, for example, research institutions towards research subjects. Some may be substantive (balancing health research advances against subject protection); others may be procedural (promoting greater clarity for researchers or promoting greater equity for subjects). While such disputes may become quite technical and legal, they are at heart about who is best positioned to protect specific interests that are at risk.

Disputes about standards and management processes seem almost inevitable given that they are often designed to be 'prophylactic' and mitigate future problems. These are similar to disputes about environmental protection and food safety ('How safe is safe enough' and the precautionary principle). In these, issues of onus and evidence loom large. Where does the onus lie to show that particular types of interests are problematic? What evidence is persuasive enough for policy changes or for showing that someone has acted problematically? Such debates highlight the importance of seeking meaningful evidence about conflicts and their management.

Earlier we explained why conflict of interest is on the health research ethics agenda in a way that it had not been before. We want to close with a question about its prominence on this agenda – is it an ethical preoccupation of the already overprivileged or is it an essential protection of the integrity of the scientific research system and human subjects protection? Optimistically, concerns about conflict of interest in health research can be seen as involving a more ethically acute awareness of systemic distorting factors that have impact on research integrity, the evaluation of research quality and human subject protections. More pessimistically, one could argue that these concerns will likely result in greater protection for those who are already well privileged economically and socially. In effect, they get additional safety nets in the form of conflict of interest protections; whereas those worst off globally lack any effective safety nets. And, to continue the metaphor, when the worst off do get fiduciary safety nets, they get them more or less adventitiously, dependent on the fickle attention and interests of developed world researchers and research sponsors.

That concerns about conflicts of interest only address a limited range of ethical concerns in global healthcare and health research should not be used as an excuse for ignoring or playing down such concerns. As we have seen, the conduct of health research involves the creation of a complex web of fiduciary relations. When distorting interests weaken that web, then there is serious risk to the moral capital of such research – the advancement of healing knowledge and the trust of research subjects and the general public.

NOTES

1 This anatomical discussion of conflict of interest is based largely on Michael Davis's discussion in volume 1 of the *Encyclopedia of Applied Ethics*. Davis (1998) breaks down the concept into four parts: relationship, judgment, interest, and proper exercise (of that judgment).

2 See, for example, Industry Canada's website at http://www.ic.gc.ca/epic/site/ic1.nsf/en/h_00007e.html, wherein it is stated that the 'Department's mission is to foster a growing, competitive, knowledge-based Canadian economy'.

3 'Financial relationships and interests in research involving human subjects: Guidance for human subject protection', *Federal Register*, Wednesday 12 May 2004/notices, 69 (92): 26393–7.

4 For example, (AAMC) Association of American Medical Colleges Task Force on Financial Conflicts of Interest in Medical Research, 2001, 2002; Shapiro and NBAC, 2001.

5 World Medical Association, *Declaration of Helsinki* adopted by the 18th WMA General Assembly, Helsinki, Finland, June 1964, and last amended by the 59th WMA General Assembly, Seoul, October 2008. http://www.wma.net/e/policy/b3.htm

6 Other relevant international guidelines in this area include, for example, the International Guidelines for Biomedical Research Involving Human Subjects (CIOMS 2002 [1993]); particularly article 5(17)). The ICH-GCP guideline stresses the importance of independent review – but is quite quiet in discussing the review of funding source/institutional affiliations, etc.

7 It is interesting to note, however, that some estimates suggest that the amounts spent on drug marketing and administration are over twice what is spent on research and development (Relman and Angell, 2002).

8 This is outlined in Stark's book, *Conflict of Interest in American Public Life* (Stark, 2000) and is cited by Sheldon Krimsky (2003; 2006).

9 This example is not without its complications, however. The REB may well in fact actually feel pressured at the institutional level to adopt a review process that will favor ongoing industry business. Where this is the case, the institution itself is in a conflict of interest (see Emanuel et al., 2006).

REFERENCES

Association of American Medical Colleges Task Force on Financial Conflicts of Interest in Medical Research (AAMC) (2001) *Report on Individual Financial Interest in Human Subjects Research*. Washington DC: Association of American Medical Colleges.

Association of American Medical Colleges Task Force on Financial Conflicts of Interest in Medical Research (AAMC) (2002) *Protecting Subjects, Preserving Trust, Promoting Progress II: Principles and Recommendations for Oversight of an Institution's Financial Interests in Human Subjects Research*. Washington DC: Association of American Medical Colleges.

Association of American Universities (AAU) (2001) *Report on Research Accountability: Report on Individual and Institutional Financial Conflict of Interest*. Washington DC: Association of American Universities.

Barnes, M. and Florencio, P.S. (2002) 'Financial conflicts of interest in human subjects research: The problem of institutional conflicts', *Journal of Law, Medicine & Ethics*, 30 (3): 390–402.

Bekelman, J.E., Li, Y.L. and Gross, C.P (2003) 'Scope and impact of financial conflicts of interest in biomedical research', *Journal of the American Medical Association*, 289 (4): 454–65.

Blumenthal, D. (2002) 'Conflict of interest in biomedical research', *Health Matrix: Journal of Law-Medicine*, 12 (2): 377–392.

Brown, J.R. (2006) 'Self-Censorship', in T. Lemmens and D.R. Waring (eds), *Law and Ethics in Biomedical Research: Regulation, Conflict of Interest and Liability*. Toronto: University of Toronto Press, pp. 82–95.

Buchanan, A. (1996) 'Toward a theory of the ethics of bureaucratic organizations', *Business Ethics Quarterly*, 6 (4): 419–40.

Canadian Institutes of Health Research (CIHR) (2005) Report: Institutional conflicts of interest invitational meeting. Available at http://www.cihr-irsc.gc.ca/e/28076.html.

Caulfield, T. (2001-2) 'Globalization, conflicts of interest and clinical research: An overview of trends and issues', *Widener Law Symposium Journal*, 8: 31–45.

Caulfield, T. and Griener, G. (2001) 'Conflicts of interest in clinical research: Addressing direct payment to investigators', unpublished manuscript, Edmonton, AB.

Davidson, R.A. (1986) 'Source of funding and outcome of clinical trials', *Journal of General Internal Medicine*, 1 (3): 155–8.

Davis, M. (ed.) (1998) *Encyclopedia of Applied Ethics*, Vol. 1. London: Academic Press.

DeAngelis, C.D. and Fontanarosa, P.B. (2008) 'Impugning the integrity of medical science: The adverse effects of industry influence', *Journal of the American Medical Association*, 299 (15): 1833–5.

DeAngelis, C.D., Drazen, J.M., Frizelle, F.A., Haug, C., Hoey, J., Horton, R. et al. (2004) 'Clinical trial registration: A statement from the International Committee of Medical Journal Editors', *Journal of the American Medical Association*, 292 (11): 1363–4.

Dickson, M. and Gagnon, J.P. (2004) 'Key factors in the rising cost of new drug discovery and development', *Nature Reviews Drug Discovery*, 3 (5): 417–29.

DiMasi, J.A., Hansen, R.W. and Grabowski, H.G. (2003) 'The price of innovation: New estimates of drug development costs', *Journal of Health Economics*, 22 (2): 151–85.

Downie, J., Baird, P. and Thompson, J. (2002) 'Industry and the academy: Conflicts of interest in contemporary health research', *Health Law Journal*, 10: 103–22.

DuVal, G. (2004) 'Institutional conflicts of interest: Protecting human subjects, scientific integrity, and institutional accountability', *Journal of Law, Medicine & Ethics*, 32 (4): 613–25.

Emanuel, E.J., Lemmens, T. and Elliot, C. (2006) 'Should society allow research ethics boards to be run as for-profit enterprises?', *PLoS Medicine*, 3 (7): 941–4.

Ferris, L.E. and Naylor, C.D. (2006) 'Promoting integrity in industry-sponsored clinical drug trials: Conflict of interest for Canadian Academic Health Sciences Centres', in T. Lemmens and D.R. Waring (eds), *Law and Ethics in Biomedical Research: Regulation, Conflict of Interest and Liability*. Toronto: University of Toronto Press, pp. 95–132.

Friedberg, M., Saffran, B., Stinson, T.J., Nelson, W. and Bennett, C.L. (1999) 'Evaluation of conflict of interest in economic analyses of new drugs used in oncology', *Journal of the American Medical Association*, 282 (Oct): 1453–7.

Harris, G. and Carey, B. (2008) 'Researchers fail to reveal full drug pay', *New York Times*, 8 June, front page.

International Committee of Medical Journal Editors (ICMJE) (2007) 'Uniform requirements for manuscripts submitted to biomedical journals: Writing and editing for biomedical publication'. Available at http://www.icmje.org/.

Krimsky, S. (2003) *Science in the Private Interest: Has the Lure of Profits Corrupted Biomedical Research?* Lanham, MD: Rowman & Littlefield.

Krimsky, S. (2006) 'The ethical and legal foundations of scientific "conflict of interest"', in T. Lemmens and D.R. Waring (eds), *Law and Ethics in Biomedical Research: Regulation, Conflict of Interest and Liability*. Toronto: University of Toronto Press, pp. 63–82.

Labonte, R. and Torgerson, R. (2005) 'Interrogating globalization, health and development: Towards a comprehensive framework for research, policy and political action', *Critical Public Health*, 15 (2): 157–79.

Lemmens, T. (2004) 'Leopards in the temple: Restoring scientific integrity to the commercialized research scene', *Journal of Law, Medicine & Ethics*, 32: 641–57.

Lemmens, T. and Freedman, B. (2000) 'Ethics review for sale? Conflict of interest in commercial review boards', *Milbank Quarterly*, 78: 547–84.

Lemmens, T. and Miller, P.B. (2006) 'The human subjects trade: Ethical, legal and regulatory remedies to deal with recruitment incentives and to protect scientific integrity', in T. Lemmens and D.R. Waring (eds), *Law and Ethics in Biomedical Research: Regulation, Conflict of Interest and Liability*. Toronto: Toronto University Press, pp. 132–83.

Lemmens, T. and Waring, D.R. (eds) (2006) *Law and Ethics in Biomedical Research: Regulation, Conflict of Interest and Liability*. Toronto: University of Toronto Press.

MacDonald, C., McDonald, M. and Norman, W. (2002) 'Charitable conflicts of interest', *Journal of Business Ethics*, 39 (1/2): 67–74.

McDonald, M. (1999) *Ethics and Conflict of Interest*. University of British Columbia, Centre for Applied Ethics. Available at http://www.armsdeal-vpo.co.za/special_items/reading/ethics.html.

McDonald, M. (ed.) (2000) *The Governance of Health Research Involving Human Subjects* (HRIHS). Ottawa: Law Commission of Canada.

Michalos, A.C. (2005) 'The loyal agent's argument', in D.C. Poff (ed.), *Business Ethics in Canada*, 4th ed. Toronto: Pearson Education.

Moreno, J.D. (2001) 'Goodbye to all that: The end of moderate protectionism in human subjects research', *Hastings Center Report*, 31 (3): 9–17.

Ogbogu, U. (2007) 'Canada's approach to conflict of interest oversight', *Canadian Medical Association Journal*, 177 (4): 375–6.

Relman, A.S. and Angell, M. (2002) 'America's other drug problem' (cover story), *New Republic*, 227 (25): 27–41.

Ross, J.S., Hill, K.P., Egilman, D.S. and Krumholz, H.M. (2008) 'Guest authorship and ghostwriting in publications related to Rofecoxib: A case study of industry documents from Rofecoxib litigation', *Journal of the American Medical Association*, 299 (15): 1800–12.

Saunders, R. and Savulescu, J. (2008) 'Research ethics and lessons from Hwanggate: What can we learn from the Korean cloning fraud?' *Journal of Medical Ethics*, 34: 214–21.

Shapiro, H.T. and National Bioethics Advisory Commission (NBAC) (2001) *Report: Ethical and Policy Issues in Research Involving Human Participants*. Bethesda, MD: National Bioethics Advisory Commission.

Stark, A. (2000) *Conflict of Interest in American Public Life*. Cambridge, MA: Harvard University Press.

Stelfox, H.T., Chua, G., O'Rourke, K. and Detsky, A.S. (1998) 'Conflict of interest in the debate over calcium-channel antagonists', *New England Journal of Medicine*, 338: 101–6.

Thompson, D. (1993) 'Understanding financial conflicts of interests', *New England Journal of Medicine*, 329: 573–6.

Thompson, T.G. (2004) 'Financial relationships and interests in research involving human subjects: Guidance for human subject protection', *Federal Register*, 69 (92): 26393–7.

Warner, T.D. and Gluck, J.P. (2003) 'What do we really know about conflicts of interest in biomedical research?', *Psychopharmacology*, 171: 36–46.

Weinfurt, K.P.P., Dinan, M.A., Allsbrook, J.S., Friedman, J.Y., Hall, M.A., Schulman, K. A. et al. (2006) 'Policies of academic medical centers for disclosing financial conflicts of interest to potential research participants', *Academic Medicine*, 81 (2): 113–18.

Westra, L. (1986) 'Whose "loyal agent"? Towards an ethic of accounting', *Journal of Business Ethics*, 5: 119–28.

27

International Research

Volnei Garrafa[1]

INTRODUCTION

This chapter begins with a provocative question – *International research?* – which allows different interpretations. The line of ideas to be presented below will stick to the clinical research developed around the world during the second half of the twentieth century that, from the nature of this book, seems to be most appropriate.

This question puts forward some doubts regarding international research within the field of healthcare – particularly multi-centre clinical trials – and its relationship with ethics. This relates especially to the last decades of the twentieth century, from the rapid progress of scientific and technological development that was experienced and the commercial interests of the globalised world that were seen. The first doubt directly relating to this question that arises is whether international investigations of this type should necessarily be developed. The response is resoundingly affirmative, in the name of the scientific search for improvements in quality of life and the future wellbeing of individuals and communities.

However, because of some problems that have historically been registered over recent decades, and as a natural consequence of the first doubt, a second question arises, of the same importance as the first doubt or even more so with regard to ethics: Are such studies – or should they be – equally rigorous in their methodological designs in rich or developed (central) countries and in poor or developing (peripheral) countries? There are many doubts and intense discussions in this regard. To analyse this question in as unbiased a manner as possible is the purpose of this chapter. The reflections presented below are based on a study that is taken as a reference point in the courses on ethics in research on human beings of the Continuing Distance Education Programme promoted by UNESCO's Latin American and Caribbean Bioethics Network (Garrafa and Lorenzo, 2006) and their viewpoint is therefore constructed around peripheral countries.

BRIEF HISTORY OF CLINICAL RESEARCH

The first reports on clinical research date from the end of the eighteenth century. With the use of probabilistic knowledge, each fact observed in examining and following up a patient started to be correlated with a set of facts that had been revealed through examining other patients, in a random manner, from which it would become possible to measure and compare occurrences of signs and symptoms. Individuals ceased to be simply people who were suffering and came to represent reproducible pathological events; subjects for constructing medical knowledge. This epistemological transformation brought clinical science close to exact sciences and opened the doors to experimentation (Foucault, 1972). In the beginning, when clinical science entered the field of experimentation, it did not have any model available; it was obliged to deal directly with human beings in their full complexity. On the other hand, the exact sciences had always used preconceived models or simulations, from which hypotheses were examined and reference was made to interpretations of the results relating to other natural phenomena.

In what is considered to be the pioneering work on clinical experimentation, Claude Bernard (1865 [1984]) stated that physicians had the right to conduct research whenever the result from such research might produce a direct benefit for its subject, and that this right would be lost whenever an experiment were to cause harm to the patient, even if the result might come to be useful for other people or for society. This reference point has become consolidated and has come to form part of most regulatory documents relating to research ethics that have emerged since the middle of the twentieth century, following the publication of the Nuremberg Code.

The emergence of regulatory documents and research ethics committees thus does not represent the beginning of ethical questioning relating to clinical research, but the recognition by society that ethical control over such activities cannot depend exclusively on the researchers' moral consciences. In a general manner, this veritable awareness-raising process relating to clinical research was also consequent to the profound transformations in human societies experienced following the Second World War.

Clinical research was transformed from an amateur activity in the eighteenth century into a university activity in the nineteenth century and, finally, into an industrial activity in the twentieth century (Ravetz, 1971). The acceleration of the market globalisation process over the last three decades of the past century has internationalised clinical research and has influenced both the way in which it is funded and the development and application of research practices.

Today, private funding seems to have supremacy over public investments relating to clinical research. This has been responsible for the decline in state power, both for establishing priorities for research within the field of healthcare and for controlling the ethical guidelines relating to this research. In this respect, peripheral countries without consolidated systems for ethics assessments are particularly at a disadvantage, since they do not have objective conditions under which to safely analyse the methodological proposals for complex studies coming from better developed countries and funded by large multinational pharmaceutical companies.

Over recent years, international multi-centre randomised clinical trials have become the model *par excellence* for research on new medications. In Brazil alone, to give an example of a developing country – although since 1997 it has had a consolidated national regulatory model for ethics in biomedical research – in 2008, around 250,000 people participated as subjects in research of this type. Such trials generally involve different countries with very distinct socioeconomic and cultural realities, which of course may generate conflicts relating to the ethical acceptance of the studies.

The power of the market in the field of medications and clinical research is a fact of life. According to Moynihan (2003) there are around 80,000 pharmaceutical industry representatives in the United States. In Germany, according to Willerroider (2004), there are 17,000 laboratory representatives for approximately 130,000 physicians, thus giving a ratio of 7.64 physicians for every sales representative. This relationship is similar to what is found in Great Britain, France and the United States. These numbers, which are very significant, make it possible to glimpse some ethical questions (conflicts of interest) relating to the pharmaceutical industry, physicians and researchers, given that the industry sponsors the studies and the physicians and researchers carry them out. On the other hand, it needs to be mentioned that the number of investigations conducted by multinational laboratories with the aim of producing medications to meet the epidemiological needs of poorer countries, such as malaria, Chagas disease or schistosomiasis, among others, is proportionally small because the financial return does not make this worthwhile (Angell, 2007).

The globalisation process has worsened the social problems of peripheral countries and their dependence on foreign capital. The research capacity of these countries has also been influenced by this new world order. A country's 'research capacity in the biomedical field' is taken to mean the set of the following requisites: its capacity to define research priorities according to the main health problems of its population; its financial independence for investing in priority research; and its ability to assess and supervise the ethical regulations for research conducted within its own territory (Sithi-amorn and Somronthong, 2000). The response to the question *International research?* would certainly be positive if international research were developed in countries with a full capacity to meet the above requirements. However, as is known, objective conditions for this to become a concrete and feasible rule do not exist in most of these countries, at least over the short and medium term.

ETHICAL QUESTIONS IN INTERNATIONAL RESEARCH

The internationalisation of research may, without doubt, be beneficial for poor and developing countries if sustainable programmes for developing the investigative capacity of the countries hosting such research projects can be added to the profit requirements of the funding institutions. This is possible through bilateral agreements between the funding institutions and the host countries, bearing in mind two objectives: (1) that the research should seek therapeutic, preventive or diagnostic methods relating to the resolution of health problems that are a priority for the populations of the participating countries; and (2) that accomplishing the research should enable technology transfer and development of skills of advanced investigative practices that can contribute towards achieving independence for the country regarding knowledge production. Under such conditions, the research can certainly be called cooperative.

On the other hand, instead of being cooperative in nature, such research may come to present unbalanced characteristics under certain situations, when it is seen that: (1) the aim in having participation from peripheral countries is only to avoid the more rigorous supervision that exists in the countries originating the research (central countries); (2) economically disadvantaged research subjects are used with the aim of either accelerating the recruitment stages or having them undergo procedures that would not be accepted in the countries of origin; or (3) the benefits generated at the end of the study are unavailable for the subjects or social groups that took part in it.

This line of reasoning becomes indispensable to the present discussion for two reasons: problems reported over recent years regarding clinical trials developed in peripheral countries that may have harmed the subjects involved in them (Lurie and Wolf, 1997; Angell, 2000; Garrafa and Lorenzo, 2008); and the attempts, now successful through the modified Declaration of Helsinki 2008 (WMA, 2008), to change the Declaration regarding its old items 19, 29 and 30, which relate to the use of placebos and the care required in this and to sponsors' responsibility towards subjects once the study has been concluded. For all these reasons, it is convenient to add to the context of this analysis an appropriate interpretation of what is conventionally called 'social vulnerability' within the fields of geopolitics, sociology and public health.

The concept of social vulnerability

Within the context of the above-mentioned disciplines, the concept of social vulnerability signifies the degree to which there is a risk that an undesirable event with the potential to cause damage particular to a given individual, community or social stratum might occur because of socioeconomic and/or cultural circumstances. The undesirable event could have a physical origin (natural catastrophes, nuclear accidents, etc) or a social origin (criminality, drugs, etc.), or it could result from interactions between physical, biological and social causes (hunger). Taking hunger as an example for reflection, the United Nations has recommended that its studies should be adapted to the methodology for analysing and mapping out vulnerability, as a means for better organisation of the actions for combating this problem worldwide (Commission Économique pour l'Amérique Latine et Caraïbe, 2003).

Despite the variety of interpretations, *social vulnerability has been accepted – especially in Latin American countries – as a phenomenon determined by the structure of people's and communities' daily lives.* There is a consensus regarding the factors determining it: lack of resources like income, information, knowledge and technology; lack of access to the public authorities and other types of social representation; limited network of social relationships; diversity of beliefs and customs among the majority of the population; advanced age; and physical deficiencies (Wisner, 1993).

Within the field of ethics in clinical research, the concept of vulnerability was at first understood to be the limit of the capacity to consent, caused by immaturity (children) or by functional disorders (elderly people and mentally ill individuals). This led the efforts for protecting vulnerable individuals to be concentrated on obtaining consent statements from third parties who were responsible for such individuals. However, criticism of cases of deviations in international research involving legally autonomous subjects and, in many cases, a demonstration of the weakness or even insufficiency of informed consent as an instrument for real ethical safety, have contributed towards bringing the concept of vulnerability in research ethics closer to the concept used by human sciences. All of this seems to show the importance of implementing procedures to minimise the risks within these specific populations and the need for fair distribution of the benefits, in determining the ethical validity of international research.

Today, the difference between vulnerability caused by the limits to the capacity to consent and vulnerability resulting from the limits observed among physically and mentally disabled individuals is well defined. It is also recognised that the legal implications in the relationships of subjects and social groups with these two forms of vulnerability are very different, as are the protection mechanisms needed.

In this respect, states of social vulnerability are taken to lie beyond the limit of self-determination and they correspond to significantly increased exposure to risks caused by situations of social exclusion. Individuals or groups whose limits of self-determination are caused by a form of disability that is recognised by law are not included in the extent of this concept.

This definition of vulnerability leads to contexts of fragility, lack of protection, debility, disadvantaged states (disadvantaged populations) and even to neglect or abandonment, encompassing various forms of social exclusion or isolation of certain population groups from the advances, discoveries or benefits that may already be underway within the dynamic process of world development (Garrafa and Prado, 2001).

By reviewing the specific literature on ethical conflicts within international biomedical research in poor and developing countries, some contextual situations that generate social vulnerability can be identified: a low capacity for research in the country; socioeconomic disparities among the population; low educational level among the population; difficulty in accessing healthcare; vulnerability relating to female gender; vulnerability relating to racial and ethnic questions; among others.

The profound cultural diversity, different political traditions and various stages of economic development seen among peripheral countries around the world have a direct influence not only on these countries' relationships with international biomedical research, but also on the creation of efficient systems for ethical assessment of investigations in these regions. The ethical conflicts stemming from the great social disparities in countries at intermediate levels of industrialisation, such as Chile and Mexico, on the other hand, present particular characteristics regarding questions of risk minimisation and benefit distribution that are very different from those of countries with a more basic level of development and more homogenous expression of poverty among the population, as seen in most African countries. It is therefore presumptuous to lump all the peripheral countries of the world at the same level for assessments and scheduling with regard to clinical research.

Likewise, the differences in the quality of government actions, capacity for research development and democratic participation of organised society throughout the investigation point towards strategies for developing ethical assessment systems that are also very different. The use of the expression *developing country*, which is excessively generic, makes it difficult to go more deeply into the implied questions relating to protection for vulnerable populations in different regions of the world, given that such questions deal equally with socioeconomic, cultural and political contexts that are as different and imbalanced as those of African countries or other contexts relating to Latin America, southern Asia or even eastern Europe.

With regard to the recent modifications to the content of the Declaration of Helsinki that were mentioned earlier, time and the results and discussions that will certainly follow over the coming years will tell whether these modifications have adequately addressed this expanded – and necessary – concept of social vulnerability.

The topic of double ethical standards in clinical research

The expression 'double standards', in relation to clinical research, arose within the international scientific context from two papers published in the late 1990s that made reference to studies that had earlier been sponsored by the National Institutes of Health (NIH) of the United States. These two papers generated heated debate around the world. Historically, there were already some known cases relating to the topic of social or circumstantial vulnerability among subjects who were taking part in clinical studies, such as the barbaric projects developed by the Nazis in the German concentration camps during the Second World War; the Tuskegee case, which occurred in Alabama, in the United States, in which black men with syphilis were kept without any treatment between the years 1930 and 1972; and a report on 22 cases of ethical abuse that had been committed in clinical studies but had nonetheless been published in internationally recognised scientific journals (Beecher, 1966).

An article published in 1997 detonated the more recent controversy, now involving the topic of so-called double standards in clinical research on human beings. This paper evaluated 15 clinical trials that had been set up to study the prevention of vertical transmission of HIV/AIDS from pregnant mothers to their babies, in developing countries, using control groups treated with placebo, and it denounced this use of placebo as serious ethical misconduct (Lurie and Wolf, 1997). The Editor-in-Chief of the *New England Journal of Medicine*, the journal that published the article, signed an editorial supporting these authors' position and comparing the 15 clinical trials in question with the Tuskegee case. He stated that, in the same way that the Tuskegee study denied penicillin to sick subjects, even after the efficacy of this drug had been proven, these 15 investigations on HIV denied antiretroviral medications to one of the groups of participants. This criticism was based on the understanding that these studies had violated informed consent, extrapolated the question of placebo and taken advantage of poor and uninformed populations (Angell, 1997).

The directors of the NIH, which had sponsored the original investigations, immediately defended the studies in question, stating that the conduct in those situations had been correct, since 'the scientific, social and economic complexities of each investigation needed to be taken into account' (Varmus and Satcher, 1997). Their central argument was that the ethical standards for research on human subjects are universal but not absolute. In other words, their position was that there are some general ethical principles that can be applied to all cases of research on humans, but that the application of these principles also needs to consider factors that are inherent to particular situations, which vary according to the social and economic contexts, in addition to the scientific conditions of such investigations (Resnik, 1998). However, other authors refuted these arguments and took the view that such arguments went completely against the progress in universal political and civil rights that had so far been achieved (Schüklenk, 1998; Thomas, 1998).

Through this, the question that has become part of major international events on clinical research, with vehement positions adopted for and against it, is the following: Are differentiated standards for research protocols and participants ethically justifiable? Or, translating this into more academic terms: Would differentiated methodologies be ethically acceptable under socioeconomic conditions that are also differentiated?

Less than a year after the episode recounted above, another investigation on HIV/AIDS that was developed in a poor country again created strong polemics. This project was developed in rural areas of Uganda with the aim of delineating the risk factors associated with heterosexual transmission of HIV type 1. It sought to determine whether sexually transmittable diseases increased the risk of infection by the virus (Wawer et al., 1999) and also to find the relationship between viral load and heterosexual transmission of HIV-1 (Quinn et al., 2000). In these studies, hundreds of people with HIV were observed for up to 30 months but were not treated. Furthermore, the participants in the sample were not provided with complete and precise information (Angell, 2000). Because of these facts, the topic reached the pages of some of the most important large-circulation newspapers that are available internationally, such as the *New York Times, Washington Post* and others, thereby further stoking up the discussion.

The debate resulting from the above-mentioned research took place because a project of this nature would not have gained approval in the United States (the country sponsoring the study) or in any other developed country, where these patients with HIV or other sexually transmittable diseases would have been alerted and treated. It was evident that the ethical standards were different for Uganda and that, therefore, many investigations developed in peripheral countries may be limited to making observations on subjects in order to monitor results that could have been prevented, as occurred in the case of the studies on pregnant women mentioned earlier. One significant detail in this question, which cannot be left out from this analysis, is that such studies are generally approved by ethical review committees both in the countries where they are conducted and in the country that sponsors them.

Brief history of recent modifications to the Declaration of Helsinki

This matter ended up coming out at the General Assembly of the World Medical Association (WMA), which is held every year and where, when necessary, the content of the Declaration of Helsinki is re-discussed. The discussions were especially heated at the Assembly of October 2000, which was held in Edinburgh and included on the agenda the possibility of modifying the content of the Declaration precisely with regard to items 19, 29 and 30, as mentioned earlier. The idea espoused by some of the plenary members was to approve the notion that the ethical standards for research and access to medical care should become the achievable standards in the country where the trial was held, thereby also providing justification for the use of placebo, even if a well established effective treatment existed internationally. The preliminary text for these modifications to the Declaration of Helsinki was published on the internet by the WMA at that time, to seek broader participation in the discussion. The proposed changes were subtle and most of the participating countries took the view that they could provide different interpretations for the same statement. Among the discussions held, a symposium held in London by the *Bulletin of Medical Ethics* and by the *European Forum for Good Clinical Practice*, with participation by 40 countries, can be highlighted. This came to the conclusion that, because of the worldwide acceptance of the Declaration at that time, it would be a serious mistake to rewrite it at that time (Nicholson, 2000). Finally, the annual meeting of the WMA in Edinburgh ended up unanimously approving some small modifications that did not substantially change the line of thought that had until then been followed by the Declaration of Helsinki regarding the points analysed here.

However, some directors of the WMA did not fail to state on that occasion that, because of the significant changes that were taking place within the field of medical research, it would be essential for the ethical guidelines to be reviewed in the future, including changes to the structure of the Declaration, in order to more clearly define that certain additional standards would be needed in situations in which the investigations were combined with medical care. In other words, they insisted on leaving the proposal for modifications open in two respects: the question of access to and quality of medical care that should be offered to research participants; and the use of placebo in control groups.

However, despite the review already mentioned conducted in the year 2000, the expression *best proven prophylactic, diagnostic and therapeutic methods* remained in the document. Moreover, two other expressions appeared in the old paragraph 30: *at the conclusion of the study* and *identified by the study*. Thus, the Declaration ceased to refer to *which* interventions should be provided to the participants *during* the investigation, which signified the introduction of a certain degree of flexibility into the rules that had until then been in force. According to some critics, the aim was to use differentiated ethical standards in order to reduce costs (Greco, 2000); while according to others, the modifications had created more confusion (Forster et al., 2001).

Thus, at the 2003 meeting of the WMA, again held in Helsinki, almost 40 years after the pioneering assembly of 1964, new proposals for amendments to the Declaration came back on to the agenda. In relation to the topic of 'access to healthcare' in places where this access was deficient, the measure would change to allow investigators and sponsors to be exempted from the responsibility to offer the necessary treatment to the volunteers in the study, provided that this possibility were spelled out to the participants. On this occasion, a group of Latin American countries defended the opposite position: that patients participating in research had the right to the best treatment *existing* and not to the best treatment *available* in the place where the study was being conducted, as recommended in the amendment to item 30 of the Declaration. With regard to item 19, they advocated that the medical investigation would only be justifiable if there was a reasonable expectation that the populations among which the research was being developed might obtain benefits from the research results (Greco, 2003). The conflict again centred on the application of differentiated methodologies to different countries, which according to some peripheral countries and also some voices from developed nations, would validate the double standards.

The burning questions therefore again related to items 19, 29 and 30 of the Declaration. To recall what these stated: item 19 said that the research would only be justified if there was an expectation that the population involved were benefited by the results; item 29 determined that the use of placebo in control groups would only be justified if there was known effective treatment for the problem in question; and item 30 was about the commitment that at the end of the study, all the participants were assured access to the proven best prophylactic, diagnostic and therapeutic methods identified by the study. The Assembly therefore decided to nominate a subcommittee that would have the task of bringing a proposal for settling this matter, to the fifty-sixth World Medical Assembly, which was scheduled to be held in Tokyo in October 2004.

With this further moratorium, the subject continued to flare up around the world. In an editorial with the title *One standard, not two*, published immediately after the meeting in Helsinki in 2003, the journal *The Lancet* stated that the WMA had missed the chance to make concrete progress for patients who underwent experiments in poor countries. According to this journal, the position adopted would only reinforce the idea that there were two ethical standards for research: one for the rich countries and another for the poor countries (Editorial, 2003a). Two months later, the *Canadian Medical Association Journal* was also outspoken, stating that the Declaration was being 'dismantled' and criticising the *United States Department of Health and Human Services* and the *British Medical Association* for the strong pressure they had exerted. This journal also criticised its own entity for remaining silent in relation to the proposal that the matter should not be taken as concluded in view of the creation of the above-mentioned subcommittee (Editorial, 2003b). Some months later, the official journal of the *International Association of Bioethics* opened its editorial space to analyse the unilateral way in which the developed countries funded research in poor nations, with standards imposed and difficulties created regarding cultural contextualisation (Chadwick and Schüklenk, 2004).

During this period, the manifestations in favour of changes continued predominant. After the international meeting which took place in Chile with support of the World Health Organization, some authors, as Lie et al. (2004), declared that at that moment there was an international consensual position with regard to standards for medical care in clinical research. Nevertheless, these always received prompt responses with contrary arguments (Schüklenk, 2004), thus demonstrating that the positions remained divided.

At the fifty-fifth World Medical Assembly in Tokyo in 2004, the debate persisted, but once again, the attempt to bring in changes was defeated. Only a 'clarifying' note was added to paragraph 30, without greater repercussions. Because of this result, the United States, through the NIH, officially withdrew its recognition from the Declaration of Helsinki, and formalised the position that, from that date onwards, American researchers and research funded by companies in that country would need to follow rules laid down by the United States itself, based on the so-called ICH-GCP guidelines (*International Conference on Harmonization – Good Clinical Practices*) and the CIOMS-2002 version. The ICH-GCP guidelines reflect the tripartite consensus agreed in 1997 between the United States, Europe and Japan, the principal worldwide producers of medications, who had wanted since that time to replace the original concept of the Declaration. In turn, the CIOMS-2002 version already brought in some favourable changes to assuage American anxieties. Even so, some researchers in that country still continued to be against the use of placebo as an effective therapy for problems known to science (Michels and Rothman, 2003).

The panorama of positions for and against the changes in the Declaration continued between 2005 and 2008, with the arguments favouring changes gaining increasing public visibility through the significant number of articles published in international scientific journals over these last few years.

THE WORLD MEDICAL ASSEMBLY, IN SEOUL, 2008

Finally, in October 2008, at the fifty-ninth Annual Assembly of the WMA in Seoul, and after several prior preparatory meetings, the changes debated here were ratified (WMA, 2008). In addition to substantive changes in the items in dispute, the intention of changing the structure of the document, as already advocated by some directors of the WMA since Edinburgh 2000, was implemented. Thus, the well known paragraphs 19, 29 and 30 changed their numbering within the context of the document, thus losing a little of their 'visibility'. The significant identifiable changes were the following.

- At the end of the new paragraph 14, in the part of the Declaration that deals with the 'Principles for all medical research', the following phrase was included. 'The protocol should describe arrangements for post-study access by study subjects to interventions identified as beneficial in the study or access to other appropriate care or benefits.'
- In the chapter dealing with 'Additional principles for medical research combined with medical care', in the second part of the new paragraph 32, the use of placebo came to have the following interpretation. 'Where for compelling and scientifically sound methodological reasons the use of placebo is necessary to determine the efficacy or safety of an intervention and the patients who receive placebo or no treatment will not be subject to any risk of serious or irreversible harm.' This is very different from the previous wording.
- Paragraph 33, with changes emphasised in italics to make it easier for readers to understand them, became the following. 'At the conclusion of the study, patients entered into the study are entitled to be informed about the outcome of the study and to share any benefits that result from it, for example, access to interventions identified as beneficial in the study or to *other appropriate care or benefits.*'
- Finally, the last paragraph of the Declaration of Helsinki, 2008 version, was amended as follows, again with the changes highlighted in italics. 'In the treatment of a patient, where proven interventions do not exist or have been ineffective, the physician, after seeking expert advice, with informed consent from the patient or a legally authorised representative, may use an unproven intervention *if in the physician's judgement* it offers hope of saving life, re-establishing health or alleviating suffering. Where possible, this intervention should be made the object of research, designed to evaluate its safety and efficacy. In all cases, new information should be recorded and, *where appropriate*, made publicly available.'

In Table 27.1 is presented the comparison between the text of the Declaration of Helsinki, in the versions of Edinburgh 2000 (in the paragraphs 19, 29 and 30) and Seoul 2008, with the changes emphasised in italics.

This entire long and detailed history is indispensable for better understanding of the events and of what was finally decided by the World Medical Association at its Assembly in 2008. Over the coming years, it is very likely that this subject will not remain unnoticed and at rest, without criticism. On the contrary, since this is a decision by an Assembly of a professional association (of physicians), regardless of how important it is, it does not have the weight of law or even of the non-binding official international norms constructed between countries through international organisations. Because of the historical strength that the Declaration of Helsinki has achieved, it has ended up becoming a worldwide technical document that is taken as a moral reference and often placed above countries' own legislation, based on its unanimous worldwide acceptance. What is feared with

Table 27.1 Declaration of Helsinki – Comparison between the versions of years 2000 and 2008

(With the changes emphasised in italics)

SUBJECT	EDINBURGH 2000		SEOUL 2008	
	Paragraph	Text	Paragraph	Text
USE OF PLACEBO	29	*The benefits, risks, burdens and effectiveness of a new method should be tested against those of the best current prophylactic, diagnostic and therapeutic methods. This does not exclude the use of placebo, or no treatment, in studies where no proven prophylactic, diagnostic or therapeutic method exists.*	32	The benefits, risks, burdens and effectiveness of a new intervention must be tested against those of the best current proven intervention, except in the following circumstances: • The use of placebo, or no treatment, is acceptable in studies where no current proven intervention exists; or • *Where for compelling and scientifically sound methodological reasons the use of placebo is necessary to determine the efficacy or safety of an intervention and the patients who receive placebo or no treatment will not be subject to any risk of serious or irreversible harm.* Extreme care must be taken to avoid abuse of this option.
POST-STUDY ACCESS	30	*At the conclusion of the study, every patient entered into the study should be assured of access to the best proven prophylactic, diagnostic and therapeutic methods identified by the study.*	14	The design and performance of each research study involving human subjects must be clearly described in a research protocol. The protocol should contain a statement of the ethical considerations involved and should indicate how the principles in this Declaration have been addressed. The protocol should include information regarding funding, sponsors, institutional affiliations, other potential conflicts of interest, incentives for subjects and provisions for treating and/or compensating subjects who are harmed as a consequence of participation in the research study. *The protocol should describe arrangements for post-study access by study subjects to interventions identified as beneficial in the study or access to other appropriate care or benefits.*
			33	At the conclusion of the study, patients entered into the study are entitled to be informed about the outcome of the study and to share any benefits that result from it, for example, access to interventions *identified as beneficial in the study or to other appropriate care or benefits.*
JUSTIFICATION FOR CONDUCTING A MEDICAL RESEARCH	19	Medical research is only justified if there is a reasonable likelihood that the populations in which the research is carried out stand to benefit from the results of the research.	17	*Medical research involving a disadvantaged population or community is only justified if the research is responsive to the health needs and priorities of this population or community and if there is a* reasonable likelihood that this population or community stands to benefit from the results of the research.

the decision in Seoul in 2008 is that, because of all the historical divergences recounted, it may become contested and thus lose the moral authority achieved over all these 40 years in which it has been the reference point in clinical research, for researchers, universities, laboratories, companies, scientific journals and even countries, all around the world.

Brazil, for example, through a Resolution from its National Health Board (*Conselho Nacional de Saúde*) with homologation from the Ministry of Health, immediately contested the position adopted by the WMA against the use of placebo in research involving human beings, in cases in which there is a proven preventive, diagnostic or therapeutic method for the problem in question. According to the position advocated officially by the Brazilian government, 'the benefits, risks, difficulties and effectiveness of a new method should be tested by comparing them with the best present methods' (Brasil, 2008). It is very likely that countries such as South Africa, Portugal and Uruguay, which also voted against the new text, will also soon express their views on this matter, as will other nations in the southern hemisphere that are known to have similar positions.

SOME FINAL CONSIDERATIONS REGARDING PERIPHERAL COUNTRIES' OWN REGULATION AND SOCIAL CONTROL SYSTEMS

International research should continue to be carried out. It is also indispensable that the documents and mechanisms created internationally to control and develop such research should be produced and implemented. However, for the process to be as transparent and fair as possible, and to dismiss any doubt regarding undesirable external interference or influences that disregard the social vulnerabilities that exist, the most appropriate way forward is for poor and developing countries to create their own autonomous regulatory systems, with transparent social control mechanisms that are operated democratically at all levels. International standards and guidelines are indispensable for providing the direction to be followed in developing clinical research in each place around the world. However, the peculiarities of each country's regulatory systems should definitively be constructed in accordance with each country's particular characteristics and needs. Autonomy is related to the independence to decide and is also related to the technical and intellectual capacity that peripheral nations must cooperatively put in place, in order to achieve this level of autonomy and development, with support from the more advanced nations and from international organisations, for constructing ethical control rules and systems for their biomedical investigations.

In accordance with the proposal presented in the courses provided by UNESCO's Bioethics Network for Latin America and the Caribbean, the construction of a social control and regulation system for research in the peripheral countries of the world, with the capability to promote international studies of cooperative and independent nature, takes place through adaptation of the whole organic system, on two main planes: (1) Formulation of norms appropriate to the socioeconomic and cultural context of these countries, involving three lines of protection for research ethics (obtaining of consent, minimisation of risks and maximisation of benefits); and (2) sociopolitical issues relating to the creation of normative regulatory instruments, represented by laws and ethical norms for research and by opening up democratic spaces for social control, as embodied by institutional or regional committees and by national commissions for trials (Garrafa and Lorenzo, 2006; Garrafa and Lorenzo, 2008).

With regard to plane 1, there are three levels to be considered: (a) adequate processes for obtaining informed consent statements, through reducing the importance of the formal contractual or bureaucratic approach and increasing the importance of a communitarian vision of autonomy for populations with low educational levels; (b) adequate procedures aimed at minimising risks, to ensure equity for all subjects participating in a clinical trial; and (c) adequate procedures to maximise benefits, for the same reason just mentioned.

With regard to plane 2, there are also three levels to be considered: (a) stimulation of sociopolitical participation in document production, within independent and interdisciplinary discussion forums, with the aim of obtaining a national consensus on the ethical limits in research; (b) creation of national or institutional spaces for evaluating the ethical aspects of protocols, with independent decisions and ethical supervision of research development; and (c) construction of adequate capacity for the members of ethics committees and commissions.

NOTE

1 Volnei Garrafa, PhD – Chair of UNESCO's Cathedra of Bioethics and Coordinator of the Post-graduate Program in Bioethics of the University of Brasília, Federal District, Brazil. [volnei@unb.br]

REFERENCES

Angell, M. (1997) 'The ethics of clinical research in third world', *New England Medical Journal*, 337: 847–9.

Angell, M. (2000) 'Investigator's responsibilities for human subjects in developing countries', *New England Journal of Medicine*, 342: 967–9.

Angell, M. (2007) *A Verdade sobre os Laboratórios Farmacêuticos.* Rio de Janeiro: Record.

Beecher, H.K. (1966) 'Ethics and clinical research', *New England Journal of Medicine*, 274: 1354–60.

Bernard, C. (1865 [1984]) *Introduction à l'étude de la médicine expérimentale.* Paris: Flammarion.

Brasil, Ministério da Saúde-Conselho Nacional de Saúde (2008) 'Resolução 404/2008'. http://conselho.saude.gov.br/resolucoes/2008/Reso_404.doc.doc, accessed 30 October 2008.

Chadwick, R. and Schüklenk, U. (2004) 'Bioethics colonialism?', *Bioethics*, 18 (5): iii–iv.

Commission Économique pour l'Amérique Latine et Caraïbe (2003) *Panorama Social de América Latina 2002–2003.* Document disponible sur: http://www.eclac.cl/cgi-bin/getProd.asp?xml=/publicaciones/xml/0/12980/P12980.xml& xsl=/dds/tpl/p9f.xsl.

Editorial (2003a) 'One standard, not two', *The Lancet,* 362 (9389): 27 September.

Editorial (2003b) 'Dismantling the Helsinki Declaration', *Canadian Medical Association Journal,* 169 (10/November): 997.

Forster, H., Emanuel, E. and Grady, E. (2001) 'The 2000 revision of The Declaration of Helsinki: A step forward or more confusion?' *The Lancet,* 365: 2983–5.

Foucault, M. (1972) *Naissance de la clinique: une arqueologie du regard médicale.* Paris: PUF.

Garrafa, V. and Lorenzo, C. (2006) *Ética e Investigación Clínica en los Países en Desarrollo – Aspectos Conceptuales, Técnicos y Sociales.* Córdoba, Argentina. Red Latinoamericana y del Caribe de Bioética de Unesco – Programa de Educación Permanente a Distancia; Tercer Curso de Ética de la Investigación con Seres Humanos, http://www.redbioetica-edu.com.ar.

Garrafa, V. and Lorenzo, C. (2008). 'Moral imperialism and multi-centric clinical trials in peripheral countries', *Cadernos de Saúde Pública*, 24 (10): 2219–26.

Garrafa, V. and Prado, M.M. (2001) 'Tentativas de mudanças na Declaração de Helsinki: fundamentalismo econômico, imperialismo ético e controle social', *Cadernos de Saúde Pública*, 17 (6): 1489–96.

Greco, D. (2000) 'A cure at any cost?' *New Scientist*, 1 July: 42–3.

Greco, D. (2003) 'A Associação Médica Mundial propõe mudanças no parágrafo 30 da Declaração de Helsinque 2000, diminuindo o acesso aos cuidados de saúde para os voluntários de ensaios clínicos', *Boletim Sociedade Brasileira de Bioética*, 7–9: 04–5.

Lie, R.K., Emanuel, E., Grady, C. and Wendler, D. (2004) 'The standard of care debate: The Declaration of Helsinki *versus* the international consensus opinion', *Journal of Medical Ethics*, 30 (2): 190–3.

Lurie, P. and Wolfe, S. (1997) 'Unethical trials of interventions to reduce perinatal transmission of the human immunodeficiency virus in developing countries', *New England Journal of Medicine*, 337: 853–6.

Michels, K.B. and Rothman, K. (2003) 'Update on unethical use of placebos in randomized trials', *Bioethics*, 17 (2): 188–204.

Moynihan, R. (2003) 'Who pays for the pizza? Redefining the relationship between doctors and drug companies. 1: Entanglement', *British Medical Journal*, 326: 1189–92.

Nicholson, R.H. (2000) 'If it ain't broke, don't fix it', *The Hastings Center Report*, 30 (I/January-February): 6.

Quinn, T.C., Wawer, M.J., Sewankambo, N.K. et al. (2000) 'Viral load and heterosexual transmission of human immunodeficiency virus type 1', *New England Journal of Medicine*, 342: 921–9.

Ravetz, J. (1971) *Scientific Knowledgement and its Social Problems*. Oxford: Oxford University Press.

Resnik, D.B. (1998) 'The ethics of HIV research in developing nations', *Bioethics*, 12: 286–306.

Schüklenk, U. (1998) 'Unethical perinatal HIV transmission trials establish bad precedent', *Bioethics*, 12: 312–8.

Schüklenk, U. (2004) 'The standard of care debate: Against the myth of an "international consensus opinion"', *Journal of Medical Ethics*, 30 (2): 194–7.

Sithi-amorn, C. and Somronthong, R. (2000) 'Strengthening health research capacity in developing countries: A critical element for achieving health equity', *British Medical Journal*, 321: 813–5.

Thomas, J. (1998) 'Ethical challenges of HIV clinical trials in developing countries', *Bioethics*, 12: 320–7.

Varmus, H. and Satcher, D. (1997) 'Ethical complexities of conducting research in developing countries', *New England Journal of Medicine*, 337: 1000–5.

Wawer, M.J., Sewankambo, N.K., Serwadda, D., Quinn, T.C., Paxton, L.A., Kiwanuka, N. et al. (1999) 'Control of sexually transmitted diseases for AIDS prevention in Uganda: A randomised community trial', *The Lancet*, 353: 525–35.

Willerroider, M. (2004) 'Making the move into drug sales', *Nature*, 430: 486–7.

Wisner, B. (1993) 'Disaster vulnerability: Scale, power and daily life', *Geojournal*, 30 (32): 127–40.

World Medical Association (WMA) (2008) 'Ethical principles for medical research involving human subjects – 59th WMA General Assembly, Seoul, October, http://www.wma.net, accessed 25 October 2008.

28

Ethical and Scientific Issues in Gene Therapy and Stem Cell Research

Kenneth Cornetta and Eric M. Meslin

INTRODUCTION

The ethical issues surrounding gene therapy and stem cell research have been an area of intense interest for investigators, research regulators and the public for many years. While traditionally discussed as distinct issues, particularly since the former burst on to the science scene many years before the latter, gene therapy and stem cell research share a number of common ethical challenges. Of course each has their share of particular issues – these will be noted as well. Our emphasis on the common issues is not to disguise or otherwise minimize issues that one has and the other does not – for example, gene therapy does not invoke discussions about the moral status of the embryo as research involving embryonic stem cells does – but rather to acknowledge that the science in both areas is moving toward clinical therapies and we hope to highlight these in particular. Therefore, this chapter will outline the ethical issues facing patients, investigators, clinicians and society as these novel therapies become technically feasible. We will also review the regulatory oversight that currently exists to help manage clinical implementation of these therapies.

STEM CELLS, CELL THERAPY

Cell therapy uses cells or whole tissues to treat disease. The source of cells may be from oneself (autologous) or from other humans (allogeneic). Cell therapy from other species also has been explored (xenotransplantation) and raises its own unique set of issues. Blood transfusion is the most commonly performed cell therapy but as blood cells are terminally differentiated, the benefit is measured in days or weeks. To provide more lasting effects, organ transplantation has developed in which a combination of organ-specific stem cells and terminally differentiated cells are used to provide long-term disease amelioration.

Stem cells are unique in that they differentiate into cells of different lineages while retaining the ability to self-renew, thereby maintaining the stem cell pool. As an example, clinical bone marrow transplantation uses hematopoietic stem cells that are capable of differentiating into a wide variety of blood cell types while maintaining a pool of undifferentiated hematopoietic stem cells for the life of the transplant recipient.

Organ-specific stem cells can be found throughout the body (e.g. bone marrow, neurons, liver, muscle, skin and adipose – fat – tissue). While these tissue-specific stem cells can self-renew, in humans it appears that they generally remain committed to the organ in which they are found. While hematopoietic stem cell can repopulate blood organs, it is unclear whether other stem cells (e.g. neuronal stem cells) will be able to regenerate functioning organs in an adult. Organ-specific stem cells may also be limited in number or reside in organs that are not amenable to biopsy. This has led investigators to research whether organ-specific stem cells can be reprogrammed. Recent research suggests that stem cells may be able to be reprogrammed *in vitro* to resemble cells of other lineages (for example, an adipose stem cell may be reprogrammed to become a liver cell), but whether these cells will function *in vivo* remains to be determined.

For this reason, there has been intense interest in exploring embryonic stem (ES) cells. Ever since researchers first isolated ES cells from embryos (Thomson et al., 1998) and fetal tissue (Shamblott et al., 1998), scientists have known of the capacity of these cells to form any cell, tissue, or organ within an organism. The promise of ES cell therapy is generation *ex vivo* or *in vivo* of cells for tissue regeneration and potentially whole organs. While organ-specific stem cells are obtained from adult tissues, ES cells are obtained from fertilized eggs, developing embryos, or in the case of embryonic germ cells, from the tissue found in the fetal gonadal ridge. Beginning with the US National Bioethics Advisory Commission (NBAC, 1999) major research groups, regulatory bodies, advocacy groups (of all types) and advisory committees have contributed to an intense public conversation about the ethical issues arising from the derivation and use of ES cells. Since obtaining ES cells requires the destruction of the human embryo, moral objections were often based on the moral status of the embryo and the commensurate harm that embryo destruction entails a debate that some consider to be both endless and irresolvable. In the US, President Bush's restrictive policy limited federal support to research that involved ES cells that had been derived prior to 8 August 2001 – a policy that permitted private sector development but did little to resolve the intense ethical and policy discussion (Meslin, 2008).

Other countries have adopted both more permissive and more restrictive policies. Indeed, rather than manipulate embryos, many laboratories have been exploring whether differentiated cells or organ-specific stem cells might be reprogrammed back into ES cells. Recent work using forced-expression of a combination of transcription factors and growth regulatory genes normally expressed in ES cells has provided preliminary evidence that mature cells, such as murine fibroblasts and human mesenchymal cells, may be reprogrammed into ES-like cells (referred to as induced pluripotent stem cells, or iPS cells) (Okita et al., 2007; Wernig et al., 2007; Yu et al., 2007). Since the long-term expression of these factors raises safety concerns, they will need to be addressed before iPS cell therapy can be moved into clinical practice. Moreover, while it may open the possibility of ending the protracted debate over the ethics of embryonic stem cell research, it will not eliminate all moral concerns. Indeed, a premature switch to iPS cells might run the risk of slowing the pace of progress toward the goal of preventing and curing disease (Schwartz and Meslin, 2007).

Interestingly, the conversion of differentiated cells into iPS cells used gene transfer to express the transcription factors required for de-differentiation (Okita et al., 2007; Wernig et al., 2007; Yu et al., 2007). This illustrates how the development of some stem cell therapies may require engineering of the stem cells with gene transfer. Likewise, genes do not function outside a cell so all gene therapy is a form of cell therapy. In time, patients and clinicians may weigh the pros and cons of cell or gene therapy as they seek to treat a disorder. For example, if one sustains bone marrow damage due to toxin exposure the current treatment is often infusion of allogeneic bone marrow stem cell. This treatment can have severe, and even lethal, side effects owing to incompatibility issues between host and donor immune systems. A theoretical alternative could be the reprogramming of the patient's own adipose stem cells into hematopoietic stem cells, allowing reconstitution of the blood elements. As the cells are of autologous origin, the patient would not be at risk for tissue incompatibility.

In a second scenario, bone marrow disorders due to a genetic defect could be treated by allogeneic transplant (as it is today), or through gene therapy approaches under development in which genetic modification of autologous stem cells provides correction of the genetic defect. Moreover, recent evidence suggests that differentiated cells can be altered without the need for stem or progenitor cells. In a recent paper, Zhou et al. utilized adenoviral vectors to express developmental regulators to induce differentiated pancreatic exocrine cells to function as ß-cells restoring insulin production in a murine model of diabetes (Zhou et al., 2008).

These scenarios demonstrate that as gene transfer technologies mature, the risk–benefit ratio for gene therapy will likely require an assessment of available cell therapies. As novel stem cell therapies mature, the converse is likely to be true.

GENE THERAPY AND GENE TRANSFER TECHNOLOGY

As with stem cell research, the history of gene therapy, including early research in recombinant DNA technology stimulated considerable discussion about the social and ethical acceptability of working on and manipulating human genetic material. In 1973–1974, researchers met at the Asilomar Conference Center in California and also at the Cold Spring Harbor Laboratories in New York to discuss, among other things, a proposed experiment by Paul Berg and colleagues in which a monkey virus (SV40) would be spliced together with a bacterial virus and then inserted into a bacterium. This was being discussed around the time that Herbert Boyer and Stanley Cohen first accomplished a successful recombinant DNA (rDNA) experiment to treat diabetes. Concerns about the possibility of an escaping pathogen lead many to carefully consider the risk–benefit ratio in such experiments. Philosopher Stephen Stich argued for *regulating* this type of research, rather than adopting the two extremes of absolute prohibition or unfettered free inquiry, was among the first to rely on what would soon become known as the precautionary principle: 'If we do not know with considerable assurance that the probability of an activity leading to disastrous consequences is very low, then we should not allow the activity to continue' (Stich, 1978).

Among the many important outcomes from Asilomar was a moratorium on rDNA research until the risks could be assessed, and a set of guidelines developed by the scientific community, which were eventually adopted by the NIH. These guidelines were modified and later used by the NIH recombinant DNA Advisory Committee, a committee with national authority to review rDNA projects. This remains one of the few national research advisory bodies in the US and stands as an important example of science and ethics collaborating for the public good. Indeed, this early rDNA work laid the groundwork for one of the most exciting and challenging areas of genetic medicine: human gene therapy (Cook-Deegan, 1995).

While there is no agreed-upon definition of gene therapy, it can be loosely defined as the transfer of genetic material with therapeutic intent. Initially, gene therapy was conceptualized in the context of a single gene defect. The field has now grown and is exploring the expression of many genes unrelated to the underlying genetic defect. For example, cancer cells are being transduced with genes that elicit an immune response as a means of stimulating anti-tumor immunity. In other trials, investigators are exploring gene transfer of ribozymes and inhibitory RNAs to protect T cells from infection with HIV. To recognize the broad scope of diseases being treated, many now use the term *gene transfer* in place of gene therapy.

The methodology used for gene transfer influences the risks and potential benefits of this technology and is therefore important when considering ethical issues related to this novel therapy. First, there are a variety of vehicles, or vectors, that are currently used to transfer genetic material. The simplest vectors used DNA plasmids to introduce the genetic material of interest (transgene) into a cell. This method is not suited to many clinical applications, owing to the inefficiency of gene transfer and the relatively rapid degradation of the genetic material. To meet these technical challenges, the majority of current clinical trials have used engineered viruses (viral vectors) to facilitate the transfer of genetic material. Vectors are engineered by replacing much of the viral genome with transgene sequences. Deletion of the viral genes prevents viral replication while using the virus to do what it does best: deliver genetic material. Almost every type of virus is being evaluated as a potential gene transfer vector and each viral vector brings with it unique risks and advantages. For example, adenoviral vectors can provide high levels of gene expression. They generally do not integrate and are degraded over time. These properties make adenoviral vectors attractive vehicles for immunization strategies. While they are not suited to long-term expression, their degradation also decreases the risk of long-term complications. In contrast, vectors based on retroviruses are attractive vectors for stem cells that are destined to multiply extensively and persist over the lifespan of the patient.

Unfortunately, retroviral insertion occurs in a wide variety of locations throughout the genome and in rare circumstances can activate oncogenes leading to cancer (Hacein-Bey-Abina et al., 2003; Dave et al., 2004). In addition, certain vectors are well suited to *in vivo* administration but this brings along with it the threat of severe, possibly lethal immune responses (Raper et al., 2003). It should be pointed out that the adverse events mentioned above were related to the vector used to deliver the gene, rather than the gene itself. Investigators are actively redesigning vectors to avoid these unintended consequences or seeking to deliver vector to tissues outside the body, thereby significantly decreasing the chance of a severe immune reaction. Therefore, understanding the vector type, intended target cell and route of administration all become critical in framing the ethical discussion regarding a specific gene therapy application. The basic science and vector development field is also moving rapidly so the risk–benefit ratio requires constant re-evaluation as new information comes to light.

A second consideration when assessing gene therapy safety is gene *addition* versus gene *correction*. In gene addition, new genetic material is introduced into a cell, often along with bacterial or viral sequences contained within the vector. This raises concern about the potential short-term and evolutionary consequences of adding DNA into the genome, both in terms of the type of DNA added and the location into which the DNA is inserted. A developing approach uses homologous recombination technology to alter the sequences of gene *in situ* using recombinases and endogenous DNA repair pathways (Urnov et al., 2005; Lombardo et al., 2007). Most clinical trials have used gene addition because of the efficiency of gene transfer. If the efficiency of homologous recombination technology improves and 'defective' genes can be altered, the concerns regarding the random additional of foreign genetic material into the gene pool may no longer be valid.

Finally, the cellular targets for gene transfer are also important for any ethical discussion. To date, all clinical gene therapy protocols have targeted somatic cells. While genetically altered somatic cells may reconstitute a cell lineage or an organ, the genetic material cannot be passed on to the patient's progeny. In contrast, germ-line gene therapy has not been attempted owing to technical and ethical concerns about transmission to offspring. In this scenario, the genetic material is introduced into cells at the egg, sperm, or embryo stage such that the genetic make-up of the individual and all of their progeny will be altered.

SOMATIC GENE THERAPY

Somatic gene therapy is an alternation of a cell's phenotype with therapeutic intent. Much of the current ethics literature views gene therapy in the context of single recessive gene disorders that can be treated through the introduction of a wild-type copy of the missing gene. Diseases that have been in clinical trial and have attracted the interest of bioethicists include severe-combined immunodeficiency ('bubble baby' disease), hemophilia and cystic fibrosis.

Even before human gene therapy trials began, statements indicating favorable views of this new therapeutic approach were published in the early 1980s by the US President's Commission on Ethical Problems in Medicine and Biomedical and Behavioral Research (PCSEPMBBR, 1982) and the Parliamentary Assembly of the Council of Europe (CoE, 1982). In a review of 28 policy statement from religious, governmental and medical societies published between 1980 and 1993, Walters and Palmer found public support and a notable consensus regarding the ethical merit of somatic gene therapy for the treatment of disease (Walters and Palmer, 1997). As discussed by Fuchs, the explanation for this acceptance relates to a view that this treatment approach is an extension of other techniques currently used to treat disease (Fuchs, 2006). Indeed, early discussions of gene therapy invoked the analogy of organ transplantation to explain to the public with an analogy that has historically enjoyed acceptance.

According to *The Journal of Gene Medicine* database in May 2008 (www.wiley.co.uk/ genmed) there are over 1300 approved gene therapy clinical trials. While the majority have been initiated in the US (67.3 percent) and Europe (26.8 percent), there have been 37 trials approved in Asia and 29 in Australasia. While much of the ethics literature focuses on treatment of genetic disease, this represents a small percentage of the patient populations participating in gene therapy trials, as 66.5 percent of trials seek to treat cancer patients while only 8.2 percent target monogenic diseases. To date, 80.4 percent of clinical trials have been for Phase I or Phase I/II trials (trials in which the objective is safety assessment and determining the maximally tolerated dose). Only 2.7 percent are reported to be Phase III trials (i.e. studies assessing efficacy) and China is the only country that has a licensed gene therapy product on the market. Not unexpectedly, as discussed below, many of the current controversies in somatic gene therapy reflect the challenges of bringing novel therapies into clinical practice.

Certain ethical issues involved with conducting early phase clinical trials were brought to the forefront after the tragic death of Jesse Gelsinger, a patient participating in Phase I clinical trial for ornithine transcarbamylase deficiency at the University of Pennsylvania (Puttagunta et al., 2002; Raper et al., 2003; Edwards et al., 2004; Kong, 2005). Many of the issues raised about this incident are not unique to gene therapy, such as the 'therapeutic misconception' or the tendency of patients to overestimate the benefit of investigational therapies, even when consent documents and verbal communications indicate that no benefit is promised nor should any be anticipated (Arkin et al., 2005). Kimmelman and Palmour reviewed 277 informed consent documents on file with the NIH Office of Biotechnology Activities and suggested that the therapeutic misconception was common in Phase I gene therapy documents (Kimmelman and Palmour, 2005). The Gelsinger case also raised a number of conflict of interest issues between the investigators and commercial interests involved with the clinical trial (Lemmens and Waring, 2006: 4).

A particular ethical challenge for Phase I studies is the need to ensure that the informed consent process communicate an accurate risk–benefit ratio, a goal that can never been attained with certainty because a goal of a Phase I studies is the discovery of unanticipated adverse events not detected or predicted from preclinical studies. This has led Kimmelman to suggest that patients with stable disease should rarely be eligible for early gene therapy (Kimmelman, 2007). We are concerned about whether this position might devalue quality of life issues, long-term disease sequelae and the risk of standard therapies. The latter issue was brought into focus after the recent death of a patient undergoing treatment for rheumatoid arthritis using an adeno-associated viral vector expressing tumor necrosis factor. A few days after the second intra-articular injection, the patient developed fever and bleeding and later died of multi-organ failure. The adverse event was made public in compliance with an NIH disclosure policy for reporting gene therapy adverse events (a policy unique to gene therapy clinical trials). This disclosure led to a series of articles in the press and in academic publications discussing informed consent and the risks of gene therapy before the cause of death was known (Weiss, 2007; Caplan, 2008;

Kahn, 2008; Pattee, 2008; Silber, 2008). It was subsequently found that the patient's death was due to infectious complications secondary to FDA-approved immunosuppressant therapy she was receiving for systemic arthritis (Anklesaria et al., 2008). There is currently no evidence that the gene therapy was involved with her illness. This case serves as a reminder that all therapies have inherent risks, and novel products cannot be judged in isolation but in reference to the alternative therapies available. It also calls to question the advisability of disclosing information about adverse events prematurely.

GERM-LINE GENE THERAPY

Germ-line gene therapy seeks to alter cells that can be passed on to subsequent generations. This involves introduction into sperm or egg cells in adults that would alter the genetic make-up of their progeny. A second scenario would be the manipulation of embryos at very early stages of development so that the genetic modification is incorporated into the developing fetus. In either scenario, the modification would be included in the germ line, into subsequent progeny, and in turn the gene pool. As such, the genetic modification affects more than the individual but society as a whole.

Today there is a moratorium on germ-line gene therapy. One argument for refraining from altering the germ line is in line with the precautionary principle. Most current gene therapy technology with non-viral and viral vectors insert genetic material into the genome and we do not know the consequences of what is inserted and what genetic sequences the insertion may disrupt. As homologous recombination technology improves and can alter the genome without adding sequences, the impact of this technical concern will likely be lessened.

Baylis and Robert have identified a number of arguments against germ-line gene therapy including transgression of divine and natural law, misuse of the technology and fear of unintended consequences (Baylis and Robert, 2004). Others have argued that individuals have the right to a genetic heritage that should not be altered by medical interventions. Sometimes referred to as a 'right to an open future' (Feinberg, 1980), this raises concerns about manipulating a person's genome so that future generations are affected by these changes. The potential for eugenic programs or for increasing disparity or favoring those already advantaged is an additional concern.

Others have argued that once the technical and safety issues surrounding germ-line gene therapy are addressed, the correction of disease will likely be the main objective, both medically and ethically (Baylis and Robert, 2004). Walters and Palmer (1997) and Resnik and Langer (2001) each provide a detailed description of the scientific and ethical issues involved with germ-line gene therapy, including scenarios where the case for germ-line gene therapy will be compelling. Examples are the rare cases where both parents are homozygous for a mutation such that all offspring will develop disease or when a mutation is lethal to the fetus or causes irreversible damage to organs in the fetus (Waddington et al., 2005). If such treatment becomes the safest or only option to cure diseases, it is argued that withholding such treatment would not be ethically acceptable.

While one can define theoretical scenarios where the justification for germ-line gene therapy will be compelling, and therefore may be ethical, the majority of genetic diseases are autosomal recessive. In this case, the parents are unaffected carriers but approximately 25 percent of their children will be affected by the disease. In this scenario, there may be desire by the parents to ensure that their children, and offspring in subsequent generations, will not be at risk of disease. Here the support for germ-line gene therapy faces additional challenges. Implementing gene therapy in autosomal recessive diseases has raised a number of concerns.

One challenge is that we may not be able to predict with complete (or even substantial) certainty the unintended consequence of a genetic manipulation. For example, individuals with two copies of a mutant globin gene may develop sickle cell anemia, while those heterozygous (i.e. with only one copy) appear to have increased protection from malaria. For most diseases we do not know if there are evolutionary advantages to maintaining recessive mutations. A second challenge is the use of gene transfer to eliminate genetic disease in the same way that public health officials use vaccination to eliminate infectious diseases from the population. This assumes gene therapy technology advances to the point where it has a safety and efficacy profile similar to today's vaccinations. As most genetic diseases are recessive, the pool of carriers greatly exceeds those with disease, so any such disease elimination program would require large-scale treatment of the population. Those who see germ-line alterations to prevent disease as acceptable do generally agree that any attempt to mandate such treatments on the population would also be ethically unacceptable.

Intertwined with deliberations of germ-line gene therapy are the many moral challenges that emerge from reproductive medicine including embryo selection, embryo screening, prenatal diagnosis, abortion and assisted reproduction (Resnik and Langer, 2001). These and other ethical issues arising from genetic testing are addressed more fully in other chapters in this book.

The discussion above assumes that the germ-line modification was done for disease treatment where the genetic basis of the disease is clear-cut. Unfortunately, our understanding of many disease traits is limited. This raises the question, 'Would genetic alterations of susceptibility genes be appropriate?' In this case, increased risk of disease does not necessarily mean the disease will occur. Susceptibility genes are influenced by other modified genes, so until our understanding advances it will be hard to predict the outcome of such a modification. Resnik and Langer have suggested that the distinction between therapy, prevention and enhancement is problematic since it requires a definition of normalcy that is often lacking (Resnik and Langer, 2001). They suggest the term 'human germ-line genome modification' better describes the procedure while avoiding misleading labels and should be used in place of germ-line gene therapy.

GENETIC ENHANCEMENT

The debate over the use of genetic technology to enhance 'favorable' traits has predated the technology itself and even the discovery of DNA. A concern that genetic manipulations could be used to foster eugenics is warranted given the historical record. Muller described the potential to enhance traits through genetic means in 1939. Walters and Palmer have detailed the three categories most discussed, specifically the enhancement of physical, intellectual and moral traits (Walters and Palmer, 1997). Kiuru and Crystal recently published a review of preclinical studies that use gene transfer to enhance stature, endurance, muscle mass, weight, memory, learning rate and even hair follicle growth (Kiuru and Crystal, 2008).

A key challenge underlying most ethical discussions of gene enhancement is the difficulty in differentiating medical conditions from 'cosmetic' treatments. For example, many would argue that genetic interventions increasing height for patients with short stature arising from a medical condition should be considered a form of somatic gene therapy. In contrast, interventions that increase height so individuals may perform better in sport raises a variety of issues. Melman et al. presented an interesting Phase I clinical study whereby a DNA plasmid vector expressing the *hSlo* gene, a sub-unit of an ion channel, was evaluated in patients with erectile dysfunction(Melman et al., 2006). While some would question whether the use of gene transfer in this setting is ethical since this is not a life-threatening disorder, Arthur Caplan presented a commentary on the article asserting that quality of life is an important goal of gene therapy (Caplan, 2006). As he points out, a number of patients offered curative therapy for prostate cancer reject the cure when learning that a radical prostatectomy leads to impotence. Serious medical conditions are not always ones that have lethal consequences. Moreover, society will be faced with deciding who is the arbiter of quality of life, if it moves to restrict gene transfer or other treatments.

Genetic enhancements raise questions about fairness and access since those of privilege are mostly likely to have access to these treatments, which may then further their privilege status. Buchanan and co-authors argue that given the potential of gene transfer to improve the wellbeing of an individual, such research should be explored. (Buchanan et al., 2000) Some have questioned these conclusions because they may be based on a presumption of a fair society, but when placed in the context of a real society (such as the US which lacks universal health coverage), there is 'enormous justice-impairing potential' of genetic enhancements (Wenz, 2005). The concerns for increasing disparity are at several levels. First, there is concern that only those with financial means are likely to be able to seek such treatment. Second, if the treatments provide improved mental or physical capability, it will add additional advantage to those already advantaged. Thirdly, there is concern that enhancements will reset what is normal into an unattainable goal. For example, tall individuals will seek to become taller as the rest of society seeks genetic height enhancement. Moreover, it can redefine normal such that an individual currently considered normal could be considered disabled when compared to enhanced individuals.

A counterargument is the restriction of individual rights, specifically the right for an individual to improve their health or general status. Harris and Chan provide an interesting commentary in which they suggest that enhancement which betters the individual is good, 'whether it brings you level with others, sets you ahead or leaves you still behind but better off than you were' (Harris and Chan, 2008). They raise the question as to whether it is ethical to restrict an individual from making such a decision on their own behalf.

As with much of the other ethical issues in gene therapy, genetic enhancement arguments reflect wider struggles within society. In those countries where gene therapy projects are undertaken, society already regulates enhancement procedures; specifically government and insurance companies deny coverage for cosmetic procedures and other interventions that are not justified on medical grounds. In suggesting that gene transfer should be viewed differently than other medical and cosmetic procedures, some have argued that genetic interventions are lifelong and irreversible. These arguments have not taken into account that many types of gene transfer technologies, especially to somatic cells, are transient or that vectors have the potential to be designed with fail-safe mechanisms that can turn off their function.

Beginning with the earliest discussions of genetic enhancement, there has been concern that the technology will be used to alter intellect and moral behavior. As reviewed by Shamoo and Cole, the arguments put forward to ban genetic manipulation of these traits face ethical challenges if such treatments were banned outright (Shamoo and Cole, 2004). It would be hard to argue to ban genetic enhancements if there was no other treatment for medical conditions that result in decreased intellectual capacity or self-destructive behavior. As with other areas of debate regarding gene therapy, the discussion involves the distinction between disease and trait, or the concept of treating illness or promoting health (Shamoo and Cole, 2004; Malmqvist, 2006). When considering the use of gene transfer to increase intelligence or generate 'moral' individuals, the debate is theoretical. Even if the technology existed to provide gene transfer in a safe and effective manner, we would be many years away from understanding the genetic basis of intellect and morality. This disconnect between what is technically feasible and the science fiction scenarios' discussed by some bioethicists has led Guyer and Moreno to suggest focusing the ethical discussion on practical issues relevant to protecting patients (Guyer and Moreno, 2004).

SUMMARY

This chapter focuses on the ethical issues arising from two of the most exciting and ethically challenging areas of genetic research. These topics were often treated separately. We think the time has come to recognize that since both areas will be moving toward clinical application and therapy, there is a benefit to considering both from the perspective of safety, effectiveness and risk–benefit assessment.

ACKNOWLEDGEMENT

We are grateful for the helpful comments of Mervin C. Yoder, M.D., Ph.D. on an earlier version of this chapter.

REFERENCES

Anklesaria, P., Heald, A.E. , Mease, P.J., and Group, G.S. (2008) 'Intra-articular administration of a recombinant adeno-associated vector containing a TNF antagonist gene was safe, well tolerated and demonstrated trend in clinical response in subjects with inflammartory arthritis', *Molecular Therapy*, 16 (Supplement 1): S111.
Arkin, L.M., Sondhi, D., Worgall, S., Suh, L., Hackett, N., Kaminsky, S. et al. (2005) 'Confronting the issues of therapeutic misconception, enrollment decisions, and personal motives in genetic medicine-based clinical research studies for fatal disorders', *Human Gene Therapy*, 16: 1028–36.

Baylis, F. and Robert, J.S. (2004) 'The inevitability of genetic enhancement technologies', *Bioethics*, 18: 1–26.

Buchanan, A., Brock, D.W., Daniels, N. and Winkler, D. (2000) *From Chance to Choice, Genetics and Justice.* New York: Cambridge University Press.

Caplan, A. (2006) 'Commentary: Improving quality of life is a morally important goal for gene therapy', *Human Gene Therapy*, 17: 1164.

Caplan, A. (2008) 'If it's broken, shouldn't it be fixed? Informed consent and initial clinical trials of gene therapy', *Human Gene Therapy*, 19: 5–6.

Cook-Deegan, R. (1995) *The Gene Wars: Science, Politics, and the Human Genome.* New York: Norton & Co.

Council of Europe (CoE) (1982) *Parliamentary Assembly Recommendation 934 on Genetic Engineering.* Strasbourg: Council of Europe.

Dave, U.P., Jenkins, N.A. and Copeland, N.G. (2004) 'Gene therapy insertional mutagenesis insights', *Science*, 303: 333.

Edwards, S.J.L., Kirchin, S. and Huxtable, R. (2004) 'Research ethics committees and paternalism', *Journal of Medical Ethics*, 30: 88–91.

Feinberg, J. (1980) 'The child's right to an open future', in W. Aiken and H. LaFollette (eds), *Whose Child? Parental Rights, Parental Authority and State Power.* Totowa, NJ: Rowman and Littlefield, pp. 124–53.

Fuchs, M. (2006) 'Gene therapy. An ethical profile of a new medical territory', *Journal of Gene Medicine*, 8: 1358–62.

Guyer, R.L. and Moreno, J.D. (2004) 'Sloughing toward policy: Lazy bioethics and the perils of science fiction', *American Journal of Bioethics*, 4: W14–W17.

Hacein-Bey-Abina, S., von Kalle, C., Schmidt, M. et al. (2003) 'LMO2-associated clonal T cell proliferation in two patients after gene therapy for SCID-X1', *Science*, 302: 415–19 [erratum appears in *Science*, 2003; 302: 568].

Harris, J. and Chan, S. (2008) 'Understanding the ethics of genetic enhancement', *Gene Therapy*, 15: 338–9.

Kahn, J. (2008) 'Informed consent in human gene transfer clinical trials', *Human Gene Therapy*, 19: 7–8.

Kimmelman, J. (2007) 'Stable ethics: Enrolling non-treatment-refractory volunteers in novel gene transfer trials', *Molecular Therapy*, 15: 1904–6.

Kimmelman, J. and Palmour, N. (2005) 'Therapeutic optimism in the consent forms of phase 1 gene transfer trials: An empirical analysis', *Journal of Medical Ethics*, 31: 209–14.

Kiuru, M. and Crystal, R.G. (2008) 'Progress and prospects: Gene therapy for performance and appearance enhancement', *Gene Therapy*, 15: 329–37.

Kong, W.M. (2005) 'Legitimate requests and indecent proposals: Matters of justice in the ethical assessment of phase I trials involving patients', *Journal of Medical Ethics*, 31: 205–8.

Lemmens, T. and Waring, D.R. (eds) (2006) *Law and Ethics in Biomedical Research: Regulation, Conflict of Interest and Liability.* Toronto: University of Toronto Press.

Lombardo, A., Genovese, P., Beausejour, C. et al. (2007) 'Gene editing in human stem cell using zinc finger nucleases and integrase-defective lentiviral vector delivery', *Nature Biotechnology*, 25: 1298–306.

Malmqvist, E. (2006) 'The notion of health and the morality of genetic intervention', *Medicine, Healthcare & Philosophy*, 9: 181–92.

Melman, A., Bar-chama, N., McCullough, A., Davies, K. and Christ, G. (2006) 'hMaxi-K gene transfer in males with erectile dysfunction: Results of the first human trial', *Human Gene Therapy*, 18: 1165–76.

Meslin, E.M. (2008) 'The stem cell decade. What have we learned?', *Journal of Cardiovascular Translational Research*; doi: 10.1007/s12265-008-9027-z.

National Bioethics Advisory Commission (NBAC) (1999) *Ethical Issues in Human Stem Cell Research: Volume 1: Report and Recommendations.* Rockville, MD: NBAC. Available at http://bioethics.georgetown.edu/nbac/stemcell.pdf.

Okita, K., Ichisaka, T. and Yamanaka, S. (2007) 'Generation of germline-competent induced pluripotent stem cells', *Nature*, 448: 313–17.

Pattee, S.R. (2008) 'Protections for participants in gene therapy trials: A patient's perspective', *Human Gene Therapy*, 19: 9–10.

President's Commission for the Study of Ethical Problems in Medicine and Biomedical and Behavioral Research (1982) *Splicing Life: The Social and Ethical Issues of Genetic Engineering with Human Beings.* Washington, DC: PCSEPMBBR.

Puttagunta, P.S., Caulfield, T.A. and Griener, G. (2002) 'Conflict of interest in clinical research: Direct payment to the investigators for finding human subjects and health information', *Health Law Review*, 10: 30–2.

Raper, S.E., Chirmule, N., Lee, F. et al. (2003) 'Fatal systemic inflammatory response syndrome in an ornithine transcarbamylase deficient patient following adenoviral gene transfer', *Molecular Genetics and Metabolism*, 80: 148–58.

Resnik, D.B. and Langer, P.J. (2001) 'Human germline gene therapy reconsidered', *Human Gene Therapy*, 12: 1449–58.

Schwartz, P.H. and Meslin, E.M. (2007) 'New technique is a promising pathway to cures', *Indianapolis Star*, 23 December, p. E1.

Shamblott, M.J., Axelman, J., Wang, S., Bugg, E.M., Littlefield, J.W., Donovan, P.J. et al. (1998) 'Derivation of pluripotent stem cells from cultured human primordial germ cells', *Proceedings of the National Academy of Sciences USA*, 95: 13726–31.

Shamoo, A.E. and Cole, J. (2004) 'Ethics of genetic manipulations of behavior', *Accountability in Research: Politics and Quality Assurance*, 11: 201–14.

Silber, T.J. (2008) 'Human gene therapy, consent, and the realities of clinical research: Is it time for a research subject advocate?', *Human Gene Therapy*, 19: 11–13.

Stich, S.P. (1978) 'The recombinant DNA debate', *Philosophy and Public Affairs*, 7 (3): 187–205.

Thomson, J.A., Itskovitz-Eldor, J., Shapiro, S.S., Waknitz, M.A., Swiergiel, J.J., Marshall, S. et al. (1998) 'Embryonic stem cell lines derived from human blastocysts', *Science*, 282: 1145–7.

Urnov, F.D., Miller, J.C., Lee, Y-L. et al. (2005) 'Highly efficient endogenous human gene correction using designed zinc-finger nucleases', *Nature*, 435: 646–51.

Waddington, S.M., Kramer, M.G., Hernandez-Alcoceba, R. et al. (2005) 'In utero gene therapy: Current challenges and perspectives', *Molecular Therapy*, 11: 661–76.

Walters, L. and Palmer, J.G. (1997) *The Ethics of Human Gene Therapy*. New York: Oxford University Press.

Weiss, R. (2007) 'Patient in gene therapy study dies', *Washington Post*, 17 August, p. A12.

Wenz, P. (2005) 'Engineering genetic injustice', *Bioethics*, 19: 1–11.

Wernig, M., Meissner, A, Foreman, R. et al. (2007) 'In vitro reprogramming of fibroblasts into pluripotent ES-cell-like state', *Nature*, 448: 318–24.

Yu, J., Vodyanik, M.A., Smuga-Otto, K., et al. (2007) 'Induced pluripotent stem cell lines derived from human somatic cells', *Science*, 318: 1917–20; doi: 10.1126/science.1151526.

Zhou, Q., Brown, J., Kanarek, A. Rajagopal, J. et al. (2008) 'In vivo reprograming of adult pancreatic exocrine cells to ß-cells', *Nature*, 455: 627–32; doi: 10.1038/nature07314.

29

Ethics of Screening

Kris Dierickx

We are under no illusion that preventive strategies will be easy to implement. For a start, the costs of prevention have to be paid in the present, while its benefits lie in the distant future. And the benefits are not tangible – when prevention succeeds, nothing happens. Taking such a political risk when there are few obvious rewards requires conviction and considerable vision.

(Kofi Annan, Secretary General of the United Nations, 2000)

DEFINITION AND CHARACTERISTICS

The first official screenings took place at the end of the nineteenth century. At that time, a law was passed in the United States to reduce the immense immigration influx. This law excluded criminals, the poor, the insane and other unwanted people. The latter category also included the ill, which led to a rapid screening process by the Marine Hospital Service, the later US Public Health Service (Wilson, 1994). This initial screening was not accompanied by a final examination. The examination was conducted as scientifically as possible, in that the participants were not aware of the examination and they were not allowed to carry luggage at the moment of observation. Still the examination was to a certain extent inaccurate, resulting in a high amount of false positives and false negatives. There was equilibrium between the costs and benefits for the government, and an effective 'treatment' for the people with a positive test result, as they were sent back to their country of origin. Finally, most participants accepted the screening as the condition of entry set by the government. This cruel example of prescriptive screening for the benefit of the state contrasts sharply with the screening programs after the Second World War. The immigrant screening is in fact an example of multiple screening: one observer executed simultaneously a couple of subjective tests. The later so-called phased screening (for example, the screening of employees through blood and urine samples and through X-raying) is primarily focused on the wellbeing of the individual.

The example described in the previous paragraph already shows at least three important characteristics that are extremely relevant for our theme: (1) the importance of an accurate test (2) that is acceptable for the target group and (3) the importance of sensible proceedings. It is also clear that the term 'screening' covers different grounds. On the one hand, it can refer to tests carried out ad hoc on one individual in the context of a latent disease, if early detection can offer life-saving advantages. On the other hand, it can also refer to one single test applied to a population. We can now distinguish two kinds of screening. On the one hand, we distinguish systematic screening. In this situation, people from a larger population are encouraged to be screened for a particular disease at predetermined intervals, and follow-up procedures are offered to those who test positive. On the other hand, people can contact health services for screening not necessarily in the context of a health problem. In general, a screening of the general population is the responsibility of the public health services. However, the distinction between the two types of screening is not always clear.

There is no universally accepted definition of medical screening. However, according to Wald (1994) there is consensus on the following three elements. (1) It is a selection process to trace individuals with sufficiently high risk to acquire a certain condition to warrant further examination or (sometimes) immediate prevention. Often it is followed by a diagnostic test. (2) It is offered systematically to people who did not yet ask for medical assistance for the symptoms. When a medical screening is concerned, the initiative is most often taken by the health professionals of a country or a region and not by a patient with a medical complaint. (3) A medical screening's main aim is the wellbeing of the screened individuals. Therefore large-scale activities, for example examinations for recruitment, are usually not considered as medical screening. Because of the first characteristic many authors think there is an ethical difference between everyday medical practice and screening. If a patient asks a physician for help, the latter will do whatever she can to find the cause and help the patient. When a screening is concerned, the doctor is in an entirely different situation. She must be able to adequately proof that the screening can significantly change the natural development of the condition. The instance starting up a screening program has the moral duty to do good for the patient who participates in the program because of promises made (Cochrane and Holland, 1971; McCormick, 1994).

In this contribution we follow the definition of the Health Council of the Netherlands (2008): screening is a medical examination offered to people who initially have no health complaints, with, as an aim, the early detection or preclusion of a latently present condition, a genetic disposition or risk factors that increase the risk of a disease. Hence, we shall primarily focus on the ethical aspects of *population* screening (for examples of screening programs: see Table 29.1). Certainly, the ethical discussion surrounding ad hoc on-demand screenings is equally important. The possibilities for early detection and risk assessments that are offered to civilians outside the public health system are rising, specifically predictive medical assessments in the form of self-test. Moreover, there are important similarities between offering medical examination to an initially complaint-free population and the marketing of self-tests.

Table 29.1 Examples of screenings at several moments in life (Holland et al., 2006)

Period	Characteristic
Antenatal	Anaemia, blood group, RhD status, hepatitis B, spina bifida Down's syndrome
Neonatal	Phenylketonuria, bloodspot, congenital hypothyroidism, hearing impairment
Adults	Cervical cancer, breast cancer
Varia	Hypertension, vision loss, incontinence

THE WHO NORMATIVE FRAMEWORK AND ITS CRITICS

The central idea of early disease detection and treatment is essentially simple. However, the path to its successful achievement (on the one hand, bringing to treatment those with previously undetected disease and, on the other, avoiding harm to those persons not in need of treatment) is far from simple though sometimes it may appear deceptively easy. For this reason the World Health Organisation (WHO) published already in 1968 a number of principles (no dogmas) to be followed by screening programs (Wilson and Jungner, 1968) (see Table 29.2).

These criteria for a screening program have been developed and adapted by many authors and authoritative organisation, particularly with a view to developments in genetic and reproductive screening (e.g. American College of Medical Genetics, 2005; Andermann et al., 2008; Comité Consultatif, 1995; Council of Europe, 1994; Danish Council of Bioethics, 2001; Health Council of the Netherlands, 1994; Nuffield Council, 1993; UK National Screening Committee, 2009). All this work has produced a normative framework for the assessment of population studies that has broad international support, although some elements remain the subject of debate. These general principles can be summarised in five main ideas. First, screening must be focused on an important health problem. In literature it has often been emphasised that 'significance' can relate both to prevalence (common illnesses or conditions) and to severity. Second, the benefit: the purpose of screening is not the actual outcome of the test, but rather the ensuing health gain or other benefit to the person being tested. This means that the drawbacks that always exist as well should be smaller than the benefits. Third, the screening needs reliable and valid test methods.

Table 29.2 WHO principles for screening (Wilson and Jungner, 1968: 26–7)

1. The condition should be an important health problem.
2. There should be a treatment for the condition.
3. Facilities for diagnosis and treatment should be available.
4. There should be a latent stage of the disease.
5. There should be a test or examination for the condition.
6. The test should be acceptable to the population.
7. The natural history of the disease should be adequately understood.
8. There should be an agreed policy on who to treat.
9. The total cost of finding a case should be economically balanced in relation to medical expenditure as a whole.
10. Case-finding should be a continuous process, not just a 'once and for all' project.

Reliable means that that repetition of the test must give the same outcome (reproducibility); the validity means that the test must measure what it is supposed to measure. A distinction is made between analytical validity and clinical or diagnostic validity. The former is a description of the performance in a trial design in the laboratory, for example how often a test produces a positive (abnormal) result in the presence of the genetic mutation which is being sought (the genotype). The latter is important to see how often the test gives a positive result for individuals who have or develop the condition in question (the phenotype) and how often does it produce a negative (normal) result for people without that phenotype? Four, the respect for the autonomy as the actual translation of the requirement that the screening should be acceptable to the population. In the 1960s, the WHO did not mention the informed consent as a separate topic. However, most, if not all recent reformulations explicitly mention the importance of autonomy as the central concept in the contemporary field of medical ethics and law. Finally, there is the responsibility in terms of cost-effectiveness: it is important that the balance between the proceeds of a screening program, in terms of health gain or other worthwhile courses of action for those affected, and the costs incurred comes down on the positive side.

Researchers and authoritative organisations agree that more than four decades later this normative framework, as developed by Wilson and Jungner (1968), is future-proof. However, it is important that this normative framework as a whole should not be considered as a decision model that easily can be 'applied' and then will automatically lead to the right conclusion. The assessment of screening programs remains a complex exercise with room for different positions and hermeneutical approaches (Potter et al., 2008). Recent adaptations of these criteria have addressed ELSIs more directly by specifying additional issues such as psychosocial benefits and harms, impact on stakeholder groups, information choice, equity, discrimination and human dignity. Given the ethics perspective of this contribution, we will focus on the three following topics that are the object of discussion in the literature: benefit and harms, informed consent and autonomy.

FOR THE BENEFIT OF THE PARTICIPANT?

One of the basic principles of medical ethics is *primum non nocere*: at least do no harm. This principle of non-maleficence is one of the core elements of the WHO normative framework; the provision of screening can only be justified if it has been established that the benefits to the participants outweigh the ever-present drawbacks. This applies regardless of whether this is being provided through public or private channels. That principle requires continual, active confirmation.

Participation rates, often used as one of the markers of success of screening programs, are not an adequate marker of the success of a screening program (Irwig et al., 2006). The reason is that when screenings are accompanied by incentive payments to practitioners (such as in the UK and Australian cervical screening programs), they may undermine the provision of genuine choice to consumers. Also insurance companies give financial discounts for screening programs (Wald, 2007). Wald states that there is a culture in which judgements on medical screening are being made in the absence of evidence that a particular screening method is an effective and safe way of reducing morbidity and mortality from a specific disorder, as if one is unaware of publications on the principles of screening and the criteria for a worthwhile screening test. However, it is important that screening is subject to professional scientific assessment before it is promoted to the public. Identifying beneficial screening programs by appraising the evidence can be considered as the core of the WHO normative framework.

This is *a fortiori* true in the context of the following statement: all screening programs do harm; so do good as well, and, of these, some do more good than harm at reasonable cost (Gray et al., 2008). It is too often assumed that early detection always leads to a better prognosis. Or that, even if that is not necessarily the case, 'being informed as soon as possible' cannot do any harm. But the truth is that screening can do harm, and in most cases it does. In Malm's (1999) opinion there are at least three problems with the assumption that the earlier a disease is detected, the better it is for the patient. The first problem is that in some cases that assumption is false. For example for diseases with no, or only rarely successful, treatments very early detection may actually be worse for the patient because it forces him/her to know for a longer period of time that he/she has a disease about which little can be done. Second, even for diseases for which we know that very early detection facilitates treatment, one cannot determine whether this early detection is actually better *for the patient* until we take into account the double extra risks it involves. On the one hand, the risks of receiving unnecessary treatment or over-treatment: treatment the patient never would have received had he/she not been screened and from which he/she gained no benefit. Studies on prostate cancer, for example, indicate that +/– 75 percent of the cancers detected through PSA screening will never cause symptoms. So it might be worse for the patient by leading to surgery from which he/she derives no benefit. On the other hand the risk of receiving a procedure that, although it is the preferred method at the time of diagnosis, is later shown to be more aggressive or more damaging than was actually needed. For prostate cancer, for example, the standard surgery until recently left the patient frequently impotent and sometimes incontinent. Newly developed methods, however, have a much better chance of avoiding both outcomes.

The third and most significant problem for Malm is that even when the assumption is true, it cannot justify a screening recommendation. The reason is that the assumption only focuses on the benefits for the sick. But screening recommendations are given to vast numbers of people most of whom are not going to be *patients*. Thus the crucial question is whether any given person in the target population is better off being screened now rather than investigated later if but only if symptoms of disease appear. These latter risks and harms are far more likely to occur, but they are frequently ignored by proponents of screening. These risks are many and varied: the very minor risks and costs of the tests (physical discomfort, time lost, etc.); the psychological costs of screening that are difficult to calculate; the costs in terms of the time, money, and resources that divert from other medical endeavours, including research to improve available treatments.

These three problems do not imply that early detection via a screening is not meaningful. However, it is important to be aware that it cannot automatically be concluded that a particular screening program is beneficial on balance just because we know that a given disease is more successfully treated when it is detected in its pre-symptomatic stages. Offering screening is only responsible if it has been ascertained that the individuals being tested will definitely benefit.

In recent literature, there is a discussion on what should count as a benefit. The WHO states that screening for a condition for which there is no treatment is not beneficial and should not be offered. Later reformulations, however, do not exclude screening programs for conditions that are not treatable. Sometimes, as in the case of a genetic screening, the benefit of a screening can also lie in the 'reproductive choice based on an improved risk assessment' (Dutch Health Council, 1994; European Society of Human Genetics, 2003). The idea that 'benefit' also can mean that meaningful courses of action should be open for the participants implies a break with the initial normative framework of the WHO (Dutch Health Council, 2008). Referring to the central assumption that the benefits for the participants should outweigh the drawbacks, it is a reality. But in practice, in a screening with serious untreatable conditions, the balance will not easily shift to the 'benefits' side.

INFORMED CONSENT

Sound evidence that screening reduces mortality is necessary but not sufficient to justify screening. High-quality evidence that a reasonable proportion of participants would see the benefits as outweighing the harms is also important to decide to offer screening. Participants and professional practitioners should therefore receive balanced information about the different aspects of the screening. In what follows we will discuss the major aspects of this *informed* consent: whether doctors should inform patients about a screening; how much (and which) information has to be provided.

Around the world, different countries have screening programs for many diseases. Each one is surrounded by controversy. As already mentioned, much current information over-emphasises the benefits of screening, minimises the harms and does not clarify that there is a choice to be made about whether screening is worthwhile for them. Health information about screening tests provided by brochures often gives incomplete information and varies widely in quality (Schwartz and Meslin, 2008; Wald, 2006). Consequently, informed choice is difficult to achieve and screening has overwhelming uncritical public support (Burger and Kass, 2009). Before becoming a patient, a healthy individual deserves fully informed consent, with information provided at the individual and population level (Editorial, 2009). This is not always evident, as a screening program frequently entails many different and complicated aspects. Screening makes use of risk-assessment tests. They require considerable amounts of information and counseling, given the inability of many people (not only patients and consumers, but also professionals (Doukas, 2009) to deal with probability information. In the case of screening that tests for diverse conditions at the same time, and sometimes for a very large number of such conditions (multiplex testing), it soon becomes unfeasible to provide information about the individual conditions and results. This is not only for practical reasons, but also because of the problem of information overload. Little if any empirical research has been done into the feasibility of actual informed consent for multiplex screening. There are also several ways to describe the risks and benefits using absolute probabilities (absolute risk reduction, relative risk reduction)

(Schwartz and Meslin, 2008). In cases where there is no robust evidence, the participant may simply ask the physician: 'What would you recommend me to do?' However, the ethical basis for such a recommendation is unclear. It cannot be based on a judgement of beneficence because in many cases there is no proof of net benefit, and it cannot be based on patient autonomy, because the patient has not made a decision. And the professionals also have their own assumptions. Authors (Marshall, 1996) have categorised physicians' attitudes towards screening procedures as maximalist ('if in doubt, screen') or minimalist ('if in doubt, don't screen'). Schwartz (2007) states that in this situation it may be ethical in some cases for physicians to make a silent decision not to mention, for example, the PSA screening for prostate cancer to healthy men in the target group.

Given these complex issues, it is not surprising that the quality of the information is a challenge in many screening programs. There has been for example criticism of the quality of the informed consent in France's national program for serum screening for Down's syndrome ever since it was introduced in 1997. Recommendations for 'improving information to pregnant women' did not appear until 2005. But a recent publication indicates that information is still not up to standard (Favre et al., 2007).

It is recommended to enhance the precision with which invitations to participate in a screening program provide potential participants with information (Goyder, 2000; Haddow, 2000). Because there is rarely time to explain this information to patients one-to-one, one solution is to use teaching aids as an adjunct to the oral discussion (Marshall, 1996). Leaflets and other materials should provide information that individuals who are considering whether they wish to be screened *need* to know, so that they can make a fair decision. Providing details on what they *want* to know is necessary but secondary. The information should be quantitative and precise rather than general. In Wald's (2006) opinion, the six items probably needed in most information materials on screening are:

- the medical disorder being screened for, specifying the disorder in terms of the adverse health outcome that matters, and including background information, for example how common and serious the disorder is;
- the screening test: what is it, how is it done, whether it is painful of dangerous, the percentage of cases that are detected, and the percentage of unaffected individuals who will have positive results;
- the next steps: what happens if the screening test is positive (another screening test, a diagnostic test or direct preventive action);
- the health gain from screening in terms of the reduction in the risk of the specified medical disorder (e.g. breast cancer deaths, not that mammography detects most breast cancers);
- the adverse effects of the screening;
- the phone number of the local helpline.

Unless the patient has adequate understanding of these key aspects, he or she cannot give adequate informed consent. Some authors sail around these challenges regarding the information and state that one should give participants relatively little information, based on benevolent paternalism: physicians know what is best for their patients and giving too much information may cause them to reject a screening program that is good for them (Marshall, 1996). However, in most Western cultures a paternalistic approach is ethically unacceptable. Instead, it is generally accepted that patients should receive sufficient information to allow informed autonomous decisions.

FREE CONSENT

This free consent is one of the central principles of medical ethics. This principle of 'respect for autonomy' is on the one hand a condition of duty of care: the party providing screening must ensure that the informed consent requirement is met. But on the other hand, respect for autonomy is also important in terms of the screening provision itself. There are two sides on this. On the one hand, approaches from the health service offering a screening test can be perceived as a violation of personal integrity. The direct and personal invitation *per se* risks changing the individual's self-image: from the feeling of being healthy to the fear of being ill. The individual may also perceive the actual approach as compelling, as 'an offer you can't refuse' (Danish Council, 2001: 46). On the other hand, screening produces knowledge about an individual's health that will be useful to them in terms of the way they want to live their life. Looked at from this point of view, the value of screening is not limited to the health gain or other benefits that may result. From a broader perspective, another aspect of screening is that it increases individual autonomy (Dutch Health Council, 2008).

In the context of a screening program it should be recognised that the obtaining of apparently informed consent does not remove any responsibility for harm from those who offer screening (Shickle and Chadwick, 1994). The more one is responsible for the occurring of an event, the more one is responsible for the outcomes of the event (Malm, 1999). This responsibility expresses also one of the particular features of screening, as articulated by Cochrane and Holland (1971): 'We believe there is an ethical difference between everyday medical practice and screening. If a patient asks a medical practitioner for help, the doctor does the best he or she can. He/she is not responsible for defects in medical knowledge. If, however, the practitioner initiates screening procedures he/she is in a very different situation. He or she should, in our view, have conclusive evidence that screening can alter the natural history of disease in a significant proportion of those screened'.

SCREENING, SOCIETY AND ETHICS: WORK IN PROGRESS

Since the original formulation of the WHO criteria for screening, many evolutions have taken place. We already mentioned that originally informed consent was not explicitly listed in the normative framework. Today it is not only a key element that should be considered, it is by some also called the goal of a screening. This idea was amongst others expressed in the work done by the Dutch Health Council's genetic screening committee (1994), which stated that a condition of screening must be: 'to enable the participants to determine the presence or the risk of a disorder or carrier status, and [to enable them] to take a decision on the basis of that information'. This phraseology makes respect for autonomy much more than a condition of duty of care: it is the very purpose of screening, and so at the heart of the normative framework. We do not find this emphasis in the WHO the normative framework. But this refinement is an extension of the central tenet, which is implicitly present in the WHO work, that screening must on balance be favorable to the participants. The moral counterpart of the autonomy is personal responsibility for the individual's health. In Germany, for example, insurance providers are given the opportunity to offer financial incentives to policyholders who always attend the screening test appointments to which they are invited. Individuals who fail to do so and fall ill have to pay a higher contribution to their medical care (Schmidt, 2007).

In addition to the government-funded screenings new forms of screening are being offered such as CT scans that aim to detect specific diseases, and whole-body CT screening examines that aim to search for a wide range of possible diseases, health checks, general medical check-ups and home-collecting laboratory tests. These are individually-requested screenings that have not been recommended at the population level, but which are nonetheless sought by individuals or offered by physicians on an ad hoc basis. The demand for new tests and the growth of provision are not always, and certainly not for all parties concerned, accompanied by the thought (or even just the awareness) that screening can be harmful too. In the recent scientific and ethical literature attention is drawn to the inevitable conflict that arises between a professional and scientific (evidence-based) assessment of the benefits of screening and an attitude based on the views of the market and consumers (Burger and Kass, 2009).

These new forms of screening take place in a changing landscape where one observes an evolution from a governance-regulated healthcare to a healthcare that is increasingly driven by market forces. One of the major consequences of this move is that the different stakeholders do not necessarily have a common vision on how screening can contribute to a better healthcare, and how and by whom this can be achieved in the best way (Dutch Health Council, 2008; Rosenberg, 2009). It is not unthinkable that commercial interests would push a screening without any certain benefit and with unnecessary consumption of healthcare. Independent of the institutional healthcare sector, the Web offers all kinds of self-tests and home-collecting tests. The individual citizen is being approached as a consumer on healthcare. Consumers of healthcare with the ability to choose are likely to demand increasing amounts of screening tests, but this is unlikely to push provision towards cost-effectiveness and quality (Hoedemaekers, 2000).

CONCLUSION

More than four decades after the publication of the WHO normative framework on screening the discussion on the ethical aspects of screening is more than ever actual. The number of screenings is still increasing and many individuals have a growing interest in a screening. The fight against disease and pain is high on the agenda these days. Whether this attention and the massive deployment of resources devoted to it are objectively justified, currently remains an open question. These societal dynamics rather have to be considered as arising from society's obsession with uncertainty in late modernity. Ulrich Beck (1992: 49) thinks of these as typical symptoms of a risk society. Such a society, he argues, 'is no longer concerned with obtaining something "good", but rather with preventing the worst'. In this way of reasoning, the rise of preventive and predictive medicine fulfils a deep need of individuals and society. Health-risk knowledge is expected to give opportunities to prevent health problems in the future or to be able to manage health problems better, essentially by reducing the risk: the number of public and private screening initiatives is endless (Palmboom and Willems, 2009). However, risks are indissolubly connected with the human condition; since all living creatures are vulnerable and have a limited lifespan there will always be ten leading causes of death (Becker, 1993).

This need for reassurance as a motivation for the participation in screenings should not necessarily be considered as irrational or blind. Most persons participate in a screening because they hope to find nothing, or in the case of a positive result they certainly hope to hear that fortunately it has been picked up in time. However, a main challenge is constituted by the observation that screening might work as a system with no negative feedback so that a reasonable assessment of the drawbacks and benefits would not take place and participants and professional practitioners could think that screening only has benefits (Dutch Health Council, 2008). Therefore a responsible attitude of the initiators and a free and well-informed choice of the participants remains a condition *sine qua non* for a good screening. Hereby it is important on the one hand that the discussed normative framework is confirmed in practice, and on the other hand that the framework is kept appropriate and up to date by means of critical reflection and debate.

REFERENCES

American College of Medical Genetics (2005) *Newborn Screening. Toward a Uniform Screening Panel and System.* Washinton, DC: US Department of Health and Human Services, Maternal and Child Health Bureau.

Andermann, A., Blancquaert I., Beauchamp S., Déry, V. (2008) 'Revisiting Wilson and Jungner in the genomic age: A review of screening criteria over the past 40 years', *Bulletin of the World Health Organisation,* 86: 317–19.

Beck, U. (1992) *Risk Society: Towards a New Modernity.* London: Sage.

Becker, M.H. (1993) 'A medical sociologist looks at health promotion', *Journal of Health and Social Behavior,* 34: 1–6.

Burger, I.M. and Kass, N.E. (2009) 'Screening in the dark: Ethical considerations of providing screening tests to individuals when evidence is insufficient to support screening programmes', *American Journal of Bioethics,* 9: 3–14.

Cochrane, A.C. and Holland, W.W. (1971) 'Validation of screening procedures', *British Medical Bulletin,* 27: 3–8.

Comité consultatif national d'éthique pour les sciences de la vie et de la santé (1995) *Génétique et médecine: de la prédiction à la prévention. Avis. Rapports n° 46,* Paris.

Council of Europe (1994) *Screening as a Tool of Preventive Medicine,* No. R (94) 11. Strasbourg: Council of Europe.

Danish Council of Ethics (2001) *Screening: A Report.* Copenhagen: Danish Council of Ethics.

Doukas, D.J. (2009) 'Professional integrity and screening tests', *American Journal of Bioethics,* 9: 19–21.

Editiorial (2009) 'The trouble with screening', *The Lancet,* 373: 1223.

European Society of Human Genetics (2003) 'Population genetic screening programmes: Technical, social and ethical issues. Recommendations of the European Society of Human Genetics', *European Journal of Human Genetics,* 11: S5–S7.

Favre, D., Duchange, N., Vayssière, C., Kohler, M., Bouffard, N., Hunsinger, M.C. et al. (2007) 'How important is consent in maternal serum screening for Down syndrome in France? Information and consent evaluation in maternal serum screening for Down syndrome: A French study', *Prenatal Diagnosis,* 27: 197–205.

Goyder, E., Barratt, A. and Irwig, L.M. (2000) 'Telling people about screening programmes and screening test results: How can we do it better?', *Journal of Medical Screening,* 7: 123–6.

Gray, M., Patnick, J. and Blanks, R. (2008) 'Maximising benefit and minimising harm of screening', *British Medical Journal,* 336: 480–3.

Haddow, J.E. (2000) 'In search of better ways to transmit information about screening tests', *Journal of Medical Screening,* 7: 122.

Health Council of the Netherlands (1994) *Genetic Screening.* The Hague: Health Council of the Netherlands.

Health Council of the Netherlands (2008) *Screening: Between Hope and Hype.* The Hague: Health Council of the Netherlands.

Hoedemaekers, R. (2000) 'Commercial predictive testing: The desirability of one overseeing body', *Journal of Medical Ethics*, 26: 282–6.

Holland, W.W., Stewart, S. and Masseria, C., for the European Observatory on Health Systems and Policies (2006) *Screening in Europe*. Available at http://www.euro.who.int/Document/E88698.pdf.

Irwig, L., McCaffery, K., Salkeld, G., Bossuyt, P. (2006) 'Informed choice for screening: Implications for evaluation', *British Medical Journal*, 332: 1148–50.

McCormick, J. (1994) 'Health promotion: The ethical dimension', *The Lancet,* 344: 390–1.

Malm, H.M. (1999) 'Medical screening and the value of early detection. When unwarranted faith leads to unethical recommendations', *Hastings Center Report*, 29: 26–37.

Marshall, K.G. (1996) 'Prevention. How much harm? How much benefit? The ethics of informed consent for preventive screening programmes', *Canadian Medical Association Journal*, 155: 377–83.

Nuffield Council on Bioethics (1993) *Genetic Screening. Ethical Issues*. London: Nuffield Council on Bioethics.

Palmboom, G. and Willems, D. (2009) 'Risk detection in individual health care: Any limits?, *Bioethics,* epub ahead of print.

Potter, B.K., Avard, D., Graham, I.D., Entwistle, V.A., Caulfield, T.A., Chakraborty P. et al. (2008) 'Guidance for considering ethical, legal, and social issues in health technology assessment: Application to genetic screening', *International Journal of Technology Assessment in Health Care,* 24: 412–22.

Rosenberg, L. (2009) 'Does direct-to-consumer marketing of medical technologies undermine the physician–patient relationship?', *American Journal of Bioethics*, 9: 22–3.

Schmidt, H. (2007) 'Personal responsibility for health-developments under the German Healthcare Reform', *European Journal of Health Law*, 14: 241–50.

Schwartz, P.H. (2007) 'Silence about screening', *American Journal of Bioethics*, 7: 46–8.

Schwartz, P.H. and Meslin, E.M. (2008) 'The ethics of information: Absolute risk reduction and patient understanding of screening', *Journal of General Internal Medicine*, 23: 867–70.

Shickle, D. and Chadwick, R. (1994) 'The ethics of screening: Is "screeningitis" an incurable disease?', *Journal of Medical Ethics*, 20: 12–18.

UK National Screening Committee (2009) 'Criteria for appraising the viability, effectiveness and appropriateness of a screening programme'. Available at http://www.nsc.nhs.uk.

Wald, N.J. (1994) 'Guidance on terminology', *Journal of Medical Screening*, 1: 76.

Wald, N.J. (2006) 'Information leaflets in medical screening', *Journal of Medical Screening*, 13: 109.

Wald, N.J. (2007) 'Screening a step too far. A matter of concern', *Journal of Medical Screening*, 14: 163–4.

Wilson, J.M.G. (1994) 'Medical screening: From beginnings to benefits: A retrospective', *Journal of Medical Screening*, 1: 121–3.

Wilson, J.M.G. and Jungner, G. for the World Health Organisation (WHO) (1968) *Principles and Practice of Screening for Disease*. Geneva: World Health Organisation. Available at http://whqlibdoc.who.int/php/WHO_PHP_34.pdf.

30

Ethics of Clinical Telemedicine

Kenneth V. Iserson

INTRODUCTION

Telemedicine refers to the practice of medicine over a distance, including interventions, diagnostic and treatment decisions and recommendations. It can be in real time (e.g., emergency medical system (EMS), surgery) or delayed (e.g., radiology, dermatology, pathology). It includes separate or combined audio and video transmissions and can be performed either through mechanical (e.g., signal flags or lights) or electronic (e.g., telecommunications) means. The similar terms 'telecare' and 'telehealth' refer to the use of telecommunications, especially ongoing monitoring, to provide nursing and community support, as well as other public health services.[1][2]

As with many other new medical technologies, telemedicine has been put into service while it is still being evaluated for efficacy and safety. Yet it has not progressed as rapidly as expected. Its most common use is still the basic consultation via telephone and emergency medical system radios. Telemedicine will, however, inevitably progress as the technology becomes less complex, more commonly available, and less costly. By the time we understand many of the benefits and problems associated with telemedicine, technology will have stretched its reach far beyond current expectations and telemedical practice may have become, for better or worse, an integral part of biomedicine. This is why, while we still have time, we should assess and codify ethical behaviors associated with telemedical practice.[3]

Currently, little thought has been given to ethically based protocols to guide and regulate telemedical practice. Yet these issues represent some of the most significant barriers to telemedicine's widespread implementation. In part, this has been because those most involved in pursuing technological advances have actively pushed ethical issues aside. Said one telemedicine proponent, 'Up until now, [we] have been so impressed with what we could technically do that we had stopped thinking about how we should ethically be doing it.'[4] This attitude is not without precedent: As J. Robert Oppenheimer said,

'When you see something that is technically sweet, you go ahead and do it and you argue about what to do about it only after you have had your technical success. That is the way it was with the atomic bomb.'[5]

In this chapter, I will briefly review telemedicine's history and current status, highlighting some of the most rapidly evolving applications for closer examination. These include email communications between patients and clinicians; the transmission of visual media in specialties such as radiology, dermatology, pathology and ophthalmology; the use of telesurgery and robotic surgery; the telemonitoring of home-bound patients; and the use of telephone call centers and decision-support software.[6] Next, I will discuss telemedicine's unique aspects and the associated moral principles and ethical norms. Finally, we will arrive at these questions: Where should we go with telemedicine ethics? What action guides do we need, based on moral principles?

TELEMEDICINE: HISTORY AND FUTURE

Telemedicine has a fascinating history. In the early twentieth century, telephones were used to transmit electrocardiograms (ECGs) and electroencephalograms (EEGs); in 1920, the first medical advice service for seafarers using Morse code and voice radio was established.[7] The 1960s saw the use of two-way closed-circuit television to transmit medical images such as radiographs and for consultations between healthcare practitioners and patients. Other applications followed, including the transmission of pathology slides (telepathology), images of skin lesions, rashes and tumors (teledermatology) and radiographic images (teleradiology).[8 9 10 11 12 13 14] The monitoring of home-bound patients by telephone has become common, especially for geriatric patients.[15] Such transmissions may take place in 'real time' or via a 'store-and-forward' system. Recently, telesurgery, performing surgery in a remote operating room with the supervision of surgeons via video-conferencing systems,[16] and robotic surgery, performing surgical procedures using robots guided by real surgeons at the same or from a remote site, have become more common.[17 18]

Telemedicine in the industrialized world has had patchy success. Many pilot projects fail to sustain themselves once their seed funding runs out. This has impeded the widespread use of telemedicine. The most ambitious programs are costly to run, have low reimbursement and are highly complex. For example, most EMS and video-link telemedicine systems other than voice and email are pilot projects that collapse as soon as the funding erodes. (EMS has long used voice only, but that is not considered 'telemedicine.') For the most part, existing telemedicine services: (1) rely on volunteer specialist expertize; (2) perform only a few hundred cases per year; and (3) have stable referral rates.[19]

Successful telemedicine systems, meaning high use over time, use commonly available equipment and techniques, and thus are low-cost or well reimbursed. One system, emailing between patients and physicians, has become so common that it is often not considered telemedicine. Other successful applications are image store-and-forward systems (e.g., teleradiology, telepathology, teledermatology) and the use of call centers, where patients can discuss their symptoms with nurses who rely on computer-based decision algorithms to provide advice. All these systems use simple technologies and are financially viable: everyone involved profits from them (or seems to).

How has telemedicine fared in the developing world? In such countries there are many barriers to obtaining health care, so it is reasonable to suppose that telemedicine would be a useful technique. Yet only a fraction (0.1 percent in one estimate) of the potential demand for telemedicine is being met at present, and although much more system capacity is available, the demand is not growing rapidly. Given that it is often difficult in developing countries to obtain a second opinion, and that telemedical networks in these regions generally offer a free and often rapid service, why isn't the demand for this service accelerating?[20] Ethical elements inherent in current telemedical systems, including a possible lack of cultural sensitivity, might hold some of the answers, as described below.

TELEMEDICINE ETHICAL CODES

One barrier to the development of ethical codes specific to telemedicine is the belief that codes for telehealth personnel should be the same as those for all other healthcare workers.[21] And in practice, most telepractitioners today rely on their organizations' existing ethical codes or legal guidelines. Yet there are elements in telemedicine that are unique to this method of delivering medical services. This provides compelling reasons to have specific ethical codes for telehealth.

There are several oaths, codes and policies describing the ethics of telemedicine whose scopes extend beyond the local or regional level,[22][23][24][25][26] and we will refer to elements of these documents as we discuss specific ethical values. It is unclear, however, what effect ethical codes have had or are having on telemedical practice, especially if most are not mandatory. For example, the head of the European Commission charged with reviewing telemedicine policies, Professor Jean Claude Healy, said that Europe could not establish an overarching telemedicine code, although they could develop a code with the help of multiple partners to which practitioners could voluntarily subscribe.[27]

Ethical aspects unique to telehealth involve the use of informed consent (perhaps not always necessary), protection of confidentiality by professionals and non-professionals and privacy/security related to the handling of confidential electronic information.[28] We will review these aspects, as well as issues that fall under the rubric of non-maleficence: adequate equipment, competent practitioners and cultural sensitivity. Other topics include those related to beneficence (actually helping patients); autonomy (informed consent); professionalism, including patient–physician relations and licensing and oversight; medical practice on the receiving end of a telemedical transmission; and distributive justice (cost/financial viability).

CONFIDENTIALITY AND PRIVACY/SECURITY

The terms confidentiality and privacy are often confused and/or misused when discussing telemedical ethics. Confidentiality, as noted in the Hippocratic Oath, means to refrain from divulging information (personally or electronically) to others not involved with a patient's care. Privacy, which overlaps with security in telemedicine, means to keep information secure from those without right of access, during both transmission and storage.

In general, the practice of telemedicine does not appear to raise any new policy issues regarding confidentiality. Healthcare facilities should have a confidentiality policy in place, and this policy should include a clear statement of the confidentiality expectations of all staff providing telehealth services. It should address access to, and the transmission of, patient and staff information, and cover not only clinicians, but also the non-clinical staff, such as technicians, camera operators, etc., whose participation is a unique aspect of telemedicine. This statement should also detail the consequences of breaching confidentiality and of misusing patient or staff information. The policies and procedures must continually be updated to reflect changes in technology and in telehealth practices.[29] [30] [31]

The privacy and security of telemedical information is a major concern for patients, medical organizations, and governments.[32] [33] [34] [35] Britain's General Medical Council, for example, stated that when clinicians are responsible for confidential electronic information, they must make sure that it is effectively protected against improper disclosure when it is transmitted, received, disposed of or stored.[36] Storage or transmission methods may be used only where confidentiality and security can be guaranteed.[37] [38]

Unique privacy elements include doing telecare in a private area away from a shared patient care area; maintaining security while sending information across organizational, facility and system boundaries; and restricting the people present during telecare while also assuring that essential non-clinical, technical personnel will maintain patient privacy and confidentiality.[39]

Each transmission mode presents its own challenges in developing technical privacy safeguards and is vulnerable to security breaches. For example, one telegeriatric system found that as technology advanced, best attempts at security failed, and practitioners had to implement additional technological safeguards to protect their information.[40] Unfortunately, at present there are no uniform privacy standards that everyone can follow. Such standards should be developed in keeping with the total electronic communication environment.[41]

Security stems from organizational policies and practices. Organizations need, and usually have, policies governing the privacy, confidentiality and security of health information. These policies should clearly state the types of information considered confidential, the people authorized to release information, the procedures that must be followed in making a release, and the types of people who are authorized to receive this information. The policy should include the use of anonymized health information for research and public health needs.[42]

Two additional policy elements are vital: patient recourse for privacy breaches and system-wide security assessments. Patients have the right to recourse when they suspect a breach in the privacy of their health information. Moreover, most hospitals have not instituted routine assessments to determine whether their existing telehealth service security is adequate.[43] Failure to protect privacy should result in sanctions imposed by professional organizations and institutions. The lack of such enforcement mechanisms has fueled skepticism about telemedicine's legitimacy as a means of patient care.[44]

NON-MALEFICENCE: EQUIPMENT, COMPETENCY AND CULTURAL SENSITIVITY

Equipment

The clinician directing a telemedical encounter is responsible for ensuring that the systems are adequate to the task, function properly and provide accurate data.[45] [46] These include systems for history taking and viewing the patient, monitoring and examining patients (remote blood pressures, digital stethoscopes, digital ECG monitors and pulse-oxymeters), and transmitting static data (ECG, radiographs, photographs and slide images).[47] Telesurgery and robotic surgery require a higher level of consistently accurate and uninterrupted function.

Telemedicine need not involve cutting-edge, sophisticated technology. Combining the telephone with the use of computer algorithms has interposed patient call centers between physicians and their patients. The risks to patients from using computers with algorithm-based clinical protocols to make clinical decisions are still unknown. Any decision-support software that guides recommendations to patients must be demonstrably accurate. Clinicians using or providing this information should treat it no differently than information obtained from any other piece of diagnostic equipment – that is, as a tool for maximizing their ability to receive and process information. The imperfect nature of human–machine interaction and the limitations of the information made available in a distant medical encounter all conspire to make the use of decision-support systems, particularly within call centers, problematic.[48]

Telesurgery, the cutting edge of telemedical treatment, is when a surgeon participates in a surgical case without being physically present in the operating room. While still uncommon, this can be accomplished by giving voice or video instructions to a less experienced surgeon while he is performing the procedure or to a preprogrammed or responsive surgical robot without another surgeon in the room. The latter process was dramatically demonstrated in 2001 when a surgeon in New York performed a cholecystectomy on a patient in Strasburg, France, in faster than normal time and without complications. Since robotic surgery with an operating surgeon in the room is becoming more common in cardiac, gastric, urologic and neurosurgery, we may eventually perform telesurgery using robots at distant sites in these specialties as well.

The ultimate goal of telesurgery is to make surgical expertize available to patients who, for whatever reason, are inaccessible geographically (e.g., in a remote rural area or in outer space), environmentally (e.g., a battlefield or the scene of a nuclear accident), or due to danger to the surgical team or to the patient (e.g., radioactive contamination, contagious disease, or an immunodeficient patient).[49]

The primary ethical stricture is that doctors who perform medical interventions via telemedical techniques are responsible for those interventions, including the equipment's operation and the presence of sufficient and adequately trained personnel to care for the patient during and after the procedure.[50] They must also ensure that all personnel, including non-physician providers and technicians, are adequately supervised and have the competence and qualifications to work in a telemedicine system.[51]

Competence

Success with telemedicine depends as much upon the clinician's skills as it does upon the reliability and suitability of the technical parts of a telemedicine system.[52] A doctor practicing telemedicine is responsible for the appropriate quality of his/her services.[53] Yet in developing countries, telemedical advice is usually provided by experts from elsewhere, who often lack local knowledge of a particular disease or condition.[54] The ethical rule-of-thumb for teleconsultants is to give only advice of which they are certain, to admit when they lack sufficient knowledge or information, and to be willing to direct recipients to other sources if necessary.[55]

Cultural sensitivity

Telemedical practitioners must be sensitive to the cultures of patients and their families and of other clinicians with whom they interact. During such interactions, telemedical clinicians should always disclose who is in the room; maintain respect for all present; remember that they are guests in the patients' homes (e.g. tele-homecare); withhold personal opinions; reserve unnecessary questions; respect patients' readiness to receive information; respect cultural diversity; and practice good manners, such as not interrupting or talking to others during presentations.[56]

When interacting with other clinicians, and especially when providing international consultations to the developing world, teleclinicians must be sensitive to the situations of the clinicians with whom they work. A lack of sensitivity may be one reason why the demand for telemedical services is stagnant in the developing world. Teleconsultants may not understand: (1) the problematic nature of asking for help, which may be viewed as a 'failure' by the physician and his patient; (2) the requesting physician's busy, if not overwhelming, schedule; (3) the requesting physician's (or the country's) perceived loss of control over medical care; and (4) a perceived lack of respect due to cultural and economic differences. Whether telemedical systems and practitioners are culturally sensitive may determine whether or not the system survives and grows.[57]

BENEFICENCE: ACTUALLY HELPING PATIENTS?

All other ethical questions pale beside that of whether telemedicine interactions or systems actually help patients. Home health care using telemedicine, for example, has been shown to benefit patients by reducing the length of hospital stays, avoiding unnecessary admissions, reducing the need for elderly patients to make what are often arduous journeys to clinics and hospitals for evaluation – and likewise limiting the need for clinicians and ambulances to visit homes.[58] [59] Good evidence also confirms the effectiveness of home-healthcare telemedicine in managing patients with heart failure and other cardiac conditions, and patients with psychiatric diseases. It may also help with high-risk pregnancy monitoring and smoking cessation; the data on patients with diabetes are mixed.[60] [61]

The availability of new technologies, however, should not preclude their thoughtful application. Highly technical telemedicine interventions may waste scarce healthcare resources that could better be used elsewhere. For example, after the 1988 Armenian earthquake, tel-ecommunications equipment and personnel benefitted approximately 54 patients in a region with more than 100,000 casualties. The reasonable question is: might these resources have produced a greater health benefit if they had been used in more conventional ways?[62]

AUTONOMY: INFORMED CONSENT

The issue of patient autonomy is often raised when discussing telemedical ethics. Informed consent for health care via telehealth is unique; it requires a specifically adapted form of telehealth-specific consent. Organizations should have procedures to explain to the patient what is going to happen; how medical expertize will be used; that they will be in front of a television; that they have a right not to do this via telehealth; who might be participating at the other end; and whether they consent to the taping of the proceedings.[63]

Although informed consent is often spoken of as being generic for telemedicine, the following scenarios will, necessarily, lead to either informed consent, presumed consent or no consent.[64]

- Providers doing a consultation or performing an elective procedure via telemedicine remain the paradigm models of telemedicine. These require informed consent, which recognizes the unique risks involved. This should include a disclosure of everyone present in both studios, and the identification of all members participating in the consultation at both sites (those not directly involved should leave).[65]
- When the consultation is done under emergency circumstances, such as during a disaster or in the field by EMS personnel, there is no requirement other than implied consent, i.e., the patient does not try to flee or stop the consultation.
- When a patient makes direct contact with a provider for information or consultation by telephone (but increasingly via email), this action constitutes presumed consent, i.e., their actions demonstrate their willingness to proceed.
- Physicians or other healthcare providers transmitting data, such as radiographic, dermatologic or pathology images for consultation with other physicians, require no consent if it is in the course of providing patient care. This is no different from one clinician asking another in geographic proximity for an expert opinion. If the images are being transmitted for other purposes, such as teaching or research, informed consent is required consistent with the purpose. The doctor who asks for another doctor's advice remains responsible for treatment options and other recommendations given to the patient.[66]

OTHER ISSUES

Five additional issues may ultimately determine the role of telemedicine within healthcare: (1) the physician–patient relationship; (2) oversight of practitioners and systems; (3) system and practitioner responsiveness; (4) competence levels on the receiving end of telemedical consults; and (5) costs and financial viability.

Physician–patient relationships

What clinician–patient relationship exists in telemedical encounters? When practicing telemedicine directly with the patient, the doctor involved in giving his or her expert opinion assumes responsibility for the case in question.[67] Telesurgery, whether through another surgeon or a surgical robot, involves an explicit relationship. Similarly, email and telephonic communications between clinicians and their patients establish this relationship.

Unfortunately, telemedical encounters for history taking do not necessarily enhance the physician–patient relationship. They are generally short, one-sided physician discourses that reinforce patient marginalization. To counter this, we should develop telemedical guidelines emphasizing the importance of doctors establishing a face-to-face relationship with patients before resorting to telemedical interactions.[68 69]

The existence of a physician–patient relationship is less clear when working through other requesting clinicians, especially in cases when only data (radiographs, images) are being interpreted. One question that has still to be answered – and is seldom raised – is whether providing a telemedical consultation establishes enough of a physician–patient relationship that the consultant must accept the patient in transfer if that is appropriate.

Licensure/oversight

New medical techniques and technologies often lack appropriate oversight to maximize patient safety.[70] That has led to the often confusing discussion of physician licensure for telemedicine. Licensing telemedicine practitioners is important to ensure adequate oversight. Some questions that arise in the debate are: Should such licensing be specific for telemedicine or is a clinician's general medical license sufficient? Should licenses be valid locally, regionally (state, province), nationally or internationally?

One medical association incorporated these ideas, writing:

> Physicians practicing telemedicine must be authorized to practice medicine in the country or state in which they are located and must be competent in the field of medicine in which they are practicing it. When practicing telemedicine directly with the patient, the doctor must be authorized to practice medicine in the state where the patient is normally resident or the service must be internationally approved.[71]

Another telemedicine code encourages appropriate oversight, credentialing and licensing of telemedicine practitioners, including promptly reporting any misuse of telemedical services.[72]

Professionalism

For telemedical systems to be professional, to survive and to meet users' needs, practitioners must give reasonable priority to these consultations, giving telemedicine patients at least the same priority as they would receive in more traditional treatment systems.[73 74]

Receivers

The ethical duty of non-maleficence requires that clinicians who supervise systems which provide complex clinical advice have some assurance that the receiving clinicians accurately receive and are competent to safely use the information. Ethical rules governing this are: (1) patient treatment information must be easily retrievable;[75] (2) information should be transmitted only to those who have the capability of carrying out the necessary interventions, or to ensure safe and reliable patient transfers; (3) receivers must use the information provided in a responsible manner, without overstating their capabilities or understanding of the facts; and (4) initial receivers must make telemedicine information available to others caring for the patient.[76]

Distributive justice and system viability

The most complex telemedical systems are often financially non-viable without external support – usually because they follow ethical rules related to distributive justice. These include: (1) promoting telemedicine services only to those who need them; (2) not using telemedicine services to promote unnecessary transfers to the base institution; (3) rejecting exorbitant reimbursement for telemedicine services or any kickbacks for getting or giving referrals; (4) promoting wide access to telemedicine services for those areas in need of them; (5) providing telemedicine services without charge to those who cannot pay; and (6) providing telemedicine services and information without regard for a receiving practitioner's or patient's race, creed or nationality.[77] With the vast number of people lacking access to quality health care, fairness suggests that external support should be provided in situations in which telemedicine is beneficial and necessary.

CONCLUSION

Before initiating or continuing a telemedical system, we must ask whether a clear case can be made for its implementation based upon clinical need, cost-benefit analysis or improving the quality of a health service. In the past, we have made the mistake of rushing to adopt technologies without considering their moral implications. Today, we have the time – but not much time – to reflect.

While telemedicine's future remains obscured behind the hazy promise of future developments, we must look at the ethical implications of using both existing and potential technologies now. By doing this, we attain three goals: (1) we can have reasoned discussions before the practices are so entrenched that they cannot be easily changed and before vested interests are so strong that finance outweighs reason; (2) we can seek optimal ways to attain telemedicine's benefits for patients and practitioners; and (3) we can find ways to advance the technology while avoiding potential pitfalls that may corrupt and diminish our profession and our society.

We have opened the genie's bottle of telemedicine. Before we proceed further, we owe it to our patients and our profession to set ethical standards to guide our future as we use this powerful technology. Doing so may enable us to answer, for telemedicine, a basic question of modern bioethics: Just because we can, should we?

NOTES

1 Stanberry, B. (2001) 'Legal ethical and risk issues in telemedicine', *Computer Methods and Programs in Biomedicine*, 64: 225–33.

2 Iserson, K.V. (2000) 'Telemedicine: A proposal for an ethical code', *Cambridge Quarterly of Healthcare Ethics,* 9 (3): 404–6.

3 Ibid.

4 Stanberry, B. (2000) 'Telemedicine: Barriers and opportunities in the 21st century', *Journal of Internal Medicine*, 247: 615–28.

5 Oppenheimer, J.R. (1954) *In the Matter of J. Robert Oppenheimer*, USAEC Transcript of Hearing before Personnel Security Board, p. 81.

6 Stanberry, B. (2000) 'Telemedicine: Barriers and opportunities in the 21st century', *Journal of Internal Medicine*, 247: 615–28.

7 Amenta, F. and Rizzo, N. (1999) 'Maritime radiomedical services', in R. Wootton (ed.), *European Telemedicine 1998–99*. London: Kensington Publications, pp. 125–6.

8 Allaert, F.A., Weinberg, D., Dusseree, P., Yvon, P.J., Dusseree, L., Retaillau, B. et al. (1996) 'Evaluation of an international telepathology system between Boston (USA) and Dijon: Glass slides versus telediagnostic television monitor', *Journal of Telemedicine and Telecare*, 2 (1): 27–30.

9 Della Mea, V., Forti, S., Puglisi, F., Bellutta, P., Dalla Palma, P., Mauri, F. et al. (1996) 'Telepathology using Internet multimedia electronic mail: Remote consultation on gastrointestinal pathology', *Journal of Telemedicine and Telecare*, 2: 28–34.

10 Sanders, J.H. and Bashshur, R.L. (1995) 'Challenges to the implementation of telemedicine', *Telemed Journal*, 1 (2): 15–23.

11 Kirby, B., Lyon, C. and Harrison, P. (1998) 'Low-cost teledermatology using Internet image transmission', *Journal of Telemedicine and Telecare*, 4 (1): 107 [10] P.; Harrison, P., Kirby, B., Dickinson, Y. and Scholfield, R. (1998) 'Teledermatology – high technology or not?', *Journal of Telemedicine and Telecare*, 4 (1): 31–2.

12 Franken, E.A. Jr, Berbaum, K.S., Smith, W.L., Chang, P.J., Owen, D.A. and Bergus, G.R. 'Teleradiology for rural hospitals: Analysis of a field study', *Journal of Telemedicine and Telecare*, 1: 202–8.

13 Agius, A.A. and Mahmoud, M.S. (1996) 'A simple worldwide teleradiology system', *Journal of Telemedicine and Telecare*, 2 (1):109–11.

14 Eng, J., Mysko, W.K., Weller, G.E., Renard, R., Gitlin, J.N., Bluemke, D.A. et al. (2000) 'Interpretation of emergency department radiographs: A comparison of emergency medicine physicians with radiologists, residents with faculty, and film with digital display', *American Journal of Roentgenology*, 175 (5): 1233–8.

15 Doughty, K., Cameron, K. and Garner, P. (1996) 'Three generations of telecare of the elderly', *Journal of Telemedicine and Telecare*, 2 (2): 71–80.

16 Gul, Y.A., Wan, A.C.T. and Darzi, A. (1995) 'Use of telemedicine in undergraduate teaching of surgery', *Journal of Telemedicine and Telecare*, 5: 246–8.

17 Vanderheyden, L. (1999) 'Telesurgery: Surgery of the future?', in R. Wootton (ed.), *European Telemedicine 1998–99*. London: Kensington Publications, pp. 174–5.

18 Stanberry, B. (2001) 'Legal ethical and risk issues in telemedicine', *Computer Methods and Programs in Biomedicine*, 64: 225–33.

19 Wootton, R. (2008) 'Telemedicine support for the developing world', *Journal of Telemedicine and Telecare*, 14: 109–14.

20 Ibid.

21 Yeo, M. and Jennett, P. (2006) *National Initiative for Telehealth Guidelines Environmental Scan of Organizational, Technology, Clinical and Human Resource Issues – Section 3: Organizational Leadership Environmental Scan*. Calgary, Canada: Health Telematics Unit, Faculty of Medicine, University of Calgary.

Hogenbirk, J.C., Brockway, P.D., Finley, J., Jennett, P., Yeo, M., Parker-Taillon, D. et al. (2006) 'Framework for Canadian telehealth guidelines: Summary of the environmental scan', *Journal of Telemedicine and Telecare*, 12 (2): 64–70.

22 Iserson, K.V. (2000) 'Telemedicine: A proposal for an ethical code', *Cambridge Quarterly of Healthcare Ethics*, 9 (3): 404–6.

23 Finnish Medical Association (1997) *Ethical Guidelines in Telemedicine*. Available at www.laakariliitto.fi/e/ethics/telemed.html, accessed 16 May 2008.

24 American Medical Association (1996) *The Promotion of Quality Telemedicine* (Policy H-160.937). Available at www.wma.net/e/ethicsunit/whats_new.htm, accessed 16 May 2008.

25 World Medical Association (2007) *Statement on the Ethics of Telemedicine*. Adopted by the WMA General Assembly, Copenhagen, Denmark, October. Available at www.wma.net/e/policy/t3.htm, accessed 16 May 2008.

26 Yeo, M. and Jennett, P. (2006) *National Initiative for Telehealth Guidelines Environmental Scan of Organizational, Technology, Clinical and Human Resource Issues – Section 3: Organizational Leadership Environmental Scan*. Calgary, Canada: Health Telematics Unit, Faculty of Medicine, University of Calgary.

Hogenbirk, J.C., Brockway, P.D., Finley, J., Jennett, P., Yeo, M. et al. (2006) 'Framework for Canadian telehealth guidelines: Summary of the environmental scan', *Journal of Telemedicine and Telecare*, 12 (2): 64–70.

27 Stanberry, B. (2000) 'Telemedicine: Barriers and opportunities in the 21st century', *Journal of Internal Medicine*, 247: 615–28.

28 Yeo, M. and Jennett, P. (2006) *National Initiative for Telehealth Guidelines Environmental Scan of Organizational, Technology, Clinical and Human Resource Issues – Section 3: Organizational Leadership Environmental Scan*. Calgary, Canada: Health Telematics Unit, Faculty of Medicine, University of Calgary.

Hogenbirk, J.C., Brockway, P.D., Finley, J., Jennett, P., Yeo, M., Parker-Taillon, D. et al. (2006) 'Framework for Canadian telehealth guidelines: Summary of the environmental scan', *Journal of Telemedicine and Telecare*, 12 (2): 64–70.

29 Ibid.

30 World Medical Association (2007) *Statement on the Ethics of Telemedicine*. Adopted by the WMA General Assembly, Copenhagen, Denmark, October. Available at www.wma.net/e/policy/t3.htm, accessed 16 May 2008.

31 American Medical Association (1996) *The Promotion of Quality Telemedicine* (Policy H-160.937). Available at www.wma.net/e/ethicsunit/whats_new.htm, accessed 16 May 2008.

32 Stanberry, B. (2001) 'Legal ethical and risk issues in telemedicine', *Computer Methods and Programs in Biomedicine*, 64: 225–33.

33 *Ethical Guidelines in Telemedicine* (1997) Approved by the Executive Board of the Finnish Medical Association in 1997. Adopted by the Comité Permanent 12 April 1997. Available at www.laakariliitto.fi/e/ethics/telemed.html, accessed 16 May 2008.

34 Yeo, M. and Jennett, P. (2006) *National Initiative for Telehealth Guidelines Environmental Scan of Organizational, Technology, Clinical and Human Resource Issues – Section 3: Organizational Leadership Environmental Scan*. Calgary, Canada: Health Telematics Unit, Faculty of Medicine, University of Calgary.

Hogenbirk, J.C., Brockway, P.D., Finley, J., Jennett, P., Yeo, M., Parker-Taillon, D. et al. (2006) 'Framework for Canadian telehealth guidelines: Summary of the environmental scan', *Journal of Telemedicine and Telecare*, 12 (2): 64–70.

35 Tachakra, S., Mullett, S.T.H., Freij, R. and Sivakumar, A. (1996) 'Confidentiality and ethics in telemedicine', *Journal of Telemedicine and Telecare*, 2 (Supp. 1): 68–71.

36 General Medical Council (GMC) (UK) (1995) *Confidentiality – Guidance from the General Medical Council*. London: GMC.

37 *Ethical Guidelines in Telemedicine* (1997) Approved by the Executive Board of the Finnish Medical Association in 1997. Adopted by the Comité Permanent 12 April 1997. Available at www.laakariliitto.fi/e/ethics/telemed.html, accessed 16 May 2008.

38 Yeo, M. and Jennett, P. (2006) *National Initiative for Telehealth Guidelines Environmental Scan of Organizational, Technology, Clinical and Human Resource Issues – Section 3: Organizational Leadership Environmental Scan*. Calgary, Canada: Health Telematics Unit, Faculty of Medicine, University of Calgary.

Hogenbirk, J.C., Brockway, P.D., Finley, J., Jennett, P., Yeo, M., Parker-Taillon, D. et al. (2006) 'Framework for Canadian telehealth guidelines: Summary of the environmental scan', *Journal of Telemedicine and Telecare*, 12 (2): 64–70.

39 Ibid.

40 Pallawala, P.M.D.S. and Lun, K.C. (2001) 'EMR-based TeleGeriatric system', in V. Patel et al. (eds), *MEDINFO 2001*. Amsterdam: IOS Press.

41 Yeo, M. and Jennett, P. (2006) *National Initiative for Telehealth Guidelines Environmental Scan of Organizational, Technology, Clinical and Human Resource Issues – Section 3: Organizational Leadership Environmental Scan*. Calgary, Canada: Health Telematics Unit, Faculty of Medicine, University of Calgary.

Hogenbirk, J.C., Brockway, P.D., Finley, J., Jennett, P., Yeo, M., Parker-Taillon, D. et al. (2006) 'Framework for Canadian telehealth guidelines: Summary of the environmental scan', *Journal of Telemedicine and Telecare*, 12 (2): 64–70.

42 Ibid.

43 Ibid.

44 Silverman, R.D. (2003) 'Current legal and ethical concerns in telemedicine and e-medicine', *Journal of Telemedicine and Telecare*, 9 (Supp. 1): 67–9.

45 *Ethical Guidelines in Telemedicine* (1997) Approved by the Executive Board of the Finnish Medical Association in 1997. Adopted by the Comité Permanent 12 April 1997. Available at www.laakariliitto.fi/e/ethics/telemed.html, accessed 16 May 2008.

46 Iserson, K.V. (2000) 'Telemedicine: A proposal for an ethical code', *Cambridge Quarterly of Healthcare Ethics*, 9 (3): 404–6.

47 Pallawala, P.M.D.S. and Lun, K.C. (2001) 'EMR-based TeleGeriatric system', in V. Patel et al. (eds.), *MEDINFO 2001*. Amsterdam: IOS Press.

48 Stanberry, B. (2000) 'Telemedicine: Barriers and opportunities in the 21st century', *Journal of Internal Medicine*, 247: 615–28.

49 Ibid.

50 *Ethical Guidelines in Telemedicine* (1997) Approved by the Executive Board of the Finnish Medical Association in 1997. Adopted by the Comité Permanent 12 April 1997. Available at www.laakariliitto.fi/e/ethics/telemed.html, accessed 16 May 2008.

51 Iserson, K.V. (2000) 'Telemedicine: A proposal for an ethical code', *Cambridge Quarterly of Healthcare Ethics*, 9 (3): 404–6.

52 Stanberry, B. (2000) 'Telemedicine: Barriers and opportunities in the 21st century', *Journal of Internal Medicine*, 247: 615–28.

53 *Ethical Guidelines in Telemedicine* (1997) Approved by the Executive Board of the Finnish Medical Association in 1997. Adopted by the Comité Permanent 12 April 1997. Available at www.laakariliitto.fi/e/ethics/telemed.html, accessed 16 May 2008.

54 Wootton, R. (2008) 'Telemedicine support for the developing world', *Journal of Telemedicine and Telecare*, 14: 109–14.

55 Iserson, K.V. (2000) 'Telemedicine: A proposal for an ethical code', *Cambridge Quarterly of Healthcare Ethics*, 9 (3): 404–6.

56 Yeo, M. and Jennett, P. (2006) *National Initiative for Telehealth Guidelines Environmental Scan of Organizational, Technology, Clinical and Human Resource Issues – Section 3: Organizational Leadership Environmental Scan*. Calgary, Canada: Health Telematics Unit, Faculty of Medicine, University of Calgary.

Hogenbirk, J.C., Brockway, P.D., Finley, J., Jennett, P., Yeo, M., Parker-Taillon, D. et al. (2006) 'Framework for Canadian telehealth guidelines: Summary of the environmental scan', *Journal of Telemedicine and Telecare*, 12 (2): 64–70.

57 Wootton, R. (2008) 'Telemedicine support for the developing world', *Journal of Telemedicine and Telecare*, 14: 109–14.

58 Ibid.

59 Pallawala, P.M.D.S. and Lun, K.C. (2001) 'EMR-based TeleGeriatric system', in V. Patel et al. (eds.), *MEDINFO 2001*. Amsterdam: IOS Press.

60 Bensink, M., Hailey, D. and Wootton, R. (2007) 'A systematic review of successes and failures in home telehealth. Part 2: Final quality rating results', *Journal of Telemedicine and Telecare*, 13 (Supp. 3): 10–14.

61 DelliFraine, J.L., Kathryn, H. and Dansky, K.H. (2008) 'Home-based telehealth: A review and meta-analysis', *Journal of Telemedicine and Telecare*, 14: 62–6.

62 Houtchens, B.A., Clemmer, T.P., Holloway, H.C., Kiselev, A.A., Logan, J.S., Merrell, R.C. et al. (1993) 'Telemedicine and international disaster response: Medical consultation to Armenia and Russia via a Telemedicine Spacebridge', *Prehospital and Disaster* Medicine, 8: 57–66.

63 Yeo, M. and Jennett, P. (2006) *National Initiative for Telehealth Guidelines Environmental Scan of Organizational, Technology, Clinical and Human Resource Issues – Section 3: Organizational Leadership Environmental Scan*. Calgary, Canada: Health Telematics Unit, Faculty of Medicine, University of Calgary.

Hogenbirk, J.C., Brockway, P.D., Finley, J., Jennett, P., Yeo, M., Parker-Taillon, D. et al. (2006) 'Framework for Canadian telehealth guidelines: Summary of the environmental scan', *Journal of Telemedicine and Telecare*, 12 (2): 64–70.

64 Iserson, K.V. (2000) 'Telemedicine: A proposal for an ethical code', *Cambridge Quarterly of Healthcare Ethics*, 9 (3): 404–6.

65 Yeo, M. and Jennett, P. (2006) *National Initiative for Telehealth Guidelines Environmental Scan of Organizational, Technology, Clinical and Human Resource Issues – Section 3: Organizational Leadership Environmental Scan*. Calgary, Canada: Health Telematics Unit, Faculty of Medicine, University of Calgary.

Hogenbirk, J.C., Brockway, P.D., Finley, J., Jennett, P., Yeo, M., Parker-Taillon, D. et al. (2006) 'Framework for Canadian telehealth guidelines: Summary of the environmental scan', *Journal of Telemedicine and Telecare*, 12 (2): 64–70.

66 *Ethical Guidelines in Telemedicine* (1997) Approved by the Executive Board of the Finnish Medical Association in 1997. Adopted by the Comité Permanent 12 April 1997. Available at www.laakariliitto.fi/e/ethics/telemed.html, accessed 16 May 2008.

67 Ibid.

68 Irvine, R. (2005) 'Mediating telemedicine: Ethics at a distance', *Internal Medicine Journal*, 35: 56–8.

69 World Medical Association (2007) *Statement on the Ethics of Telemedicine*. Adopted by the WMA General Assembly, Copenhagen, Denmark, October. Available at www.wma.net/e/policy/t3.htm, accessed 16 May 2008.

70 Iserson, K.V. and Chiasson, P.M. (2002) 'The ethics of applying new medical technologies', *Seminars in Laparoscopy*, 9 (4): 222–9.

71 *Ethical Guidelines in Telemedicine* (1997) Approved by the Executive Board of the Finnish Medical Association in 1997. Adopted by the Commité Permanent 12 April 1997. Available at www.laakariliitto.fi/e/ ethics/telemed.html, accessed 16 May 2008.

72 Iserson, K.V. (2000) 'Telemedicine: A proposal for an ethical code', *Cambridge Quarterly of Healthcare Ethics*, 9 (3): 404–6.

73 Yeo, M. and Jennett, P. (2006) *National Initiative for Telehealth Guidelines Environmental Scan of Organizational, Technology, Clinical and Human Resource Issues – Section 3: Organizational Leadership Environmental Scan.* Calgary, Canada: Health Telematics Unit, Faculty of Medicine, University of Calgary.

Hogenbirk, J.C., Brockway, P.D., Finley, J., Jennett, P., Yeo, M., Parker-Taillon, D. et al. (2006) 'Framework for Canadian telehealth guidelines: Summary of the environmental scan', *Journal of Telemedicine and Telecare*, 12 (2): 64–70.

74 Iserson, K.V. (2000) 'Telemedicine: A proposal for an ethical code', *Cambridge Quarterly of Healthcare Ethics*, 9 (3): 404–6.

75 Yeo, M. and Jennett, P. (2006) *National Initiative for Telehealth Guidelines Environmental Scan of Organizational, Technology, Clinical and Human Resource Issues – Section 3: Organizational Leadership Environmental Scan.* Calgary, Canada: Health Telematics Unit, Faculty of Medicine, University of Calgary.

Hogenbirk, J.C., Brockway, P.D., Finley, J., Jennett, P., Yeo, M., Parker-Taillon, D. et al. (2006) 'Framework for Canadian telehealth guidelines: Summary of the environmental scan', *Journal of Telemedicine and Telecare*, 12 (2): 64–70.

76 Iserson, K.V. (2000) 'Telemedicine: A proposal for an ethical code', *Cambridge Quarterly of Healthcare Ethics*, 9 (3): 404–6.

77 Ibid.

31

Ethical, Legal and Social Issues in Brain Death and Organ Transplantation: a Japanese Perspective

Tsuyoshi Awaya

INTRODUCTION: BRAIN DEATH AND ORGAN TRANSPLANTATION AS A PANDORA'S BOX

Brain death and organ transplants have generated not just medical issues but various other controversies including philosophical questions directly linked to life, or general or specific ethical, legal and social issues.[1] These issues highlight important principle questions such as the following: What is life and death? This is an age-old question. Is brain death human death?[2] Should we promote organ transplantation?[3] Where does the limit of organ transplantation lie? In other words, up to what extent can we allow organ transplantation?[4] Can we use organs that are collected from special sources such as anencephalic infants, people who have died from euthanasia, people who killed themselves or executed prisoners? Can we set a proprietary right on organs?[5] Is the selling or buying of organs allowed? How should we consider 'resourcialization' and commodification of the human body?[6] The issues have also generated practical questions such as the following: How can we prevent organ shortage? How should we distribute organs? What is the appropriate method to express willingness to donate organs: 'opting in' or 'opting out'?

Brain death and organ transplantation have been a veritable Pandora's box and thus created various kinds of problems. I leave aside thorough discussion of these general issues in other articles; but against this backdrop, I present the ethical, legal and social issues surrounding brain death and organ transplantation, particularly in Japan.

HISTORICAL BACKGROUND AND LEGISLATIVE PROCESS OF ORGAN TRANSPLANTATION IN JAPAN

In Japan, organ transplantation began with a cornea transplant in 1949, although the cornea was not medically recognized as an organ. In 1957, cornea transplantation was criticized by society, and the ophthalmic surgeon who performed the operations faced a criminal charge but was exempted from prosecution. This triggered the enactment of the Law on Cornea Transplantation in 1958. The law set the conditions and procedures for eyeball removal from cardiac dead bodies, which did not require the consent of donors but simply that of bereaved family members, if any.

Kidney transplantation was first performed in 1955 and the Law on Cornea and Kidney Transplantation was enacted in 1979. This Law on Cornea and Kidney Transplantation extended the Law on Cornea Transplantation to cover kidney transplantation from cardiac dead bodies, but still did not ask for the donor's consent and required only the bereaved family's written permission.

Cardiac transplant was first performed in 1968. At first, society positively accepted the operation, but later raised huge social problems regarding, for example, the certainty of the death of the donor or the necessity of the transplant for the recipient. A criminal charge was filed against the surgeon who performed the operation, but the case was dropped because of lack of evidence.[7] For about 30 years after that, cardiac transplantation was not carried out in Japan and only in 1999 was it resumed. Lung transplantation was first performed in 1965 and liver transplantation in 1989.

The law for the regulation of donation and transplantation of general organs such as heart, lung, liver and kidney was enacted in 1997 and that is the current Law on Organ Transplantation. The law allowed organ removal from dead bodies, including brain dead bodies (as explained below). According to the Law on Organ Transplantation, organ transplantation requires the donor's consent, as well as the absence of refusal by the donor's family (Section 6, Subsection 1: The exact wording is given in the next part). The law also prohibits the selling and buying of organs, i.e. receipt or provision of financial profit for the donation of organs (including organs from living bodies) for transplantation (Section 11). It imposes a penalty on violators, namely imprisonment for up to 5 years, fines up to 5 million yen, or both (Section 20, Subsection 1). Japanese citizens who violate the law in foreign countries can also be punished (Section 20, Subsection 2).

With regard to willingness to donate organs, the 'Guideline for the Operation of the Law on Organ Transplantation' states that the expression of the will of people aged 15 or older shall be deemed effective. According to this rule, in Japan it was impossible for children under 15 years of age to donate their organs. However, this age limit was abolished by the amendment in July 2009 of the Law on Organ Transplantation (enforcement: July 2010). To be precise, according to an additional, so-called 'opting-out' system, the consent of parents alone, without the consent of children, became sufficient to enable pediatric donation.

LAWMAKING AND DISCUSSIONS IN JAPAN ABOUT BRAIN DEATH

Lawmaking in Japan about brain death

As mentioned above, the current Law on Organ Transplantation in Japan was enacted in 1997. In enacting the law, discussions focused not on transplantation itself but mostly on brain death issues, i.e. whether or not brain death is human death. Brain death issues have probably been discussed more actively in Japan than anywhere else in the world. As a result of these discussions, the final form of the law was enacted as follows:

> In cases where a deceased person has, during his/her lifetime, expressed his/her will in writing to donate his/her organs for the purposes of transplantation, a physician may remove organs from the dead body (including the body of a brain dead person; the same shall apply hereinafter) in order to carry out transplantation in accordance with this law if the bereaved family of the deceased, receiving notice of the said expression, are not opposed to such removal, or if the deceased has no bereaved family. (Section 6, Subsection 1) The body of a brain dead person, as referred to in the previous subsection, means the body of a person whose organs are to be removed for the purposes of transplantation and the functions of whose entire brain, including the brain stem, have been determined to have ceased irreversibly. (Section 6, Subsection 2)

(In July 2009, the phrase 'whose organs are to be removed for the purposes of transplantation [and]' was deleted by the amendment of the Law on Organ Transplantation.)

> The determination referred to in the previous subsection in connection with organ removal can be performed if the person concerned, in addition to having expressed his/her will in accordance with Subsection 1, has expressed his/her will in writing in accordance with determination by the previous subsection and insofar as the family of the person concerned, receiving notice of the said expression, are not opposed to the aforementioned determination, or if the person concerned has no family. (Section 6, Subsection 3)

Here, Subsection 1 states that the dead body includes the body of a brain dead person, indicating that brain death is human death. Tremendously long discussions in Japan on brain death have been distilled into this single sentence. Subsection 2 states that the concept of brain death shall be the death of the entire brain and the cessation of functions. Subsection 3 states that all people shall in principle have the right to select their criteria for human death, which gives consideration to those who do not think of brain death as human death.

In July 2009, the Law on Organ Transplantation was amended, as mentioned above. An added point about Section 6 is as follows.

> Except in cases where a deceased person has, during his/her lifetime, expressed his/her will in writing to donate his/her organs and cases where he/she has, during his/her lifetime, expressed no will to donate his/her organs for the purposes of transplantation, a physician may remove organs from the dead body in order to carry out transplantation if the bereaved family of the deceased has expressed its will in writing to donate his/her organs. (Section 6, Subsection 1, Text and Paragraph 2)

Here, the 'opting-out' system regarding the said person was added. This is the biggest change in this current amendment of the Law on Organ Transplantation.

Discussions in Japan about brain death

As mentioned above, there were tremendously long discussions on brain death in Japan. However, many of the stances proved to be illogical.[8] Four of them are summarized below:

- Discussions on whether brain death is human death or not must eliminate specific intent or purpose such as the facilitation of medical organ transplantation and the termination of life-support treatment. The logic that we cannot remove organs from living bodies and so therefore we should define brain death as human death is like 'putting the cart before the horse', that is to say, it confuses the natural order of things. The reverse logic, that organ removal from dead bodies sounds like part replacement and organs should only be received from living bodies in a way which allows the donor's life to continue, which is why brain death should not be judged as human death, also confuses the natural order of things.

- The expression 'wavering concept of death' (i.e. the concept of death becoming uncertain) was frequently used, but the 'concept' of death never wavers according to the brain criterion of human death. What the criterion causes to waver is the 'image' of death. The brain criterion does not change the concept of death but the image of death. Also, the expression 'two deaths' was often used, but there is only one kind of death. Although it is a tautology, death is the impossibility of resuscitation. There are not two deaths, but two criteria of death, which are the cardiopulmonary criterion of human death and the brain criterion. In other words, the brain criterion is not the 'concept of death' itself, but it is, like the cardiopulmonary criterion, a criterion of death.
- Although it was said that the brain death issue is a highly advanced ethical issue, it is not, at least not primarily. It is a logical issue. Whether medical transplantation should be promoted or not is a value judgment and is certainly an ethical issue. However, whether brain death is human death or not is primarily a matter of factual judgment.
- Although it has been said that brain death is human death from the viewpoint of medical science, medical science as a natural science cannot in principle judge whether brain death is human death. What is medically judged is whether a person is brain dead, not whether the person has reached human death.

WHY HAS ORGAN-TRANSPLANT MEDICINE MADE LITTLE PROGRESS IN JAPAN?

In Japan, although legal and social conditions for organ transplantation were developed, organ transplant medicine has made little progress. The main cause is the lack of organs voluntarily donated from dead bodies, including brain dead bodies. So, why is there a shortage of organ donations from dead bodies in Japan? Some people say the shortage is due to the severe legal restrictions in the Law on Organ Transplantation, 1997. But this does not seem to be the fundamental cause. There is room for improvement in the circumstances surrounding organ transplant medicine; but again, this is not the fundamental factor.

On this issue, it has been said that in Japan the main reason for people's reluctance to donate organs is because the Japanese have a strong sense of attachment to dead bodies. However, it is not so clear that the Japanese have a stronger sense of attachment to a corpse, when compared with people of other countries. Basically, it is difficult to compare customs that originate from different cultures: for instance, the practice of sky burials in Tibet and Nepal does not indicate a lesser sense of attachment to the corpse. It seems that the main reason in Japan for the small number of organ donations from dead bodies is because cultural concepts such as altruism or philanthropy, which are seen more in Europe, America, and other areas with Christian backgrounds, have not been developed in Japan.[9]

Although the total number of organ transplants from cardiac dead or brain dead donors is small, live related organ donation (between parent and child, between husband and wife, between brother and sister, etc.) is comparatively popular in Japan. Japanese traditionally tend to differentiate relatives ('Miuchi') from strangers ('Tanin') in many situations. It may be the case that most Japanese are not willing to donate their organs to strangers, who are very different proposition from their own relatives.

In addition, in Japan a general mistrust of medical doctors has indirectly led to many opinions against the brain criterion of human death and organ transplantation itself. These opinions seem to have led to a low rate of organ donations.

TRANSPLANTATION BY GOING ABROAD

As mentioned above, cadaveric organ donation in Japan is extremely rare, compared with the situation in many Western countries. Some patients who have no chance of having an organ transplant in Japan go to Western countries in order to receive organs. With a worldwide shortage of organs, this is causing a so-called 'organ conflict', in which some Western countries restrict organ transplants for Japanese patients. Moreover, there are some Japanese patients who have received organs through some sort of organ trade in the Philippines or organs from executed prisoners in China. These incidences have caused not just organ conflict, but have also stirred up serious and varied ethical, legal and social concerns.

The case of the Philippines

In the Philippines, live non-related organ transplantation is possible, as is well known. Most cases have involved the buying and selling of organs.[10] Formerly, organs were sold mostly by prisoners,[11] but now they are being sold by poor people living in slums.[12]

The Organ Donation Act[13] was enacted in 1992 in the Philippines, but it does not prohibit the buying and selling of organs.[14] The Act is an existing law. With regard to the prohibition of the buying and selling of organs, an administrative order, the 'National Policy on Kidney Transplantation from Living Non Related Donors (LNRDs)' released in 2002, states that 'the sale and purchase of "kidney organs" by kidney vendors is prohibited.' However, it does not carry a penalty; it is just an advisory provision.

In addition, the Anti-Trafficking in Persons Act of 2003[15] ordains that:

> it shall be unlawful for any person, natural or juridical, to commit any of the following acts: to recruit, hire, adopt, transport or abduct a person, by means of threat or use of force, fraud, deceit, violence, coercion, or intimidation for the purpose of removal or sale of organs of said person. (Section 4, Text and Paragraph (g))

Violation attracts 'imprisonment of 20 years and a fine of not less than one million pesos (P 1,000,000.00) but not more than two million pesos (P 2,000,000.00) (Section10, Text and Paragraph (a)). However, this regulation is applied only when demanding organ donations by means of threat, use of force, fraud, etc., and hence does not apply to normal organ trading in the Philippines.

In this situation, some Japanese patients have received organs through the organ trade in the Philippines, as mentioned above. When I conducted a survey study[16] at a prison in the Philippines in 1992, I found the names of Japanese people in the prison hospital records.

As mentioned above, there is no law to punish people for the buying and selling of organs in the Philippines. On the other hand, the Law on Organ Transplantation in Japan does prohibit the buying and selling of organs and carries a penalty. The Japanese law also punishes Japanese citizens who violate the law in foreign countries, as mentioned above.

Thus, Japanese patients who are involved in the buying and selling of organs may not be punished under any laws in the Philippines, but may be punished under the law on Organ Transplantation in Japan for their violation of the prohibition code, although no one has ever been charged by the authorities.

During my research into the buying and selling of organs since 1992, I have met many donors and patients and found that they have had to make difficult choices. The Filipinos who sell organs suffer from poverty and the Japanese patients who buy them suffer from disease. They could not be criticized lightly.

The case in China

In China, as we already know, organ transplantation has been carried out using organs from executed prisoners. After execution by shooting or lethal injection, their organs are removed and then transplanted into patients.[17] In 2007, the Human Organ Transplantation Act was enacted in China;[18] however, this does not directly prohibit or regulate the removal and transplantation of organs from executed prisoners, so that this is not necessarily illegal. However, since the law requires the donor's or their family's consent for the donation of organs from the dead body of the donor, the removal of organs from executed prisoners without their consent is illegal.

With regard to the necessity for donor's or family's consent, to be precise, the law states:

> When a person does not agree to provide his/her organs before he/she died, no organization or individual shall provide or remove his/her organs. However, when he/she does not express disapproval of organ donation, his/her spouse, adult child and parents can cooperatively express approval of his/her organ donation in a written form. (Section 8)

As for the penalty, the law states that anyone removing organs from a dead body shall be charged with criminal liability in accordance with the law if the donor subject has not previously approved of the removal of his/her organs when he/she was alive (Section 25, Paragraph (2)).

It goes without saying that the removal of organs from executed prisoners who express no consent for transplantation is, in general, saddled with human rights issues.[19] Also, even if they show their consent, the voluntariness of the consent can be problematic.

The Chinese Human Organ Transplantation Act prohibits the buying and selling of organs. Namely, it states that 'no organizations or individuals are allowed to buy or sell organs in any way and to be engaged in any activities of the buying and selling of organs' (Section 3). The law calls for a penalty against the buying and selling of organs by citizens, confiscating illegal income and imposing a fine of eight to 10 times as much as the income (Section 26).

Under such conditions, some Japanese patients have received organs that had been removed from executed Chinese prisoners.[20] Generally speaking, organ transplantation for Japanese patients performed in China is not illegal under either the Chinese Human Organ Transplantation Act or the Japanese Law on Organ Transplantation, as long as the patients are not engaged in the buying of organs. But there is nevertheless a problem with the human rights of prisoners, as mentioned above. However, as in the case of the Philippines, it seems that we should not be too quick to criticize patients' difficult decisions.

TRANSPLANTS IN JAPAN USING DISEASED KIDNEYS[21]

'Medical adequacy'[22]

In Japan in 2006, it was discovered and widely reported that a hospital was involved in kidney transplantation through the buying and selling of organs. Triggered by the scandal, 42 diseased kidney transplants have since been uncovered in several institutions.[23] Kidneys affected by cancer were used in 16 cases.[24]

Diseased kidney transplantation has been strongly denounced by critics all over Japan, including the general public, mass media and the medical community. In 2007, in a joint statement released by the Japan Society for Transplantation and related societies, it was maintained that transplants for diseased kidneys were medically inadequate. The Ministry of Health, Labour and Welfare also announced that diseased kidney transplantation is 'not medically adequate at the present moment' and therefore should be prohibited in principle.[25] The primary reason they gave was a lack of 'medical adequacy' in the treatment of both donor and recipient. The statement raises the question of whether medical inadequacy can be a sufficient reason for banning diseased kidney transplantation.[26] Should diseased kidney transplantation be ethically unjustified because it is medically inadequate?

PATIENTS WHO HAVE KIDNEYS REMOVED

The medical adequacy of the complete removal of a diseased kidney, for example a cancerous kidney, depends on various factors. From the point of view of 'patient self-determination', even if there is no medical adequacy, removal could be justified in principle if the patient whose kidney is to be removed is well informed and consents to the removal, namely, if there is informed consent. For example, if a doctor explains to a patient: 'Your kidney is cancerous and needs to be removed. But complete removal is not necessary', the patient may decide nevertheless to have his/her diseased kidney removed completely because the cancer may spread; in any case, having one kidney is sufficient. Even if the patient's determination is not rational from a medical point of view, the patient's wishes should take priority in the long run. This is in accordance with the patient's right to self-determination.

PATIENTS WHO RECEIVE KIDNEYS

Is the transplantation of a diseased kidney, for example a cancerous kidney, unjustifiable ethically because of its medical inadequacy? Not necessarily. Even without medical adequacy, the transplantation could be accepted in principle if the patient is well informed, fully understands and consents to the transplantation; or put simply, if there is informed consent. If a patient decides to risk having a transplant to avoid undergoing painful dialysis, knowing that the transplanted kidney could spread cancer at a probability of several tens of percentiles,[27] the patient's wishes should take priority. This is based on the principle of self-determination and involves the freedom to take a risk.

When evaluating a (restored) cancerous kidney transplant, it is not appropriate to say, 'Cancerous kidney transplantation is justified because of the lack (or low probability) of the recurrence of cancer'. (Lack of the recurrence of cancer is of course preferable.) Even if the cancerous kidney transplantation has a high risk of recurrence of cancer, the transplantation could be justified with the above-mentioned informed consent.

MEDICAL PATERNALISM

The Supreme Court in Japan handed down a judgment in the case of a Jehovah's Witness who refused a blood transfusion at the Institute of Medical Science, University of Tokyo, and granted compensation giving priority to the patient's self-determination (more exactly, 'decision making'), irrespective of the medical adequacy of the transfusion.[28] My argument is that it is ultimately necessary to prioritize the patient's self-determination over 'medical adequacy' in every medical field. Disrespecting the patient's self-determination on the grounds of a lack of medical adequacy is medical paternalism.

In principle, paternalism should clear the field for individual self-determination. This should also be respected in diseased kidney transplantation. It would not be truly ethical if diseased kidney transplantation were to be denied due to a lack of medical adequacy, and as a result patients who could be saved, are not saved.[29] (Sick kidney transplantation in Japan was resumed in clinical research on 30 December 2009.)

CONCLUSION

As mentioned above, the Law on Organ Transplantation in Japan was amended in July 2009. After its enforcement, organ removal from a dead body in order to carry out transplantation will be legal with the consent of the bereaved family of the deceased, even where there is no consent on the part of the deceased. It will also be legal with the consent of parents, even where there is no consent on the part of their deceased child.

There remains some room for debate over the justice of removing organs from people who have not expressed their will to donate. According to this legal amendment, there will be no problem in such organ removal. However, there may well be a problem from an ethical viewpoint.

Basically, whether undergoing an operation and other medical treatments, undergoing an organ transplant, and donating one's organs or not are in the category of patient's or donor's self-determination. This 'self-determination' is at the centre of bioethics. Now, under this legal amendment, the possibility is created that organs may be removed from someone who had no self-determination.

From another point of view, this legal amendment becomes to indirectly compel an expression of one's own will to 'donate or not' to those people not interested in organ donation, unable to reach one's own decision about donation, reluctant for such donation, etc. Here, this expression of one's own will becomes a kind of legal obligation. Thus, all the people of the nation become involved in organ-transplant medicine one way or another, whether they like it or not.

Thus far, at least in Japan, the very basic premise in organ transplants is that 'no one has the right to receive an organ from anyone else, and no one is obliged to donate his/her organs'.[30] However, this legal amendment will now probably demolish this premise and strongly enhance another one, namely that 'organs are part of the public medical resources.' We may be heading towards a society where a parent of a seriously sick child may accuse someone else, saying, 'My child is dying because you are not donating your organ!'

NOTES

1 Technologies (and the market economy), including medical transplant technology, are 'Manufacturing Machines' which create ELSI (ethical, legal and social issues), and we already have 'Technology Dependence Syndrome (TDS)'. On these points, see Awaya, T. (2001) 'Ningen kaizo no seiki: Yokubo big bang' [A century of human remodeling: Big bang of desires], *Shiso no hiroba* [*Forum of Thought*], 13: 77–89; Awaya, T. (2003) 'Saisei-iryo no mohitotsu no rinri mondai' [Common ethical issues in regenerative medicine], *Saisei-iryo* [*Regenerative Medicine*], 22 (2): 249–52. (In 2005, this article was translated into English and appeared in the *Journal International De Bioethique*, 16: 69–75); Awaya, T. (2005) 'Noshi to zoki-ishoku' [Brain death and organ transplantation], in Y. Kato (ed.), *Jitsumu ijiho kogi* [*Practical lecture on medical laws*], Japan: Minjiho-kenkyukai, 294–308.

2 For my point of view on this, see Awaya, T. (1991) 'Shi no gainen: Noshi-setsu no ichiduke' [The notion of death: An assessment of brain death theory], *Tokuyama University Review*, 36: 1–13; Awaya, T. (1994) 'Noshi-setsu to shi no gainen' [Brain death theory and the notion of death], *Seimeirinri* [*Journal of the Japan Association for Bioethics*], 4 (1): 21–4.

3 Criticisms of medical transplantation, whether strong or weak, include the ideas that the origin of organ transplantation is cannibalism; that organ transplantation is a road to changing the human body into a resource; and that organ transplantation derives from 'human desire'. Modern civilization is a 'desire' fulfilling system led by technologies and the market economy on earth. Precisely speaking, modern civilization is a system by which human desires are stimulated, fulfilled and subsequently extinguished, and this cycle is repeated. Transplant technology must be understood in this context. On this point, see Awaya, T. (1998) 'Zoki-ishoku to gendai bunmei' [Organ transplantation and modern civilization], in K. Yamaguchi (ed.), *Ayatsurareru sei to shi: Seimei no tanjo kara shuen made* [*Manipulating life and death: From birth to the end*], Japan: Shogakukan, 153–72; Awaya, T. (1999) 'Organ transplantation and the human revolution', *Transplantation Proceedings*, 31: 1317–19.

4 Hands and faces have already been transplanted. The simultaneous transplant of eight organs has also already been performed. The theoretical limit of transplantation could be the entire body of a brain-dead person. On the issue of this theoretical limit of transplantation, see Awaya, T. (1999) *Jintai buhin bijinesu* [*Human body parts business*], Japan: Kodansha, 1–260 (151).

5 For the issue on the ownership rights of organs removed for transplantation in Japan, judicial precedents and commonly accepted theories of the civil laws in Japan admit the ownership of body parts such as hair or teeth separated from bodies (see Supreme Court Judgment on 25 July 1921 [Supreme Court Judgment Record, 27: 1408–12]). Based on this, the ownership of removed organs would be accepted by the judicial courts and common theories.

6 For my point of view, see Awaya, T. (1999) 'The human body as a new commodity', *Tokuyama University Review*, 51: 141–7; Awaya, T. (2001) 'Medical technologies vs human dignity: Commodification of the human body and the moral cost', *Formosan Journal of Medical Humanities*, Taiwan, 2 (1/2): 99–105.

7 Kawai, N., Hirano, K. and Oguro, J. (1998) *Kogoreru shinzo [A frozen heart]*, Japan: Kyodo News, 1–303.

8 See Awaya, T. (2000) 'Noshi-rongi ni miru botsu-ronri' [Illogicality in the discussions on brain death], *Shukan-dokushojin* [*weekly newspaper for book reviews*], 4 February.

9 I mentioned this opinion to the *Los Angeles Times* (Lazarowitz, E. (1997) 'Japan's brain-death bill fuels debate – and hope for the ill', 2 May).

10 I performed field research on the actual condition of organ sales in the Philippines from 1992 to 1993. The details are described in my article, Awaya, T. (1993) 'Zoki-baibai: Philippine New Bilibid keimusho no jirei' [The sale of human organs; Philippine's New Bilibid Prison case], *Tokuyama University Review*, 39: 1–15; Awaya, T. (1993) 'Philippine ni okeru zoki-baibai' [The sale of human organs in the Philippines], *Hogaku Seminar* (*law journal*), 462: 26–30 and in my book, *Jintai buhin bijinesu* (see note 4).

11 See my articles and book in n. 10.

12 My research team, including professors at the University of the Philippines, interviewed 311 kidney donors (sellers) in the Philippines between May 2007 and April 2008 (see Awaya, T., Siruno, L., Toledano, S., Aguilar, S., Shimazono, Y. and Castro, L. (2009) 'Failure of informed consent in compensated non-related kidney donation in the Philippines', *Asian Bioethics Review*, 1 (2). Available at http://www.asianbioethicsreview.com/ojs/index.php?journal=abr_sbc1.

13 The precise name of this law is 'An Act Authorizing the Legacy or Donation of All or Part of a Human Body after Death for Specified Purposes'.

14 In the Philippines, no prohibition rule was created in case it might hinder the development of medical transplantation. To my question of why a prohibition code was not added, the late Senator Narciso Monfort, who drafted the bill, answered,

'It is a fact that organs save a patient's life no matter whether it involves money. We have a serious shortage of donors. A prohibition code will enhance the shortage. I don't want to cut down the chance of medical transplantation which has been proceeding on the track to development.' (See also my two articles in n. 10.)

15 The precise name of this law is 'An Act to Institute Policies to Eliminate Trafficking in Persons Especially Women and Children, Establishing the Necessary Institutional Mechanisms for the Protection and Support of Trafficked Persons, Providing Penalties for Its Violations, and for Other Purposes'.

16 See my articles and book in n. 10.

17 In China, I researched this phenomenon from 1995 to 1997. The details are described in my article, Awaya, T. (1996) 'Chugoku shikeishu-ishoku' [Transplantation of organs from executed prisoners in China], *Horitsu jiho* (*law journal*), 68 (9): pp. 28–34. In addition, in 1997, I have been to China with Japanese patients and with a Japanese broker.

18 Organ transplantation has been performed in China without legal support. The details are described in my article, Awaya, T. (2007) 'Asia shokoku ni okeru seitai-zoki no teikyo/ishoku ni kansuru hosei' [Legislation about the donation and transplantation of living organs in Asian countries], *Horitsu jiho* (*law journal*), 79 (10): 71–5. The Chinese Human Organ Transplant Act does not mention brain death. Issues of the brain criterion of human death in China are discussed, for example in Awaya, T. (2007) 'Chugoku shikeishu-ishoku to seimeirinri: Noshi to chushasatsu no kumiawase ha nani wo motarasuka' [Transplantation of organs from executed prisoners in China and bioethics: What does a combination of the brain criterion of human death and execution by lethal injection bring?], *Nicchu Igaku* [Bulletin of the Japan–China Medical Association], 22 (1): 10–13.

19 It is sometimes considered in China that human rights suppression is a necessary evil. Some in China also believe that the donation of organs from executed prisoners is payment for their crimes. The details are described in my article in n. 17.

20 I testified before the International Relations Committee and Government Reform & Oversight Committee of the United States House of Representatives about organ transplants in China to Japanese patients (4 June 1998). The details are described in my article, Awaya, T. (1998) 'Chugoku Shikeishu-ishoku ni tsuite no America renpo-gikai-shogen' [Testimony at the US Congress on the transplantation of organs from executed prisoners in China], *Tokuyama University Review*, 50: 177–89. Also available at http://commdocs.house.gov/committees/intlrel/hfa73452.000/hfa73452_0f.htm.

21 Usually kidneys are used (i.e. implanted) after the removal of the diseased/damaged parts. Therefore some people say we should use the term 'restored kidney transplantation' instead of 'diseased kidney transplantation'.

22 'Medical adequacy' means the adequacy of medical treatment, including surgical operation, from the point of view of medicine itself.

23 For a fuller picture of diseased kidney transplantation in Japan, see Muraguchi, T. (2007) *Hitei sareta jin-ishoku* [Denied kidney transplantation], Japan: Soufusha-shuppan, 1–271.

24 Of course, kidneys were used (i.e. implanted) after the removal of the cancerous parts. So here we may say 'restored cancerous kidney transplantation'.

25 See 'Revision of the Guideline for the Operation of the Law on Organ Transplantation'. Notification No. 0712001 (12 July 2007) from Director General, Health Service Bureau, Japan.

26 I shall not detail other reasons for condemning diseased kidney transplantation (e.g. experimental medical treatment or informal avoidance of ethics committee discussion) to clarify this controversial point.

27 According to Dr. Emanuela Taioli, USA, in reality, in most cases, transplanted cancerous kidneys do not spread cancer (Taioli, E. (2007)'Kokei-zoki ishoku go no gan-hassho' [Cancer occurrence after solid organ transplant], *Doctor's Network* [Japan], 32: 17–19).

28 The Japanese Supreme Court's judgment on 29 February 2000 (*Hanrei Times* (law report), 1031: 158–61).

29 As for this point of view, the details are described in my article, Awaya, T. (2007) 'Byojin-ishoku no "igakuteki datosei" to kanja no jikokettei: Seimeirinri no shiten kara' [Medical adequacy of sick kidney transplantation and patient's self-determination: From the point of view of bioethics], *Seijinbyo to seikatsushukanbyo* [Journal of Adult Diseases and Lifestyle Diseases], 37 (12): 1333–7; Awaya, T. and Takagi, M. (2009) 'Is the use of so called "restored kidneys" for transplantation ethically unjustified?', *Biomedical Law & Ethics* [Korea], 3 (1): 69–80; Awaya, T. (2009) 'Cases of sick kidney transplantation in Japan and patients' self-determination', in A. Covic, N. Gosic and L. Tomasevic (eds), *From New Medical Ethics to Integrative Bioethics: Dedicated to Ivan Segota on the Occasion of His 70th*, Croatia: Pergamena, 281–7.

30 Awaya, T. (1991) 'Risaikuru yuaserufu: Noshi, zoki-ishoku no tou mono' [Recycle yourself: Questions posed to us by brain death and organ transplantation], in Ho to seikatsu kenkyukai [Society for the Study of Law and Life] (ed.), *Ho to seikatsu* [*Law and life*], Japan: Sogensha, 6 (add.): 11–18.

32

Ethical Issues in Nanotechnology

Bert Gordijn, Rob de Vries and Dónal P. O'Mathúna

INTRODUCTION

Recently, numerous bioethicists have become actively engaged in two new fields of ethical inquiry: neuroethics and nanoethics. We will focus on the latter, seeking a balance between a complete and thus somewhat superficial review of the ethical issues in nanotechnology and an in-depth analysis of one particular topic.[1] Accordingly, after briefly explaining the technology itself, we present three urgent ethical concerns currently being debated. These concerns pertain to the risks of nanotechnology, the fear that nanotechnology might contribute to injustice and the possibility that this technology will enable monitoring and surveillance equipment that will infringe on our privacy. Nanotechnology raises many other ethical issues, but they seem less acute than the three we selected. Moreover, we examine whether the ethical issues in nanotechnology are novel. Finally, we address the procedural question of how nanotechnology should be governed.

NANOTECHNOLOGY

One nanometer equals one billionth of a meter. Hence, nanotechnology is the technology of very little things. However, as with any other emerging technology, much discussion has focused on the precise demarcation of the field of nanotechnology. We will apply a definition that most contemporary nanotechnologists appear to have adopted.[2] According to this definition nanotechnology refers to the study, creation and application of structures with *at least one* dimension between 1 and 100 nm.[3]

Most current research in nanotechnology focuses on the production, study and application of a wide array of different nanoscale structures.[4] It uses both bottom-up approaches, where one organizes smaller components into more complex assemblies, and top-down approaches, where smaller devices are created by using larger ones to direct their assembly. These nanostructures have interesting applications in fields as different as materials and manufacturing, electronics and computer technology, medicine, aeronautics and space exploration, environment and energy, biotechnology and agriculture as well as security. New nanotechnology-influenced products are already being introduced onto the market, including more protective sunscreens, stronger sports equipment and anti-graffiti paint (Project on Emerging Nanotechnologies, 2008). Hence, many authors argue that nanotechnology will profoundly change the world as we know it (see Sparrow, 2007).[5]

Inspired by the seemingly limitless applications of nanotechnology, many national governments around the world have set up programs to financially support its further development. Worldwide government R&D investments have increased five-fold in 5 years. From about $825 million in 2000 they had reached about $4.1 billion in 2005 (Roco, 2007). Moreover, private companies are rapidly becoming more interested in investing in nanotechnology development projects. All in all, the nanotechnology industry might be worth $1 trillion by the year 2012 (Service, 2004).

RISKS

Currently, research on nanotechnology risk focuses on the possible detrimental health and environmental effects of nanoparticles. This research has turned out to be quite challenging. The central problem is that the material properties and toxicological effects of microparticles may be completely different when the same material exists as nanoscale particles.[6] For several reasons, nanoparticles can act differently, giving rise to novel beneficial properties but unknown detrimental effects. First, quantum effects can become quite prominent at the nanoscale (Shrader-Frechette, 2007). Second, nanoparticles are much smaller than microparticles and can access almost every hidden niche of the body. This poses new health risks. They can, for instance, cross the blood–brain barrier and might cause brain damage (Lenk and Biller-Andorno, 2007).[7] Third, the larger surface-to-volume ratio enhances the reactivity of nanoparticles compared to larger particles of the same material (Shrader-Frechette, 2007). We are just beginning to appreciate the complexity of predicting the detrimental effects of nanoparticles.

The unpredictability of the negative effects of nanoparticles not only raises the question of how to prevent these effects, but also how to deal with unknown risks. Pivotal in the debate about the latter question is the so-called precautionary principle, which became quite important in debates about emerging technologies in general through the *Rio Declaration on Environment and Development*, a brief document produced at the 1992 United Nations Conference on Environment and Development. It contains 27 principles intended to direct future sustainable development. Principle 15 refers to 'the precautionary approach'.

'In order to protect the environment, the precautionary approach shall be widely applied by States according to their capabilities. Where there are threats of serious or irreversible damage, lack of full scientific certainty shall not be used as a reason for postponing cost-effective measures to prevent environmental degradation' (Rio Declaration, 1992).

Unfortunately, the precautionary principle as formulated in the Rio Declaration is too vague to be practically usable as a policy instrument. Nonetheless, the precautionary principle has since been included in various multilateral agreements, policy statements and international law. As a result, the precautionary principle currently appears in a wide range of different formulations adding to confusion about its precise meaning.[8] According to Sandin (1999) the different versions retain a common appeal that in the face of some potentially dangerous activity some action should be undertaken. However, this proposition is almost meaningless.

Phoenix and Treder (2004) make a helpful distinction between two forms of the precautionary principle: the 'strict form' and the 'active form'. The former 'requires inaction when action might pose a risk.' The latter, in contrast, 'calls for choosing less risky alternatives when they are available, and for taking responsibility for potential risks.' Several non-governmental organizations (NGOs) seem to use a strict form of the precautionary principle to inform their position on nanotechnology risks. The ETC Group, for example, has called for a global moratorium on the production and use of synthetic nanoparticles in view of the uncertainties regarding their health and environmental effects (ETC, 2003). Likewise, Greenpeace (2004) has called for a moratorium on the release of nanoparticles into the environment until the hazards are characterized and understood. In contrast, Phoenix and Treder reject the strict form. Since every action inherently entails a certain degree of risk, following the strict principle might stifle scientific endeavors in general (see Holm and Harris, 1999). What is more, inaction might pose an even greater risk. Therefore, they prefer the active form that calls for an appropriate effort to mitigate the risk of nanotechnology (Phoenix and Treder, 2004).

According to the latter interpretation of the precautionary principle, further toxicological research should urgently be done into the nature and magnitude of the hazards associated with different types of nanoparticles.[9] After all, nanomaterials are already present in hundreds of consumer products.[10] After identifying the potential for nanoparticles to cause harm, the probability of exposure to the hazard and the associated consequences should be assessed. On this basis adequate strategies to control and reduce the risks should be developed. Feasible options of effectively dealing with risks might, for example, involve substituting dangerous nanoparticles with less dangerous ones or reducing exposure to dangerous particles. At the same time, the public should be informed about nanotechnology products to enable them to give or withhold their consent to using these products, and also to prevent inaccurate risk perception and irrational public backlash (Shrader-Frechette, 2007).

JUSTICE

In debates about nanotechnology and justice the most common concern is that nanotechnology could lead to a widening of economic inequalities. This might indeed be unjust from the viewpoint of at least two influential theories of justice.

According to utilitarian theory, economic distribution is just as long as it contributes to the promotion of overall social wellbeing or happiness. Against this background a strong argument can be made for the reduction of the great disparities that characterize wealth distribution within most societies and between different societies globally. The argument is based on the observation that, in general, successive additions to one's income produce less happiness than did earlier additions. With the first additions to our income we purchase goods of the highest priority. Goods we purchase with further additions have a lower priority, thus adding less to our happiness. Consequently, money tends to have a declining marginal utility. Therefore, distributions of income that lift up the lowest incomes will tend to boost total happiness more than situations where the rich get richer and resources are unequally distributed (Shaw, 2008).

Also from the viewpoint of Rawls' *Theory of Justice* (1971) a reinforcement of economic inequality caused by nanotechnology might be problematic. Rawls' second principle of justice states that social and economic inequalities must be to the greatest expected benefit of the least advantaged members of society (Rawls, 1971). Thus, if nanotechnology leads to bigger economic inequalities, this can only be just if the least advantaged members of society benefit from this development.

On a global scale Rawls' 'maximin' rule implies that nanotechnology will only advance justice if it benefits poor countries. Whether nanotechnology will benefit poorer countries and satisfy the Rawlsian condition remains to be seen. However, even if there is an absolute improvement in the situation of the poor, the divide between them and the rich might continue to widen, thus worsening the relative position of the poor (Swierstra and Rip, 2007). Approaches based on rights and duties also raise concerns about justice and world poverty (Pogge, 2008).

Against the backdrop of these ethical considerations, we would like to point out how nanotechnology could lead to increased economic inequalities through cognitive enhancement technologies. Many authors expect that nanotechnology will contribute to the development of technologies that enhance cognitive abilities.[11] Since intelligence is a decisive factor in achieving a professional career, material wealth and social prestige, many would be interested in these enhancement systems. However, given the present shortage of resources in the health sector, these nanotechnological systems are unlikely to be made available to everybody. In contrast it is more likely they would be available only to those who could afford them. Only those members of society who already enjoy considerable material wealth would profit from them, making additional opportunities for social and professional improvement available to precisely those people already at the top of the social hierarchy. This would further exacerbate the already unequal distribution of goods between the rich and the poor.

In addition, nanotechnology is likely to increase the gap between the developed and the developing world (Schummer, 2006). In the Western world there has been a shift from public to private knowledge as universities have started to file and market their own patents. This has contributed to increased costs of industrial research that builds on existing knowledge. Poorer countries often cannot afford the licensing fees, while in rich countries R&D budgets are generally higher. Thus, the further development of nanotechnology is expected to add to the economic gap between affluent and poor countries (Schummer, 2006). Moreover, industrial nanotechnology will have a substantial effect on the world metals markets. Most interesting metals are mined and produced in developing countries. If industrialized countries produce new nanostructured materials and no longer require traditional metals such as platinum, palladium, tungsten, gallium, germanium, selenium, cadmium, etc., this would have serious impact on the economies of developing countries. This will make developed countries more independent of the resources of developing countries, thus increasing the economic gap (Schummer, 2006). Potentially, nanotechnology could provide substantial benefits to the developing world by developing, for example, better systems for water purification, solar energy and healthcare. Unfortunately, however, many poorer countries may be unable to afford these developments (Allhoff, 2007). Justice concerns also pertain to possible detrimental environmental and health effects of nanotechnology. The distribution of burdens and risks caused by nanotechnology might be unequal. Typically these burdens fall heaviest on poor people, children, minorities and workers (Shrader-Frechette, 2007). Risky research that primarily benefits developed countries should not be moved to poor countries (see Lenk and Biller-Andorno, 2007; Mnyusiwalla et al., 2003).

PRIVACY

The term 'privacy' will be used here to refer to the possibility of withdrawing oneself or keeping information about oneself from others. Privacy is widely held to be important, strongly supported by two moral reasons: prevention of information-based harm and respect for autonomy. However, nanotechnology will enable radically miniaturized tracking, tracing, monitoring and surveillance technologies that might make protection of privacy increasingly difficult.[12] This concern is not just for the future as miniaturization is well underway already.

Radio frequency identification (RFID) is a good example (Allhoff, 2007; Grunwald, 2007). RFID tags contain a minute chip for storing and processing information, and a tiny radio antenna for receiving and transmitting radio signals. These tags are already widely used for tracing individual consumer products (Van den Hoven and Vermaas, 2007). The uniqueness of RFID tags allows individual products to be tracked as they move from one place to another, permitting companies to combat product loss. Tags are placed on artifacts, but animals and human beings may be labeled as well. Monitoring capabilities might be greatly improved using wireless and portable communication amenities, with links to the Internet and computer networks. Nanotechnology will make RFID tags even smaller than they are already, thus becoming undetectable by ordinary means. As a result nanotechnology might produce RFID gadgets that spy on us without us being able to notice their presence.

Another example is smart dust, a sensor/communication system that is basically a network of minuscule wireless sensors, robots and other devices that can detect whatever they are programmed to spot. They might, for example, be used as defense-related sensor networks for battlefield surveillance purposes. Other possible functions include inventory control and product quality monitoring. Smart dust is already causing privacy concerns. Kris Pister, the developer of smart dust, acknowledges that 'personal privacy is getting harder and harder to come by' (Pister, 2001). However, he believes that the potential benefits of smart dust far outweigh the loss of personal privacy: 'If I thought that the negatives of working on this project were larger than or even comparable to the positives, I wouldn't be working on it' (Pister, 2001).

A third example is nanomedicine.[13] Much research is being conducted into various nanotechnological diagnostic methods. Tests that measure the presence or activity of particular substances become faster and more sensitive with the help of nanoscale particles that function as tags or labels. Magnetic nanometric particles, for example, can be used as substitutes for the radioactive or fluorescing markers currently used to detect certain diseases. Another development is the lab-on-a-chip, a device that integrates various laboratory functions on a single chip (Grunwald, 2007). Nanotechnology could even further miniaturize this technology. Nanotechnological diagnostic devices will facilitate new methods of fast and comprehensive medical diagnosis and screening. This will create increasingly elaborate personal health and genetic profiles. However, employers, insurance companies or the judicial system will probably try to find ways to access this information, creating privacy concerns. Hence, strict standards for data protection will be needed (see Bawa and Johnson, 2007; European Commission, 2007; Grunwald, 2007; RS/RAE, 2004). In addition to this traditional threat to privacy, the use of nanotechnology in medicine presents novel challenges as well. An example is the privacy problem that might be generated by the convergence of nanotechnology, biotechnology, information technology and cognitive science (NBIC convergence). NBIC enabled technological enhancement of the human body and its functions might seriously infringe privacy. Standard use of neuroimplants to improve cognitive ability might facilitate brain–computer links as well as intensive links to other human beings by establishing brain-to-brain interfaces. This excessive networking of human brains would enable easy access to all areas of human privacy, even the most intimate (visual impressions, thoughts, emotions and so on) (Gordijn, 2006).

These three examples demonstrate that the development of better ways to gather, store and distribute data, personal or otherwise, is driven by concerns for important goods such as economic, intelligence and medical purposes. While pursuing those goods, privacy may come under increasing threat from more invasive and ubiquitous monitoring and surveillance devices enabled by nanotechnology. Balancing the protection of privacy against the above-mentioned goods is a significant ethical challenge.[14]

NOVELTY

Much debate has arisen about whether the ethical issues raised by nanotechnology are novel or unique (see Allhoff, 2007; Godman, 2008; Grunwald, 2004, 2005, 2007; Litton, 2007; Swierstra and Rip, 2007). Proponents of nanotechnology sometimes argue that, since the ethical issues that nanotechnology triggers are not new, it is not necessary to invest time and energy discussing them. However, we believe that to a large extent the question of novelty is a pseudo-problem. After all, the answer depends greatly on the level of abstraction with which one analyses a particular ethical issue.

Let us take the issue of privacy as an example. If framed on a high level of generalization – as a threat to privacy triggered by a new technology – one can positively argue that this issue is not new. For example, the very same threat has often been associated with advances in genetics and information technology. Therefore one could argue that many of the privacy and personal data issues associated with nanotechnologies are not new but will only be intensified by the application of sophisticated nanotechnological monitoring and surveillance gadgets.

However, if we leave the high ground of abstraction, and analyze the privacy issue associated with nanotechnology as a real world issue, certain new aspects appear. For example, it could be argued that nanoscale surveillance devices have a novel and unique capacity to make the abusers of this technology less accountable (Rodrigues, 2006). Furthermore, Van den Hoven and Vermaas (2007) argue that nanotechnology will facilitate stealthy *in situ* information gathering using local and transient databases. This significantly differs from the more classical information flows to and from permanent centralized databases. They argue that as a result the focus in privacy debates is likely to shift 'from constraints on the processing of the information itself and the management of the databases in which it is stored, to constraints on the design of nano-artifacts which enable these flows of information' (Van den Hoven and Vermaas, 2007).

When the ethical issues with nanotechnology are framed in a more contextualized way, suddenly novel aspects pop up in the analysis. Therefore, the novelty of the ethical issues hinges on the extent to which they are contextualized. Against this backdrop, we agree with the view expressed in the report published by Britain's Royal Society and Royal Academy of Engineering (RS/RAE) (2004) that it does not really matter whether the arising social and ethical issues are new or not: they urgently need to be analyzed either way (RS/RAE, 2004; cf. Godman 2008).

GOVERNANCE

The three examples of ethical issues in nanotechnology illustrate the necessity to reflect carefully on nanotechnology to help steer further development in a responsible direction. However, who should make decisions about the future direction of nanotechnology? And what kind of citizen involvement is desirable in the decision-making process? Schummer (2006) identifies three governance models of emerging technologies: the *autocratic* model, the *information-plus-debate* model and the *democratic* model.

In the autocratic model decisions about the development, application and regulation of a technology are made by governments or corporations. Public debate and information about the technology and its expected effects on society are negligible or entirely absent. Thus, citizen engagement is minimal.

In the information-plus-debate model, information about all R&D activities is provided and debate may occur. However, involvement of citizens in the actual decision-making processes that shape the future of the technology is minimal.

In the democratic model, citizens are not only informed about the new technology but are actively involved in the political decision-making process from the earliest stage. Most countries have a mix of the first two models, differing in the degree of information and public debate (Schummer, 2006).

Without analyzing the ethical questions relating to these models in depth, we would like to make the following few remarks. Surely, the autocratic model is not acceptable in a democratic society with a well-educated citizenry. It is not respectful of the autonomy of the population and is likely to generate mistrust and rejection of emerging technologies.[15] Moreover, the information-plus-debate model has the disadvantage that it is rather frustrating to debate questions without having any effect on the decision-making process. On first sight, therefore, the democratic model seems the most desirable one, at least in a democratic culture with a sufficiently educated public. Public participation is also likely to enhance public trust and confidence in the policymaking process (Rogers-Hayden, 2007). Accordingly, the idea of involving the public more upstream in the R&D process of emerging technologies has steadily become more popular in Europe and North America (Rogers-Hayden, 2007).

An example of existing models of involvement is the citizens' jury. This is a forum, at which a citizens' panel of between 10 and 20 people questions experts on a particular topic. After assessment of the responses and in depth discussion of the topics the panel presents its findings at a press conference. Consensus conferences have been held in countries such as Denmark, The Netherlands, the UK, New Zealand, Norway, Austria, France and Switzerland. Some of these events are said to have had a direct effect on parliamentary decision making.[16]

In general, we applaud attempts to move public debate upstream. A citizens' jury is a useful instrument to increase involvement of the public. However, it triggers difficult questions too. How are the members of the panel recruited or selected? Are they in any way representative of the general public? What kind of guarantee, if any, is there that the work of the citizens' panel will indeed affect parliamentary decision making?

Finally, upstream public policymaking engagement on emerging technologies creates the following problem. For the panel to impact the development of a technology, it must do its work early on in the R&D process. However, it would then be addressing applications of a technology which are largely yet to come, which does not make reflection and analysis particularly easy. This reminds us of the dilemma described by Collingridge (1980): If the assessment of a new technology is completed before the technology is applied in practice and has shown its effects, there is an information problem. After all, it is not easy to predict what those effects will be. However, if the assessment is done after the technology has been developed, it may be easier to know the facts about the impact of the technology, but now there is a power problem. It is hard to control or change a technology after the technology has become well established.

The idea of upstream public engagement involves prospective discussions early in the research and development phases of an emerging technology. Accordingly, the model has to cope with the problems inherent to prospective ethics. Horner (2005), for example, is quite pessimistic about prospective nanoethics based on skeptical analysis of the feasibility of technological forecasting. We agree that it is impossible to see all the consequences of an emerging technology at an early R&D stage. However, prospective thinking about the potential future impact of a technology can still be very useful. Ethical reflection will have to be organized as a dynamic enterprise that develops as the technology moves downstream, constantly open for reassessment of the situation on the basis of new findings, predictions and considerations (see Moor, 2005).

CONCLUSION

Amongst the most acute ethical concerns raised by the fast development of nanotechnology are the risks of nanoparticles, the further exacerbation of the gap between the rich and the poor and the possibility of extremely small monitoring and surveillance equipment that might infringe on our privacy. When analyzed on a high level of generalization these issues hardly appear to be new. However, when looked at in more detail, novel aspects pop up in the analysis. Be this as it may, these ethical issues urgently need to be analyzed to guarantee an ethically sound development of nanotechnology. Models of upstream public policymaking engagement will have to be further explored as useful tools of technology governance.

NOTES

1 See Gordijn, 2005; Kjølberg and Wickson, 2007 for analyses of the early literature on social and ethical aspects of nanotechnology.

2 It is also used in conjunction with the US National Nanotechnology Initiative (NNI), a program established in 2001 to coordinate US Federal nanotechnology R&D (NNI, 2007).

3 There is also debate about the distinction between nanoscale technology, engineering and science. Although interesting in its own right, we will not engage with this discussion here.

4 Examples are buckminsterfullerenes, nanotubes, nanoparticles, nanocapsules, nanopores, nanomembranes, molecular motors, biomolecules, quantum dots and quantum wires.

5 Sparrow (2007) gives an interesting analysis of public discourse about nanotechnology involving contradictory narratives. For example, nanotechnology is simultaneously depicted as revolutionary and familiar.

6 See Shrader-Frechette (2007) for more elaborate analysis and references pertaining to this extrapolation problem.

7 On the other hand, the ability to cross the blood–brain barrier might be useful for the delivery of therapeutic molecules into the brain.

8 Against this backdrop, further work on the policy level has been done. For example, UNESCO has published a most useful booklet on the precautionary principle, which provides member states with a solid base for further discussion. It endeavours to clarify the principle in a pragmatic way thus informing decision-makers about possible uses and misuses of this principle (see UNESCO, 2005).

9 See Schulte and Salamanca-Buentello (2007) for a review of the current state of knowledge about the risks and hazards of nanotechnology.

10 According to Alpert (2008) there are already 580 different consumer products, a number that has more than doubled in the last 18 months.

11 Such views have recently have been advanced about the convergence of nanoscience, biotechnology, information technology and cognitive science (Roco and Bainbridge, 2003; Roco and Montemagno, 2004). See Gordijn (2006) and Grunwald (2007) for an elaborate ethical and conceptual analysis of these views.

12 See Allhoff, 2007; Grunwald, 2007; Gutierrez, 2004; Mehta, 2002; Mnyusiwalla et al., 2003; Toumey, 2007; Van den Hoven and Vermaas, 2007.

13 See Freitas (2005) for a good review of different research endeavors within nanomedicine. See Bawa and Johnson (2007), Gordijn (2007) and Lenk and Biller-Andorno (2007) for more elaborate surveys of the ethical problems in nanomedicine.

14 Similar questions have already been discussed, especially in relation to what privacy infringements are necessary for enhanced security. This subject has been fiercely debated since the September 11th terrorist attacks and the subsequent US Patriot Act, which clearly increases surveillance at the expense of privacy.

15 However, in case of the development of military technologies the autocratic model may very well be adequate for national security reasons.

16 In general, it is difficult to demonstrate a direct impact. However, in 1987, the first Danish citizens' panel opposed genetic modification of animals. Thereupon, the Danish Parliament decided not to support such projects in the first biotechnology R&D program (1987–1990) (see Einsiedel et al., 2001).

REFERENCES

Allhoff, F. (2007) 'On the autonomy and justification of nanoethics', *NanoEthics*, 1: 185–210.
Alpert, S. (2008) 'Neuroethics and nanoethics: Do we risk ethical myopia?', *Neuroethics*, 1: 55–68.

Bawa, R. and Johnson, S. (2007) 'The ethical dimensions of nanomedicine', *Medical Clinics of North America,* 91: 881–7.

Collingridge, D. (1980) *The Social Control of Technology.* New York: St. Martin's Press.

Einsiedel, E.F., Jelsøe, E. and Breck, T. (2001) 'Publics at the technology table: The consensus conference in Denmark, Canada, and Australia', *Public Understanding of Science,* 10 (1): 83–98.

ETC (2003) *The Big Down: Technologies Converging at the Nano-scale.* Available at http://www.etcgroup.org/documents/TheBigDown.pdf, accessed 25 May 2008.

European Commission (EC) (2007) Group on Ethics in Science and New Technologies. Opinion No. 21. *Opinion on the Ethical Aspects of Nanomedicine.* Available at http://ec.europa.eu/european_group_ethics/activities/index_en.htm, accessed 25 May 2008.

Freitas, R.A. Jr (2005) 'What is Nanomedicine?', *Nanomedicine: Nanotechnology, Biology, and Medicine,* 1: 2–9.

Godman, M. (2008) 'But is it unique to nanotechnology? Reframing nanoethics', *Science and Engineering Ethics,* (online first), 14 (3): 391–403.

Gordijn, B. (2005) 'Nanoethics. From apocalyptic nightmares and utopian dreams towards a more balanced view', *Science and Engineering Ethics,* 114: 521–33.

Gordijn, B. (2006) 'Converging NBIC technologies for improving human performance: A critical assessment of the novelty and the prospects of the project', *Journal of Law, Medicine & Ethics,* 34 (4): 726–32.

Gordijn, B. (2007) 'Ethical issues in nanomedicine', in H.A.M.J. Ten Have (ed.), *Nanotechnologies, Ethics and Policies.* Paris: UNESCO, pp. 99–123.

Greenpeace (2004) *Nanotechnology.* Available at www.greenpeace-org.uk, accessed 25 May 2008.

Grunwald, A. (2004) 'Ethische Aspekte der Nanotechnologie. Eine Felderkundung', *Theorie und Praxis,* 13 (2): 71–8.

Grunwald, A. (2005) 'Nanotechnology – A new field of ethical inquiry?', *Science and Engineering Ethics,* 11: 187–201.

Grunwald, A. (2007) 'Converging technologies: Visions increased contingencies of the conditio humana, and search for orientation', *Futures,* 39: 380–92.

Gutierrez, E. (2004) *Privacy Implications of Nanotechnology.* Electronic Privacy Information Center (EPIC), Technical Report. Available at www.epic.org/privacy/nano, accessed 25 May 2008.

Holm, S.and Harris, J. (1999) 'Precautionary principle stifles discovery', *Nature,* 400: 398.

Horner, D.S. (2005) 'Anticipating ethical challenges: Is there a coming era of nanotechnology?', *Ethics and Information Technology,* 7: 127–38.

Kjølberg, K. and Wickson, F. (2007) 'Social and ethical interactions with nano: Mapping the early literature', *NanoEthics,* 1: 89–104.

Lenk, C. and Biller-Andorno, N. (2007) 'Nanomedicine – Emerging or re-emerging ethical issues? A discussion of four ethical themes', *Medicine, Health Care and Philosophy,* 10: 173–84.

Litton, P. (2007) '"Nanoethics"? What's new?', *Hastings Center Report,* (Jan/Feb): 22–5.

Mehta, M.D. (2002) 'On Nano-panopticism: A sociological perspective', *Interfaces, Canadian Chemical News,* 31–3. Available at http://chem4823.usask.ca/?cassidyr/OnNano-Panopticism-ASociologicalPerspective.htm, accessed 17 May 2007.

Mnyusiwalla, A., Daar, A.S. and Singer, P.A. (2003) 'Mind the gap: Science and ethics in nanotechnology', *Nanotechnology,* 14: R9–R13.

Moor, J.H. (2005) 'Why we need better ethics for emerging technologies', *Ethics and Information Technology,* 7 (3): 111–19.

National Nanotechnology Initiative (NNI) (2007) *Strategic Plan.* Available at http://www.nano.gov/NNI_Strategic_Plan_2007.pdf, accessed 25 May 2008.

Phoenix, C. and Treder, M. (2004) *Applying the Precautionary Principle to Nanotechnology.* Available at http://www.crnano.org/precautionary.htm, accessed 25 May 2008.

Pister, K. (2001) *Smart Dust: Autonomous Sensing and Communication in a Cubic Millimeter.* Available at http://robotics.eecs.berkeley.edu/~pister/SmartDust/, accessed 25 May 2008.

Pogge, T. (2008) *World Poverty and Human Rights,* 2nd ed. Cambridge: Polity.

Project on Emerging Nanotechnologies (2008). Available at http://www.nanotechproject.org/inventories, accessed 30 May 2008.

Rawls, J. (1971) *A Theory of Justice.* Cambridge, MA: Harvard University Press.

Rio Declaration on Environment and Development (1992). Available at http://www.unep.org/Documents.Multilingual/Default.asp?DocumentID=78&ArticleID=1163, accessed 25 May 2008.

Roco, M.C. (2007) *National Nanotechnology Initiative – Past, Present, Future*. Available at http://www.nsf.gov/crssprgm/nano/nni_past_present_future_update_tables.pdf, accessed 25 May 2008.

Roco, M.C. and Bainbridge, W.S. (eds) (2003) *NBIC Convergence for Improving Human Performance. Nanotechnology, Biotechnology, Information Technology and Cognitive Science*. Dordrecht/Boston/London: Kluwer Academic Publishers.

Roco, M.C. and Montemagno, C.D. (eds) (2004) 'The coevolution of human potential and converging technologies', *Annals of the New York Academy of Sciences*, 1013. Available at http://www.annalsnyas.org, accessed 25 May 2008.

Rodrigues, R. (2006) 'The implications of high-rate nanomanufacturing on society and personal privacy', *Bulletin of Science, Technology & Society*, 26 (1): 38–45.

Rogers-Hayden, T., Mohr, A. and Pidgeon, N. (2007) 'Introduction: Engaging with nanotechnologies – engaging differently?' *NanoEthics*, 1 (2): 123–30.

Royal Society and Royal Academy of Engineering (RS/RAE) (2004) *Nanoscience and Nanotechnologies: Opportunities and Uncertainties*. Available at http://www.nanotec.org.uk/finalReport.htm, accessed 25 May 2008.

Sandin, P. (1999) 'Dimensions of the precautionary principle', *Human and Ecological Risk Assessment*, 5 (5): 889–907.

Schulte, P. and Salamanca-Buentello, F. (2007) 'Ethical and scientific issues of nanotechnology in the workplace', *Environmental Health Perspectives*, 115 (1): 5–12.

Schummer, J. (2006) 'Cultural diversity in nanotechnology ethics', *Interdisciplinary Science Reviews*, 31 (3): 217–30.

Service, R.F. (2004) 'Nanotechnology grows up', *Science*, 304 (5678): 1732–4.

Shaw, W. H. (2008) *Business Ethics*, 6th ed. Belmont, CA: Thomson Wadsworth.

Shrader-Frechette, K. (2007) 'Nanotoxicology and ethical conditions', *NanoEthics*, 1: 47–56.

Swierstra, T. and Rip, A. (2007) 'Nano-ethics as NEST-ethics: Patterns of moral argumentation about new and emerging science and technology', *NanoEthics*, 1: 3–20.

Toumey, C. (2007) 'Privacy in the shadow of nanotechnology', *NanoEthics*, 1: 221–2.

UNESCO (2005) *The Precautionary Principle. Report of UNESCO's Expert Group on the Precautionary Principle*, adopted by COMEST at its fourth session (March 2005). Available at http://unesdoc.unesco.org/images/0013/001395/139578e.pdf, accessed 25 May 2008.

Van den Hoven, M.J. and Vermaas, P.E. (2007) 'Nano-technology and privacy: On continuous surveillance outside the panopticon', *Journal of Medicine and Philosophy*, 32 (3): 283–97.

33

Ethics of Environmental Health

Michiel Korthals

INTRODUCTION: ETHICAL ISSUES OF ENVIRONMENTAL HEALTH

The ways societies are organized contribute in numerous ways to the health of individuals. By producing highways, factories, nature parks, airports, cycling paths and elevators, society promotes or harms, intentionally or unintentionally, the health of individuals. These societal factors go of course hand-in-hand with physical factors, such as weather, soil characteristics on which crops are cultivated and volcanoes. All these factors contribute to the environment of healthy and unhealthy individuals.

The research and policy field of environmental health is therefore extremely complex and interdisciplinary and has many connections with other types of health research and policies (see for example Lawrence and Worsley, 2007). The ethics of environmental health gets its inspiration from the general task of ethics, i.e. to inquire first, about the presuppositions and consequences of actions with respect to the interests and wellbeing of living beings; second, what the most desirable distribution of benefits and losses between individuals and groups is; and last but not least, what the opportunities are of living in accordance with the values people have that represent a good life (Korthals, 2004).

With these notions in mind, we can discern at least four significant types of ethical issues in the complex relationship of environmental factors and human health. The first concerns the identification of what environmental factors count as a problem (and what type of problem) in causing unhealthy consequences, and where the environmental causes can be located. Second, policy measures with respect to and doing research into environmental factors determining adverse effects on human health raises many ethical issues: e.g. what is better, ringing alarm bells or keeping silent about the problem? Third, the responsibility of the agencies involved is always at stake and often contested; and fourth, these agencies assume the right to intervene to reduce unhealthy conditions; moreover, the methods of intervention themselves demand ethical attention.

First, the *identification of problematic adverse* effects of environmental factors on human health that should be tackled raises ethical questions. Exposure to potentially hazardous substances and processes is often difficult to identify and document, not only because of the complexity of their interactions and their long-term risks, but also because individuals can experience differing susceptibilities to their harmful effects (Sharp, 2001; Paulson, 2006). This complexity shows that research into all these interwoven factors is quite expensive and often controversial. Is society willing to pay for this and to prioritize this problem rather than others (Resnik and Roman, 2007)?

The uninitiated, moreover, can often see a direct connection between a toxic waste location and living in houses near such places; or between motorways and a higher occurrence of asthma, for example. Many think that when on-street eateries such as McDonald's, KFC, Fish'n'chips and Ben and Jerry's are tolerated not only in cities, but also in mass media advertising and sponsorship, it should not be surprising that the numbers of obese persons are greatly increasing, as they still are in Britain, along with increased instances of concomitant diseases, such as type-two diabetes, cancer of the intestines and cardiovascular diseases. However, one of the most powerful food companies, for example, McDonald's, thinks otherwise and acts accordingly. Third, environmental risks to health are for the most part not equally distributed, so that rich people tend to live in healthier environments than do poor people.

These three different factors challenge us with the ethical issue of justifying the identification of adverse environmental effects and the corresponding selection of research topics and research trajectories. Should one start research and policies with the most difficult cases or on the cases that are easier to deal with? What power play is involved in identifying the problems? Should one give priority to the environmental health problems of the poor and powerless (Sharp, 2001; Lavery et al., 2003)?

Second, *research into and policy measures* with respect to environmental factors that are identified as responsible for a decline in public health confronts us with new ethical issues. When researchers identify environmental toxicants like dioxin in waste locations and step up research about their effects, ethics come to the fore, because the decision to pursue research in certain areas can interfere with power relations, people's concerns about safety and other expectations, for example. Moreover, research and policy measures can encourage the use of animals for testing purposes, which is problematic from an animal ethics point of view.

Third, the *responsibilities* different people and organizations have vis-à-vis any adverse effects of the environment on human health are at stake (Minkler, 2000; FEC, 2005). How far are the people involved accountable and can they, from an ethical point of view, be prevented in one way or another from repeating similar actions that contribute to those adverse effects?

Finally, new ethical issues are raised by the *type of interventions* that should be followed after research has identified adverse effects and studied the precise effects on health. It is possible to distinguish between the more personal types of intervention and more collective social regulations, as well as between more expert or community based intervention (Sharp, 2001; Paulson, 2006). Estimates of cost on the basis of value perspectives do play an important role here, and identification of susceptible sub-populations can lead to a discriminating attitude when ineffective precautions are taken, a question which is also connected with the issue of responsibility.

In this chapter, I will first discuss these four ethical types of issues in general and then discuss one of them in depth, an important environmental health problem: the occurrence of obesity in the West.

HISTORICAL DISCUSSION

Well known cases of environmental health demonstrate most of these four types of ethical issues very clearly. A very famous case started in 1978 in Love Canal, a suburban town in the state of New York that was built over the waste-disposal site of a former chemical factory Citizens suffered all kinds of health problems such as asthma and urinary track infections, due to the presence of many toxic substances, some of which were carcinogenic. Government scientists made many mistakes in identifying the exact causes of the health problems that these citizens had, and resisted the data and findings of citizen activists. Even a Hollywood movie (*A Civil Action*) was made about these events (Brown, 2008). The exact identification of the problem was at stake here and was determined from differing normative backgrounds, including the more conservative taxonomy that a place is safe until it is proved unsafe, or the opposite taxonomy that a place is unsafe until it is proved otherwise.

The type of research to be carried out and the policy measures connected to these research efforts were also controversial and value laden. The government scientists researched only the locations near to the waste-disposal site; however, the citizen activists analysed the locations near old drainage ditches. Different estimations of carcinogenic effects were made, and the ensuing uncertainty was a good excuse for some of the participants to do as little as possible. Not only was the question of the responsibility of the owners of the former factory addressed, but also that of the government and their scientists. Communication of the research results caused a lot of consternation. Eventually, intervening in the structure of the property structure was seen by some as an infringement, and by others as necessary actions inspired by more basic values.

There are many other cases in which environmental health has been at stake, resulting in attempts, for example, to have lead identified as severely toxic, and to remove it from the vicinity of children; or to link cases of cancer or asthma to the proximity of factories. In most of these cases, environmental justice activists achieved much in getting these problems formulated and onto the agendas of researchers and policymakers. Identifying environmental toxicants involves many ethical choices (Sharp, 2001). The establishment of research agendas achieves ethical outcomes; identification of a problem that is up against a balance of power and entrenched positions often encounters many difficulties. Second, data that are indeterminate due to their complexity and dynamics often result in different and opposing interpretations upheld by rival groups. Data can be interpreted in multiple ways, depending on theoretical assumptions and normative perspectives. Sometimes, an answer is found by using very detailed research, which often means that more animal testing is required.

New types of research also challenge traditional research methods, applications and practices. For example, genomics (scientific research into the relation between genes and their environment) can have an important role to play in improving environmental health and environmental health research (Darnton-Hill et al., 2004; Khoury and Mensah, 2005; Brand et al., 2008). Genomics can contribute to insight into genetic predispositions that mean certain groups of people have a higher risk of certain environmental health hazards than other groups. Some lifestyles are more vulnerable to adverse environmental influences on health than others (Cockerham and Rutten, 1997). In such cases, screening and testing involve important ethical decisions, because they often tend to discriminate against the chosen group; however, they also provide opportunities for new professions and new allocations of responsibilities (FEC, 2005).

Controversies over how to interact with the people involved do influence their reactions. There are strategies that assume the right to intervene in unhealthy practices and to impede certain practitioners, and this raises new ethical questions. Often, a distinction is made between three types of paternalism: hard paternalism, soft paternalism and maternalism (Haÿry, 1991; Bayer and Fairchild, 2004). The first type comprises direct coercion and denies autonomy of choice, the second one involves cancelling some options for action; or less drastic, offering unwanted information (such as 'smoking kills'). Maternalism involves psychological control by addressing moral feelings such as guilt. Often, there is a mixture of two or three to implement the strategy. For example, with respect to obesity, certain types of unhealthy food can be made more expensive (soft paternalism) or certain persons may be prevented from purchasing fatty foods (hard paternalism). However, ethical considerations, such as autonomy, the right to determine your own life, and the cost–benefit analysis or utilitarian arguments, play a role here (Korthals, 2004).

Improving environmental health requires attributing responsibility to people, institutions, networks and policy agents, which is often connected with differences in power and interests (Minkler, 2000). Responsibilities of different stakeholders are at stake: when environmental health effects are severe, there is an effort to blame others; or by referring to the complexity of the issue by raising the problem of 'many hands' (a situation where so many people are involved that it is impossible to trace back to individual actors or groups what their responsibility is) (Myers, 2002).

FOCUS: DIET-RELATED HEALTH AND OBESITY

Somehow, even without modern science, people have been aware for a long time of the relationship between food, environment and health. For example as early as 1500 BC, probably the first nutritional deficiency disease to be clearly recognized was night blindness, treated by the Egyptians and Greeks with the ingestion or local application of cooked liver. It was not until 1915 and beyond that experimental work identified vitamin A as the relevant factor and paved the way for its inexpensive production and use in the prevention of vitamin A deficiency. However, the intricacies of nutrient–environment interactions are difficult to unravel and many think that our ability to more accurately pinpoint nutrient requirements, as well as define the contribution of other dietary constituents to disease prevention and health, is now growing.

One of the most complex and urgent environmental health problems is that of obesity. Obesity is an extreme imbalance of energy input and energy output. Everyone with a body mass index (bodyweight in kilograms divided by height squared in metres) higher than 30 is classed as obese. However, this simple formula hides many complicating factors. In the complex and dynamic case of obesity, four ethical types of problems are also present. The first concerns identifying what type of problem this is and how far the environment plays a role in determining it. Second, having defined the problem of obesity, and researching and devising policies to deal with it, ethical issues of discrimination and justice are encountered. Third, obesity presupposes and impacts on the responsibilities of those involved; fourth, it is ethically debatable how far one might have the right to intervene in reducing unhealthy factors and with what type of intervention.

FIRST: IDENTIFICATION OF THE PHENOMENON OF OBESITY

Is obesity a problem at all? And what type of a problem is it? These important ethical questions are typically asked in identifying the problem. Obesity is seen by many as a huge social health problem and even as a disease; that there is a problem is not questioned – something has to be done! Indeed, it is common knowledge that food influences the health of consumers and the intake of too much food can cause obesity. The complex and interactive factors that are responsible for this relationship and for obesity are however far from clear.

The environment in the West over the last fifty years has changed into one that promotes the intake of excessive energy-rich food and discourages physical activity. Many argue that we live in an obesogenic environment. The World Health Organization (WHO) published a report in 2004 in which it was stated that by 2020, 50 per cent of the world population could be overweight (WHO, 2004). It demonstrated that diet strongly influenced obesity, cancer, diabetes, hypertension, atherosclerosis and other non-communicable chronic diseases. For instance, in the USA 15-20 per cent of adults in some States are obese and in some others, even more than 25 per cent of inhabitants have a BMI >30. In the Netherlands, 13 per cent of boys are overweight and 0.9 per cent obese (BMI >30 kg/m²); and of the girls, 14 per cent are overweight and 1.5 per cent obese (Roth et al., 2004; Lawrence and Worsley, 2007). Many practitioners are involved and held responsible; consequently, many blame each other.

However, the most fundamental ethical question is why, how far and in what way should obesity be identified as a disease or even as a social problem at all (Council of the Obesity Society, 2008). In an article entitled 'Is obesity a disease?', Stanley Heshka and David Allison critically remark that in recent years obesity is often labelled a disease by authoritative organizations such as NIH or WHO, but that an explicit rationale for such labelling is seldom given. They concede that obesity may be associated with and contribute to increased risks for hypertension, coronary heart disease, type-two diabetes, dyslipidemia, cancer and cholelithiasis, but insist that 'being a risk factor for other diseases is not an accepted definition of disease' (Heshka and Allison, 2001: 1401). The condition that a purported disease should exhibit a set of identifiable signs and symptoms is met in this particular case, 'but only in a circular or tautological sense: the only characteristic (pathonomic), identifiable sign of obesity is also the characteristic which defines obesity, i.e. fatness' (Heshka and Allison, 2001: 1402).

Heshka and Allison hold that discrepancies in the usage of the disease label for obesity may reflect a process of social negotiation in which different organized lobbies and interest groups take part, rather than being a scientific dispute about evidence. Those who propound the disease label usually want to relieve obese persons from responsibility for their condition and to assign responsibilities to others for providing treatment and reimbursing costs (compare Chang and Christakis, 2002). Those who oppose the disease label, by contrast, may consider obesity a self-inflicted condition brought about by 'wilful' overeating or the result of behavioural choice, with no obligations placed on others to provide treatment or cover costs.

The financial stakes in the debate about the disease status of obesity are considerable. As in other areas, corporations have found that they can influence public opinion and promote their interests more effectively by working through seemingly independent organizations. Thus the American Obesity Association (AOA), formed in 1995, is nominally 'a lay advocacy group representing the interest of the 70 to 80 million obese American women and children and adults afflicted with the disease of obesity'. However, the Association 'receives most of its funding – several hundred thousand dollars in all – from the pharmaceutical industry, including Interneuron, American Home Products, Roche Laboratories, Knoll Pharmaceuticals Ltd, and Servier – all of which market or develop diet pills' (CSPI, 2003: 17).

In particular, associations of obese persons contest the obesity 'disease' or even 'epidemic'; they show that many of the findings in respect of obesity are controversial, contest claims concerning the health risks and show counterclaims of medical knowledge that put other claims in perspective. It becomes apparent that, because the search for medical solutions to obesity is the trillion dollar thing, many scientists are exaggerating the risks and costs. Furthermore, they often promote the opposite of the 'normal', dominant body culture, by claiming 'fat is beautiful' and 'fat but fit'.

Such considerations should make us careful in defining the obesity problem, in particular when obese persons themselves are not allowed to make themselves heard (and they aren't; see Council of the Obesity Society, 2008). However, from the data and trends it is also clear that obese persons have many problems in living with their vulnerability. In particular, obese children and adolescents may not have been instrumental in achieving their condition, one which they very often see as quite problematic; and they find it extremely difficult to eliminate the obese conditions that were inflicted on them during childhood. Obese persons may in addition have an adverse influence on their social environment, for example by claiming more space; but they can also harm the environment because these claims are connected to increased use of scarce resources, such as energy, health care and food. These considerations should indeed justify seeing obesity as a serious social problem that deserves policies and research.

The formal definition (when bodyweight in kilograms divided by height in metres squared is higher than 30 one is classed as obese) covers many social and ethical issues. In looking at the field of obesity research and those connected professionally with it, as well as the views of policymakers, one can distinguish at least three perspectives: (1) that obesity has essentially to do with the individual behaviour of the obese; (2) that the social contexts of obese persons are dominant; and (3) that great attention should be paid to the body of obese persons (including interaction between genes and the environment). Three different social and ethical networks are connected with these groups: one that emphasizes individual responsibility and action; one that holds social environments responsible and proposes social regulations; and a third one that proposes surgical, genetic and other medical solutions.

These perspectives have a practical point in so far as their diagnoses locate responsibilities and accountabilities, and indicate the direction for finding solutions to the problem. Although all agree that obesity constitutes a pressing problem, they then continue by focusing on the different causes of and solutions to the problem. The first perspective centres around individual actions (behaviour); the second gives centre stage to environmental influences; and the third perspective focuses on biological and genetic causes in the body. As a result, the first individualizes and moralizes; the second moralizes but does not individualize; and finally, the third individualizes but does not moralize.

The individual perspective

Most people see the individual behaviour of obese persons as the most important cause of their condition and blame them personally for it. The general formula, imbalance of energy output and input, seems to support this premise. If people don't move about, watch TV all day, drink and eat too much and pay no attention to the guidelines for healthy food that are communicated everywhere, and remain as obese as they are, it is down to their own way of life. This is the simplest view, due to the fact that everyone can see when someone is obese. However, it is clear that individuals are not isolated from their environment; their lifestyles are often constrained and channelled by environmental stimuli in the broadest sense.

The environmental perspective

In 1983, one of the first UK government reports from the National Advisory Committee on Nutrition Education, food companies were implicitly accused of the fact that many foodstuffs were not healthy. Since then, food industries have often been accused of contributing to obesity. According to Marion Nestlé (2002), it is in their interest to produce and sell as much food as possible, and to encourage people to eat more. So in the course of the last decades the amount of fat and salt in food products has steadily been increased. The recent row about the industry influencing World Health Organization recommendations adds evidence to Nestlé's accusation. Larger portions, super-sizing of drinks and free refills are some of strategies these industries employ to have people eat more. Offering catering contracts to schools is another strategy.

This tendency to hold corporate actors responsible for the weight problem has also taken a legal form. For example, MacDonald's was sued both in the UK and in the US. In the UK case it was argued that McDonald's deliberately misinformed its consumers (Appleson, 2002). The company asserted that Big Macs and other of their products were healthy and nutritious, and they intentionally concealed information about their nutritional value and about the health effects of continuing consumption.

An enabling environment encompasses a wide frame of reference, from the environment at school, in the workplace and in the community, to transport policies, urban design policies and the availability of a healthy diet. Furthermore, it requires supportive, legislative, regulatory and fiscal policies to be in place. Unless there is an enabling context, the potential for change will be minimal. The ideal is an environment that not only promotes but also supports and protects healthy living, making it possible, for example to cycle or walk to work or school, to buy fresh fruit and vegetables, and to eat and work in smoke-free rooms (WHO, 2003: 138)

Interaction of bodily, environmental and genetic factors

Most studies agree that genetic factors cannot account for the high occurrence of overweight and obese people in western countries. Contrary to what was predicted at the beginning of the genomics era, obesity is a multifactorial phenomenon that has many causes; only in very few cases is some monogenetic disorder at stake. However, there still are indications that, particularly in the more morbid forms of obesity (BMI higher than 35), multifactorial genetic factors that determine for example satiety, can play a role (Brand et al., 2008). But in general there have not been found any relevant genetic causes for differences in metabolism between obese and non-obese persons, although some studies show genetic differences in satiety. Loos and Bouchard (2003) conclude their study with: 'the susceptibility to obesity is partly determined by genetic factors, but an "obesogenic" environment is typically necessary for its phenotypic expression'. On the basis of Loos and Bouchard (2003), a matrix (see Table 33.1) can be constructed in which the interaction between genetic and environmental factors is shown on four different levels.

Note also that this scheme totally rules out individual variation, because it fully emphasizes the role of the environment in becoming obese. Here again ethics is prominent in the selection of the perspectives.

It is probable that the three perspectives have their respective values in different contexts, and it is therefore wise not to exclude any one of them in policy measures; but it is important to realize that they have different ethical implications of one's view on what is a good life and what is a responsibility.

SECOND: ETHICS OF PURSUING RESEARCH AND FORMULATING POLICIES

Obtaining information or carrying out research about obesity confronts one straight away with the large number of factors that are at stake. Only a brief look at the two very

Table 33.1   Different levels of interaction between genetic susceptibility and environment

Levels of genetic susceptibility	Body size in a non-obesogenic environment	Body size in an obesogenic environment
Genetic	Massively obese	Massively obese
Strong predisposition	Normal weight/overweight	Obese
Slight predisposition	Normal weight/overweight	Overweight/obese
Genetically resistant	Normal weight	Normal weight

sophisticated studies from the Government Office for Science, *Modelling Future Trends in Obesity and their Impacts on Health* (GOS, 2007a) and *Tackling Obesity: Future Choices – Building the Obesity Map* (GOS, 2007b), gives a feeling of being overwhelmed by the infinitely huge number of relationships and factors involved. Moreover, research does contradict itself, produces totally differing results and changes of time, because of the indeterminate nature of data which are often subject to opposite interpretations that are upheld by rival groups. For some stakeholders, this uncertainty is a reason to doubt all the evidence.

These uncertainties put older, more philosophical reflections on certainty in a new light. In government circles, scientific knowledge is often used to end a state of uncertainty; but in this case, science increases uncertainties. Mary Douglas, in her article 'Dealing with uncertainty', asks rhetorically 'Where do we humans get our confidence in certain knowledge? The answer is cultural learning. ... We create institutions that protect our valued ideas' (Douglas, 2001: 148). We pay a particular price for certainty: closure of debate, taboos, correctness and its institutions that try to uphold correct behaviour. Her reflections on certainty very much resemble those of Wittgenstein (1969). He stresses the importance of fundamental certainties that cannot be doubted, or which, when doubted, receive reactions such as, 'this person is nuts'. He states that the human condition begins with non-doubting: 'The game of doubting itself presupposes certainty' (Wittgenstein, 1969: para 115). A doubt requires its own grounds, i.e. a context we trust. Doubting is only possible because we are absolutely sure of certain basic propositions, as for example, 'this is my hand'; or 'it is impossible that I was on the moon yesterday'. Nevertheless, as we live in a risk society (Beck, 1990), some profit more from uncertainties and risks than others.

But although scientific evidence is indeterminate and often uncertain, it is still clear that certain connections do exist. An ethics of dealing with uncertainties is lacking to date; it should enable one to identify and be selective between important, major uncertainties and minor, unimportant ones. There are not general tools or general guidelines to deal with that process of selection, but people who feel uncertain about scientific evidence can be assisted by such procedures as consultations, deliberations and the exchange of stories and life narratives. Some ethical support can be given by Putnam's distinction between commonsense doubt, meaning the selecting of more or less certain cases; and philosophical doubt, i.e. the radical denial of all certainties (Putnam, 1995: 57–81): 'We have to remind ourselves of the distinction between common sense doubt and philosophical doubt. Finishing in believing in something is not really a human possibility. Criticism can not be a reason for universal scepsis. The fact that sometimes we are wrong is not a reason to really doubt every particular conviction' (Putnam, 1995: 75). Commonsense doubt shifts between different types of doubt that are more or less realistic. The selection of these types of doubt with respect to what is an adverse environmental influence on human health and what is really a hazard that can be prevented, can be made in public interactions and communications.

In improving environmental health there is a role for public health nutrition to play, directed at general risk profiles. Governments should regulate the food sector, improve research ethics and medical testing of health foods, and allow only affordable health foods. Its main aim in nutrition policy should be the encouragement of the (in)formal ties in pleasurable eating that has health as a fundamental. Health should be a secondary goal in eating, and consumer groups should be empowered as stakeholders (most trusted according to the Eurobarometer (2005): 33 per cent) and be given a voice not only downstream in nutrigenomics (with respect to the end products) but also upstream in the nutrigenomics research agenda.

To tackle the issue of easy expectations and hype, it is necessary to establish independent gatekeepers to safeguard the independence of testing, marketing, communicating and providing the services of nutrigenomics. With respect to *ethics for scientists*, scientists are in need of codes of practice to put forward ethically acceptable research agendas and to validate scientific claims with respect to environmental health hazards. Research focusing on common illnesses should not fall into disarray, as has that for affordable and common drugs and food stuffs. Making healthy foodstuffs easy to obtain for everyone remains an important challenge for nutrigenomics.

THIRD: WHO IS RESPONSIBLE FOR OBESITY, WHO HAS TO ACT AND HAS TO FOOT THE BILL?

Many agencies, practitioners and stakeholders are connected within a network that consists of at least three circles: one that emphasizes behaviour, a second that has the social contexts as its core and a third that centres on the body. Many actors are responsible and blame each other. According to the theory of role responsibility, you should not be doing harm by performing your job according to best practice, something that has already been established. So this theory is essentially negative (avoiding harm) and retro-active. However, the theory of public responsibility, which is reacting to new developments in a socially and ethically acceptable way, even when there is no clear best practice, is both positive and prospective. While role theory stresses being liable or even punishable for risks and dangers, the public responsibility theory concentrates on future acts that enhance trust in the professions vis-à-vis the public. It means that informing the public and stimulating the forming of opinions also belongs to a profession.

Complicated problems in confused contexts, so characteristic of obesity, such as the issue of many hands and that of the diffusion of responsibility, should be discussed. Children are more vulnerable than adults, meaning that parents have great responsibility for their health. Often, new technologies and practices (such as genomics) create new public responsibilities and new distributions of responsibility, but also new types of responsibility for food professionals. How can obese persons (adults, children and their caretakers) move on in this jungle of new responsibilities? Who is held responsible/ accountable for the causes of obesity, and for its remedies? Is the current distribution of responsibilities adequate, fitting for the task in hand in the new circumstances created by the introduction of genomics?

Currently, most people blame the obese. The famous ethicist Peter Singer states: 'others just eat too much and should show more restraint. Along with the old-fashioned virtue of frugality, the idea that it is wrong to be a glutton is in urgent need of revival' (Singer, 2006: 278). However, this moralizing should be restricted by one important condition. Individuals can only be held responsible for their own weight when they are adequately informed about their food and are able to act accordingly. Otherwise, their choices are not really autonomous. As in medical practice, in questions related to food the principle of *informed consent* plays a role.

Most ethicists will agree with Immanuel Kant who tells us in his *Metaphysics of Morals* (Kant, 1983) that stuffing oneself with food incapacitates a person 'for actions that would require him to use his powers with skill and determination' and because putting oneself in such a state violates one's duty to oneself. However, Kant emphasizes that the enjoyment of eating and drinking together with others is nevertheless a moral event. 'Although a banquet is a formal invitation to excess in both food and drink, there is still something in it that aims at a moral end, beyond mere physical well-being: it brings a number of people together for a long time to converse with one another.' Even if it is a moral problem it doesn't necessarily mean that the responsibilities are suddenly apparent. When parents do raise obese children, this implies that they restrict freedom of space for children to choose their own lifestyle.

From an environmental point of view one might raise arguments in favour of taking care of one's own body weight. Taking up a disproportionate share of resources such as health care, meat, crops and all the other material resources that are necessary, such as water and pesticides, has severe environmental and north–south implications, because most of these resources are processed in the south and their production processes strengthen existing power and unsustainable relationships. These arguments are not confined to obese persons, but they contribute in high measure to these problems.

Responsibility for complex problems in complex societies reveals all kinds of mechanisms to escape from responsibility, in particular in contexts of widespread responsibility (Myers, 2002). Either too many are held responsible, or even more simply too many people cause practitioners to step back from taking responsibility and *social idling* (social ignorance) takes place. This can also happen in cases where one person or institution is held responsible, with the consequence that everyone else can cease to feel responsible. In such cases it appears that the allocation of responsibility is like water: it has the dynamism of communicating vessels, and it is diluted when too many are held responsible.

Because of their vulnerability, children in particular should get special attention in the prevention of obesity; practitioners have special responsibilities with respect to them; but how to structure the field in order to prevent the spreading of the epidemic? In cases of social idling and dilution of responsibility, the remedy is to install clear structures of responsibility, to identify the big players in the field and to define the spots where responsible action can make a difference. These big players are primarily food companies, retailers, governments (and governmental agencies) and food scientists and technologists – all can make a difference. Where is the weakest link that promises the most efficient outcome and requires the least effort? It can be a combination of several short- and long-term measures, of preventive and curative measures, of social structures and material products.

FOUR: IS THERE JUSTIFICATION FOR INTERVENTION, BY WHOM AND IN WHAT WAYS?

Who should intervene? As we have seen, obesity is an extremely complex phenomenon, with many practitioners involved. Should governments take the lead and discourage obesity by making healthy foodstuffs easily accessible and cheaper? Does that mean that contributors to the rise of obesity, like food industries and computer companies, have to take part in their share of intervention strategies? In most countries governments do indeed take the lead, often giving assistance to companies to facilitate for example the reduction of salt and fat.

What type of intervention is ethically acceptable?

There is little evidence for the effectiveness of one strategy versus another (Lawrence and Worsley, 2007: 206). Those who think that genetics and genomics can play a role propose screening or tests to find particularly vulnerable groups. Criteria for screening in the low-risk population were developed as early as 1968 by the WHO. These so-called Wilson and Jungner criteria mention several aspects to balance the pros and cons of screening possibilities, and to evaluate whether benefits outweigh the disadvantages. A central criterion is the availability of treatment (Wilson and Jungner, 1968). However, there is not one effective treatment for obesity. Moreover, identifying individuals or groups of individuals who show higher risks of certain vulnerability for environmentally induced diseases through screenings can produce discrimination.

Often, all the emphasis of health and food experts in both personal and collective programmes is put on to dietary intake and they propose special diets. For example in Japan under a national law, Japanese citizens between the ages of 40 and 74 must measure their waistlines. If they exceed a certain limit, they will receive dietary education (Onishi, 2008). This looks like rather forceful intervention into personal life, rather dubious when viewed from the standpoint of autonomy. Moreover, as we have seen, eating is an institution comprising activities that have many aspects, one of which is eating together, that has a huge social impact and contributes in high measure to the improvement of the informal ties of society. Dieting is often connected with fear, feeling humiliated and guilt, which do not contribute well to a healthy life. To discourage eating is therefore a very tricky affair, and is moreover ineffective in the main. Also, dieting creates mostly adverse effects of feelings of guilt, with temporary but strong cravings, or even binge eating activities. Many interventions incorporate the idea that obese persons are somehow immoral (Prose, 2003).

Therefore, strategies directed at increasing energy output are one-sided; they should be complemented by social and medical strategies directed at energy input, such as radical changes in the supply chain to produce healthier foods, and in the built environment. Plans of action to prevent obesity should cover a broad portfolio of promising interventions. The growing number of obese persons implies that a growing investment in health is needed to manage the health problems of the more than one billion people who are overweight and obese.

OUTLOOK AND CONCLUSION

Most problems of environmental health are, when identified, extremely complex and difficult to tackle, either in research, or in policy measures or in communication. From an ethical point of view at least four issues of environmental factors deserve ethical attention. First, the identification of what type of problem is an environmental factor causing unhealthy influences, and where the problem is located. Second, there is the ethics of doing research into the factors that produce environmental hazards. Third, responsibility for managing and increasing the environmental health of the various practitioners involved is in need of ethical attention. Fourth, the right to intervene to reduce unhealthy factors and the type of intervention require ethical analysis. In all four of these types of problems, in the main it is not the case that ethicists have a box of tools ready to be used. But ethicists can, in cooperation with social and communication scientists, contribute to an ethical analysis of the issues where it really impacts, and try to offer proposals to reduce ethical damage as much as possible.

These contributions require a more transparent role for interdisciplinary ethicists in government and science circles that focus on environmental health. But continuous research is also required on the different ethical methods and in how far they can improve the ethical status of the complex and multifactorial problems that are so prototypical for problems of environmental health.

REFERENCES

Appleson, G. (2002) 'McDonald's tries to spit out obesity lawsuit', *Reuters/Yahoo! News*, 20/11. Available at www.mcspotlight.org.

Bayer, R. and Fairchild, A.L (2004) 'The genesis of public health ethics', *Bioethics*, 18 (6): 473–92.

Beck, U. (1990) *Risk Society*. London: Sage.

Brand, A., Brand, H. and den Baumen, T.S. (2008) 'The impact of genetics and genomics on public health', *European Journal of Human Genetics*, 16 (1): 5–13.

Brown, P. (2008) *Toxic Exposures, Contested Illnesses and the Environmental Health Movement*. New York: Columbia University Press.

Center for Science in the Public Interest (CSPI) (2003) *Lifting the Veil of Secrecy: Corporate Support for Health and Environmental Professional Associations, Charities, and Industry Front Groups*. Washington, DC: CSPI.

Chang, V.W. and Christakis, N.A. (2002) 'Medical modelling of obesity: A transition from action to experience in a 20th century American medical textbook', *Sociology of Health & Illness*, 24: 151–77.

Cockerham, W., Rutten, A., and Abel, T. (1997) 'Conceptualizing contemporary health lifestyles', *Sociological Quarterly*, 38 (2): 321–42.

Council of the Obesity Society (Chair: D.B.Allison) (2008) 'Obesity as a disease: A White Paper on evidence and arguments commissioned by the Obesity Society', *Nature*, 16 (6):1161–77.

Darnton-Hill, I., Margetts, B. and Deckelbaum, R. (2004) 'Public health nutrition and genetics: Implications for nutrition policy and promotion', *Proceedings of the Nutrition Society*, 63 (1): 173–85.

Douglas, M. (2001) 'Dealing with uncertainty', *Ethical Perspectives*, 8: 145–55.

European Commission, Special Eurobarometer 225 (2005) *Social Values, Science and Technology*. Available at http://ec.europa.eu/public_opinion/archives/ebs/ebs_225_report_en.pdf.

Food Ethics Council (FEC) (2005) *Getting Personal: Shifting Responsibilities for Health*. Brighton: FEC.

Government Office for Science (GOS) (2007a) *Tackling Obesities: Future Choices. Modelling Future Trends in Obesity and the Impact on Health*. London: Department of Innovation, Universities and Skills.

Government Office for Science (GOS) (2007b) *Tackling Obesities: Future Choices. Obesity System Atlas*. London: Department of Innovation, Universities and Skills.

Haÿry, H. (1991) *The Limits of Medical Paternalism*. London: Routledge.

Heshka, S. and Allison, D.B. (2001) 'Is obesity a disease?', *International Journal of Obesity*, 25: 1401–4.

Kant, I. (1983) 'The metaphysics of morals', in I. Kant (ed.), *Ethical Philosophy*, trans. J.W. Ellington. Indianapolis, IN: Hackett.

Khoury, M.J. and Mensah, G.A. (2005) 'Genomics and the prevention and control of common chronic diseases: Emerging priorities for public health action', *Preventing Chronic Disease* (serial online). Available at http://www.cdc.gov/pcd/issues/2005/apr/05_0011.htm.

Korthals, M. (2004) *Before Dinner.* Dordrecht: Springer.

Lavery, J.V., Upshur, R., Sharp, R. and Hofman, K. (2003) 'Ethical issues in international environmental health research', *International Journal of Hygiene and Environmental Health*, 206: 453–63.

Lawrence, M. and Worsley, T. (eds) (2007) *Public Health Nutrition: From Principles to Practice.* Maidenhead/New York: Open University Press/McGraw-Hill.

Loos, R.J. and Bouchard, C. (2003) 'Obesity – is it a genetic disorder?', *Journal of Internal Medicine*, 254: 401–25.

Minkler, M. (2000) 'Personal responsibility for health: Contexts and controversies', in D. Callahan (ed.), *Promoting Healthy Behavior.* Washington, DC: Georgetown University Press, pp. 1–22.

Myers, D.G. (2002) *Social Psychology,* 7th ed. Boston, MA: McGraw Hill.

Nestle, M. (2002) *Food Politics: How Food Industry Influences Nutrition and Health.* Berkeley, CA: University of California Press.

Onishi, N. (2008) 'Japan, seeking trim waists, measures millions', *New York Times*, 13 June.

Paulson, J.A. (2006) 'An exploration of ethical issues in research in children's health and the environment', *Environmental Health Perspectives*, 114 (10): 1603–9.

Prose, F. (2003) *Gluttony. The Seven Deadly Sins.* New York: Oxford University Press.

Putnam, H. (1995) *Pragmatism: An Open Question.* Oxford: Blackwell.

Resnik, D.B. and Roman, G. (2007) 'Health, justice, and the environment', *Bioethics*, 21 (4): 230–41.

Roth, J., Qiang, X., Marbán, S.L., Redelt, H. and Lowell, B.C. (2004) 'The obesity pandemic: Where have we been and where are we going?', *Obesity Research,* 12: 88S–100S.

Sharp, R. (2001) 'Ethical issues in environmental health research', *Environmental Health Perspectives*, 111 (14): 1786–8.

Singer, P. (2006) *Eating.* London: Penguin.

Wilson, J.M.G. and Jungner, G. (1968) *Principles and Practice of Screening for Disease*, Public Health Papers, nr 34. Geneva: WHO.

Wittgenstein, L. (1969) *On Certainty* [Uber Gewissheit]. ed. G.E.M. Anscombe and G.H. von Wright; trans. D. Paul and G.E.M. Anscombe. Oxford: Basil Blackwell.

World Health Organization (WHO) (2003) *Diet, Nutrition and the Prevention of Chronic Diseases.* Geneva: WHO.

World Health Organization (WHO) (2004) 'Global strategy on diet, physical activity and health', Fifty-seventh World Health Assembly, WHA57.17, 22 May, Geneva.

34

Pharmaceuticals[1]

Margit Sutrop and Kadri Simm

INTRODUCTION

The past 100 years have seen major improvements in length and quality of life. While in the year 1900 only one quarter of people were able to see their sixty-fifth birthday, now three-quarters of us can expect to reach this age in good health (Winnacker, 2000).[2] This dramatic change has become possible, among other things, through progress in medicine and technology. Several former killer diseases, such as diphtheria, polio and smallpox have been virtually eliminated, at least in the so-called developed countries. It was only as recently as 1929 that Alexander Fleming discovered the antibacterial effect of penicillin; since that time, the use of antibiotics has saved millions of lives.

Complete sequencing of the human genome and other advances in biomedical science and bioinformatics are expected to once again revolutionize the face of medicine. Over the past 50 years there have been rapid advances in our understanding of the involvement of genetic polymorphisms in response to drug therapies. There is clear evidence of considerable variability in drug response depending on the genetic make-up of the patient. The emergence of pharmacogenetics heralds a new era in which genotype-based therapies are expected to reduce drug-induced morbidity and mortality.

Today, adverse reaction to medicines is an important cause of hospital admissions (Lazarou et al., 1998; Guyer et al., 2000; Davies et al., 2009). Ineffective drug treatment is a big burden on the health-care system. It is hoped that pharmacogenetics will improve drug efficacy and safety, and at the beginning of the twenty-first century there is widespread optimism that the development of personalized medicine is only a matter of time.

On the other hand, optimism about the increasing curability of diseases is justified only in some parts of the world. In emerging and developing countries, major killer diseases are under-researched, and access to available medicines is lacking due to grave poverty. Difficult debates are raging over intellectual property rights, generic drug manufacturing and pricing for AIDS drugs in developing countries. Ever-rising drug prices also raise the issue of affordability for the health-care systems of the developed world. The growing gap between profits and public health interests causes damage to the reputation of the pharmaceutical industry. It has been pointed out that while during the second half of the twentieth century the pharmaceutical industry was praised for delivering miracles, at the beginning of the twenty-first century 'there is growing controversy and even hostility in the relationship between the pharmaceutical industry and the public' (Santoro, 2005: 1). Despite the drug companies' notable contributions to the production of life-saving and life-enhancing drugs, the public tends to mistrust the pharmaceutical industry.[3]

Journalists, researchers, physicians and government officials criticize the pharmaceutical industry for not fulfilling its social obligations. How can public trust in the pharmaceutical industry be restored? Part of the problem lies in the complexity of the relationships involved. The industry engages the worlds of science, medicine and healthcare, economics, human rights, governance and social welfare. It is no wonder there are tensions between different stakeholders with their vastly differing aims: whereas industry is profit-driven, scientists seek to advance knowledge, and physicians aim to cure patients' diseases and promote public health. How can one find a sustainable path for the pharmaceutical industry to thrive economically while also serving the needs of society and individuals? Balancing these different interests is difficult, but communication and an open debate on the many ethical and social issues is surely necessary if we ever hope to find common ground between the disparate discourses of profit-driven market rationale and the centrality of human needs and vulnerabilities that traditionally character the sphere of healthcare.

This paper is concerned with analyzing transformations in the development, marketing, prescription, and access issues of pharmaceuticals, paying special attention to a variety of ethical and social aspects. A major focus of the article is on pharmacogenetics – a rapidly developing discipline which in the near future might well have a major effect on both drug development and clinical medicine.

DRUG DEVELOPMENT

Pharmaceuticals are mostly produced by pharmaceutical companies. Over the past decades, many mergers, acquisitions and buyouts have resulted in there being a limited number of large pharmaceutical corporations dominating the trade (the top six companies having almost 38 percent and the fifteen largest companies having nearly 64 percent world market share).[4] Globalization has also stimulated the formation of various non-profit organizations and partnerships for drug development – for example, the TB Alliance that includes public and private sector partners to accelerate the treatment of tuberculosis, or the Path Malaria Vaccine Initiative that has a similarly diverse range of collaborators. International organizations like the World Health Organisation and the Joint United Nations Programme on HIV/AIDS are working globally and in cooperation with local authorities to control, treat and eradicate diseases.

The focus of the latter programmes is mostly on diseases prevalent in the poorer areas of the world, whereas the for-profit pharmaceutical companies focus their research more on the diseases and conditions of the developed world. Such a 'division of labour' is reflected in the infamous 90/10 gap, meaning that 90 percent of investment in medical research is spent on the health-care issues of 10 percent of the world population.[5] Of the 1233 drugs approved for market between 1975 and 1999, only 13 were designed specifically for tropical diseases (and six of these were sponsored by international organizations).[6] Thus most current research is carried out on diseases prevalent in industrialized countries, and, sadly, much less scientific attention is paid to the health-care problems of the majority of the world population. This disproportionate R&D investment highlights the fact that drug development is increasingly market-driven.

The drug development process starts with drug discovery, in which a certain chemical component is discovered that is identified as potentially beneficial in curing a targeted condition. Further research will have to establish the efficacy and safety of the drug before it is finally allowed to proceed to human clinical trials; these are divided into three phases. The first phase, usually undertaken with healthy volunteers, aims to establish the safety of the drug and its pharmacokinetic and pharmacologic properties. The second phase involves patients suffering from the condition that the new drug should target; in the course of the trial the efficacy and side-effects of the new drug are determined. Should this phase be successful, a wider group of patients is enrolled (anywhere from a few hundred to a few thousand people) in a third series of both controlled and uncontrolled trials to determine the efficacy and safety of the drug. After the trials, the drug needs to be approved by appropriate regulatory authorities for production. Since many of the new drugs are developed by US companies or companies that aim to market their products in the US, it is crucial that most drugs follow the Food and Drug Administration's (FDA) procedures and guidelines.

There may also be a fourth, pharmacovigilant phase in clinical trials, for monitoring any long-term or very rare effects of the drug after it has already been approved.

Since the early 1990s, an increasing amount of research has been undertaken by specialized Contract Research Organisations (CROs) that provide services to the pharmaceutical industry (Dewberry et al., 2006). The industry can outsource some or even most of its research at almost any stage of the drug development process. In fact, a considerable amount of basic research is done by academic and non-profit institutions, and the drug companies often build on the fundamental discoveries originating from these sources (Relman and Angell, 2002: 29). Drug development is truly global, as research laboratories are situated around the world: many original (re)sources – especially plants and animals, originate from the developing countries; clinical trials also take place all across the globe– increasingly moving away from the US and Western Europe to the countries of Asia (India, China), Latin-America and Central and Eastern Europe. This raises a host of ethical issues for the researchers, companies and trial participants involved.

CHALLENGES OF PHARMACOGENETICS

During the twentieth century, progress in the development of effective pharmaceuticals was achieved by focusing on large groups of patients with precisely defined diseases. This approach ensured the relative safety of a drug in relation to the expected benefits, even though efficiency was not achieved with every single patient (Melzer et al., 2003: 15). If some of the patients suffered dangerous side effects, the drug had to be discarded, although in reality it might have been unsuitable only for a small group of patients with a certain genetic profile. This made the clinical trials extremely long and costly, and sometimes ineffective and unsuccessful. The strategy of 'one size fits all' in drug development was challenged in the twenty-first century with the arrival of pharmacogenetics, offering the prospect of an era of 'personalised medicine'.

The history of pharmacogenetics has been dated back to Pythagoras, who in 510 BC recognized that the ingestion of fava beans resulted in a potentially fatal reaction in some, but not all, individuals (Nebert, 1999). The term 'pharmacogenetics' was coined by Friedrich Vogel in 1959 (Vogel, 1959). Pharmacogenetic research began in the 1950s when scientists began to document clinical observations of inherited differences in responses to drugs.[7]

Pharmacogenetics studies variability in drug responses attributed to hereditary factors in different populations. In this it differs from 'pharmacogenomics', which determines and analyzes the genome (DNA) and its products (RNA and proteins) as they relate to drug response (Roses, 2001). Pharmacogenetics and pharmacogenomics are thus 'related facets of cutting edge therapeutic research' (Badcott, 2006). Whereas pharmacogenetics is helping to find the best medicine for an individual patient in a clinical setting, pharmacogenomics will help to find the best drug candidate in pharmaceutical research (Lindpainter, 2002).

From a scientific point of view, three routes are open for studying inter-individual variation in drug response: pharmacokinetic variability (considering variation between individuals in drug processing because of genetic polymorphisms); pharmacodynamics (focusing on interactions between a drug and the proteins the drug is meant to target); and disease pathways (focusing on interactions between genetic predispositions to disease) (Delden et al., 2004: 305–8).

Pharmacogenetics may be of relevance at various stages in the development of new medicines. The application of pharmacogenetics to the development of *new medicines* offers an advantage in clinical trials of distinguishing smaller groups of genetically homogeneous participants for whom effective 'tailor-made' drugs could be produced. In the case of *existing medicines*, the application of pharmacogenetic analysis plays an important role in improving safety and efficacy. As adverse reactions to medicines have significant cost, in both human and monetary terms, pharmacogenetics has great potential.

However, it is unclear whether the cost of genotype-based drugs will rise or drop. Initially it was expected that the inclusion of pharmacogenetic testing in drug development would lower the cost of drugs and decrease the amount of time needed for research (Peakman and Arlington, 2001; Tollman et al., 2001). First, fewer participants would be needed in trial phases as drugs would be targeted to specific genotypes. Second, drugs that are only effective for certain genotypes could still be approved, while previously such drugs would not have made it to the market, since they were ineffective or even harmful to those with different genotypes. However, these hopes have been called into question (NCB, 2003: 25–6). The number of trial participants still needs to be high to determine all pertinent pharmacogenetic variants that respond to the drug (either positively or adversely). Also, more time may be needed to find and involve participants with targeted genotypes. Additional cost will come from undertaking pharmacogenetic testing and analysis. Only time will show whether pharmacogenetics lowers or raises the overall costs of drug development and consequently what its impact will be on drug accessibility.

Both the development of new drugs as well as the improvement of existing ones raises numerous ethical issues.[8] The advent of pharmacogenetics means that clinical trials will necessarily involve the collection and analysis of the genetic data of participants. Currently it is not obligatory for new drugs to go through pharmacogenetic testing, but this might well change in the near future, meaning that such testing has to be included in the clinical trials. This raises privacy concerns associated with the handling and storage of DNA. Whether and to what degree are the samples anonymized, and if they are not, should one allow feedback for participants? Do biological relatives have a right to know the test results as well as the secondary information? What type of consent should be acquired from the participants – consent solely for the ongoing research, or for any similar research or for any biomedical research? There are ongoing debates in medical ethics regarding the appropriateness of redefining informed consent to suit the needs of genetic research.[9]

The knowledge of a person's genotype raises the possibility of discrimination and stigmatization. If patients are divided into subgroups on the basis of genetic profile, there may be those who turn out to be 'non-responders', for whom the developed drug is ineffective or harmful. Although non-responses or adverse reactions already exist as problems today, the availability of this information early on will, on the one hand, help to avoid these effects, and, on the other hand might well have a serious impact on people's access to health- and life-insurance. Since information about drug response might be interesting for insurance companies, there will probably be growing pressure, especially from life insurers, to disclose information about genetic profile and drug response. Especially in systems of private healthcare, there is particular anxiety that if individuals are categorized as 'difficult to treat', they may be denied insurance.

There may also be so-called orphan indications: genotypes for which drugs are not developed because the target market is too small. Thus developments in pharmacogenetics raise additional social justice and global justice issues, and highlight the social consequences of using the categories of race or ethnicity in research and clinical care.

DRUG MARKETING AND PRESCRIPTIONS

Once a drug has been approved – after years of research, testing and trials – the marketing of the new drug to physicians and potential patients can begin. Producing a new drug is expensive, requiring vast sums of money and on average 10-15 years in development. Studies disagree on the average financial cost of a new drug, with estimates ranging from $200 million (Public Citizen, 2001) to $800 million (DiMasi et al., 2003). The costs are high because only very few drugs out of the potential pool that is researched make it through all the phases of clinical trials and the approval process. New drugs are covered by patents, meaning that a pharmaceutical company has a monopoly on a product for a certain time – usually 20 years.[10] During this time, as competitors are prohibited from producing and marketing the drug, the pharmaceutical company will be able to reap the benefits of its success. Once the patent runs out, other companies can start producing a generic version of the drug.

Marketing as well as advertising a drug has become an increasingly large proportion of the overall budget of drug development. Although it is difficult to draw the line between academic and for-profit research, especially in the early phases of fundamental research, it has been argued that the marketing and advertising budget of the drug companies is now larger than the amounts spent on R&D, totaling over 1/3 of their entire budget (Relman and Angell, 2002: 28, 34).

A number of profound ethical dilemmas characterize contemporary drug marketing practices, especially regarding the relationship between the pharmaceutical industry and the medical profession. Drug companies are known internationally to be very generous with sponsored events and travel, direct and indirect gifts, funding of educational and other events as well as research. Among medical professionals a strong correlation has been established between the acceptance of gifts and other sponsorship from the drug company and a resulting increase in prescribing that sponsor's drug (Lexchin, 1993; Wazana, 2000).

In response to these concerns, both medical professional organizations and the pharmaceutical industry have formulated codes of ethical conduct regulating and limiting the acceptable amount and level of sponsorship and gift-giving. Sometimes legislation has been introduced that requires the documenting of everything received by the physician from the company, but even in those instances, the true level of pharmaceutical industry influence on doctors is difficult to establish (Ross et al., 2007).

The continuous flow of gifts and sponsorships that surrounds health-care professionals from their early student days tends to create a 'long term sense of entitlement' (Moynihan, 2003) that might jeopardize a doctor's obligations towards their patients (Katz et al., 2003). Also, a number of studies have shown that drug company sponsored trials or studies consistently produce results that are skewed positively towards the product of that very same sponsoring company (Lexchin et al., 2003; Bhandari et al., 2004: 477–8). Patients and society at large expect medical professionals to offer unbiased expert advice, but this might prove difficult due to the serious conflict of interests that these professionals are facing.

Prescription of pharmacogenetic drugs brings additional challenges. Tailor-made medicine based on pharmacogenetics presupposes genetic testing – knowledge about the individual's genetic make-up. This creates difficult juxtapositions where, for example, a right to privacy and the right not to know conflict with the right to better healthcare. One person's right to know may conflict with his or her family members' right not to know. As a test may reveal that a patient is effectively untreatable because the medicines available are not effective or have serious side-effects, the psychological effects of pharmacogenetic testing also need to be taken into account. As such information could be distressing or restrict access to insurance, one may argue for the patient's right to refuse a pharmacogenetic test, and still receive the medicine. On the other hand, it may be argued that since health-care resources are limited, one should not waste money for treatment with medicines which may not be effective or may cause adverse reactions. This would mean that one actually has a duty to know, and that choice can only be exercised between being treated or not being treated. Our knowledge about drug reactions creates risks for discrimination and stigmatization, and puts the principle of solidarity in health-insurance under pressure.

Since the developments of pharmacogenetics relate to several fields – pharmaceutical research and development, clinical practice, healthcare, genetics, insurance, and genetic

databases – the ethical issues common to all these fields become relevant. Thus pharmacogenetics serves as a battlefield *par excellence* for bioethicists (Sutrop, 2004: V).

ACCESS AND JUSTICE ISSUES

The overwhelming majority of the new drugs and associated clinical trials target diseases
prevalent in the developed countries. However, many natural plant resources for drug
discovery are situated in the biodiversity-rich developing countries. Furthermore, clinical
trials increasingly take place in developing countries (Agres, 2005), due to a number of
factors, from the benefits of researching ethnically more diverse populations to the lower
costs of conducting a trial. Concerns of fairness arise when the burdens of clinical trials
are on the shoulders of developing countries, but the resultant drugs are not made available
for them. In a survey conducted by the US National Bioethics Advisory Commission
(NBAC), 33 percent of US researchers and 48 percent of researchers abroad were of the
opinion that the results of their research taking place in developing countries would not be
available to these populations in the foreseeable future (NBAC, 2001).

A number of international and local regulations and guidelines have been published that
aim to ensure that clinical trials are conducted ethically and that participating populations
are not solely carrying the burdens of trials; rather, research should be responsive to the
health-care needs of the population.[11] A concept of benefit-sharing has been influential in
highlighting the importance of a just balance of benefits and burdens in international
biomedical research (Simm, 2007). When individuals, communities or even populations
accept risks and provide their time and effort, for example during clinical trials, then it
should be ensured that they would also be able to benefit from the results later on.

The subject matter of post-trial obligations is an increasingly significant subset of the
benefit-sharing discussion that is largely limited to potential duties arising from clinical
trials (and thus excluding a host of other issues that benefit sharing has traditionally
addressed, such as, for example, intellectual property debates). Post-trial obligations
deal with the specific question of what, if anything, is owed to the research participants,
community or population, after the clinical trial has been completed. How are these duties,
if any, ethically justified? Who has the responsibility to fulfill these obligations?

The issue of responsibility is a difficult one in the arena of healthcare, where availability
and access to pharmaceuticals and therapies can be a question of life or death. In traditional
medical ethics the provision of healthcare has been guided by the principle of need –
treatments were due to those who were ill. In this traditional setting, medical researchers
could also count on the altruism of volunteers participating in research and clinical trials.
Indeed, attempts to offer participants anything more than something symbolic in appreciation
of their time and effort would have been viewed as undue inducement.

However, in the era of global biomedical research, with for-profit companies conducting
much of the research, medicine itself has changed considerably and is consequently not
the arena of altruism it perhaps used to be. Commercialization has meant that the main
investments in biomedical research currently originate from the private sector, and the
primary responsibility of for-profit companies lies with their shareholders. The medical

industry has become big business; the pharmaceutical trade sector has been the most profitable in the world for some time (HUGO, 2000). The stringent ethical principles traditionally associated with medical research have thus acquired a whole new background. It seems hypocritical to suggest the centrality of altruism to the many developing countries while the other half of the research relationship – the pharmaceutical industry – is cashing in some of the biggest profits in the world.

Perhaps it is time to rethink the question of responsibilities. Although it is largely accepted that it is the overarching responsibility of national governments to provide healthcare and access to medicines to their populations (NCB, 2005: 122), it can also be argued that, for example, trial participants in developing countries can justifiably expect continued access to beneficial drugs after the trial has been concluded and their government is not capable of providing it. Some international guidelines require post-trial obligations whereas others require merely that this issue should be addressed and that non-provision should be explained to research ethics committees.[12] The HUGO *Statement on Benefit Sharing* has suggested that medical enterprises might have special moral obligations. This is based on an understanding that human health is of fundamental value, and access to healthcare is a basis upon which much else in life depends. Illnesses often diminish the choices we have in life, thus linking this issue to the principle of equal opportunities (Daniels, 1985). While the fulfillment of this principle has traditionally been the responsibility of governments, the HUGO statement introduces an alternative possibility that acknowledges the increasing influence and power that non-state actors have in our globalizing world.

What is the potential impact of pharmacogenetics on justice and access issues on the global health scale? In developed countries, the promise of pharmacogenetic drugs has generally been linked to the idea of personalized medicine, stressing the importance of inter-individual differences in drug metabolism and often requiring individual pharmacogenetic testing. However, for such drugs to be accessible and affordable to developing country populations, the reliance on pharmacogenetic testing is questionable, primarily due to associated high costs. An alternative would be to rely on certain default or self-identified population categories (race, geographical or continental ancestry, ethnicity) (Daar and Singer, 2005). However, the scale of population mixture has been quite significant over the time span of human history, so it is very likely that self-identified population categories are not useful or even safe categories for pharmacogenetic drug prescription (Holm 2008: 86). The history of humankind with its massive migrations, nomadic and other travelling, colonizations, wars and also simply interracial or inter-ethnic marriages has turned the relationship between one's mirror image and genetic heritage into a very fluid one.

It is also unclear whether pharmacogenetics will change anything in making developing countries a more inviting market for pharmaceutical companies. While the markets certainly are potentially huge and the disease burden heavy, these factors have been such for the past decades and the segmentation of the markets likely to follow from applied pharmacogenetics could prove to be an even less inviting prospect.

Policy issues

Pharmacogenetics is still an emerging field in its early stages of development, with very few commercial products available.[13] At the scientific level the accumulation of pharmacogenomic data has not led to a reduction but rather to an increase of questions to be answered as things turn out to be much more complex than expected (Wolffe and Matzke, 1999; Johnson and Lima, 2003). Practical aspects also need to be addressed: the integration of pharmacogenetics into a clinical setting requires new medical infrastructure (routine genetic testing), knowledge (interpretation of the complex test results) as well as negotiation of responsibilities (NCB, 2003)

While its proponents hope that pharmacogenetics will solve the current problems of the pharmaceutical industry and lead to a paradigm shift in the practice of medicine (Lindpainter, 2002; Bunk, 2003), more critical voices point at the uncertainties and numerous ethical issues which require careful consideration and wise policy responses (Buchanan, et al., 2002). Issues of ethical concern relate to the different applications of pharmacogenetics – from the development of new drugs to the improvement of already existing ones. Several questions require reflection and debate: what type of consent, confidentiality and privacy protection measures are needed for pharmacogenetic research relying on biobanks as well as for prescriptions of 'tailor-made' drugs? How is the unsolved problem of unequal access to drugs and healthcare affected by the further stratification of patient populations in pharmacogenetics? How should responsibilities be divided between different parties in a clinical setting? Who decides whether to take a test, whether to make the drug available after the test or whether to make the drug available if the patient is unwilling to take the associated test? The effective delivery of pharmacogenetics will require the cooperation of patients, doctors and other health-care professionals, but it will also call for new regulatory frameworks to ensure that access to drugs is provided to those in need despite increased patient stratification and potential threat of orphan-populations and – diseases.

Despite the high levels of uncertainty concerning both scientific and ethical aspects of pharmacogenetics, there is pressure on policymakers to lay down regulatory and governance framework decisions (Ling and Raven, 2006).

For successful policymaking, identification of various stakeholder interests is the first step – clarification of the often opposing positions of the pharmaceutical industry, biomedical scientists, health-care providers, insurance companies and the public health sector is required. For example, genetic stratification of disease categories and patient populations will lead to the segmentation of drug markets; thus different stakeholders may have different attitudes towards these developments. While health-care providers and biotech companies may be very interested in taking advantage of the potential cost-effectiveness and innovativeness of tailor-made drugs, the pharmaceutical industry might not be too keen to fragment the markets for already existing medicines (Smart and Martin, 2006).

Identification of smaller, more narrowly defined groups of patients for whom a medicine is appropriate will have a negative effect on profitability. As drugs become more specific to genotypes, their target groups will become smaller. This is where proactive policy regulations could have an impact in negotiating existing tensions and gearing overall development. Policies to motivate the pharmaceutical industry to develop and produce drugs for smaller patient strata are needed (potential options range from novel patent policies to dedicated funds and tax regimes). Similarly to the public-private partnerships formed for the purpose of developing drugs for tropical diseases for poorer populations, potential segmentation of markets resulting from pharmacogenetic drug research requires policymakers and stakeholders to come together.

Also, successful implementation of pharmacogenetics requires the renegotiation of the interests of public health administrations, insurance companies and the users of health-care services. If drugs that are tailor-made for a smaller subgroup of patients will be more expensive than 'bulk drugs', the question arises as to which costs should be reimbursed by public health services, private insurance, and which should be paid for by the patients themselves? Insurers and patients often have conflicting interests regarding the confidentiality of the information provided by the pharmacogenetic tests.

To conclude, it is important to assess and debate the various ethical and social issues, but it is also evident that both risk assessment and regulation is only achievable in close cooperation with different stakeholders: biomedical scientists, pharmaceutical companies, health-care providers, insurance companies, ethicists and policymakers. Various public-private partnerships are one way of reconciling profit-seeking with public health interests and social justice concerns. Finally, in our globalizing era, harmonization at the international level is necessary as solutions cannot and should not be worked out for any one country alone.

NOTES

1 The following article has profited from the participation in the European Economic Area (EEA) grant "New Ethical Frameworks for Genetic and Electronic Health Record Databases" 2008-2010 and in the Estonian Ministry of Education and Research targeting funded project "Critical Analysis of Relativism and Pluralism Regarding Truth and Knowledge, Norms and Values" 2008-2013. We gratefully acknowledge their support. The authors would like to thank Dr Andres Soosaar and Prof. Tiina Kirss for their help, and Aire Vaher for research assistance.

2 For example, a summary of vital statistics of trends in the health of Americans during the twentieth century reveals two dramatic changes: first, the age-adjusted death rate declined by about 74 percent , and second, life expectancy increased 56 percent. Leading causes of death shifted from infectious to chronic diseases (Guyer et al., 2000).

3 According to the Harris Poll, between 1997 and 2004 the percentage of adults believing that the pharmaceutical industry was adequately serving its customers declined from 79 percent to 44 percent (Santoro, 2005: 3). Available at http://www.harrisinteractive.com/news/allnewsbydate.asp?NewsID.

4 Global Company Sales Summary 2006. Wood Mackenzie's Productview™ March, 2007. Available at Pharma Documentation Ring at http://www.p-d-r.com/ranking/2006_Company_Sales.pdf, accessed 12 November 2008.

5 Global Forum for Health Research, *The 10/90 Report on Health Research,* 2000; available at http://www. globalforumhealth.org/Site/002__What%20we%20do/005__Publications/001__10%2090%20reports.php, accessed 28 August 2005.

6 WHO, Genomics and World Health, pp. 30. whqlibdoc.who.int/hq/2002/a74580.pdf.

7 A good historical overview of pharmacogenetics and pharmacogenomics can be found in Pirmohamed, M. (2001).

8 See for example Thomas (2001); Buchanan et al. (2002); Consortium on Pharmacogenetics (2002); Lipton (2003); Melzer et al. (2003); NCB (2003); Paul and Roses (2003); Rothstein (ed.) (2003), a special issue of *Bioethics,* ed. by Sutrop (2004), and a special issue of Studies in *History and Philosophy of Biological and Biomedical Sciences,* ed. by Ashcroft and Hedgecoe (2006).

9 See for example, the expanding literature on the consent problem within biobanks (O'Neill 2001, 2003, 2004; Árnason, 2004; Nõmper, 2005; Shickle, 2006).

10 US Food and Drug Administration, Center for Drug Evaluation and Research. FAQ on Patents and Exclusivity http://www.fda.gov/cder/ob/faqs.htm.
11 World Medical Association (WMA), *Helsinki Declaration,* 2008. Available at http://www.wma.net/e/policy/ b3.htm, Council for International Organisations of Medical Sciences, 2002: *International Ethical Guidelines for Biomedical Research Involving Human Subjects,* 2002 guideline 10. Available at http://www.cioms.ch/ guidelines_nov_2002_blurb.htm.
12 For example, a non-binding opinion from the European Group on Ethics in Science and New Technologies states that 'there should be an obligation' to provide benefits to communities post-trial and even that drugs should be provided to participants for a lifetime, if necessary (EGESNTEC, 2003: 16). On the other hand, the binding European Directive 2001/20/EC on good clinical practice does not mention benefit sharing nor post-trial obligations (Directive 2001/20/EC).
13 There is evidence that the safety and effectiveness of some drugs can be improved by pharmacogenetic testing. Such drugs include Trastuzumab, Thiopurines, Irinotecan, Abacavir, Warfarin and Tamoxifen (Clemerson and Payne, 2008).

REFERENCES

Agres, T. (2005) 'Clinical trials trickling away', *Drug Discovery and Development,* 7. Available at http://www.dddmag.com/clinical-trials-trickling-away.aspx.

Árnason, V. (2004) 'Coding and consent: Moral challenges of the database project in Iceland', *Bioethics,* 18 (1): 27–49.

Ashcroft, R.E. and Hedgecoe, A.M. (eds) (2006) *Studies in History and Philosophy of Biological and Biomedical Sciences,* 37 (3): 195–217.

Badcott, D. (2006) 'Some causal limitations of pharmacogenetic concepts', *Medicine, Health Care and Philosophy,* 9: 307–16.

Bhandari, M., Busse, J.W., Jackowski, D., Montori, V.M., Schünemann, H., Sprague, S. et al. (2004) 'Association between industry funding and statistically significant pro-industry findings in medical and surgical randomized trials', *Canadian Medical Association Journal,* 170 (4): 477–80.

Buchanan, A., Califano, A., Kahn, J., McPherson, E., Robertson, J. and Brody, B. (2002) 'Pharmacogenetics: Ethical issues and policy options', *Kennedy Institute of Ethics Journal,* 12 (1): 1–15.

Bunk, S. (2003) 'Into the Future', *The Scientist,* 17(Suppl. 2): 38–40.

Clemerson, J. and Payne, K. (2008) 'Pharmacogenetics – current applications', *Hospital Pharmacist,* 15: 167–9.

Consortium on Pharmacogenetics (Buchanan A, McPherson E, Brody BA, Califano A, Kahn J, McCullough N & Robertson JA.). Pharmacogenetics: ethical and regulatory issues in research and clinical practice. Consortium on Pharmacogenetics 2002.

Daar, A.S. and Singer, P. (2005) 'Pharmacogenetics and geographical ancestry: Implications for drug development and global health', *Nature Reviews Genetics,* 6: 241–6.

Daniels, N. (1985) *Just Health Care.* Cambridge: Cambridge University Press.

Davies, E.C., Green C.F., Taylor, S., Williamson, P.R., Mottram, D.R. and Pirmohamed, M. (2009) 'Adverse drug reactions in hospital in-patients: A prospective analysis of 3695 patient-episodes', *PLoS ONE,* 4 (2): e4439.

Delden, J. Van, Bolt, I., Kalis, A., Derijks, J. and Leufkens, H. (2004) 'Tailor-made pharmacotherapy: Future developments and ethical challenges in the field of pharmacogenomics', *Bioethics,* 18 (4): 303–23.

Dewberry, P., DeSantis, S., Kalt, J., Gambrill, S. and Zisson, S. (2006) *Clinical Trials State of the Industry Report 2006: Market Players, Data, Drug Development, and the Future,* ed. M. J. Lamberti. Boston, CA: Center-Watch.

DiMasi, J.A., Hansen, R.W. and Grabowski, H.G. (2003) 'The price of innovation: New estimates of drug development costs', *Journal of Health Economics,* 22 (2): 151–85.

European Group on Ethics in Science and New Technologies to the European Commission (EGESNTEC) (2003) *Ethical Aspects of Clinical Research in Developing Countries.* Available at http://ec.europa.eu/european_group_ethics/ docs/avis17_en.pdf.

Guyer, B., Freedman, M.A., Strobino, D.M. and Sondik, E.J. (2000) 'Annual summary of vital statistics: Trends in the health of Americans during the 20th Century', *Pediatrics,* 106 (6): 1307–17.

Holm, S. (2008) 'Pharmacogenetics, race and global injustice', *Developing World Bioethics*, 8 (2): 82–8.

HUGO Ethics Committee (2000) 'Genetic benefit sharing', *Science*, 290 (5489): 49.

Johnson, J.A. and Lima, J.J. (2003) 'Drug receptor/effector polymorphisms and pharmacogenetics: Current status and challenges', *Pharmacogenetics*, 13 (9): 525–34.

Katz, D., Caplan, A. and Merz, J. (2003) 'All gifts large and small: Toward an understanding of the ethics of pharmaceutical industry gift giving', *American Journal of Bioethics*, 3 (3): 39–46.

Lazarou, J., Pomeranz, B. and Corey, P. (1998) 'Incidence of adverse drug reactions in hospitalized patients: A meta-analysis of prospective studies', *Journal of the America Medical Association*, 279 (15): 1200–05.

Lexchin, J. (1993) 'Interactions between physicians and the pharmaceutical industry: What does the literature say?', *Canadian Medical Association Journal*, 149 (10): 1401–7.

Lexchin, J., Bero, L.A., Djulbegovic, B. and Clark, O. (2003) 'Pharmaceutical industry sponsorship and research outcome and quality: Systematic review', *British Medical Journal*, 326 (7400): 1167–70.

Lindpainter, K. (2002) 'The impact of pharmacogenetics and pharmacogenomics on drug discovery', *Nature Reviews*, 1: 463–9.

Ling T. and Raven A. (2006) 'Pharmacogenetics and uncertainty: Implications for policy makers', *Studies in History and Philosophy of Biological and Biomedical Sciences*, 37 (3): 533–49.

Lipton, P. (2003) 'Pharmacogenetics: The ethical issues', *Pharmacogenomics Journal*, 3: 14–16.

Melzer, D., Raven, A., Detmer, D.E., Ling, T. and Zimmerman, R.L. (2003) *My Very Own Medicine. What Must I Know? Information Policy for Pharmacogenetics*. Cambridge: University of Cambridge Press.

Moynihan, R. (2003) 'Who pays for the pizza? Redefining the relationships between doctors and drug companies. 1: Entanglement', *British Medical Journal*, 326 (7400): 1189–92.

Nebert, D.W. (1999) 'Pharmacogenetics and pharmacogenomics: Why is this relevant to the clinical geneticist?', *Clinical Genetics*, 56 (4): 247–58.

Nõmper, A. (2005) *Open Consent – A New Form of Informed Consent for Population Genetic Databases*. Tartu, Estonia: Tartu University Press.

Nuffield Council on Bioethics (NCB) (2003) *Pharmacogenetics: Ethical Issues*. London: Nuffield Council on Bioethics.

Nuffield Council on Bioethics (NCB) (2005) *The Ethics of Research Related to Healthcare in Developing Countries*. London: Nuffield Council on Bioethics. Available at http://www.nuffieldbioethics.org/fileLibrary/pdf/errhdc_fullreport001.pdf.

O'Neill, O. (2001) 'Informed consent and genetic information', *Studies in History and Philosophy of Biological and Biomedical Sciences*, 32 (4): 689–704.

O'Neill, O. (2003) 'Some limits of informed consent', *Journal of Medical Ethics*, 29 (1): 4–7.

O'Neill, O. (2004) 'Informed consent and public health', *Philosophical Transactions of the Royal Society: Biological Sciences*, 359 (1447): 1133–6.

Paul, N.W. and Roses, A.D. (2003) 'Pharmacogenetics and pharmacogenomics: Recent developments, their clinical relevance and some ethical, social, and legal implications', *Journal of Molecular Medicine*, 81 (3): 135–40.

Peakman, T. and Arlington, S. (2001) *Putting the Code to Work: The Promise of Pharmacogenetics and Pharmacogenomics*. London: PricewaterhouseCoopers.

Pirmohamed, M. (2001) 'Pharmacogenetics and pharmacogenomics', *British Journal of Clinical Pharmacology*, 52 (4): 345–7.

Public Citizen (2001) *Rx R&D Myths: The Case Against the Drug Industry's R&D Scare Card*. Washington, DC: Public Citizen Congress Watch, July.

Relman, A. and Angell, M. (2002) 'America's other drug problem', *New Republic*, 227 (25): 27–41.

Roses, A.D. (2001) 'Pharmacogenetics', *Human Molecular Genetics*, 10 (20): 2261–7.

Ross, J.S., Lackner, J.E., Lurie, P., Gross, C.P., Wolfe, S. and Krumholz, H.M. (2007) 'Pharmaceutical company payments to physicians. Early experiences with disclosure laws in Vermont and Minnesota', *Journal of American Medical Association*, 297 (11): 1216–23.

Rothstein, M. (ed.) (2003) *Pharmacogenomics: Social, Ethical and Clinical Dimensions*. Hoboken, NJ: Wiley-Liss.

Santoro, M.A. (2005) 'Introduction. Charting a sustainable path for the twenty-first century pharmaceutical industry', in M.A. Santoro and T.M. Gorrie (eds) *Ethics and the Pharmaceutical Industry*. Cambridge: Cambridge University Press, pp. 1–20.

Shickle, D. (2006) 'The consent problem within DNA biobanks', *Studies in History and Philosophy of Biological and Biomedical Sciences*, 37: 503–19.

Simm, K. (2007) 'Benefit-sharing: A look at the history of an ethics concern', *Nature Reviews Genetics*, 8 (7): 496.

Smart, A. and Martin, P. (2006) 'The promise of pharmacogenetics: Assessing the prospects for disease and patient stratification', *Studies in History and Philosophy of Biological and Biomedical Sciences*, 37: 583–601.

Sutrop, M. (2004) 'Pharmacogenetics: Ethical Issues', *Bioethics*, 18 (4): III-VIII.

Thomas, S.M. (2001) 'Pharmacogenetics: The ethical context', *Pharmacogenomics Journal*, 1: 239–42.

Tollman, P., Guy, P., Altshuler, J., Flanagan, A. and Steiner, M. (2001) *A Revolution in R & D.* Boston, CA: Boston Consulting Group.

United States National Bioethics Advisory Commission (NBAC) (2001) *Ethical and Policy Issues in International Research: Clinical Trials in Developing Countries.* Available at http://bioethicsprint.bioethics.gov/reports/past_commissions/nbac_international.pdf, accessed 26 August 2005.

Vogel, F. (1959) 'Moderne Probleme der Humangenetik', *Ergebnisse der Inneren Medizin in Kinderheikunde*, 12: 52–125.

Wazana, A. (2000) 'Physicians and the pharmaceutical industry: Is a gift ever just a gift?', *Journal of American Medical Association*, 283 (3): 373–80.

Winnacker, E-L. (2000) *Gentechnik – Eingriffe am Menschen. Was wir dürfen und was wir nicht dürfen.* Bad Homburg: Herbert Quandt Stiftung.

Wolffe, A.P. and Matzke, M.A. (1999) 'Epigenetics: Regulation through repression', *Science*, 286 (5439): 481–6.

Index